THE HUMAN
NERVOUS
SYSTEM

THE HUMAN NERVOUS SYSTEM

An Anatomical Viewpoint

SIXTH EDITION

Murray L. Barr, M.D., D.Sc., F.R.C.P.(C), F.R.S.
Emeritus Professor, Department of Anatomy
Health Sciences Centre
University of Western Ontario
London, Ontario, Canada

John A. Kiernan, M.B., Ch.B., Ph.D., D.Sc.
Professor, Department of Anatomy
Health Sciences Centre
University of Western Ontario
London, Ontario, Canada

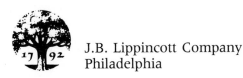
J.B. Lippincott Company
Philadelphia

Acquisitions Editor: Richard Winters
Sponsoring Editor: Jody M. Schott
Project Editor: Bridget Hannon Thatch
Indexer: John A. Kiernan
Design Coordinator: Kathy Kelley-Luedtke
Interior Designer: Ellen Dawson
Cover Designer: Jerry Cable
Production Manager: Caren Erlichman
Production Coordinator: David Murphy
Compositor: Circle Graphics
Printer/Binder: R.R. Donnelley & Sons Company

Cover illustration: A section of a fragment of choroid plexus (see Chapter 26) stained by a method that imparts yellow fluorescence to glycoproteins, here seen in the basement membranes and perivascular connective tissue and at the apical borders of the choroidal epithelial cells. Magnification, × 1000.

6th Edition

6 5 4 3 2 1

Library of Congress Cataloging-in-Publication Data

Barr, Murray Llewellyn, 1908–
    The human nervous system : an anatomical viewpoint / Murray L. Barr, John A. Kiernan.—6th ed.
        p. cm.
    Includes bibliographical references and index.
    ISBN 0-397-51243-0
    1. Neuroanatomy.   2. Human anatomy.   I. Kiernan, J. A. (John Alan)   II. Title.
    [DNLM: 1. Nervous System—anatomy & histology.   WL 101 B268h]
QM451.B27   1993
611'.8—dc20
DNLM/DLC
for Library of Congress   92-48790
                                                             CIP

The authors and publisher have exerted every effort to ensure that drug selection and dosage set forth in this text are in accord with current recommendations and practice at the time of publication. However, in view of ongoing research, changes in government regulations, and the constant flow of information relating to drug therapy and drug reactions, the reader is urged to check the package insert for each drug for any change in indications and dosage and for added warnings and precautions. This is particularly important when the recommended agent is a new or infrequently employed drug.

Preface

The first edition of this textbook (1972) was written to make life easier for those approaching the neurosciences for the first time, especially medical students and those in the allied health sciences for whom the interpretation of clinical signs and symptoms requires a sound basis of neuroanatomy. This objective remains the same, although advances in the science have necessitated much revision during the past 20 years. Textbooks are often kept for many years despite the ephemeral nature of much of their contents. The authors must therefore balance the requirement for up-to-date information against the need to conserve important facts that do not change with time. As in previous revisions, we have introduced new information when it clarifies the normal functional mechanisms or contributes to the understanding of how disease causes disordered function.

Much recently acquired neuroanatomical information relates to rodents and other animals with brains conspicuously smaller and presumably simpler than that of man. This book is about the human nervous system, so we have included recent data from animals other than primates only when there is reason to believe that they apply also to man. The most extensively revised sections are those concerned with the cells of nervous tissue, the reticular formation, sleep, the basal ganglia, the control of movement, the limbic system, memory, and the cerebral cortex. The chemical neurotransmitters in many parts of the central nervous system are now known. These are discussed briefly when there is relevance to human disease or clinical pharmacology. The plan of the book has not been changed. As in previous editions there are five major parts. General and cellular aspects of the nervous system are followed by the regional anatomy of the brain and spinal cord, with frequent references to functional systems and clinical anatomy. The major sensory and motor pathways are then reviewed, and are followed by accounts of the blood vessels and meningeal coverings of the central nervous system. Finally there are two appendices. One contains biographical information about investigators mentioned in the text, especially those whose names have been attached to parts of the nervous system. The second appendix is the glossary.

In this edition some of the text has been set in small print. This material should interest many readers but it is not essential for understanding the normal anatomy and function of the human nervous system. For example, there is clinical information that will interest medical students, but will not be needed by some readers. Some descriptive details, such as the laminae of the spinal gray matter and the positions of gyri and sulci, are also in smaller type. Anatomical features of this kind are obvious from the illustrations, and the text is there mainly for reference on those rare occasions when more precise definition is required. Other "small print" information does not apply to man but has importance for those studying neuroanatomy as a biological science.

Recommended readings at the ends of chapters seem to be consulted by teachers, but rarely by students. These lists have all been revised and most are shorter than in earlier editions. The items cited are recent review articles, chapters in more advanced texts, or recent original papers about human neuroanatomy that were useful when making the revisions. A few older "classics" are also listed, to remind readers that many important discoveries were made more than ten years ago.

Neuroanatomy is cursed with a surfeit of nomenclature and terminology. Tables and schematic diagrams are now provided for reference in some fields, including the hypothalamo-hypophysial system and the basal ganglia. The glossary has been expanded to include a greater variety of clinical and neurobiological terms. To assist the reader with more complicated matters there are now more cross-references in the text.

A number of readers have suggested the inclusion of short lists of the most important facts in each chapter. Summaries of this kind are necessarily incomplete and can never satisfy everyone's idea of what is essential knowledge. However, they are now provided in the hope that they might be useful. These lists are not always understandable without reading the text, and the student should not attempt to commit the items to memory without first learning what they mean.

Various colleagues have kindly read sections of the text, given advice, or provided new illustrations. The help of Drs. J. Ronald Doucette, Brian A. Flumerfelt, Elias B. Gammal, D. G. Montemurro, David M. Pelz, N. Rajakumar and A. Jon Stoessl is gratefully acknowledged, and we thank Louise Gadbois for preparing new illustrations and improving old ones. The staff of the J.B. Lippincott Company have, as always, been most helpful in preparing the book for print.

Contents

BLOOD SUPPLY AND THE MENINGES 377

APPENDICES

INDEX 427

THE HUMAN
NERVOUS
SYSTEM

Introduction and Neurohistology

One

The Human Nervous System: An Anatomical Viewpoint, Sixth Edition, Murray L. Barr and John A. Kiernan. J.B. Lippincott Company, Philadelphia, © 1993.

Development, Composition, and Evolution of the Nervous System

Important Facts

The nervous system is derived from the ectoderm of the embryo.

The central nervous system is formed from the neural tube, and the peripheral nervous system is formed from the neural crest.

The major divisions of the central nervous system are present from the 4th week after fertilization. They are the spinal cord, medulla, pons, midbrain, diencephalon, and cerebral hemispheres.

Abnormal development of the brain or spinal cord often is due to faulty closure of the neural tube.

The brains of vertebrate animals all have the same basic plan.

The human brain has large cerebral hemispheres with an extensive and much folded cerebral cortex. The cerebellum, an outgrowth of the brain stem, also is highly developed.

The first cells to differentiate in the nervous system are neurons, which are specialized for communication. They are followed by supporting cells known as neuroglia.

All living organisms respond to chemical and physical stimuli. The response may be a movement, or it may be the expulsion of biosynthetic products from cells. These receptive, motor and secretory functions are combined in a single cell in both unicellular organisms and the simplest multicellular animals, the sponges. In all other groups of animals, cells are able to communicate, so that the reception of a stimulus by one cell may result in motile or secretory activity of other cells. Specialized cells known as **neurons** exist to transfer information rapidly from one part of an animal's body to another. All the neurons of an organism, together with their supporting cells, constitute a **nervous system**.

To carry out its communicative function, a neuron exhibits two different, but coupled, activities. They are **conduction** of a signal from one part of the cell to another and **synaptic**

transmission, which is communication between adjacent cells. An **impulse** is a wave of electrical depolarization that is propagated within the surface membrane of the neuron. A stimulus applied to one part of the neuron initiates an impulse that travels to all other parts of the cell. Neurons commonly have long cytoplasmic processes, known as **neurites**, that end in close apposition to the surfaces of other cells. The ends of the neurites are called **synaptic terminals**, and the cell-to-cell contacts they make are known as **synapses**. The neurites in higher animals usually are specialized to form **dendrites** and **axons**, which typically conduct toward and away from the cell body, respectively. The arrival of an impulse at a terminal triggers synaptic transmission. This event normally involves the release of a chemical compound from the neuronal cytoplasm, which evokes some type of response in the postsynaptic cell. At some synapses, the two cells are electrically coupled. Another type of neuron exists that discharges its chemical products into the circulating blood, thereby influencing distant parts of the body. Neurons of the latter type, known as **neurosecretory cells**, are functionally related to endocrine gland cells.

Development of the Nervous System

The nervous system develops from the dorsal ectoderm of the early embryo. Nerve cells, together with neuroglial or interstitial cells, are derived from the outer ectodermal layer, similar to the cells of the epidermis that cover the body surface. The first indication of the future nervous system is the neuroectoderm, comprising the **neural plate**, which appears in the dorsal midline of the embryo at the 16th day after fertilization. The change in the ectoderm is induced by the nearby mesodermal cells. The neural plate changes 2 days later into a **neural groove** with a **neural fold** along each side.

NEURAL TUBE, CREST, AND PLACODES

By the end of the 3rd week, the neural folds have begun to fuse with one another, thereby

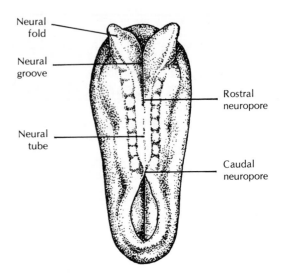

Figure 1-1. Dorsal view of a human embryo about 22 days after fertilization. Closure of the neural tube is in progress.

converting the neural groove into a **neural tube** (Fig. 1-1). The transformation proceeds rostrally and caudally, and the openings at each end (the rostral and caudal neuropores) close at about the 24th and 27th days,[1] respectively. The neural tube is the forerunner of the brain and spinal cord.

Neuroectodermal cells that are not incorporated into the tube form **neural crests**, which run dorsolaterally along each side of the neural tube. From the neural crests are derived the dorsal root ganglia of spinal nerves, some of the neurons in sensory ganglia of cranial nerves, autonomic ganglia, the nonneuronal cells (neuroglia) of peripheral nerves, and secretory cells of the adrenal medulla. Thus the cells of the neural crest are notable for their extensive migrations. Many of them even differentiate into cells of nonneural tissue, including the melanocytes of the skin and some of the bones, muscles, and other structures of the head. The connective tissue cells in nerves and ganglia are derived from the local mesoderm.

---

[1] In clinical practice, **pregnancy** is timed from the 1st day of the last menstrual period, about 14 days before fertilization. The age of an **embryo** is stated from the known or estimated time of fertilization. When it is 8 weeks old and all the organs are formed, an embryo is renamed a **fetus**.

Some peripheral nervous elements are derived from **placodes**, which are thickened regions of the ectoderm of the head's surface. Thus the olfactory neurosensory cells, the sensory cells and associated ganglia of the inner ear, and some of the neurons in the sensory ganglia of cranial nerves are derived from placodes.

PRODUCTION OF NEURONS AND NEUROGLIA

The first populations of cells produced in the neural tube are **neuroblasts**, the precursors of neurons. Most of the neurons are produced between the 4th and the 20th weeks. As the neurons form, they migrate, grow cytoplasmic processes, and form synaptic connections with other neurons. **Glioblasts**, the precursors of the nonneuronal cells of the central nervous system, are first produced at about 19 weeks. The number and complexity of synapses continue to increase until well after birth, as does the generation of neuroglial cells.

The number of neuroblasts formed in the neural tube exceeds the number of neurons in the adult brain and spinal cord. Large numbers of neuroblasts die in the normal course of development. This occurrence, known as **cell death**, is seen in many embryonic systems throughout the animal kingdom. In invertebrates, the cell death is genetically programmed. Experimental studies carried out by Hamburger in the 1930s have shown that in vertebrates, the cells that die are those that fail to make synaptic connections.

FORMATION OF THE BRAIN AND SPINAL CORD

Even before the closure of the neural folds, the neural plate is conspicuously larger at the rostral end of the embryo and irregularities corresponding to the major divisions of the developing **brain** are already visible. The remainder of the neural tube becomes the **spinal cord**. The site of closure of the caudal neuropore corresponds to the upper lumbar segments of the cord. Further caudally the spinal cord is formed by "secondary neurulation," which is the coalescence of a chain of ectodermal vesicles that becomes continuous with the lumen of the neural tube about 3 weeks after the closure of the caudal neuropore.

As described conventionally, three **primary brain vesicles** appear at the end of the 4th week: the **prosencephalon** (forebrain), **mesencephalon** (midbrain), and **rhombencephalon** (hindbrain). During the 5th week, both the first and the third vesicle change into two swellings, so that there are five **secondary brain vesicles**: the **telencephalon**, **diencephalon**, **mesencephalon**, **metencephalon**, and **myelencephalon**. In the developing mammalian brain (Fig. 1-2B), the brain vesicles are less distinct than in the chick embryo, which is a favorite subject for embryological investigation. The terminology, however, has been widely used as a general convention for many years, and the same words are used for the corresponding parts of the adult human brain. The early embryonic central nervous system also is divisible longitudinally into segments known as **neuromeres**. The neuromeres become indistinguishable as the complex structure of the brain develops, but segmental organization of the spinal cord persists throughout life.

As cellular proliferation and differentiation proceed in the neural tube, a longitudinal groove called the **sulcus limitans** appears along the inner aspect of each lateral wall. The sulcus demarcates a dorsal **alar plate** from a ventral **basal plate**; they acquire afferent and efferent connections, respectively, and are present from the rostral end of the mesencephalon to the caudal end of the spinal cord. Responding to an inductive effect of the nearby notochord (which marks the position of future vertebrae), the basal laminae of the left and right sides become separated by a thin **floor plate**. Some of the basal plate cells differentiate into motor neurons, with axons that grow out into the developing muscles. The growing axons of neurons of the sensory ganglia enter the alar plate.

DERIVATIVES OF THE BRAIN VESICLES

The regions of the brain that develop from the secondary brain vesicles acquire a distinctive structure, and some of the formal embryologi-

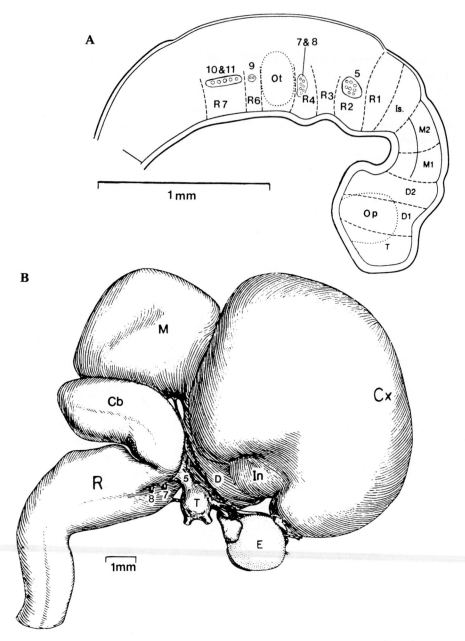

Figure 1-2. Human embryos at 4 weeks (**A**) and 7 weeks (**B**), showing the positions of the primary brain vesicles. (**A**) Midline section of a 4-week-old embryo. Some neuromeres are indicated for the telencephalon (**T**), diencephalon (**D1, D2**), mesencephalon (**M1, M2**), isthmus (**Is**), and rhombencephalon (**R1–R7**). The levels of the optic (**Op**) and otic (**Ot**) vesicles, which are lateral to the neural tube, are indicated. The numerals (**5–11**) indicate the levels of the sites of emergence of some of the cranial nerves. (*With permission, from O'Rahilly R, Müller F, Bossy J: Arch Anat Histol Embryol 72:3-24, 1989.*) (**B**) The brain of an 8-week-old embryo reconstructed from sections, showing its major parts: **Cb** = cerebellum; **Cx** = cerebral cortex; **D** = diencephalon; **E** = eye; **In** = insula; **M** = mesencephalon; **R** = rhombencephalon; **T** = trigeminal ganglion; **5** = sensory root of trigeminal nerve; **7, 8** = rootlets of facial and vestibulocochlear nerves. (*With permission, from O'Rahilly R, Müller F, Bossy J: Arch Anat Histol Embryol 69:3-24, 1986.*)

TABLE 1-1 ▬▬▬▬▬
Development of the Mature Brain from the Brain Vesicles

Primary Brain Vesicles	*Secondary Brain Vesicles*	*Mature Brain*
Rhombencephalon	Myelencephalon	Medulla oblongata
	Metencephalon	Pons and cerebellum
Mesencephalon	Mesencephalon	Midbrain, consisting of tectum and cerebral peduncles
Prosencephalon	Diencephalon	Thalamus, epithalamus, hypothalamus, and subthalamus
	Telencephalon	Cerebral hemispheres, each containing olfactory system, corpus striatum, cortex, and medullary center

cal names are replaced by others for common usage (Table 1-1 and Fig. 1-3). The myelencephalon becomes the medulla oblongata, and the metencephalon develops into the pons and cerebellum. The mesencephalon of the mature brain usually is called the midbrain. The names diencephalon and telencephalon are retained because of the diverse nature of their derivatives. A large mass of gray matter, the thalamus, develops in the diencephalon. Adjacent regions are known as the epithalamus, hypothalamus, and subthalamus, each with distinctive structural and functional characteristics. The left and right halves of the telencephalon are known as the cerebral hemispheres. These undergo the greatest development in the human brain, in respect both to other regions and to the brains of other animals. The telencephalon includes the olfactory system, the corpus striatum (a mass of gray matter with motor functions), an extensive surface layer of gray matter known as the cortex or pallium, and a medullary center of white matter.

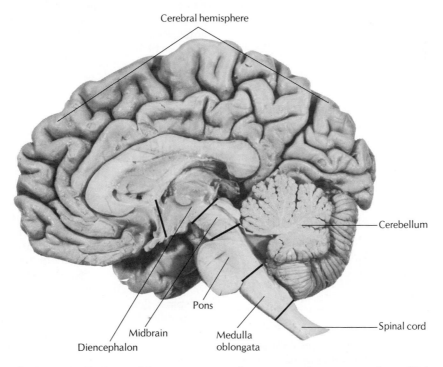

Cerebral hemisphere

Cerebellum

Spinal cord

Pons

Midbrain

Diencephalon

Medulla oblongata

Figure 1-3. Regions of the mature central nervous system, as seen in sagittal section. (× 0.5; *photograph kindly provided by Dr. D. G. Montemurro.*)

The lumen of the neural tube is converted into a lateral ventricle in each cerebral hemisphere, the third ventricle in the diencephalon, and the fourth ventricle bounded by the medulla, pons, and cerebellum. The third and fourth ventricles are connected by a narrow channel, the cerebral aqueduct, through the midbrain. The lumen also remains narrow in the caudal part of the medulla and throughout the spinal cord, where it becomes the central canal.

Flexures in the neural tube help to accommodate the initially cylindrical brain in what will eventually be a round head. The first to form are the cervical flexure at the junction of the rhombencephalon with the spinal cord, and the cephalic flexure at the level of the mesencephalon. The pontine flexure in the metencephalon soon follows. These flexures in the brain ensure that the optical axes of the eyes (which connect with the prosencephalon) are at right angles to the axis of the vertebral column. This necessary feature of the erect posture of humans contrasts with the posture of quadrupedal animals, in which there is no abrupt bend at the junction of the midbrain with the forebrain.

MENINGES

The membranous coverings of the brain and spinal cord first appear as a single mesodermally derived **primitive meninx**. This then differentiates into the three layers that constitute the meninges: the pia mater, closest to the nervous tissue; the arachnoid; and the dura mater, lining the cranial cavity and spinal canal. The subarachnoid space, which contains cerebrospinal fluid, forms between the inner two meningeal layers.

Abnormal Development of the Nervous System

Anencephaly and Spina Bifida

Congenital malformations of the central nervous system include those that result from failure of the neural tube to close normally. Developmental failure may also occur in associated bone and skin. In **anencephaly**, the neural folds do not fuse at the rostral end of the developing neural tube, so that forebrain, cranial vault, and much of the scalp are missing. The abnormal brain (the brain stem and, sometimes, the diencephalon) is exposed to the exterior. Anencephaly occurs once in about 1000 births and is incompatible with sustained life. The equivalent condition at the caudal end of the central nervous system is **myelocele**, also known as myeloschisis (cleft spinal cord), in which there is extensive exposure of nonfunctional nervous tissue in the lumbosacral region. Sometimes these two conditions coexist in the same baby.

Myelocele is the severest form of **spina bifida**. In less severe types, the spinal cord and its adjacent connective tissue ensheathment (the leptomeninges; see Ch. 26) are intact, but the overlying mesodermal derivatives are not. In **meningomyelocele**, the dura mater, vertebral arches, and skin are missing. The caudal part of the spinal cord forms a visible protrusion. If the cord remains in the vertebral canal, the lump at the surface is a **meningocele**: a cyst containing cerebrospinal fluid. These types of spina bifida can be corrected surgically, but there often is permanent paralysis or weakness of the lower limbs. **Spina bifida occulta** is a common condition in which the dura and skin remain intact, but one or more bony vertebral arches fail to develop. Usually there are no symptoms other than a dimple, a tuft of hair, or some other minor irregularity of the overlying skin.

Hydrocephalus

Cerebrospinal fluid accumulates in the ventricles of the brain if its normal flow is obstructed (see Ch. 26). Nervous tissue is destroyed by the pressure, and the head can become greatly enlarged. Causes include stenosis of the cerebral aqueduct in the midbrain and the Chiari malformation, in which the medulla and part of the cerebellum are located not in the skull, but in the upper cervical spinal canal. This abnormal anatomy can obstruct the flow of cerebrospinal fluid out of the ventricular system. Spina bifida is also present in many infants with Chiari malformations. Hydrocephalus is treated by installing an alternative pathway for drainage of the ventricular system of the brain.

Summary of Main Regions of the Central Nervous System

Certain features of the main regions are noted in the following summary by way of introduction and to provide a first acquaintance with some neuroanatomical terms.

SPINAL CORD

The spinal cord is the least differentiated component of the central nervous system. The segmental nature of the spinal cord is reflected in a series of paired spinal nerves, each of which is attached to the cord by a dorsal sensory root and a ventral motor root. The central **gray matter**, in which nerve cell bodies are located, has a roughly H-shaped outline in transverse section. **White matter**, which consists of nerve fibers running longitudinally, occupies the periphery of the cord. The spinal cord includes neuronal connections that provide for spinal reflexes. There are also pathways that convey sensory data to the brain and other pathways that conduct impulses, typically of motor significance, from the brain to the spinal cord.

MEDULLA OBLONGATA

The fiber tracts of the spinal cord are continued in the medulla, which also contains clusters of nerve cells called nuclei. The most prominent of these, the inferior olivary nuclei, send fibers to the cerebellum through the inferior cerebellar peduncles, which attach the cerebellum to the medulla oblongata. Of the smaller nuclei, some are components of cranial nerves.

PONS

The pons consists of two distinct parts. The dorsal portion has features shared with the rest of the brain stem. It therefore includes sensory and motor tracts, together with some nuclei of cranial nerves. The basal (ventral) portion of the pons is special to this part of the brain stem. Its function is to provide for extensive connections between the cortex of a cerebral hemisphere and that of the contralateral cerebellar hemisphere. These connections contribute to maximal efficiency of motor activities. A pair of middle cerebellar peduncles attaches the cerebellum to the pons.

MIDBRAIN

Like other parts of the brain stem, the midbrain contains sensory and motor pathways, together with nuclei for two cranial nerves. There is a dorsal region, the roof or **tectum**, which is concerned principally with the visual and auditory systems. The midbrain also includes two prominent motor nuclei, the **red nucleus** and the **substantia nigra**. The cerebellum is attached to the midbrain by the superior cerebellar peduncles.

CEREBELLUM

The cerebellum is especially large in the human brain. Receiving data from most of the sensory systems and the cerebral cortex, the cerebellum eventually influences motor neurons that supply the skeletal musculature. The function of the cerebellum is to produce changes in muscle tonus in relation to equilibrium, locomotion and posture as well as nonstereotyped movements based on individual experience. The cerebellum operates behind the scenes at a subconscious level.

DIENCEPHALON

The diencephalon forms the central core of the cerebrum. The largest component of the diencephalon, the **thalamus**, consists of several regions or nuclei, some of which receive data from sensory systems and project to sensory areas of the cerebral cortex. Part of the thalamus has connections with cortical areas that are concerned with complex mental processes. Other regions participate in neural circuits related to emotions, and certain thalamic nuclei are incorporated into pathways from the cerebellum and corpus striatum to motor areas of the cerebral cortex. The **epithalamus** includes small tracts and nuclei, together with the pineal gland, an endocrine organ. The **hypothalamus** is the principal autonomic center of the brain and, as such, has an important controlling influence over the sympathetic and parasympathetic systems. In addition, neurosecretory cells in the hypothalamus synthesize hormones that reach the bloodstream by way of the neurohypophysis or influence the hormonal output of the adenohypophysis through a special portal system of blood vessels. The **subthalamus** includes sensory tracts that proceed to the thalamus, nerve fibers that originate in the cerebellum and corpus striatum, and the subthalamic nucleus (a motor nucleus). The retina is a derivative of the diencephalon; the optic nerve and the visual system are, therefore, intimately related to this part of the brain.

TELENCEPHALON (CEREBRAL HEMISPHERES)

The telencephalon includes the cerebral cortex, corpus striatum, and medullary center. Small areas of the **cerebral cortex** have an ancient lineage (**paleocortex**) and receive data from the olfactory system, which dominates the cerebrum of lower vertebrates. Other areas of cortex that appeared early in vertebrate evolution are called **archicortex**. These are included in the limbic system, which is involved with memory and the influence of emotions on visceral function through the autonomic nervous system. Nine-tenths of the human cerebral cortex is **neocortex**. This includes areas for all modalities of sensation (except smell), motor areas, and large expanses of association cortex, in which the highest levels of neural function presumably take place, including those inherent in intellectual activity.

The **corpus striatum** is a large mass of gray matter with motor functions situated near the base of each hemisphere. It consists of caudate and lentiform nuclei, the latter being subdivided into a putamen and a globus pallidus. The **medullary center** of the hemisphere consists of fibers that connect cortical areas of the same hemisphere, fibers that cross the midline (in a large commissure known as the corpus callosum) to connect cortical areas of the two hemispheres, and fibers that pass in both directions between cortex and subcortical centers. Fibers of the last category converge to form a compact internal capsule in the region of the thalamus and corpus striatum.

SIZE OF THE HUMAN BRAIN

At birth, the average brain weighs about 400 g. Further increase in size is due to continuing formation of synaptic connections, production of neuroglial cells, and thickening of the myelin sheaths around axons. The most rapid growth of the brain occurs in utero and during the first 20 postnatal weeks. By age 3, the average weight (1200 g) is almost that of the adult, although slow growth continues until age 18. After age 50, there is a slow decline in brain size. This decrease in size does not lead to intellectual deterioration unless there is considerable atrophy caused by disease.

The weight of the mature brain varies with age and stature. The normal range in the adult man is 1100 to 1700 g (average 1360 g). The lower figures for the adult woman (1050–1550 g, average 1275 g) are due mainly to the smaller stature of women compared with men. There is no evidence of a relation between brain weight, within normal limits, and a person's level of intelligence.

Evolution of the Nervous System

The embryology and components of the human nervous system have been briefly discussed. It will be useful now to present some evolutionary background regarding the comparative anatomy of the invertebrate and vertebrate nervous systems.

Invertebrates

The simplest Cnidaria, such as the hydra, are branched tubular animals. A netlike arrangement of neurons, each with two or more processes, is interposed between the epithelium that covers the outside of the animal and the epithelium that lines the digestive cavity. A stimulus applied to any part of the animal causes the propagation of signals among the neurons of the nerve net and results in contraction or bending of the tubular body and its tentacles. The site and intensity of the stimulus determine the strength and direction of the response. With this simple nerve net, the hydra may move about, vary its length, and use its tentacles to push food particles into its mouth. Occasional strong contractions of the whole animal serve to expel indigestible material from the same orifice, which also serves as an anus.

In the higher Cnidaria, such as the jellyfish, and in all other invertebrate animals, the neurons are not uniformly distributed in the wall of the body but are collected together in aggregates known as **ganglia**. In invertebrates, only the cytoplasmic processes (neurites) of the neurons are involved in synaptic contacts. The cell bodies usually lie in the outer rind of the ganglion. Many neurites synapse with one another in the central core, whereas others travel in bundles called **connectives** to other ganglia or in **nerves** to receptor and effector organs. Receptor cells are located mainly on the body's surface, often in highly differentiated organs such as the eyes. In bilaterally symmetrical animals, such as worms and arthropods, pairs of ganglia are arrayed along the length of the body, joined longitudinally and across the midline by connectives. Most creatures of this type have a distinct head that bears special sensory organs for the perception of light and chemical stimuli. This concentration of important functions in the head is associated with the presence there of ganglia larger and more complex than those in the more posterior parts of the body. Such ganglia may be said to constitute a **brain**.

Vertebrates

Vertebrates are thought by biologists to have evolved from simpler animals that lacked backbones. Their lowly ancestors may never be known because they must be extinct, but they might have resembled the modern worm-like nemerteans or primitive chordates such as the amphioxus. These are all bilaterally symmetrical creatures with brains in their heads.

The nervous systems of all vertebrate animals—fishes, amphibians, reptiles, birds, and mammals—are of similar construction. The brain is a hollow structure that extends posteriorly toward the tail as a tubular spinal cord. The brain is encased in the skull, and the spinal cord is encircled intermittently by the vertebrae of the vertebral column. Ganglia are associated with nerves that connect the spinal cord and the caudal parts of the brain with the skin, other

sense organs, muscles, and viscera. A second system of neurons, which forms a plexus within the wall of the alimentary canal, is connected with the main nervous system but also can function independently. There is thus a **central nervous system** composed of the brain and spinal cord, a **peripheral nervous system** composed of the spinal and cranial nerves, and an **autonomic nervous system** that innervates smooth muscle and gland cells, together with cardiac muscle.

The structural plan of the spinal cord and of its associated nerves and ganglia is essentially the same in all vertebrates. The size, vascularity, variety of nonneuronal cells, and complexity of neuronal circuitry in the central nervous system all increase with the phylogenetic advance from the primitive fishes to the mammals. The most conspicuous differences among the nervous systems of vertebrates are found in the relative sizes of the various parts of the brain (Fig. 1-4).

The rhombencephalon and mesencephalon contain groups of neurons that are connected with most of the **cranial nerves**. These nerves are similar to the spinal nerves, although their segmental organization is less obvious. The cranial nerves supply structures in the head as well as large parts of the cardiopulmonary and alimentary systems and, in aquatic animals, the lateral line sensory organs. The last named are sensory receptors that detect vibrations and electric signals under water. Fishes and amphibians have 10 pairs of cranial nerves, numbered rostrocaudally. Two additional pairs of cranial nerves are found in reptiles, birds, and mammals. In addition to the cranial nerve nuclei, the brain stem contains many groups of neurons whose synaptic connections are related to other parts of the central nervous system. These vary in size and complexity in the different vertebrate classes, generally becoming larger and more diverse as the phylogenetic scale is ascended.

The **cerebellum** in fishes receives most of its input from the vestibular and lateral line receptors, with smaller contributions from the optic system, the spinal cord, and some sensory nuclei of the cranial nerves. Spinal afferents are more numerous in reptiles and birds. In mammals, there are also extensive indirect connections with the cerebral cortex, which attain their greatest development in humans. The increasing importance of the cerebellum is apparent

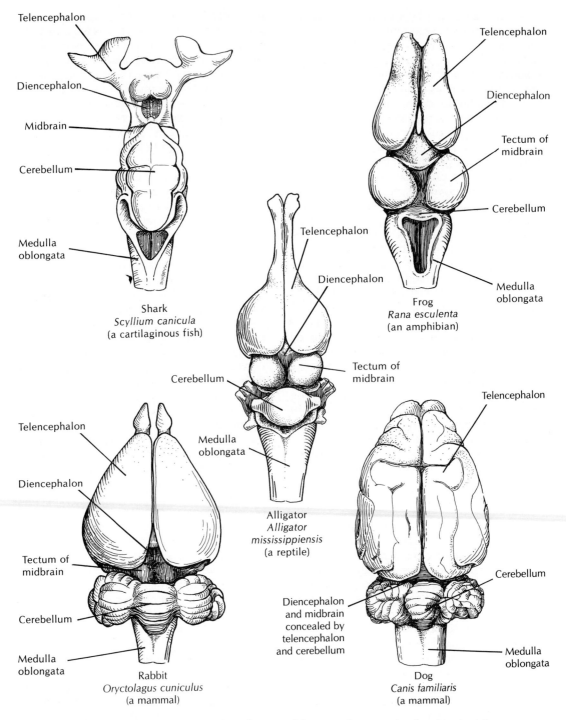

Telencephalon

Diencephalon

Midbrain

Cerebellum

Medulla
oblongata

Shark
Scyllium canicula
(a cartilaginous fish)

Telencephalon

Diencephalon

Tectum of
midbrain

Cerebellum

Medulla
oblongata

Frog
Rana esculenta
(an amphibian)

Telencephalon

Diencephalon

Cerebellum

Tectum of
midbrain

Medulla
oblongata

Alligator
*Alligator
mississippiensis*
(a reptile)

Telencephalon

Diencephalon

Tectum of
midbrain

Cerebellum

Medulla
oblongata

Rabbit
Oryctolagus cuniculus
(a mammal)

Telencephalon

Cerebellum

Diencephalon
and midbrain
concealed by
telencephalon
and cerebellum

Medulla
oblongata

Dog
Canis familiaris
(a mammal)

Figure 1-4. Dorsal views of the brains of five vertebrate animals, showing the relative sizes of the main regions.

from its greater size in the more advanced animals.

The dorsal part of the mesencephalon reaches its highest degree of development, relative to other parts of the brain, in bony fishes and amphibians. In these forms, the **optic tectum** is a many-layered structure of great synaptic complexity that forms prominent bilateral bulges on the dorsal surface of the brain. In addition to receiving most of the output of the retina, it is significantly involved in other modalities of sensation and in the control of movement. In mammals, the relatively small tectum consists of a **superior** and an **inferior colliculus** on each side. The superior colliculus, homologous with the optic tectum, is an important visual center in lower mammals, such as rodents, but is of lesser importance in humans. The inferior colliculus is part of the polysynaptic pathway by which auditory sensation is relayed to the forebrain.

The diencephalon has four parts which are present in all vertebrates. The **epithalamus** is the largest part in the most primitive fishes, in which, as in higher vertebrates, it forms a link between the telencephalon and the midbrain. The **hypothalamus** is the largest division of the diencephalon in both cartilaginous and bony fishes. It retains its functional importance in higher animals but is relatively smaller because of the increased size of the **thalamus** (the "dorsal thalamus" of comparative anatomists). The size and complexity of the thalamus increase in association with the evolution of the telencephalon. The **subthalamus** (also known as the "ventral thalamus") is always the smallest part of the diencephalon.

The telencephalon consists of the two **cerebral hemispheres**, each containing a lateral ventricle, derived from the bifurcated neural tube. In fishes and amphibians, the most rostral part of the hemisphere is the **olfactory lobe**, which receives the olfactory nerves. The olfactory lobe is joined to the diencephalon by a simple tubular structure in which the ventricular cavity is surrounded by gray matter, external to which is a layer of nerve fibers; this arrangement is similar to that of the spinal cord. The nervous tissue dorsal to the ventricle is the **pallium**, that ventrolateral to the ventricle is the **striatum**, and that ventromedial to the cavity is the **septum**. All these regions receive input from the olfactory lobe. In these lower vertebrates, the telen-

cephalon is implicated in decisive, as distinct from purely reflex, responses. Decisions and judgments in these animals are strongly influenced by olfactory stimuli and are important in relation to the recognition and treatment of potential food, mates, and enemies. In reptiles, all parts of the telencephalon are larger than in amphibians, and the striatum is especially prominent. Reciprocal connections with the thalamus and with lower levels of the nervous system also are more developed.

In mammals, the cerebral hemispheres are even larger. The olfactory bulb, equivalent to the olfactory lobe of lower vertebrates, projects mainly to the ventral and medial parts of the forebrain. The striatum forms a large mass of gray matter, the **corpus striatum**, inside each hemisphere, and the pallium forms an outer covering of gray matter, the **cerebral cortex**. The more complex behavioral patterns are observed in those mammals in which the area and therefore the volume of the cerebral cortex are greater. The increased area is accommodated by the development of convolutions in the cortical surface, which are most numerous in primates, including humans.

The ratio of the size of the brain to the size of the whole body is related to dietary and other habits. Thus the ratio is smallest in animals that live on the ground and eat grass and leaves. This is true even in the case of the African elephant, whose brain weighs 5000 g. The largest brain-to-body weight ratios are found in animals that live in trees or that eat seeds, fruits, or other vertebrates.

SUGGESTED READING

FitzGerald MJT: Human Embryology: A Regional Approach. Hagerstown, MD, Harper & Row, 1978

Harvey PH, Krebs JR: Comparing brains. Science 249:140–146, 1990

Lemire RJ, Loeser JD, Leech RW, Alvord EC: Normal and Abnormal Development of the Human Nervous System. Hagerstown, MD, Harper & Row, 1975

Lumsden, A: Motorizing the spinal cord. Cell 64: 471–473, 1991

LeDouarin NM: The Neural Crest. New York, Cambridge University Press, 1982

McNab BK, Eisenberg JF: Brain size and its relation to the rate of metabolism in mammals. American Naturalist 133:157–167, 1989

Northcutt RG: Evolution of the vertebrate central nervous system: Patterns and processes. Am Zool 24:701–716, 1984

O'Rahilly R, Müller F, Bossy J: Atlas des stades du développement des formes exterieures de l'encéphale chez l'embryon humain. Arch Anat Histol Embryol 69:3–39, 1986

O'Rahilly R, Müller F, Bossy J: Atlas des stades du développement de l'encéphale chez l'embryon humain étudié par des reconstructions graphiques du plan médian. Arch Anat Histol Embryol 72:3–24, 1989

Purves D, Lichtman JW: Principles of Neural Development. Sunderland, MA, Sinauer & Associates, 1985

Sarnat HB, Netsky MG: Evolution of the Nervous System, 2nd ed. New York, Oxford University Press, 1981

Two

The Human Nervous System: An Anatomical Viewpoint, Sixth Edition, Murray L. Barr and John A. Kiernan. J.B. Lippincott Company, Philadelphia, © 1993.

Cells of the Central Nervous System

Important Facts

Neurons are cells specialized for rapid communication. Most of the cytoplasm of a neuron is in long processes, the neurites (dendrites and axon), which conduct signals toward and away from the cell body, respectively.

In the central nervous system, neuronal cell bodies and dendrites occur in gray matter. White matter consists largely of axons, most of which have myelin sheaths that serve to increase the velocity of conduction.

A neuronal surface membrane has a resting potential of -70 mV, maintained by the sodium pump. This is reversed to $+40$ mV in an axon during the passage of an action potential.

The fastest signals, known as impulses or action potentials, are carried in the surface membrane of the axon. There is rapid (saltatory) conduction in myelinated axons because the ion channels in the axolemma are confined to the nodes.

The surface membrane of the perikaryon and dendrites does not conduct impulses. Potential changes move more slowly and are graded. An action potential is initiated when the region of the axonal hillock is depolarized to a threshold level.

Neurons communicate with one another at synapses. Chemical transmitters released by axonal terminals evoke changes in the membrane of the postsynaptic cell, which may be either stimulated or inhibited. The effect depends on the transmitter and the type of receptor molecule in the postsynaptic membrane.

Local reductions of membrane potential (excitatory postsynaptic potentials) add together and may result in initiation of an action potentials. Hyperpolarization (inhibitory postsynaptic potentials) reduces the likelihood of initiation of an impulse.

Proteins and other substances are transported within axons at different speeds and in both directions.

The neuroglial cells of the normal central nervous system are astrocytes, oligodendrocytes, ependymal cells (derived from neural tube ectoderm), and microglia (derived from mesoderm). Oligodendrocytes produce myelin.

There are two classes of cells in the central nervous system in addition to the usual cells found in blood vessel walls. **Nerve cells**, or **neurons**, are specialized for excitation (or inhibition) and nerve impulse conduction and are therefore responsible for most of the functional characteristics of nervous tissue. **Neuroglial cells**, collectively known as the **neuroglia** or simply as **glia**, have important ancillary functions.

The central nervous system consists of gray matter and white matter. **Gray matter** contains the cell bodies of neurons, each with a nucleus, embedded in a **neuropil** made up predominantly of delicate neuronal and glial processes. **White matter**, on the other hand, consists mainly of long processes of neurons, the majority being surrounded by myelin sheaths; nerve cell bodies are lacking. Both the gray and the white matter contain large numbers of neuroglial cells and a network of blood capillaries.

The Neuron

Neurons are cells specialized for sending and receiving signals. The part of the cell that includes the nucleus is called the **cell body**, and its cytoplasm is known as the **perikaryon. Dendrites** are typically short branching processes that receive signals from other neurons. Most neurons of the central nervous system have several dendrites and are therefore multipolar in shape. By reaching out in various directions, dendrites increase the ability of a neuron to receive input from diverse sources. Each cell has a single **axon**. This process, which varies greatly in length from one type of neuron to another, typically conducts impulses away from the cell body. Some neurons have no axons, and their dendrites conduct signals in both directions. Axons of efferent neurons in the spinal cord and brain are included in spinal and cranial nerves. They end on striated muscle fibers or on nerve cells of autonomic ganglia. The term **neurite** refers to any neuronal process, axon or dendrite.

The fact that each neuron is a structural and functional unit is known as the **neuron doctrine**, proposed in the latter part of the 19th century in opposition to the then prevailing view that nerve cells formed a continuous reticulum or syncytium. The unitary concept, conforming to the cell theory, was advanced by His on the basis of embryological studies, by Forel on the basis of the responses of nerve cells to injury, and by Ramón y Cajal from his histological observations. The **neuron doctrine** was given wide distribution in a review by Waldeyer of the whole subject of the individuality of nerve cells.[1] The lack of cytoplasmic continuity between neurons at synapses was conclusively demonstrated in the 1950s when it became possible to obtain electron micrographs with sufficient resolution to show the structures of intimately apposed cell membranes.

Different Shapes and Sizes of Neurons

Although all neurons conform to the general principles outlined above, there is a wide range of structural diversity. The size of the cell body varies from 5 μm across for the smallest cells in complex circuits to 135 μm for the largest motor neurons. Dendritic morphology, especially the pattern of branching, varies greatly and is distinctive for neurons that constitute a particular group of cells. The axon of a local circuit neuron may be as short as 100 μm, less than 1 μm in diameter, and devoid of a myelin covering. On the other hand, the axon of a motor neuron that supplies a muscle in the foot is nearly 1 m long, up to 10 μm in diameter, and encased in a myelin sheath up to 5 μm thick. (Much longer axons are present in large animals such as giraffes and whales.)

Neurons occur in **ganglia** in the peripheral nervous system and in either **laminae** (layers) or groups called **nuclei** in the central nervous system. The large neurons of a nucleus or comparable region are called Golgi type I or **principal cells**; their axons carry the encoded output of information from the region containing

---

[1] For brief biographical details, see "Investigators Mentioned in the Text," at the end of the book.

their cell bodies to other parts of the nervous system. The dendrites of a principal cell are contacted by axonal terminals of several other neurons. These neurons include principal cells of other areas and nearby small neurons. The latter are known variously as Golgi type II, internuncial, or local circuit neurons, or, more simply, as **interneurons**, and they greatly outnumber the principal cells.

Examples of large and small neurons are shown in Figure 2-1, which shows the cells as they might appear in specimens stained by the Golgi method.

Neurohistological Techniques

The neuron, although made from the same basic components as other cells, has some specialized characteristics that are not apparent in sections prepared by general-purpose staining methods such as the alum-hematoxylin-eosin beloved of pathologists. Information about neurocytology has accumulated over the past century, first from the application of specialized staining methods for light microscopy, later with the aid of the electron microscope, and most recently from studies in which functionally significant chemical compounds are localized in the cells and parts of cells in which they are synthesized or stored.

Cationic dyes, such as thionine, toluidine blue, neutral red, and cresyl violet, are called "Nissl stains" when applied to nervous tissue. They bind to nucleic acids and, therefore, demonstrate the nuclei of all cells as well as the cytoplasmic Nissl substance (ribonucleic acid [RNA]) of neurons (Fig. 2-2).

Reduced silver methods produce dark deposits of colloidal silver in various structures, notably the proteinaceous filaments inside axons (Fig. 2-3). The most widely used techniques for axons are those of Ramón y Cajal, Bielschowsky, Bodian, and Holmes. Other methods, notably those developed by Ramón y Cajal, del Rio Hortega, and Penfield, are available for selective demonstration of different types of neuroglial cell.

Stains for myelin rely on the affinities of certain dyes for protein-bound phospholipids. They are valuable to teachers and students of neuroanatomy because they reveal the major tracts of fibers. Some of the photographs in this book (eg, in Ch. 7) are of sections stained by Weigert's method for myelin. At low magnification, the bundles of myelinated fibers are blue-black, whereas cellular areas such as nuclei usually are colorless. Combined myelin and Nissl stains commonly are used in research and neuropathology.

The **Golgi method**, which has many variants, is valuable for the study of neuronal morphology, especially of dendrites (Fig. 2-4). In the original method, pieces of tissue are treated sequentially over several days with solutions that contain potassium dichromate and silver nitrate, after which sections 100 to 200 μm thick are prepared. Some of the neurons, including the finest branches of their dendrites, stand out in brown or black against a clear background. Occasional neuroglial cells are similarly displayed, but axons (especially if myelinated) are typically unstained. An important feature of these methods is the staining of only a small proportion of the cells. If all were blackened, it would be impossible, in the dense forest of neurites, to resolve the structural details of individual cells.

Filling techniques provide pictures similar to those obtained by the Golgi method, but for individual neurons that have been studied physiologically. A histochemically demonstrable ion (such as cobalt), fluorescent dye (procion yellow or lucifer yellow), or enzyme (usually horseradish peroxidase) is injected into the neuron through a micropipette that has been used for intracellular electrical recording. Also available are fluorescent dyes that move laterally in the cell membranes. These can be applied to fresh or even fixed tissue and used to trace neuronal connections over distances of up to 5 mm. Filling techniques are reminiscent of the tract-tracing methods described in Chapter 4, but the latter are based on activities of the living nervous system.

Histochemical and immunohistochemical methods are available for localizing substances contained in specific populations of neurons. These substances include putative neurotransmitters (eg, noradrenaline, dopamine, serotonin, glutamate, and numerous peptides) and enzymes involved in the synthesis or degradation of neurotransmitters (eg, dopamine-β-hydroxylase, choline acetyltransferase, and acetylcholinesterase). Several previously unrecognized systems of neurons have been identified by the use of these methods in laboratory

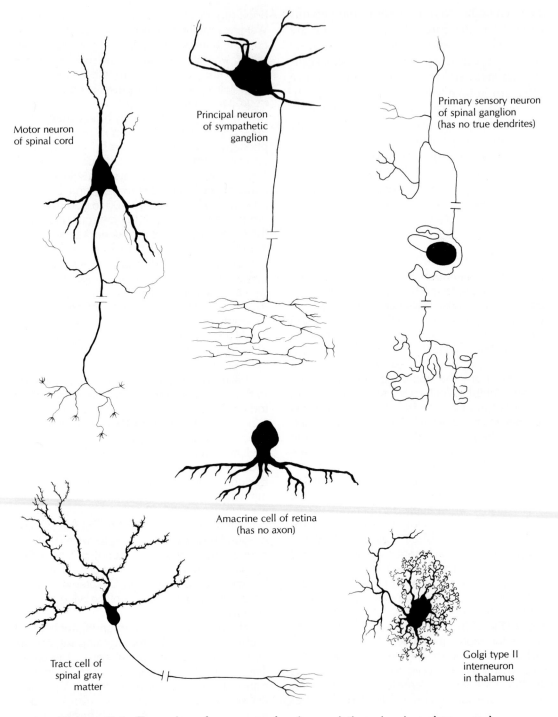

Figure 2-1. Examples of neurons, showing variations in size, shape, and branching of processes.

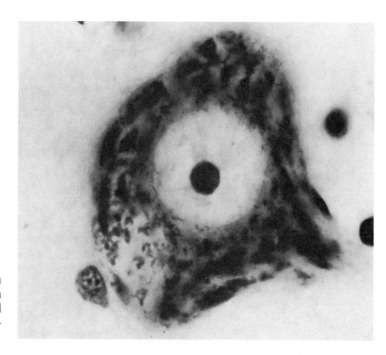

Figure 2-2. Motor neuron in the spinal cord, stained with cresyl violet, showing the Nissl bodies and a prominent nucleolus. (× 100)

animals, and it is reasonable to surmise that equivalent systems exist in humans.

Electron microscopy reveals the detailed internal structure of neurons and the specializations that exist at synaptic junctions. The necessity of using very thin sections makes it difficult to reconstruct in three dimensions. Electron microscopy may be combined with staining by Golgi methods or with immunohistochemical procedures.

Cytology of the Neuron

The parts of a generalized multipolar neuron are shown in Figure 2-5.

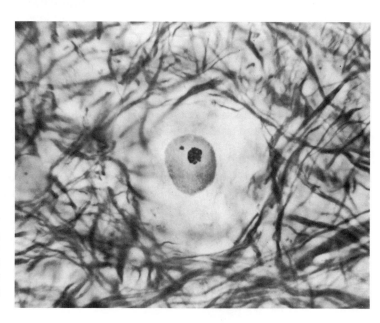

Figure 2-3. Nerve cell surrounded by axons. In addition, the nucleolus and a small accessory body of Cajal are seen in the nucleus. (Stained by one of Cajal's silver nitrate methods, × 1000)

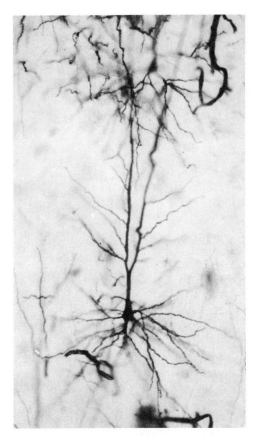

Figure 2-4. Pyramidal cell of the cerebral cortex, stained by the Golgi technique. The cell body is in the lower one-third of the picture, and dendrites extend up toward the cortical surface as well as laterally. (× 90; *courtesy of Dr. E. G. Bertram*)

CELL SURFACE

The surface or limiting membrane of the neuron assumes special importance because of its role in the initiation and transmission of nerve impulses. The plasma membrane, or plasmalemma, is a double layer of phospholipid molecules whose hydrophobic hydrocarbon chains are all directed toward the middle of the membrane. Embedded in this structure are protein molecules, many of which pass through the whole thickness. Some transmembrane proteins provide hydrophilic **channels** through which inorganic ions may enter and leave the cell. Each of the common ions (Na^+, K^+, Ca^{2+}, Cl^-) has its own specific type of molecular channel. The channels are voltage-gated, which means that they open and close in response to changes in the electrical potential across the membrane. Nerve impulses are propagated (conducted) along the cell membrane of the neuronal surface. A simplified account of this process follows.

CONDUCTION

Extracellular fluid has a high concentration of sodium ions (Na^+) and a low concentration of potassium ions (K^+), whereas in neuronal cytoplasm, there is a high concentration of K^+ and a low concentration of Na^+. In the resting state, K^+ ions can leave the cell by diffusion through their channels in the membrane. Only small numbers of Na^+ ions diffuse in through the membrane because at rest, the Na^+ channels are closed. Larger quantities of sodium enter when impulses are being conducted. The entry of Na^+ and the loss of intracellular K^+ are opposed by another membrane protein, the **sodium pump**. A **pump** is a molecule that uses energy (from adenosine triphosphate) to move ions through a membrane against a concentration gradient. The ionic concentrations in the cytoplasm are maintained, with expenditure of energy, largely as a result of the activity of the sodium pump. The resulting differences in concentrations of ions impart to the membrane a **resting potential**, with the inside of the cell at about -70 mV with respect to the outside.

During excitation, which may be due to any of a variety of chemical or physical stimuli, there is a reduction of the membrane potential, and the membrane is said to be **depolarized**. The reduction of potential spreads laterally in the plane of the membrane, declining in magnitude with distance from its site of initiation. This graded potential change is the only type of signaling in the dendrites and cell body. Stimuli of sufficient number and intensity may reduce the membrane potential of the initial segment of the axon by as much as 10 to 15 mV. This is a threshold value that triggers the opening of the voltage-gated sodium channels of the axonal membrane. Na^+ ions surge locally from the outer to the inner surface, moving

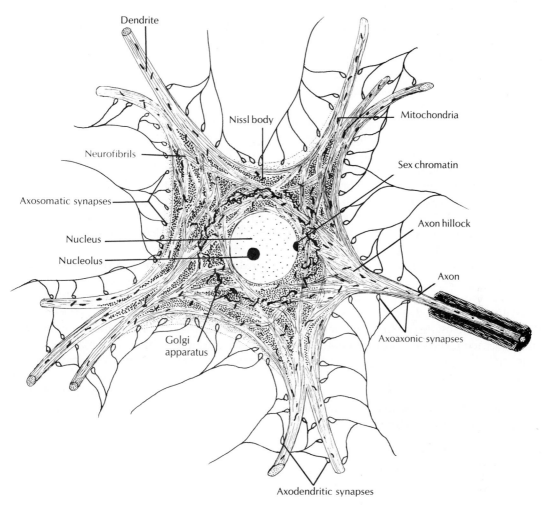

Figure 2-5. Diagrammatic representation of the constituents of a nerve cell in a female animal. The associated neuroglial cells (see Fig. 2-9) are not included.

down a concentration gradient and also being attracted by the excess of negative charge in the axoplasm. The inside of the axon is transiently some + 40 mV with respect to the outside. This change is called an **action potential**, or **nerve impulse**. Once generated, the action potential is self-propagated along the membrane by local circuits of electric current, which open the nearby sodium channels. It can be recorded from the outer surface of the nerve fiber as a wave of negative potential.

Stimuli that reduce the neuronal membrane potential are said to be excitatory because sufficient numbers of them will sum-

mate to cause depolarization and thereby initiate an action potential. Some stimuli have the opposite effect of **hyperpolarization**, in which the membrane potential exceeds its resting value of − 70 mV. Stimuli that cause hyperpolarization inhibit the generation of action potentials because they oppose the effects of depolarizing stimuli.

NUCLEUS

The spherical nucleus of a neuron is usually in the center of the cell body. In large neurons, it is vesicular (ie, the chromatin is finely dispersed), whereas in most small neurons, the chromatin is in coarse clumps. There are a few binucleate neurons in sympathetic ganglia. The nuclear envelope has the usual double-layered ultrastructure with numerous pores. Typically there is a single prominent **nucleolus**.

In females, one of the two X chromosomes of the interphase nucleus is compact (heterochromatic) rather than elongated (euchromatic) like the remaining 45 chromosomes of the complement. The compact X chromosome is evident as the **sex chromatin body**. This occurs in all cells but was first recognized in neurons. It is normally situated at the inner surface of the nuclear membrane.

Within the nuclei of some neurons, intranuclear rods and fibrillogranular bodies (accessory bodies of Cajal) can be seen in sections of tissue stained by silver methods (see Fig. 2-3). These inclusions are made up of fibrils 7 nm in diameter. They are most commonly seen in sensory systems that are continuously active (olfactory and auditory) and in cells in which increased activity has been induced experimentally by electrical stimulation. Their functions are otherwise unknown.

CYTOPLASMIC ORGANELLES

NEUROFIBRILS, NEUROFILAMENTS, MICROTUBULES, AND MICROFILAMENTS. When certain reduced silver stains are used, the cytoplasm is seen by light microscopy to contain neurofibrils, sometimes grouped into bundles that run through the perikaryon and into the dendrites and axon. Electron micrographs show that the cytoplasm contains neurofilaments 7.5 to 10 nm in thickness. These are known from biochemical and immunohistochemical studies to be made of structural proteins similar to those of the intermediate filaments of other types of cell and to be components of the larger **neurofibrils** of light microscopy. The electron microscope also reveals microtubules, 25 nm in external diameter, similar to those of other cells. Microtubules are involved in the rapid transport of protein molecules and small particles in both directions along axons and dendrites. Microfilaments (4 nm) are molecules of the contractile protein actin. They occur on the inside of the plasmalemma and are

particularly numerous in the tips of growing neurites.

NISSL SUBSTANCE. Clumps of basophilic material are seen in the perikarya of most nerve cells after staining with a cationic dye. Known as Nissl bodies, they extend into the proximal parts of the dendrites but are absent from the axon and from the axonal hillock (the region in the periphery of the cell body where the axon emerges). Nissl material is sometimes called the tigroid substance because of its striped appearance in large neurons.

The electron microscope shows Nissl bodies to be orderly arrays of **granular (rough) endoplasmic reticulum** (Fig. 2-6). This is a system of flattened cisternae or vesicles that bear ribosomal particles on their outer surfaces and with polyribosomes in the adjacent cytoplasmic matrix. The ribosomes contain RNA, which accounts for their basophilia. They are the sites of synthesis of structural and enzymatic proteins. Consequently large neurons, with great quantities of cytoplasm in their long processes, have abundant Nissl substance in their perikarya.

MITOCHONDRIA. Mitochondria are cytoplasmic organelles scattered throughout the perikaryon, dendrites, and axon. They may be spherical, rod-shaped, or filamentous, measuring from 0.2 to 1.0 μm by about 0.2 μm. The mitochondria of nerve cells show the double membrane and internal folds or cristae that are present in mitochondria of cells generally. Mitochondria are the repository of enzymes involved in cellular respiration as well as the site of energy-producing chemical reactions.

GOLGI APPARATUS, SMOOTH ENDOPLASMIC RETICULUM, AND LYSOSOMES. The Golgi apparatus (or complex) is a universal cytoplasmic organelle, first described in neurons by Camillo Golgi. With the light microscope, the Golgi apparatus is demonstrable, using special staining methods, as an irregular reticulated structure that commonly surrounds the nucleus. It is seen in electron micrographs to consist of clusters of closely apposed, flattened cisternae arranged in stacks and surrounded

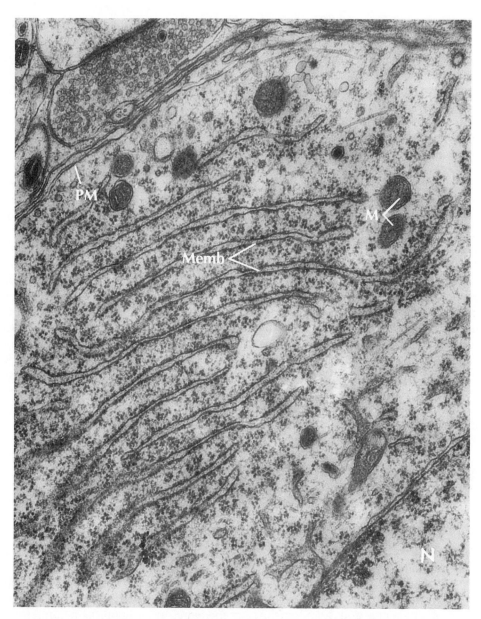

Figure 2-6. Electron micrograph of a portion of a neuron in the preoptic area of a rabbit's brain. The series of membranes, together with the free polyribosomes between the membranes, constitute the Nissl material of light microscopy. **M** = mitochondria; **Memb** = membranes of endoplasmic reticulum; **N** = nucleus; **PM** = plasma membrane. (× 36,000; *courtesy of Dr. R. Clattenburg*)

by many small vesicles. The Golgi complex is the site of the addition of carbohydrates to some proteins, which thus become glycoproteins. These substances are packed into several types of membrane-bound vesicles for trans-

port distally along the cytoplasmic processes of the neuron. The vesicles are used for the renewal of the cell membrane and for the renewal of synaptic vesicles in axonal endings.

Lysosomes, which are derived from the

smooth endoplasmic reticulum and the Golgi apparatus, are membrane-bound vesicles. They are typically slightly smaller than mitochondria and contain enzymes that catalyze the breakdown of unwanted large molecules. Lysosomes are occasionally seen in normal neurons, but they are more numerous and conspicuous in injured or diseased cells.

PIGMENT INCLUSIONS. The perikaryon may contain cytoplasmic inclusions (deposits of nonliving material, as opposed to organelles), of which the most conspicuous are pigment granules. **Lipofuscin** (lipochrome) pigment occurs as yellowish brown granules containing lipids that are so firmly bound to proteins that they are not extracted by solvents. Traces of this pigment appear in neurons of the sensory and sympathetic ganglia, spinal cord, and medulla at about age 8. The amount of pigment increases with age. Lipofuscin granules are large, old lysosomes that contain indigestible remains of cellular components. They are found in other cells, including cardiac muscle fibers, and the amount of stored pigment increases with age. Some types of neuron, of which the Purkinje cells of the cerebellar cortex are a notable example, do not accumulate lipofuscin even in old age.

The presence of black **melanin** granules in the cytoplasm is restricted to a few cell groups, the largest being the substantia nigra in the midbrain and the locus coeruleus in the pons. The metabolic precursor of this pigment is dihydroxyphenylalanine (DOPA), which is converted to melanin by a series of oxidations followed by polymerization. Dopa is also the precursor of dopamine and noradrenaline, which are neurotransmitters used by the neurons of the substantia nigra and locus coeruleus, respectively. Melanin may accumulate as a by-product of the synthesis of these amines. The pigment in the substantia nigra appears at the end of the second year, increases until puberty, and normally remains constant thereafter.

PROCESSES OF THE NERVE CELL

Dendrites taper from the cell body and branch in its immediate environs; the branching may be exceedingly profuse and intricate. The cytoplasm of dendrites resembles that of the perikaryon, with granular endoplasmic reticulum (Nissl substance) in their proximal trunks and at points of branching. In some neurons, the smaller branches bear large numbers of minute projections, called **dendritic spines** or **gemmules**, which participate in synapses. The surface of the cell body is also included in the receptive field of the neuron.

The single **axon** of a nerve cell has a uniform diameter throughout its length. In interneurons, it is a short, delicate process that branches terminally to establish synaptic contact with one or more adjacent neurons. Some interneurons have no axon, so they can conduct only graded changes of membrane potential. In principal cells, the diameter of the axon increases in proportion to its length. **Collateral** branches may be given off at right angles to the axon. The terminal branches are known as **telodendria**; they typically end as **synaptic terminals** in contact with other cells. The cytoplasm of the axon is called **axoplasm**, and the surface membrane is known as the **axolemma**. The axoplasm includes neurofilaments, microtubules, scattered mitochondria, and fragments of smooth endoplasmic reticulum.

The axon of a principal cell is usually surrounded by a myelin sheath, which begins near the origin of the axon and ends short of its terminal branching. Within the central nervous system, the myelin is laid down by oligodendrocytes and consists of closely apposed layers of their plasma membranes. The sheath, therefore, has a lipoprotein composition. Interruptions called **nodes of Ranvier** indicate those points at which regions formed by different oligodendrocytes adjoin. Voltage-gated sodium channels are present only at the nodes of a myelinated axon, so the ionic movements of impulse conduction occur only at these sites. The sheath insulates the axon between nodes, and thus there is almost instantaneous conduction of the action potential from one node to the next. This **saltatory conduction** permits much faster signaling in a myelinated than in an unmyelinated axon. The thickness of the myelin sheath and the distance between nodes are directly proportional to the axon's diameter and length. The greater the diameter of the nerve fiber, the faster is the conduction of the nerve impulse. (A nerve "fiber" in the central nervous system consists of the axon and the surrounding myelin sheath, or of the axon only in the case of unmyelinated fibers.) The formation and structure of the myelin sheath are discussed in Chapter 3 in the context of peripheral nerve fibers, in which these aspects of myelin have been studied in greater detail.

SYNAPSES

A neuron influences other neurons at junctional points, or synapses. The term *synapse*, meaning a conjunction or connection, was introduced by Sherrington in 1897. A nerve impulse can be propagated in either direction along the surface of an axon. The direction it follows under physiological conditions is determined by a consistent polarity at most synapses, where transmission is from the axon of one neuron to a dendrite or the perikaryon of another neuron. Consequently action potentials are initiated at the axonal hillock and propagated away from the cell body.

CHEMICAL SYNAPSES
AND THEIR ACTIVITIES

SYNAPTIC STRUCTURE AND CLASSIFICATION. Most synaptic junctions are of the type known as **chemical synapses**, in which a substance, the **neurotransmitter**, diffuses across the narrow space between the two cells and becomes bound to **receptors**, which are special protein molecules that reside in the postsynaptic membrane. The nature of the receptor molecule determines whether the effect produced will be excitation or inhibition of the postsynaptic cell. Some synapses are, therefore, excitatory, whereas others are inhibitory. As soon as the neurotransmitter has accomplished its purpose, it is released from the receptors and immediately inactivated. Inactivation may be effected either by chemical degradation catalyzed by an enzyme present at the synapse or by reabsorption of the neuro-

transmitter into the presynaptic terminal or the nearby neuroglial cells.

Several types of chemical synapse can be recognized at the ultrastructural level. In all of them, the presynaptic and postsynaptic cell membranes are separated by a synaptic cleft about 20 nm wide. The presynaptic terminal contains many small vesicles, usually clustered beneath the site of the functional contact, and several mitochondria. The **synaptic vesicles** contain the neurotransmitter substances. They probably discharge their contents into the synaptic cleft by fusing with the presynaptic axolemma, a process of exocytosis. At other sites, the presynaptic elements are not at the ends of telodendria, so the axons make synaptic contacts *en passant*.

The most abundant types of synapse are those designated as **Gray's type I (asymmetrical)** and **Gray's type II (symmetrical)**. In Gray's type I synapses, the vesicles are spherical and 40 nm in diameter, and the postsynaptic membrane is thickened by a deposition of electron-dense material on its cytoplasmic surface (Fig. 2-7). In Gray's type II synapses, the vesicles are of similar size but are ellipsoidal, and there are thickenings of both the presynaptic and the postsynaptic membranes. The small synaptic vesicles in types I and II synaptic boutons contain acetylcholine and amino acid neurotransmitters. It is not possible to identify the transmitter from the ultrastructural appearance of the vesicles in a presynaptic terminal. Another common type of synapse, usually with asymmetrical membrane thickenings, is one in which spherical synaptic vesicles are about 50 nm in diameter and have electron-dense cores. In these synapses, the neurotransmitters are believed to be the monoamines: noradrenaline, dopamine, and serotonin. Even larger (80–100 nm) dense-cored synaptic vesicles may contain peptide neurotransmitters. There also are synapses with mixed granular and agranular vesicles, and it is suspected that some neurotransmitters may be released by diffusion from the axoplasmic cytosol, rather than by exocytosis of vesicles.

Synapses also are classified according to the parts of the neurons that form the pre-

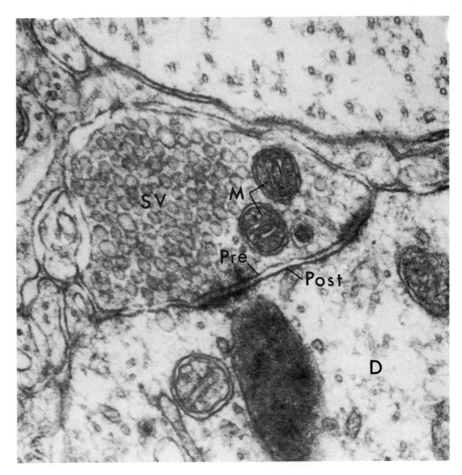

Figure 2-7. Electron micrograph of an axodendritic Gray's type I (asymmetrical) synapse in a rabbit's hypothalamus. **D** = dendrite; **M** = mitochondria; **Pre** = presynaptic membrane; **Post** = postsynaptic membrane; **SV** = synaptic vesicles. (× 82,000; *courtesy of Dr. R. Clattenburg*)

synaptic and postsynaptic components. **Axodendritic** and **axosomatic** synapses are the most abundant, but **axoaxonal** and **dendrodendritic** contacts also are present in many parts of the nervous system. Furthermore, an axonal terminal or dendritic branchlet commonly engages several other axons or dendrites. Some of the common types of synapse are shown in Figure 2-8.

SYNAPTIC TRANSMISSION. When the membrane potential of a presynaptic neurite is reversed by the arrival of an action potential (or, in the case of a dendrodendritic synapse, ade-

quately reduced by a graded fluctuation), calcium channels are opened and Ca^{2+} ions diffuse into the cell because they are present at a much higher concentration in the extracellular fluid than in the cytoplasm. Entry of calcium triggers the release of neurotransmitters and neuromodulators into the synaptic cleft.

Among the first transmitters to be recognized were **acetylcholine** at the neuromuscular junction and in the autonomic nervous system (see Ch. 24) and **noradrenaline**, used by most neurons of the sympathetic division of the autonomic system. Other neurotransmitters include amines such as **dopa-**

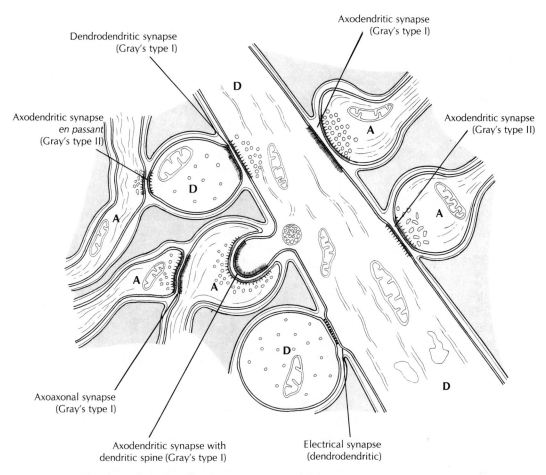

Dendrodendritic synapse
(Gray's type I)

Axodendritic synapse
(Gray's type I)

Axodendritic synapse
en passant
(Gray's type II)

Axodendritic synapse
(Gray's type II)

Axoaxonal synapse
(Gray's type I)

Axodendritic synapse with
dendritic spine (Gray's type I)

Electrical synapse
(dendrodendritic)

Figure 2-8. Ultrastructure of various types of synapse. The shaded areas represent the cytoplasmic processes of astrocytes. **A** = axons; **D** = dendrites.

mine and **serotonin**, amino acids such as **glutamic acid** and **gamma-aminobutyric acid**, and many **peptides**. **Nitric oxide**, formed enzymatically from the amino acid arginine, is a simple inorganic compound thought to serve as a neurotransmitter at some sites in the peripheral and central nervous systems. Some of these substances may be **neuromodulators** rather than classic transmitters. The modulatory action consists of making the postsynaptic membranes more or less susceptible to the action of the chief transmitter. Immunohistochemical studies show that probably all neurons, even those with well-known classical transmitters, secrete two or more substances that might be neurotransmit-

ters or neuromodulators. Having crossed the synaptic cleft, the transmitter molecules combine with receptors on the postsynaptic cell.

If the transmitter–receptor interaction is one that results in excitation, entry of Ca^{2+} ions occurs at postsynaptic sites. Inhibition, on the other hand, usually involves the opening of chloride channels in the postsynaptic membrane, which is transiently hyperpolarized as a consequence of the diffusion of Cl^- ions into the cytoplasm.

The arrival of an impulse at an excitatory synapse locally depolarizes the postsynaptic membrane, whereas an impulse arriving at an inhibitory synapse causes local hyperpolarization. These changes in the membrane potential are additive over the whole receptive surface of the postsynaptic neuron. If the net electrical change reaches a threshold level of depolarization to about -55 mV at the axon hillock, an action potential will be initiated and will travel along the axon. Thus the sum of the postsynaptic responses in the receptive field of a neuron determines whether or not, at any given moment, an impulse will be sent along the axon.

Some neurotransmitters, like acetylcholine and the glutamate ion, act rapidly (milliseconds) by combining with receptors that are directly associated with ion channels in the membrane. Other substances, notably the peptides and nitric oxide, have more protracted actions (seconds, minutes, or hours). Slowly acting transmitters or modulators combine with receptors associated with **G-proteins**. The latter are proteins that bind guanosine triphosphate and participate in intracellular second-messenger systems in the cytoplasm of the postsynaptic cell.

ELECTRICAL SYNAPSES. Electrical synapses, as opposed to the chemical synapses already described, are common in invertebrates and lower vertebrates, and have been observed at a few sites in the mammalian nervous system. They consist of a close apposition (2 nm) of presynaptic and postsynaptic membranes, across which the cytoplasms of the two cells are joined by numerous tubules or **connexons**, formed from transmembrane protein molecules of both cells. Water and small ions and molecules move freely through the connexons. An electrical synapse offers a low-resistance pathway between neurons, and there is no delay because a chemical mediator is not involved. Unlike most chemical synapses, electrical synapses are not polarized, and the direction of transmission fluctuates with the membrane potentials of the connected cells. A cluster of connexons that join cells other than neurons is known by the general term **gap junction**.

AXONAL TRANSPORT

Proteins, including enzymes, membrane lipoproteins, and cytoplasmic structural pro-

fied by studying the distribution of proteins labeled by incorporation of radioactive amino acids. Most of the protein moves distally at a rate of about 1 mm/day. This component consists largely of structural proteins, including the subunits of neurofilaments and microtubules. A smaller proportion is transported much more rapidly, at a mean velocity of 300 mm/day. Transport also occurs simultaneously in the reverse direction, from the synaptic terminals to the cell body. The retrogradely transported material includes proteins imbibed from the extracellular fluid by axonal terminals as well as proteins that reach the axon terminals by fast anterograde transport and are returned to the perikaryon. The rate of retrograde transport is variable, but most of the material moves at about two thirds the speed of the fast component of the anterograde transport.

The mechanisms of axonal transport are only partially understood. The rapid components in both directions involve predominantly particle-bound substances and require the integrity of the microtubules of the axoplasm. Particles probably move along the outside of the tubules. It is an amazing feat of biological engineering that different substances can move at different rates and in different directions at the same time within a tube as thin as an axon.

Neuroglial Cells

Although neuroglial cells are not primarily involved with excitation, inhibition, and propagation of the nerve impulse, they have their own ancillary roles. Certain of these cells are in close contact with nerve cells, leading to a high degree of metabolic interdependence. The term *neuroglia* originally referred only to cells in the central nervous system. It is now applied also to the nonneuronal cells that are intimately related to neurons and their processes in peripheral ganglia and nerves. The central neuroglia are discussed in this section. The peripheral neuroglial cells are considered in Chapter 3.

The nomenclature of neuroglial cells is

teins, are transported distally within axons from their sites of synthesis in the perikaryon. Two major rates of transport have been identi-summarized in Table 2-1, and the principal structural features of each type are shown in Figure 2-9. The developmental biology of neuroglial cells is reviewed at the end of this chapter.

Astroglia

STRUCTURE AND LOCATION

Astrocytes are variable cells with medium-size spherical or ellipsoidal nuclei, often with deep indentations, having moderately dispersed chromatin. The cytoplasm has numerous processes and contains the characteristic organelles of these cells, the gliofilaments, which are slightly finer than neurofilaments and gathered into bundles. The filaments are made of a substance known as glial fibrillary acidic protein (GFAP). Mitochondria interspersed among the bundles probably correspond to the "gliosomes" seen by light microscopy. The cytoplasm also contains numerous inclusions, 20 to 40 nm in diameter, which are composed of glycogen. Many astrocytic processes are closely applied to capillary blood vessels, where they are known as perivascular **end feet**. Other end feet are applied to the pia mater at the external surface of the central nervous system (including the outer surfaces of the perivascular spaces around larger blood vessels), forming the **external glial limiting membrane**. Astrocytic end feet also form the **internal glial limiting membrane** beneath the single layer of ependymocytes that line the ventricular system.

Two extreme types of astrocyte are easily recognized by light or electron microscopy, although intermediate forms commonly are encountered. **Fibrous astrocytes** occur in white matter. They have long processes with coarse bundles of gliofilaments. **Protoplasmic (or velate) astrocytes** are found in gray matter. Their processes are greatly branched and flattened to form delicate lamellae around the terminal branches of axons, dendrites, and synapses. Müller cells (in the retina) and pituicytes (in the neurohypophysis) are morphologically distinct varieties of protoplasmic astrocytes.

By staining immunohistochemically to demonstrate certain cell surface glycoproteins, astrocytes in laboratory animals have been classified into two types (designated as types 1 and 2) that do not correspond to the classic fibrous and protoplasmic varieties. The type 1 cells form the glial limiting membranes and have end feet on blood vessels, whereas the type 2 cells are intimately associated with neuronal surfaces around synapses and at nodes of Ranvier. Modern methods are likely to reveal yet other cell types, but the traditional classification of astrocytes as fibrous and protoplasmic cell types remains valuable for naming the cells in ordinary light and electron microscopy.

FUNCTIONS

Astrocytes, like other glial cells, fill in the spaces that would otherwise exist among the neurons and their processes. The GFAP may confer some rigidity on the cytoplasm of astrocytes, thereby providing physical support for the other cellular elements of the nervous system. The disposition of astrocytic processes with their perivascular end feet suggests that these cells may be involved in the exchange of metabolites between neurons and the blood.

Synapses and nodes of Ranvier are surrounded by the cytoplasmic processes of protoplasmic astrocytes, which can absorb some neurotransmitters, notably glutamate ions. This serves to terminate the action on the postsynaptic membrane. Potassium ions are re-

TABLE 2-1 ▬▬▬▬▬▬▬
Classification of Neuroglial Cell Types

Astroglia	Fibrous astrocytes
	Protoplasmic (velate) astrocytes
Oligodendroglia	Interfascicular oligodendrocytes
	Satellite oligodendrocytes
Ependyma	Ependymocytes
	Tanycytes
	Choroidal epithelial cells
Microglia	Resting microglial cells

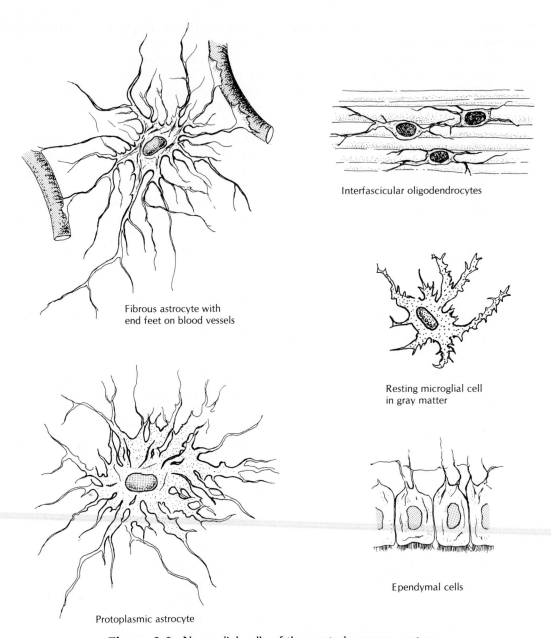

Fibrous astrocyte with
end feet on blood vessels

Interfascicular oligodendrocytes

Resting microglial cell
in gray matter

Ependymal cells

Protoplasmic astrocyte

Figure 2-9. Neuroglial cells of the central nervous system.

leased from neurons when their cell membranes are depolarized. The absorption of K^+ by astrocytes around synapses, unmyelinated axons, and nodes of Ranvier restrains the spread of electrical disturbances within bundles of axons and regions of neuropil. The dissipation of potassium ions and other small molecules is further enhanced by the existence of gap junctions between adjacent astrocytes.

Oligodendroglia

STRUCTURE AND LOCATION

The nuclei of oligodendrocytes are small and spherical, with dense chromatin. A rim of cytoplasm surrounds the nucleus and produces a few long, thin processes. The cytoplasm is conspicuous because of its high electron density and because it contains much granular endoplasmic reticulum and many polyribosomes. Gliofilaments and glycogen are absent, but there are numerous microtubules in the processes. **Interfascicular oligodendrocytes** occur in rows among myelinated axons, where their cytoplasmic processes form and remain continuous with the myelin sheaths. One cell is connected to several myelinated nerve fibers. **Satellite oligodendrocytes** are closely associated with the cell bodies of large neurons.

FUNCTIONS

Interfascicular oligodendrocytes are responsible for producing and maintaining the myelin sheaths of axons in the central nervous system. The concentrically organized membrane of the myelin is continuous with the plasmalemma of the oligodendrocyte. This function is equivalent to that of the Schwann cell in peripheral nerves. One cytoplasmic process of an oligodendrocyte provides the myelin of one internode (the myelinated interval between two nodes of Ranvier) of one axon. The fact that each oligodendrocytic process is attached to a different axon indicates that the layers of the myelin sheath could not possibly have been formed by a rotational movement of the cell around the axon. The myelin sheath enlarges because lipoprotein added to the surface of the central part of an oligodendrocyte diffuses laterally within the plasmalemma and is quickly incorporated into the whole surface of the cell. This surface includes the myelin sheaths of all the internodes associated with the oligodendrocyte.

Satellite oligodendrocytes are in contact with some neuronal cell bodies. Astrocytes also are often closely associated with neuronal cell bodies. It is thought that neuroglial cells provide essential metabolic support for the adjacent neurons, but the nature of this relation (other than absorption of potassium and glutamate ions by astrocytes) has not been determined.

Ependyma

The ependyma is the simple cuboidal to columnar epithelium that lines the ventricular system. Three cell types are recognized in the ependyma. **Ependymocytes** constitute the great majority of ependymal cells. Their cytoplasm contains all the usual organelles as well as many filaments similar to those found in astrocytes. Most ependymocytes bear cilia and microvilli on their free or apical surfaces. The bases of the cells have cytoplasmic processes that mingle with the astrocytic end feet of the internal glial limiting membrane.

Ependymocytes line the ventricular system and are thus in contact with the cerebrospinal fluid (CSF). These cells are not connected by tight junctions, and molecules of all sizes are freely exchanged between the CSF and the adjacent nervous tissue.

Tanycytes differ from ependymocytes in having long basal processes. Most of these cells are found in the floor of the third ventricle. Their basal processes end on the pia mater and on blood vessels in the median eminence of the hypothalamus (see Ch. 11).

It has been suggested that the tanycytes of the ventral hypothalamic region respond to changing levels of blood-derived hormones in the CSF by discharging secretory products into the capillary vessels of the median eminence. Such activity may be involved in the control of the endocrine system by the anterior lobe of the pituitary gland (see Ch. 11).

Choroidal epithelial cells cover the surfaces of the choroid plexuses. They have microvilli at their apical surfaces and invaginations at their basal surfaces, which rest on a basement membrane. Adjacent choroidal epithelial cells are joined by tight junctions, thus preventing the passive movement of plasma proteins into the CSF. The cells also are metabolically active in controlling the chemical composition of the fluid, which is secreted by the choroid plexuses into the cerebral ventricles.

Microglia

About 5% of the total neuroglial population is composed of **resting microglial cells**. These have small elongated nuclei with dense, but patchy chromatin. The cytoplasm is scanty, with several short branched processes that bear spiny appendages. Resting microglial cells occur in gray and white matter and are evenly spaced in the tissue, with little overlapping or intertwining of their processes.

Resting microglial cells are equivalent to the resident macrophages of other tissues, and they can acquire phagocytic properties when the central nervous system is afflicted by injury or disease. They may also be involved, although less conspicuously, in protecting the nervous tissue from viruses, microorganisms, and the formation of tumors.

Abnormal Neuroglia

When the brain or spinal cord is injured, the astrocytes near the lesion undergo hypertrophy. The cytoplasmic processes become more numerous and are densely packed with gliofilaments. There may also be a small increase in the number of the cells caused by mitosis of mature astrocytes. These changes, known as **gliosis**, occur in many pathological conditions, and sometimes the reactive astrocytes acquire phagocytic properties.

Cells with structure and staining properties similar to those of resting microglial cells appear in large numbers at the sites of injury or inflammatory disease in the central nervous system. Experimental evidence indicates that these pathological cells, known as **reactive microglial cells**, arise from monocytes that enter the nervous system by passing through the walls of blood vessels. The reactive microglial cells have a phagocytic function equivalent to that of macrophages in other parts of the body.

Development of Neurons and Neuroglial Cells ————

NEURONS AND MACROGLIA

The term **macroglia** is applied collectively to the different types of astrocyte, oligodendrocyte, and ependymal cell. No one doubts that these cells, like the neurons, are descendants of cells of the neural plate and tube. The cells that line the lumen of the neural tube of the embryo are known as neuroepithelial cells, and they constitute the ventricular zone. The first daughter cells produced in this zone are **early neuroblasts**, which migrate outward and differentiate into neurons. Other neuroepithelial cells become **radial neuroglial cells**, with long processes that cross the whole thickness of the wall of the neural tube. These processes evidently provide directional guidance for the outwardly migrating young neurons.

At a later stage, the neuroepithelium produces a population of cells in the subventricular zone in which further mitoses occur, with the formation of **late neuroblasts** and **glioblasts**. The former differentiate into neurons and the latter, into oligodendroglia and astroglia. The radial neuroglial cells persist into adult life in fishes and amphibians, but they nearly all disappear in mammals as the central nervous system grows. The old term **spongioblast** is still sometimes applied collectively to radial glial cells and glioblasts. Examination of cultured cells from the brain of the fetal rat reveals that types 1 and 2 astrocytes are derived from different precursor cells and that the type 2 precursors also give rise to oligodendrocytes. Mitosis of glioblasts continues after birth in the human brain and is conspicuous in the subventricular zone of the lateral ventricles in the first year of postnatal life.

Ependymocytes and choroidal epithelial cells are derived directly from the neuroepithelium of the ventricular zone, although some may be radial neuroglial cells that have retracted their cytoplasmic processes.

MICROGLIA

The origin of microglia has been a subject of controversy ever since these cells were recognized as distinct elements by del Rio Hortega in 1920. In stained sections, del Rio Hortega observed "fountains" of round amoeboid cells entering the nervous tissue alongside blood vessels and described their subsequent transformation into resting microglial cells. Experimental studies aimed at tracing the cells from

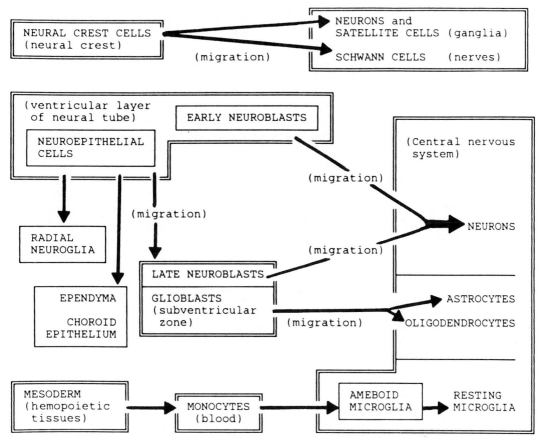

Figure 2-10. Development and differentiation of the cells of the nervous system. The cells of the peripheral nervous system (upper part of figure) are considered in Chapter 3.

sites of origin in the hematopoietic tissues to their eventual places of residence in the brain were unsuccessful, and in the 1970s and 1980s it seemed more probable that the resting microglia were the progeny of cells of the neuroectoderm, which can give rise to microglia-like cells in tissue culture. Recent histochemical investigations, in which cells have been demonstrated by virtue of characteristic enzymes in their cytoplasm and glycoproteins on their surfaces, support del Rio Hortega's contention that amoeboid cells grow cytoplasmic processes and transform into microglial cells. These events occur in the late embryonic and early fetal stages of development (7–12 weeks after fertilization).

The postulated developmental lineages of neurons, glial cells, and their precursors are set out in Figure 2-10.

SUGGESTED READING

Barr ML: The significance of the sex chromatin. Int Rev Cytol 19:35–95, 1966

Bunge RP: Glial cells and the central myelin sheath. Physiol Rev 48:197–251, 1968

Cameron RS, Rakic P: Glial cell lineage in the cerebral cortex: A review and synthesis. Glia 4:124–137, 1991

Federoff S, Doucette JR: Development of glial cells. In Meisami E, Timiras PS (eds): Handbook of Human Growth and Developmental Biology, vol I, pt A, pp. 27–44. Boca Raton, FL, CRC Press, 1988

Lasek RJ, Garner JA, Brady ST: Axonal transport of the cytoplasmic matrix. J Cell Biol 99:212s–221s, 1984

Leitch B: Ultrastructure of electrical synapses: review. Electron Microsc Rev 5:311–339, 1992

Miller RH, ffrench-Constant C, Raff MC: The macroglial cells of the rat optic nerve. Annu Rev Neurosci 12:517–534, 1989

Peters A, Palay SL, Webster HdeF: The Fine Structure of the Nervous System: Neurons and Their Supporting Cells, 3rd ed. New York, Oxford University Press, 1991

Sanders KM, Ward SM: Nitric oxide as a mediator of nonadrenergic, noncholinergic neurotransmission. Am J Physiol 262:G379–G392, 1992

Scheller RH, Hall ZW: Chemical messengers at synapses. In Hall ZW (ed): An Introduction to Molecular Neurobiology, ch 4. Sunderland, MA, Sinauer Associates, 1992

Shepherd GM: Neurobiology, 2nd ed. New York, Oxford University Press, 1988

Shepherd GM: The Synaptic Organization of the Brain, 3rd ed. New York, Oxford University Press, 1990

Somjen GG: Nervenkitt: Notes on the history of the concept of neuroglia. Glia 1:2–9, 1988

Thomas WE: Brain macrophages: Evaluation of microglia and their functions. Brain Res Rev 17:61–74, 1992

Three

The Human Nervous System: An Anatomical Viewpoint, Sixth Edition, Murray L. Barr and John A. Kiernan. J.B. Lippincott Company, Philadelphia, © 1993.

Peripheral Nervous System

Important Facts

Ganglia are the sites of all neuronal cell bodies in the peripheral nervous system. Motor and preganglionic autonomic neurons have their cell bodies in the spinal cord and brain stem.

A nerve is a bundle of axons, together with the associated glia, myelin sheaths and supporting connective tissue. A nerve fiber is one axon together with its myelin sheath and neuroglial cells.

Nerve fibers are classified according to their diameters. The largest, most rapidly conducting fibers are those innervating extrafusal muscle fibers and those serving discriminative touch, proprioception, and vibration. The smallest axons are for pain, olfaction, and visceral innervation.

There are sensory ganglia on the dorsal roots of spinal nerves and on some cranial nerves. They contain unipolar neurons with axons that enter the central nervous system.

Skin contains a variety of types of sensory nerve endings for touch, temperature, pain, and other external sensations. Muscles, tendons, and joints contain proprioceptive endings. Muscle spindles inform the central nervous system of changes in the length of a muscle; tendon receptors respond to tension.

Striated skeletal muscle is supplied by motor neurons, which have their cell bodies in the spinal cord and brain stem.

The motor end plate is the structurally specialized effector ending in striated skeletal muscle. The synaptic transmitter is acetylcholine, which makes the muscle fibers contract.

Preganglionic neurons have axons that synapse with the neurons in autonomic ganglia. Smooth muscle and glands are innervated by the neurons in autonomic ganglia.

The endings of autonomic axons are swellings (varicosities) of unmyelinated axons, containing a variety of chemical transmitter substances that stimulate or inhibit smooth muscle and secretory cells.

General Organization

Certain aspects of the peripheral nervous system are especially pertinent to a study of the brain and spinal cord. These include the sensory receptors, motor endings, histology of peripheral nerves, and structure of ganglia. The following introductory comments refer to all spinal nerves and to those cranial nerves that are not restricted to the special senses. The structures discussed in this chapter are shown in Figure 3-1, which represents a spinal nerve in the thoracic or upper lumbar region in which neurons for visceral innervation are included.

The general sensory endings are scattered profusely throughout the body. They are biological transducers, in which physical or chemical stimuli create action potentials in nerve endings. The resulting nerve impulses, on reaching the central nervous system, produce reflex responses, awareness of the stimuli, or both. Sensory endings that are superficially located, such as those in the skin, are called **exteroceptors**; they respond to stimuli for pain, temperature, touch, and pressure. **Proprioceptors** in muscles, tendons, and joints provide data for reflex adjustments of muscle action and for awareness of position and movement.

COMPONENTS OF NERVES, ROOTS, AND GANGLIA

Nerve impulses from exteroceptors and proprioceptors are conducted centrally by primary sensory neurons, whose cell bodies are located in dorsal root ganglia (or in a cranial nerve ganglion). On entering the spinal cord,

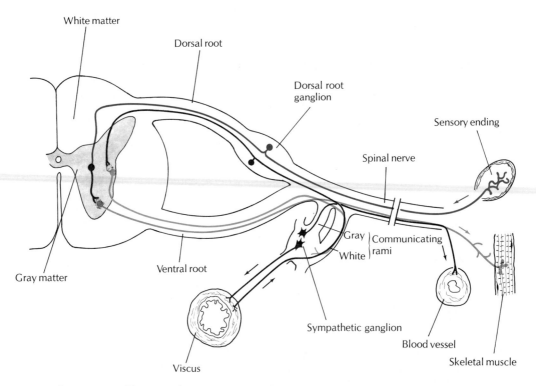

Figure 3-1. Functional components of a "typical" spinal nerve, in this case between levels T1 and L2. *Color scheme:* Red for somatic motor neurons; blue for primary sensory neurons; green for preganglionic autonomic (sympathetic) neurons; black for interneurons in the spinal cord and for postganglionic sympathetic neurons.

the dorsal root fibers divide into ascending and descending branches; these are distributed as necessary for reflex responses (of which some are considered in Ch. 5) and for transmission of sensory data to the brain (pathways are reviewed in Ch. 19).

There is a third class of sensory endings, known as **interoceptors**, in the viscera. Central conduction occurs through primary sensory neurons like those already noted, except that the peripheral process follows a different route. For a receptor concerned with pain, the fiber reaches the sympathetic trunk through a white communicating ramus and continues to a viscus in a nerve arising from the sympathetic trunk. For receptors concerned with the functional regulation of internal organs, some fibers may follow similar courses, but the best understood of the "physiological afferent" nerve fibers have their cell bodies in cranial nerve ganglia and are connected centrally with the brain stem. There are, therefore, two broad categories of sensory endings and afferent neurons: **somatic afferents**, for the skin, bones, muscles, and connective tissue that makes up most of the mass of the body (soma), and **visceral afferents**, for the internal organs of the circulatory, respiratory, alimentary, excretory, and reproductive systems.

There also are two categories of efferent or motor neurons. The cell bodies of **somatic efferent** neurons are situated in the ventral gray horns of the spinal cord and motor nuclei of cranial nerves. The axons of ventral horn cells traverse the ventral roots and spinal nerves and terminate in motor end plates on skeletal muscle fibers. The **visceral efferent** or autonomic system has a special feature, in that at least two neurons participate in transmission from the central nervous system to the viscera. In the sympathetic division of the autonomic system, for example, the cell bodies of preganglionic neurons are located in the thoracic and upper lumbar segments of the spinal cord. The axons traverse the corresponding ventral roots and white communicating rami, ending either in ganglia of the sympathetic trunk (see Fig. 3-1) or in prevertebral ganglia such as those found in the celiac and superior mesenteric plexuses of the abdomen (see Ch. 24). Axons of postganglionic neurons in these locations proceed to smooth muscle and secretory cells of some viscera, to the heart, and to neurons of the enteric plexuses in the alimentary canal. Axons from some of the cells in ganglia of the sympathetic trunk enter spinal nerves through gray communicating rami (see Fig. 3-1) for distribution to blood vessels, sweat glands, and arrector pili muscles of hairs.

Substantial numbers of unmyelinated fibers in the ventral roots originate in dorsal root ganglia. These sensory fibers approach the cord but do not enter it: they turn abruptly back and then join the mixed spinal nerve.

Sensory Endings

The sensory endings are supplied by nerve fibers that differ in size and other characteristics. This is a matter of some interest because there is a correlation between fiber diameter and the rate of conduction of the action potential and because functionally different sensory endings are supplied by fibers of specific sizes.

Classification of Nerve Fibers

A commonly used nomenclature for peripheral nerve fibers, using Roman and Greek letters, is given in Table 3-1. This includes the functions associated with the categories. The diameters of group A and group B fibers include the thicknesses of the myelin sheaths. Group A is further subdivided into alpha, beta, gamma, and delta fibers in decreasing order of size. There is some overlapping of the diameters of the A, B, and C groups because physiological properties, especially the form of the action potential, are taken into consideration when defining the groups. The smallest fibers (group C) are unmyelinated and have the slowest conduction rate, whereas the myelinated fibers of group B and group A exhibit rates of conduction that progressively increase with diameter. Group B fibers are not present in the nerves of the limbs; they occur in white rami (see Fig. 3-1) and some cranial nerves.

TABLE 3-1 ▰▰▰▰▰▰▰▰▰▰▰▰▰▰▰▰▰▰▰▰

Classification of Fibers in Peripheral Nerves and Dorsal Roots

Group	External Diameter (μm)	Conduction Velocity (m/sec)	Function
Myelinated Fibers			
Aα or Ia	12–20	70–120	Motor to skeletal muscle; sensory from annulospiral endings of muscle spindles
Aβ: Type Ib	10–15	60–80	Sensory from Golgi tendon organs and Ruffini endings of skin
Type II	5–15	30–80	Sensory from flowerspray endings of muscle spindles, Meissner's and pacinian corpuscles, and large hair follicles
Aγ	3–8	15–40	Motor to intrafusal fibers of muscle spindles
Aδ or III	3–8	10–30	Sensory from small hair follicles and free nerve endings mediating pain and temperature sensation
B	1–3	5–15	Preganglionic autonomic fibers (in sympathetic white rami, splanchnic nerves, and some cranial nerves)
Unmyelinated Fibers			
C or IV	0.2–1.5	0.5–2.5	Postganglionic autonomic fibers supplying smooth muscle, glands; sensory for pain and temperature; smell (olfactory nerves)

A second classification, also summarized in Table 3-1, uses Roman numerals. This nomenclature applies specifically to somatic afferent fibers of the dorsal roots. The table lists some of the receptors from which impulses traverse each of the four categories in this numerical system, together with their equivalents in the alternative classification.

Cutaneous Sensory Endings

On a structural basis, two classes of cutaneous and other sensory endings are recognized. **Nonencapsulated endings** are terminal branches of the axon that may either be closely applied to cells or lie freely in the extracellular spaces of connective tissue. **Encapsulated endings** have distinctive arrangements of nonneuronal cells that completely enclose the terminal parts of the axons. In the following account, the receptors are described according to location, with exteroceptors and some proprioceptors being shown in Figures 3-2 and 3-3, respectively.

Most of the skin bears hairs that vary greatly in length, thickness, and abundance from one part of the body to another. Glabrous skin, which lacks hairs, is present on the palmar surfaces of the hands and fingers, the soles, and parts of the face and external genitalia. There are different patterns of innervation in hairy and glabrous skin.

HISTOLOGY OF CUTANEOUS INNERVATION

The skin is supplied by cutaneous branches of the spinal and cranial nerves. The terminal branches of these nerves pass through the subcutaneous connective tissue into the dermis. The axons spread out horizontally to form three plexuses, which lie in the plane of the

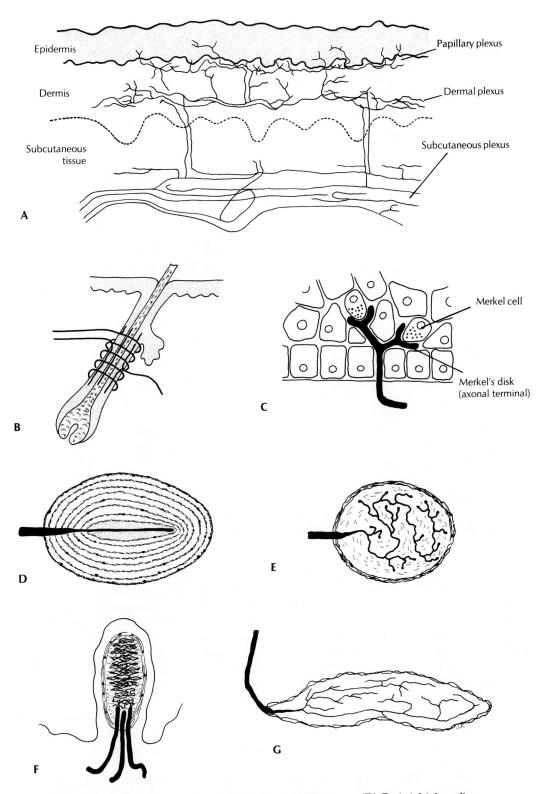

Figure 3-2. Sensory innervation of skin. (**A**) Plexuses. (**B**) Peritrichial ending. (**C**) Merkel ending in epidermis. (**D**) Pacinian corpuscle. (**E**) End bulb. (**F**) Meissner's corpuscle. (**G**) Ruffini ending.

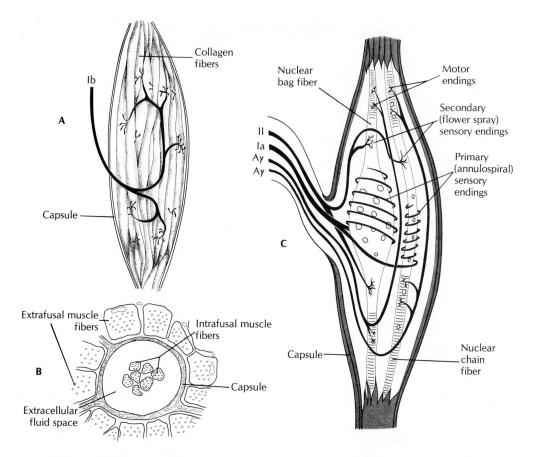

Figure 3-3. Specialized sensory endings in skeletal muscle and tendon. **(A)** Golgi tendon organ. **(B)** Neuromuscular spindle (transverse section). **(C)** Sensory and motor innervation of a muscle spindle.

skin's surface. The **subcutaneous plexus** lies in the loose connective tissue deep to the skin, the **dermal plexus** is within the densely collagenous reticular layer that constitutes the deeper part of the dermis, and the **papillary plexus** lies in the papillary layer of the dermis, which is immediately beneath the epidermis. The axons of each plexus send branches into the adjacent tissues. The density of cutaneous innervation varies considerably from one region to another. For example, the face and hands are more richly innervated than is the dorsal aspect of the trunk.

Free nerve endings occur in the subcutaneous tissue and dermis and, occasionally, extend among the cells of the epidermis. They are the terminal branches of group C fibers and

the unmyelinated terminal branches of group A fibers, and they are receptive to all modalities of cutaneous sensation. Although they are called "free endings," these axons are always invested with Schwann cells (the neuroglia of peripheral nerves) and do not contact the extracellular fluid directly. Indeed, it is impossible to identify the exact point of termination of an axon within the skin. The existence of free nerve endings is inferred from the functional sensitivity of regions of skin in which no other types of sensory ending can be recognized.

Merkel endings are found in the germinal layer (stratum basale) of the epidermis. Axonal branches end as flattened expansions that contain mitochondria and small, electron-lucent vesicles. Each axonal terminal is closely applied to a **Merkel cell**. This small cell differs from the other epidermal cells in having an indented nucleus and electron-dense cytoplasmic granules 80 nm in diameter. Merkel cells are found in glabrous skin and in the outer root sheaths of hairs. Another type of Merkel ending in hairy skin is the *Haarscheibe*, or touch-dome, an elevation about 0.2 mm in diameter associated with the follicle of a small atypical hair. The structure contains many Merkel cells supplied by branches of a single myelinated axon. The *Haarscheiben* are about 1 cm apart in human skin but are more abundant in furry animals.

Peritrichial nerve endings are cage-like formations of axons that surround hair follicles. By extensive branching, a single axon in an overlapping arrangement supplies many hair follicles, and each follicle is supplied by from 2 to 20 axons. The axons approach the follicle deep to its sebaceous gland and branch in the connective tissue outside the outer root sheath. Some branches encircle the follicle, and others run parallel to its long axis. Expanded axonal terminals are applied to Merkel cells in the outer root sheath.

Skin contains several types of encapsulated ending. The **Ruffini ending**, typically about 1 mm long and 20 to 30 μm wide, is a greatly branched array of expanded terminal branches of a myelinated axon surrounded by capsular cells. The **pacinian corpuscle** (or corpuscle of Vater-Pacini) consists of a single axon that loses its myelin sheath on entering the corpuscle and is encapsulated by several layers of flattened cells with greatly attenuated cytoplasm. The whole corpuscle is ellipsoidal, with an average length of 1 mm and a diameter of 0.7 mm. Ruffini endings and pacinian corpuscles are present in the subcutaneous tissue and dermis of both hairy and glabrous skin. **Meissner's tactile corpuscles** are present in large numbers in the dermal papillary ridges of the fingertips and are less abundant in other hairless regions. Each Meissner's corpuscle is supplied by three or four myelinated axons whose terminal branches form a complicated knot that is infiltrated with modified Schwann cells and enclosed in a capsule of cells and collagen fibers. Meissner's corpuscles are about 80 μm by 30 μm in size and are oriented with their long axes perpendicular to the skin's surface. **End bulbs** vary in size and shape, and several types have been described (eg, end bulbs of Krause, Golgi-Mazzoni endings, genital corpuscles, mucocutaneous endings), although all may be variants of the same structure. They are commonly spherical, about 50 μm across, with each containing a coiled, branching axonal terminal surrounded by a thin cellular capsule. Most end bulbs occur in mucous membranes (mouth, conjunctiva, anal canal) and in the dermis of glabrous skin close to orifices (lips, external genitalia).

PHYSIOLOGIC CORRELATES

The types of sensation that are consciously perceived from the skin are known as **modalities**. The different sensations are not always clear-cut, but in medical practice it is customary to recognize five modalities that are easily tested by clinical examination. These are fine (discriminative) touch, vibration, light touch, temperature (warmth or cold), and pain. The central pathways that process these sensations are fairly well known, but for other modalities (eg, itch, tickle, rubbing, firm pressure), they are only poorly understood. Careful testing has revealed that the human skin is a mosaic of spots, each of which responds selectively to only one of the four elementary sensations of touch, warmth, cold, and pain. The response of any one of these spots is always the same, whatever the nature of the stimulus. For example, a feeling of coldness will be experienced from a "cold spot" even if it is heated or injured. The sensitivity is greatest (or in physiologists' parlance, the threshold is lowest) for the specific modality.

Several attempts have been made to correlate the modalities of sensation in humans with the distribution of morphologically identified nerve endings, but the results have been inconclusive. Each modality-specific spot is supplied by several axons, and the qualities of the sensation perceived cannot be correlated with the distribution of microscopically identifiable nerve endings. Results of electro-physiological studies in animals, however, have shown that although no cutaneous receptors have an absolute specificity, there is a high degree of selectivity for certain end organs. Merkel endings and Meissner's corpuscles respond preferentially to tactile stimuli, and pacinian corpuscles initiate nerve impulses when they are deformed, with a special sensitivity to vibration. Ruffini endings also respond to mechanical stimuli, including pressure on and stretching of the skin. Peritrichial endings respond to mechanical displacement of the hair shaft, so that hair follicles serve as receptor organs for light touch. For some sensations, such as warmth and cold, no sensory endings have been identified. It is presumed that these modalities are transduced into nerve impulses by free nerve endings derived from the dermal and papillary plexuses. Painful sensations are also received by free nerve endings, termed nociceptors, which are stimulated by various substances released from damaged cells.

Sensory Endings in Joints, Muscles, and Tendons

Proprioceptors in the capsules of joints, muscles and tendons furnish the central nervous system with information required for the performance of properly coordinated movements through reflex action. In addition, proprioceptive information reaches consciousness so that there is awareness of the position of body parts and of their movements (**kinesthetic sense**). Pain that arises in muscles, tendons, ligaments, and bones is probably detected by free nerve endings in connective tissue. These nociceptive endings respond to physical injury and to local chemical changes, such as those that may be caused by ischemia.

JOINTS

Four types of sensory ending, each having a distinctive morphology and physiological responsiveness, are recognized within and around the capsules of synovial joints. Encapsulated formations similar to the Ruffini cuta-neous endings are present in the capsules of joints; these are derived from group A myelinated afferent fibers. Small pacinian corpuscles in the connective tissue outside the articular capsule are also supplied by group A fibers. They respond to the initiation and cessation of movement (ie, to acceleration and deceleration). The articular ligaments contain receptors identical to Golgi tendon organs and are similarly supplied by group A axons. These receptors mediate reflex inhibition of the adjacent musculature when excessive strain is placed on the joint. The importance of articular innervation is highlighted by Hilton's Law, which states that every peripheral nerve that supplies a muscle sends a branch to the joint moved by the muscle and to the skin overlying the joint.

Free nerve endings are abundant in the synovial membrane, capsule, and periarticular connective tissues. They are believed to respond to potentially injurious mechanical stresses and to mediate the pain that arises in diseased or injured joints.

MUSCLES

The proprioceptive organs contained in skeletal muscles are the **neuromuscular spindles**, often simply called muscle spindles. In addition to functioning as sensory receptors, these spindles have a significant motor role because they are components of the gamma reflex loop.

Neuromuscular spindles are a fraction of a millimeter wide and up to 6 mm long. They lie in the long axis of the muscle, and their collagenous capsules are continuous with the fibrous septa that separate the muscle fibers. The fibrous septa are in mechanical continuity with the skeletal attachments of the muscle so that the spindles are lengthened whenever the muscle is passively stretched. Spindles are typically located near the tendinous insertions of muscles and are especially numerous in muscles that perform highly skilled movements, such as those of the hand.

Each spindle (see Fig. 3-3) consists of a fusiform capsule of connective tissue, with 2 to 14 intrafusal muscle fibers. The latter differ in several respects from the main or extrafusal fibers of the muscle. Intrafusal fibers are considerably smaller than the extrafusal; the equatorial region lacks cross striations and contains many nuclei that are not in the subsarcolemmal position characteristic of mature striated muscle. The equatorial region is expanded in some intrafusal fibers (**nuclear bag fibers**) and in others it is not (**nuclear chain fibers**). Nuclear bag fibers project from the capsular investment of the spindle poles before inserting onto the extrafusal connective tissue or tendon.

A muscle spindle is supplied by two afferent nerve fibers. One of these is an Aα or Ia fiber; the axon loses its myelin covering as it pierces the capsule, and then it winds spirally around the midportions of the intrafusal muscle fibers in the form of an **annulospiral ending**. The second, slightly smaller afferent fiber (Aβ or II) branches terminally and ends as varicosities on the intrafusal muscle fibers some distance from the midregion. The latter terminals are called **flower spray endings**. The annulospiral and flower spray terminals are also known as **primary** and **secondary sensory endings** of the spindle.

The extrafusal fibers composing the main mass of a muscle are innervated by large motor cells (alpha motor neurons), whose axons are of alpha size in the A group. Smaller motor cells (gamma motor neurons), with axons of gamma size in the A group, supply the intrafusal muscle fibers within the spindle. There are motor end plates on both sides of the specialized equatorial zones of the intrafusal muscle fibers.

Neuromuscular spindles contribute to muscle function in several ways, the simplest role being that of a receptor for the stretch or extensor reflex. Slight stretching of a muscle lengthens the intrafusal muscle fibers; the sensory endings are stimulated and nerve impulses pass to alpha motor neurons that supply the main mass of the muscle. The latter thereupon contracts, in response to stretch, through a two-neuron reflex arc. Stimulation of the spindles ceases when the muscle contracts because the spindle fibers, in parallel with the other muscle fibers, return to their original lengths. The stretch reflex is in constant use in the adjustment of muscle tonus. It also forms the basis of tests for tendon reflexes, such as the knee-jerk test (extension at the knee on tapping the patellar tendon), which are standard items in a clinical examination.

The spindles also have an important role in muscle action that results from the activity of the brain. A considerable proportion of the motor fibers that originate in the brain and descend in the white matter of the spinal cord influence gamma motor neurons in the ventral gray horns, either by synapsing with them directly or through the mediation of interneurons. Contraction of the intrafusal muscle fibers in response to stimulation by gamma motor neurons lengthens the midportions and starts a volley of impulses in the sensory fibers. This causes contraction of the regular muscle fibers through reflex stimulation of alpha motor neurons. The **gamma reflex loop** consists of the gamma motor neuron, neuromuscular spindle, afferent or sensory neuron, and alpha motor neuron supplying extrafusal muscle fibers. It is an important adjunct to the more direct control of muscular activity by means of descending fibers from the brain that control the alpha motor neurons, both directly and through local circuit neurons.

TENDONS

Golgi tendon organs, also known as **neurotendinous spindles**, are most numerous near the attachments of tendons to muscles. Each receptor consists of a thin capsule of connective tissue that encloses a few collagenous fibers of the tendon, on which a nerve fiber ends. It is an Aα or Ib fiber (there may be more than one) that enters the spindle and breaks up into branches, ending as varicosities on the intrafusal tendon fibers. This type of sensory ending is stimulated by *tension* on the tendon. This specificity contrasts with that of the muscle spindle, which responds to changes in the *length* of the region containing sensory nerve endings. Afferent impulses from Golgi tendon organs reach interneurons in the spinal cord, which in turn have an inhibitory effect on alpha motor neurons, causing relaxation of the muscle to which the particular tendon is attached. The opposing functions of the neuromuscular spindles and the neurotendinous spindles are in balance in the total integration of spinal reflex activity. As constant monitors of tension, the neurotendinous spindles also provide protection against the damage to muscle or tendon that might result from an excessively strong contraction.

CONSCIOUS PROPRIOCEPTION

As already noted, the various types of proprioceptor provide essential information for neuromuscular control at the subconscious level. This includes reflexes that involve the spinal cord and brain stem, provision of proprioceptive data required by the cerebellum, and sensorimotor integration in the cerebral cortex. The role of specific proprioceptors in conscious proprioception (kinesthesia) is still debated. For many years, awareness of position and movement was attributed mainly to receptors in joints. More recent assessment of the available evidence has identified the neuromuscular spindles as the principal receptors for kinesthesia.

Sensory Endings in Viscera

Except for pacinian corpuscles, most of which are in mesenteries, the sensory endings in viscera consist mainly of nonencapsulated terminal branches of nerve fibers, some of which are quite complicated. In general, visceral afferents function in physiological visceral reflexes; in the sensations of fullness of the stomach, rectum, and bladder; and in pain caused by visceral dysfunction or disease.

Effector Endings

The nervous system acts on muscle fibers and secretory cells. Control of these nonneural cells is effected by a mechanism similar to that of chemical synaptic transmission between neurons. At the neuroeffector endings, axons terminate in relation to skeletal, cardiac, and smooth-muscle fibers and to the cells of exo-

crine and endocrine glands. When the response to a neural signal must be rapid (as in the case of contraction of skeletal muscles or secretion from the cells of the adrenal medulla), the axon terminals are closely applied to the effector cells. The distance between the two elements is often greater in hollow viscera and in exocrine glands, in which responses are somewhat slower. Many endocrine organs are controlled, directly or indirectly, by hypothalamic neurosecretory neurons that discharge their products into blood vessels for subsequent delivery to the target cells.

MOTOR END PLATES

The **motor end plates**, or **myoneural junctions**, on extrafusal and intrafusal fibers of skeletal striated muscles are synaptic structures with two components: the ending of a motor nerve fiber and the subjacent part of the muscle fiber. In regard specifically to the extrafusal fibers, the axon of an alpha motor neuron divides terminally to supply variable numbers of muscle fibers. A **motor unit** consists of a motor neuron and the muscle fibers that it innervates. The number of muscle fibers in a motor unit varies from fewer than 10 to several hundred, depending on the size and function of the muscle. A large motor unit, in which a single neuron supplies many muscle fibers, is adequate for the functions of muscles such as those of the trunk and proximal portions of the limbs. Small muscles, such as the extraocular and intrinsic hand muscles, must contract with greater precision, so their motor units include only a few muscle fibers.

Each branch of the motor nerve fiber gives up its myelin sheath on approaching a muscle fiber and ends as several branchlets that constitute the neural component of the end plate (Fig. 3-4). The end plate is typically 40 to 60 μm in diameter and is usually located midway along the length of the muscle fiber. Each peripheral nerve fiber is surrounded by two sheaths external to the myelin sheath. The neurolemmal sheath consists of the nucleated cytoplasmic portion of Schwann cells, whose cell membrane wraps around the axon or axis cylinder to form the myelin sheath. The neuro-

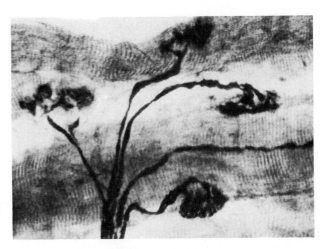

Figure 3-4. Motor end plates. (Gold chloride stain, × 800; *courtesy of Drs. R. Mitchell and A. S. Wilson*)

lemmal sheath continues around the terminal branches of the motor fiber after the Schwann cells cease to form myelin, but it does not intervene between the nerve ending and the muscle fiber. The nerve fiber is surrounded outside the neurolemma by a delicate endoneurial sheath of connective tissue. The endoneurium is continuous at the motor end plate with the thin endomysium or connective tissue sheath of the muscle fiber.

The axonal endings within the end plate contain small, spherical synaptic vesicles and mitochondria. The surface of the muscle fiber is slightly elevated at the myoneural junction. The accumulation of sarcoplasm at this site constitutes the **sole plate**, in which there are nuclei of the muscle fiber and mitochondria. Each axonal branchlet occupies a groove or "synaptic gutter" on the surface of the sole plate; there is an interval of 20 to 50 nm, constituting a synaptic cleft between the surface of the nerve terminal and that of the muscle fiber. The plasma membrane and associated basement membrane, which together constitute the sarcolemma of the muscle fiber, have a wavy outline where they appose the nerve terminal, with the irregularities being known as junctional folds. This folded region of the sarcolemma, the **subneural apparatus**, is demonstrable histochemically by its content of acetylcholinesterase, the enzyme that inactivates acetylcholine.

Acetylcholine, released from the synaptic vesicles by nerve impulses that travel along the axon, binds to receptor molecules in the folded sarcolemma of the subneural apparatus. An adequate train of nerve impulses releases enough acetylcholine to depolarize the postsynaptic membrane. The resulting action potential propagates along the sarcolemma and is carried into the muscle fiber, along the invaginations that constitute the transverse tubular system, to the contractile myofibrils.

MYASTHENIA GRAVIS

An autoimmune disease is one in which there is production of antibodies that bind to cells or proteins that are normal components of the person's own body. In myasthenia gravis, such antibodies combine with the acetylcholine receptors at motor end plates, thereby preventing the normal action of acetylcholine. In many cases, the antibody-producing cells are derived from a benign tumor of the thymus. All skeletal muscles become weak and easily fatigued, so the first signs of the disease appear in constantly used muscles, such as those that move the eyes and eyelids and those of respiration. Eventually there may be total paralysis and dependence on artificial respiration. Symptomatic relief is provided by drugs that inhibit acetylcholinesterase, allowing higher concentrations of the transmitter to accumulate in the synaptic cleft. Treatments that suppress the immune system (eg, removal of the thymus, corticosteroids and other drugs) also are valuable in the management of patients with myasthenia gravis.

POSTGANGLIONIC AUTONOMIC ENDINGS

The presynaptic effector nerve endings on smooth muscle and secretory cells are swellings along the courses and at the tips of unmyelinated axons. These swellings contain accumulations of mitochondria, together with clusters of synaptic vesicles. The terminals are applied to the effector cells, but not as closely as they are in skeletal muscle, and there are no obvious postsynaptic structural specializations. Noradrenergic terminals of the sympathetic nervous system contain electron-dense synaptic vesicles, whereas cholinergic terminals (typically parasympathetic) contain small electron-lucent vesicles. Other types of synaptic vesicles also commonly are seen, and immunohistochemical studies indicate that most autonomic nerve endings contain one or more peptides in addition to the classical neurotransmitters.

Ganglia

Spinal ganglia are swellings on the dorsal roots of spinal nerves. In humans these are in the intervertebral foramina, just proximal to the union of dorsal and ventral roots. Spinal ganglia contain the cell bodies of primary sensory neurons, mainly in a large peripheral zone. The center of the ganglion is occupied by nerve fibers, which are the proximal portions of peripheral and central processes of the nerve cells. Dorsal root ganglia and ganglia of cranial nerves involved with general sensation have the same histological structure.

These sensory neurons develop from the embryonic neural crests, which consist of neuroectodermal cells that lie along the dorsolateral borders of the neural tube. (Some of the neurons in the sensory ganglia of cranial nerves originate from placodes, which are thickened regions of the ectoderm of the surface of the head; see Ch. 1.) The cells are at first bipolar, but the two processes soon unite to form the single process of this unipolar type of neuron.[1] The processes that arise from the smaller cell bodies are short and straight, whereas those given off by larger cells often wind at first around the parent cell body. In both, the fiber divides into peripheral and central branches; the former terminates in a sensory ending, and the latter enters the spinal cord through a dorsal root. The nerve impulse passes directly from the peripheral to the central process, thereby bypassing the cell body. Both processes have the structural and electrophysiological characteristics of axons, although the peripheral process resembles a dendrite in the sense of conduction toward the cell body.

The spherical cell bodies vary from 20 to 100 μm in diameter; their processes are similarly of graded size, ranging from small unmyelinated fibers in group C to the largest myelinated fibers in group A. The large neurons are for proprioception and discriminative touch; those of intermediate size are concerned with light touch, pressure, pain, and temperature; the smallest neurons transmit impulses for pain and temperature. Each cell body is closely invested by a layer of **satellite cells**, which is continuous with the Schwann cell sheath that surrounds the axon. External to this, the neurons are supported by connective tissue fibers and vascular connective tissue.

It has been shown that in lower mammals, some of the axons in the ventral root loop into the dorsal root and form synaptic connections with the neuronal cell bodies there. This observation contradicts the long-held notion that there are no synapses in sensory ganglia. The functional significance of such synapses is unknown, and they have not yet been demonstrated in human sensory ganglia.

A common disorder involving spinal or cranial nerve ganglia is **herpes zoster (shingles)**, in which a viral infection of the ganglion

---

[1] Sometimes the term "pseudounipolar" is applied to the sensory ganglion cell, but this is a truly unipolar neuron after the two processes of the bipolar embryonic cell have fused.

causes pain and other sensory disturbances and a skin eruption in the area of distribution of the affected dorsal root or cranial nerve. The cutaneous inflammation is due in part to spontaneous antidromic conduction of impulses in the group C fibers of the nerve. These release at their terminals a peptide known as substance P, which dilates small arteries and makes small veins permeable, causing exudation of plasma.

Autonomic ganglia include those of the sympathetic trunks along the sides of the vertebral bodies, collateral or prevertebral ganglia in plexuses of the thorax and abdomen (eg, the cardiac, celiac, and mesenteric plexuses), and certain ganglia near viscera. The **principal cells** of autonomic ganglia are multipolar neurons 20 to 45 μm in diameter. The nucleus is often eccentric, and binucleate cells are occasionally encountered. The cell body is surrounded by satellite cells similar to those of spinal ganglia. Several dendrites extend and branch outside the capsule of satellite cells and are in synaptic contact with terminals of preganglionic fibers. The thin, unmyelinated axons (group C fiber) of the principal cells leave the ganglia and eventually supply smooth muscle and gland cells in some viscera, the heart, the enteric plexuses, blood vessels throughout the body, and sweat glands and arrector pili muscles in the skin.

In addition to their principal cells, autonomic ganglia also contain **interneurons**, which are small cells with no axons. Their short dendrites are postsynaptic to the axons that innervate the ganglion and presynaptic to the dendrites of the principal cells.

Peripheral Nerves

ARRANGEMENT AND ENSHEATHMENT OF NERVE FIBERS

The constituent fibers of all but the smallest peripheral nerves are arranged in bundles or fasciculi, and three connective tissue sheaths are recognized. The entire nerve is surrounded by the **epineurium**. This is composed of ordinary connective tissue, and it also fills the spaces between the fasciculi. A nerve root within the spinal canal does not have an epineurium; this ensheathing layer is acquired as the nerve pierces the dura mater on its way through an intervertebral foramen.[2]

The sheath that encloses each small bundle of fibers in a nerve consists of several layers of flattened cells, collectively known as the **perineurium**. Within the perineurium, individual nerve fibers have a delicate covering of connective tissue that constitutes the **endoneurium**, or sheath of Henle. Experiments with embryos of small animals indicate that the cells of all three connective tissue layers of peripheral nerves are derived from mesodermal cells rather than from the neuroectoderm.

NERVE FIBERS

A **nerve fiber** consists of the axon or axis cylinder, the myelin sheath (of fibers belonging to groups A and B) and the neurolemmal sheath (of Schwann). The axis cylinder has no features that are not shared with long axons in the central nervous system. Its cytoplasm (axoplasm) contains neurofilaments, microtubules, patches of smooth-surfaced endoplasmic reticulum, and mitochondria. The plasma membrane is called the axolemma.

The **neurolemma** (also spelled neurilemma) and the **myelin sheath** have several points of interest, centering around the fact that both are components of Schwann cells. The myelin has no significant intrinsic structure at the level of light microscopy (Fig. 3-5A). That it contains lipids has been obvious because the myelin is partially dissolved by lipid solvents and is stained black by osmium tetroxide, which reacts with lipids. Proteins were also known to be present in myelin; they remain as fibrillar material ("neurokeratin") after the lipids have been dissolved. The detailed chemistry of myelin became known subsequently through the results of biochemical studies.

---

[2] The dura mater is the outermost as well as the thickest and toughest of the three meninges (see Ch. 26), or layers of connective tissue that envelop the brain and spinal cord within the cranium and spinal canal.

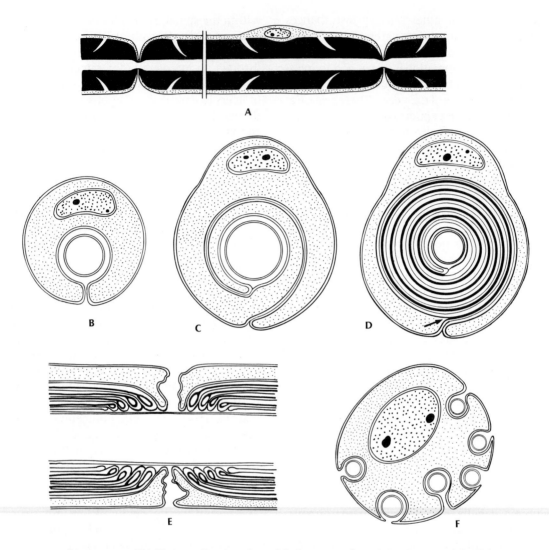

Figure 3-5. (**A**) The myelin sheath and Schwann cell as they are seen (ideally) by light microscopy. (**B**, **C**, and **D**) Successive stages in the development of the myelin sheath from the plasma membrane of a Schwann cell. (**E**) Ultrastructure of a node of Ranvier, sectioned longitudinally. (**F**) Relation of a Schwann cell to several unmyelinated axons.

The myelin sheath is interrupted at intervals by **nodes of Ranvier**; the length of an internode varies from 100 μm to about 1 mm, depending on the length and thickness of the fiber. Funnel-shaped clefts, called the **incisures of Schmidt-Lanterman**, are clearly visible in the myelin sheath in longitudinal sections of a nerve stained with osmium tetroxide. (Demonstration of these incisures in the central nervous system has been difficult, but they have been seen in large myelinated fibers in electron micrographs.) Using light microscopy, the neurolemmal sheath is seen as a series of **Schwann cells**, one for each internode. Most of the cytoplasm is in the region of the ellipsoidal nucleus, but traces of cytoplasm and the plasma membrane closely surround the myelin sheath from one node of Ranvier to the next. The Schwann cells are neuroglial cells descended from the ectodermal cells of the embryonic neural crest (see Ch. 1 and Fig. 2-10).

Observations on the growth of nerve fibers in embryos and tissue cultures and on regeneration of fibers after trauma to a peripheral nerve have established that Schwann cells are responsible for laying down the myelin sheath around the axis cylinder. Use of electron microscopy has established that the myelin consists of the plasma membrane of the Schwann cell, wrapped around the axis cylinder. The term *neurolemmal sheath* or *sheath of Schwann* is used to distinguish the nucleated cytoplasmic layer from the layer of myelin. In fact, the Schwann cell is included in both sheaths, with the cytoplasmic portion forming the neurolemma and an extensive proliferation of the plasma membrane constituting the myelin. The Schwann cells are contiguous with satellite cells that surround nerve cell bodies in cerebrospinal and autonomic ganglia. Oligodendrocytes are the comparable cells associated with neuronal cell bodies and myelinated axons in the central nervous system.

Myelin sheaths are laid down during the later part of fetal development and during the first postnatal year in the manner shown in Figure 3-5B, C, and D. The ultrastructure of the sheath is seen in Figure 3-6. To explain the alternating layers of electron-dense and less dense material, it is necessary to show the plasma membrane as a double line that represents the outer and inner electron-dense protein layers, separated by an electron-lucent interval composed of lipids.

The axon is first surrounded by the Schwann cell; the external plasma membrane is continuous with the membrane immediately around the axon through a mesaxon. New membrane lipoprotein is synthesized in the cytoplasm of the Schwann cell and added to the plasmalemma. The fluidity of the membrane ensures that newly added material quickly spreads through the whole plasma membrane, which forms itself into layers around the axon. The direction of the spiral is clockwise in some internodes and counterclockwise in others. The cytoplasm between the layers of cell membrane gradually disappears, except for surface cytoplasm that is most abundant in the region of the nucleus. The thickness of the myelin sheath of the mature nerve fiber, which is determined by the number of turns of membrane, varies in direct proportion to the diameter and length of the axon. The major dense line, 2.5 nm in thickness,

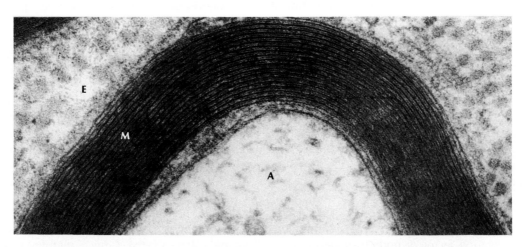

Figure 3-6. Ultrastructure of the myelin sheath (**M**) in a peripheral nerve. The dense and less dense layers alternate, and the latter includes a thin intraperiod line. **A** = axoplasm; **E** = endoneurium, with collagen fibers. (Electron micrograph, × 107,500; *courtesy of Dr. R. C. Buck*)

consists of two inner protein layers of the plasma membrane that fuse along a line indicated by the arrow in Figure 3-5D. The less dense layer, about 10 nm wide, consists of a double thickness of the lipid layer of the cell membrane. The fused outer protein layers of the membrane become exceedingly thin, forming an inconspicuous intraperiod line in the middle of the lighter lipid layer (see Fig. 3-6).

The node of Ranvier is the interval between the plasma membrane systems of two Schwann cells (Fig. 3-5E). The neurolemmal sheath portion of the adjoining Schwann cells has an irregular edge at the node, and there is a narrow space between the Schwann cells through which the axolemma at the node is bathed by tissue fluid. Voltage-gated sodium channels are present in the axolemma only at nodes. Consequently the action potential skips electrically from node to node, and the transmission of a nerve impulse along a myelinated fiber is called saltatory conduction (from the Latin *saltare*, to jump). This type of conduction depends on adequate electrical insulation—the myelin sheath—between the internodal axoplasm and the extracellular fluid. The length of internodes, therefore, has a bearing on the conduction rate of the nerve impulse, and the thicker and longer the nerve fiber, the longer the internodes, up to a maximum of about 1 mm. The Schmidt-Lanterman incisures are formed by a loosening of the plasma membrane layers of the sheath with retention of cytoplasm between the membranes. These incisures may aid the passage of materials through the myelin sheath to the axon.

With respect to unmyelinated fibers, a Schwann cell envelops several (up to 15) thin axons, as shown in Figure 3-5F. The axon is surrounded by a single layer of the Schwann cell's plasma membrane; it is, therefore, unmyelinated, and there are no nodes of Ranvier. The nerve impulse is a self-propagating action potential along the axolemma, without the accelerating factor of node-to-node or saltatory conduction. This accounts for the slow rate of conduction that is characteristic of unmyelinated fibers.

PERIPHERAL NERVE DISORDERS

The peripheral nervous system is subject to various disorders. **Peripheral neuropathy** (neuritis), the most common of these, consists of degenerative changes in peripheral nerves that produce sensory loss and motor weakness. Distal portions of nerves are affected first, with symptoms in the hands and feet. There are many causes of peripheral neuropathy, including nutritional deficiencies, toxic substances of various kinds, and metabolic disorders, notably diabetes.

Nerve injuries may or may not cause transection of axons, with resulting loss of function. The cellular changes that follow axotomy are described in Chapter 4. Damage to a peripheral nerve by a penetrating wound may be followed by an incapacitating disorder known as **causalgia**. There is severe pain in the affected limb, together with changes in skin texture. The symptoms of causalgia may be attributable, at least in part, to the formation in the injured nerve of abnormal excitatory contacts between sympathetic and sensory axons. The pain can often be relieved by surgical removal of the sympathetic ganglia that supply the affected skin. Painful sensations perceived as coming from an amputated limb (phantom limb pain) may be similarly caused.

A nerve may be pressed on where it passes over a bony prominence or through a restricted aperture; for example, the ulnar nerve is subject to pressure at the elbow, and the median nerve, in the carpal tunnel at the wrist. The resulting **entrapment syndrome** includes motor and sensory disturbances in the area of distribution of the nerve. The major plexuses, especially the brachial plexus, may be compressed (as in crutch palsy). **Nerve roots** are more fragile than nerves because they lack an epineurium. They may be irritated or compressed by inflamed meninges, by abnormally protruding parts of intervertebral disks (spondylosis), or by bony irregularities (spinal osteoarthritis). Clinical manifestations of nerve root lesions include weakness and wasting of muscles and pain in the affected cutaneous areas.

SUGGESTED READING —————

Bunge MB, Wood PM, Tynan LB, Bates ML, Sanes JR: Perineurium originates from fibroblasts: Demonstration in vitro with a retroviral marker. Science 243:229–231, 1989

Ferrell WR, Gandevia SC, McCloskey DI: The role of joint receptors in human kinesthesia when intramuscular receptors cannot contribute. J Physiol (Lond) 386:63–71, 1987

Halata Z, Grim M, Christ B: Origin of spinal cord meninges, sheaths of peripheral nerves, and cutaneous receptors including Merkel cells. An experimental study with avian chimeras. Anat Embryol 182:529–537, 1990

Iggo A, Andres KH: Morphology of cutaneous receptors. Annu Rev Neurosci 5:1–31, 1982

Kayahara T: Synaptic connections between spinal motoneurons and dorsal root ganglion cells in the cat. Brain Res 376:299–309, 1986

Matthews PBC: Where does Sherrington's muscular sense originate? Annu Rev Neurosci 5:189–218, 1982

Risling M, Dalsgaard C-J, Cukierman A, Cuello AC: Electron microscopic and immunohistochemical evidence that unmyelinated ventral root axons make U-turns or enter the spinal pia mater. J Comp Neurol 225:53–63, 1984

Schott GD: Mechanisms of causalgia and related clinical conditions. The role of the central and of the sympathetic nervous systems. Brain 109:717–738, 1986

Swash M, Fox KP: Muscle spindle innervation in man. J Anat 112:61–80, 1972

Winkelmann RK: Cutaneous sensory nerves. Seminars in Dermatology 17:236–268, 1988

Four

The Human Nervous System: An Anatomical Viewpoint, Sixth Edition, Murray L. Barr and John A. Kiernan. J.B. Lippincott Company, Philadelphia, © 1993.

Response of Nerve Cells to Injury; Nerve Fiber Regeneration; Neuroanatomical Methods

Important Facts

Most of the cytoplasm of a neuron is removed when the axon is transected. The segment that has been isolated from the cell body degenerates together with its myelin sheath, and the fragments are phagocytosed.

The neuronal cell body typically reacts to axotomy with greatly increased protein synthesis, accompanied by structural changes known as the axon reaction, or chromatolysis.

Axonal regeneration occurs when an axon is transected within the peripheral nervous system, but functional recovery is commonly imperfect because not all axons reach the correct destinations.

In mammals, axons transected within the central nervous system fail to regenerate effectively. Synaptic rearrangements, however, can occur in partly denervated regions of gray matter, and some recovery of function occurs as a result of recruitment of alternative neuronal circuitry.

The distribution of fragments of degenerating axons can provide evidence for the former existence of neuronal connections in the injured or diseased brain or spinal cord. Investigation of neuronal activities, such as axonal transport and glucose or oxygen metabolism, is now more widely used in the study of connectivity and function in the central nervous system.

Neurons may be injured by physical trauma or by involvement in pathological processes, such as infarction caused by vascular occlusion. Small interneurons are likely to suffer total destruction, whereas injury to large neurons may result either in destruction of the cell body or in transection of the axon, with preservation of the cell body. The best known change proximal to the site of axonal transection is the **axon reaction**, which may be displayed in the cell body. When the cell body of a neuron is destroyed, the axon is isolated from the synthetic machinery of the cell and soon breaks up into fragments, which are eventually phagocytosed. Similar changes occur distal to the site of an axonal injury. The degeneration of an axon that has been detached from the remainder of the cell is called **wallerian degeneration**. The process affects not only the axon, but also its myelin sheath, even though the latter is not part of the injured neuron.

Axon Reaction

Changes in the cell body after axonal transection vary according to the type of neuron. Cells in some locations undergo progressive degeneration and, ultimately, disappear. This happens to most neurons when the injury occurs before or soon after birth. Conversely, the proximal portions of some adult neurons are not significantly altered by cutting the axon. The cytological details of the classical axon reaction are best seen in large neurons, such as those supplying skeletal muscle, which contain coarse clumps of Nissl material. The following account includes the more typical aspects of the response to cutting the axon of a motor neuron.

The nerve fiber between the cell body and the lesion is not altered appreciably. The cell body, in sections stained by a cationic dye (the Nissl method), first shows signs of reaction 24 to 48 hours after interruption of the axon. The coarse clumps of Nissl substance are changed to a finely granular dispersion; this change, known as **chromatolysis**, occurs first between the axon hillock and the nucleus, gradually spreading throughout the perikaryon (Fig. 4-1). The nucleus assumes an eccentric position away from the axon hillock, and the whole cell body swells. This aspect of the reaction reaches a maximum 10 to 20 days after axonal transection, and the closer the injury is to the cell body, the severer the swelling. Electron microscopy shows disorder of the granular endoplasmic reticulum and an increase in the number of polyribosomes in the cytoplasmic matrix.

There are signs of recovery from the early effects of trauma to the axon even while these changes are occurring. The nucleolus enlarges, and dense basophilic caps are often seen on the cytoplasmic side of the nuclear membrane. Both the nucleolar enlargement and the nuclear caps are evidence of accelerated ribonucleic acid and protein synthesis, which would favor regeneration of the axon when conditions make regeneration possible. Recovery commonly takes several months, and the cell body is eventually smaller than normal if the axon does not regenerate.

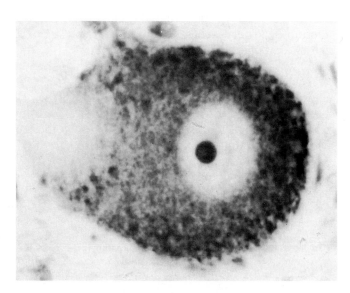

Figure 4-1. Motor neuron, showing changes in the cell body 6 days after transection of its axon. (Stained with cresyl violet, × 800). Compare this with the normal neuron in Figure 2-2.

In cells confined to the central nervous system, the axon reaction is conspicuous only in some large neurons. Changes in smaller neurons that have inconspicuous Nissl substance are not detectable by light microscopy, and large cells may exhibit no axon reaction when collateral axonal branches that arise close to the cell body are spared. Some central neurons normally have eccentric nuclei, thus giving a false impression of an axon reaction.[1] The axon reaction has been exploited in the past as a means of identifying the cells of origin of fibers in nerves and the sources of some central tracts. As a research method, it has been supplanted by more informative procedures, which are discussed later.

Wallerian Degeneration in Peripheral Nerves

The nucleus is essential for the synthesis of cytoplasmic proteins, which are transported distally in the axoplasm to replace proteins that have been degraded as part of the metabolic activity of the cell. The axon, therefore, does not survive for long when separated from the cell body. Simultaneously throughout its length, the part of the axon distal to the lesion becomes slightly swollen and irregular within the 1st day and breaks up into fragments by the 3rd to 5th day. Muscle contraction on electrical stimulation of a degenerating motor nerve ceases 2 to 3 days after the nerve is interrupted. The degeneration includes the neural components of the sensory and motor endings.

The myelin sheath is converted into short ellipsoidal segments during the first few days after interruption of the fiber and gradually undergoes complete disintegration. Meanwhile cells accumulate in the cylindrical space within the basal lamina of the column of Schwann cells associated with each nerve fiber. Most of these cells are derived from mononuclear leukocytes that emigrate through the

walls of endoneurial blood vessels. The remains of the axon and its myelin sheath (or the axon only in the case of unmyelinated fibers) are phagocytosed. Thus the distal stump of a degenerated nerve is filled with tubular formations, known as the **bands of von Büngner**, that contain phagocytes and Schwann cells.

Axonal Regeneration in Peripheral Nerves

If a neuron is envisaged as a spherical cell body 15 μm in diameter, with an axon 10 cm long and 2 μm in diameter, a calculation shows that 99.4% of the protoplasm is in the axon. If the axon of this hypothetical neuron were severed halfway along its length, the cell would lose 49.7% of its volume. This lost part of the neuron can be regrown when the injury occurs within the territory of the peripheral nervous system, a reparative process known as **axonal regeneration**. It is important to distinguish between this use of the word "regeneration" and its more usual connotation, which is the replacement of lost cells by mitosis and reorganization of tissue.

If a nerve has been severed, the regeneration of its axons requires apposition of the cut ends by placement of sutures through the epineurium. The individual fascicles of the nerve should be realigned as accurately as possible. A crushing injury (or freezing a short length of nerve in a laboratory animal) transects the axons but leaves intact the connective tissues of the nerve, including the perineurial sheaths of the fascicles. No surgical intervention is needed for this type of injury because the cells and connective tissue of the endoneurium are there to guide growing axons to their appropriate destinations.

AXONAL GROWTH

The following description applies to nerves that have been cleanly cut through and repaired. During the first few days, phagocytes and fibroblasts fill the interval between the apposed nerve ends. Regenerating fibers, accompanied by migrating Schwann cells, invade the region by about the 4th day, with

---

[1] Such cells include those of the nucleus thoracicus of the spinal cord (see Ch. 5) and the accessory cuneate nucleus of the medulla (see Chs. 7 and 10).

each axon dividing into numerous branches having enlarged tips. Each tip, known as a **growth cone**, is about the same size as a neuronal cell body and has a convoluted and constantly moving surface membrane at its leading edge. The rate of axonal growth is slow at first; 2 to 3 weeks may elapse before the growth cones traverse the region of the lesion. The fine branches may then find their way into the bands of von Büngner in the distal segments. Several filaments enter each endoneurial tube, and the invasion of a particular tube leading to a specific type of end organ appears to be determined only by chance. Many filaments miss altogether and grow into epineurial connective tissue. This is the fate of all regenerating axons if the severed ends are too widely separated or if dense collagen or extraneous material intervenes. Such fibers often form complicated whorls (spirals of Perroncito), producing a swelling or neuroma that may be a source of spontaneous pain. At the other extreme is the almost perfect regeneration of the nerve through the growth of each fiber along its original endoneurial tube. This type of regeneration may occur if the nerve is crushed just enough to interrupt axons without disruption of the endoneurial connective tissue. Experimentally, this type of "ideal" lesion can be achieved by local freezing.

After crossing the region of the lesion and entering the bands of von Büngner, the axonal filaments grow along the clefts between columns of Schwann cells and the surrounding basal laminae. Usually only one branch of each axon enters a single tube; other sprouts are drawn back into the shaft of the growing axon. The rate of growth within the nerve distal to the lesion is 2 to 4 mm per day—somewhat faster than the slow component of normal axonal transport. Regenerating fibers eventually reach motor and sensory endings; the proportion of endings that are correctly reinnervated depends on conditions at the site of the original injury. The amount of time that elapses between nerve suture and the beginning of functional return may be estimated on the basis of a regeneration rate of 1.5 mm daily. This value takes into account the time required

for the fibers to traverse the lesion and for the peripheral endings to be reinnervated.

In a human limb, the course of axonal regeneration can be followed by testing for **Tinel's sign**. When part of a nerve trunk containing regenerating axons is tapped with a small hammer, the patient reports a tingling or electric sensation in the area of skin normally supplied by the nerve.

MATURATION OF NERVE FIBERS

Meanwhile changes occur along the course of the regenerating fibers. Each axon becomes surrounded by the cytoplasm of the Schwann cells. For axons that are to be myelinated, myelin sheaths are laid down by Schwann cells (see Ch. 3 for mechanism). Myelination begins near the lesion and proceeds in a proximodistal direction. Although the myelin sheath is formed by the Schwann cells, its development is determined by the type of axon. Experimental studies indicate that all the neuroglial cells in a regenerating nerve have the potential to produce or not to produce myelin, irrespective of the nature of the axons with which they have previously been associated.

Even years after injury and repair, the diameter, internodal length, and conduction velocity of a regenerated nerve fiber are rarely more than 80% of the corresponding values for the original fiber. The motor unit for a regenerated fiber is larger than that of the preexisting motor unit; that is, the axon supplies more muscle fibers than it formerly did. These factors contribute to less precise control of reinnervated muscles and to the fact that sensory function also is inferior to that mediated by the uninjured nerve.

Axonal Degeneration and Regeneration in the Central Nervous System

The simplest lesion to visualize, although rather rare in clinical practice, is a clean incised wound of the brain or spinal cord. The space made by the knife blade fills with blood and later with collagenous connective tissue, which is continuous with the pia mater. The astrocytes in the nervous tissue on each side of the collagenous scar acquire longer and more numerous cytoplasmic processes, which form a tangled mass. The number of astrocytes in the region does not increase appreciably, but there is a large increase in the total cell population, caused mainly by the emigration of monocytes from blood vessels to form phagocytic cells known as reactive microglia. The resting microglia that had been present in the central nervous tissue also may become phagocytes, but the great majority of such cells come from the blood. Reactive microglia also appear in parts of the central nervous system remote from the lesion but occupied by axons that are degenerating in consequence of having been severed from their cell bodies. Wallerian degeneration is different from the process described for peripheral nerves because the degradation and phagocytosis of debris are carried out much more slowly in the central nervous system. Degenerating fragments of myelinated axons are frequently recognizable several months after the original injury, and the phagocytic cells that contain the debris persist in situ for many years.

A fundamental difference between the consequences of injuries to the peripheral and central nervous systems concerns the regeneration of axons. The proximal stumps of axons transected within the brain or spinal cord begin to regenerate, sending sprouts into the region of the lesion, but this growth ceases after about 2 weeks. Abortive regeneration of this type occurs in the central nervous systems of mammals, birds, and reptiles. Axonal regeneration in fishes and amphibia occurs efficiently in the central nervous system, with remarkably accurate restoration of synaptic connections.

The reasons for the failure of axonal regeneration in the central nervous systems of higher animals are unknown. Current hypotheses are concerned with axonal growth-promoting and growth-inhibiting substances, perhaps derived from the blood or from the neuroglia, which are absent from or unable to act in the adult mammalian central nervous system. Earlier hypotheses, such as the lack of Schwann cells in the brain and spinal cord and the obstruction of growing axons by scar tissue or cyst formation, although perhaps somewhat valid, fail to explain all the available experimental data.

There are a few circumstances in which axons do regenerate successfully within the mammalian brain. For example, the neurosecretory axons of the pituitary stalk (see Ch. 11) and some monoamine-containing fibers in the brain stem regenerate effectively. The failure of most axons to regenerate means that permanent disability follows destruction of any tract that cannot be bypassed by redistribution of function to alternative pathways.

Transplantation of Nervous Tissue

With some types of injury, notably gunshot wounds, substantial lengths of peripheral nerve are lost. The deficit can be repaired by inserting a graft taken from a thin cutaneous nerve that is functionally less important than the one to be repaired. Several strands of thin nerve are placed side by side, in the manner of a cable, for grafting into a large nerve. The process of axonal regeneration in a nerve graft is identical to that in a transected and sutured nerve, but the growing axons have to negotiate two sites of anastomosis. The functional recovery is, therefore, far from perfect. A nerve graft must be an autograft (derived from the same individual) or an isograft (from an identical twin or an animal that belongs to the same inbred strain), or it will be rejected by the immune system.

The neurons in pieces of adult mammalian brain or spinal cord do not survive removal and transplantation. Axons will grow, however, into and out of tiny fragments of embryonic or fetal central nervous tissue transplanted into certain parts of the adult brain. Central axons can also grow from the brain, spinal cord, or optic nerve into transplanted pieces of peripheral nerve and even into some nonneural tissues. Such experiments are contributing importantly to knowledge of growth-promoting factors that are lost with the maturation of the central nervous system. Tissues placed in the brain are partly protected from the host's immune system, so for short-term experiments, it is possible to use grafts from other individuals of the same species (allografts or homografts) or even from different species (xenografts or heterografts).

Transplanted fetal neurons can partly compensate for the effects of injuries and experimentally induced diseases in small animals. The grafts probably deliver both neurotransmitters and trophic substances that promote survival of postsynaptic neurons. In the late 1980s, many attempts were made to try such grafts in people with Parkinson's disease (see Ch. 12), but without any substantial or lasting benefits to the recipients. Transplantation into the human brain or spinal cord is unlikely to acquire therapeutic significance because (a) the numbers of neurons in the grafts are unrealistically small in relation to the corresponding parts of the recipient brain; (b) neurons deposited in what would be the normal locations of their cell bodies are unlikely to generate axons that will grow several centimeters in the right direction through the host brain into appropriate populations of postsynaptic neurons; and (c) neurons deposited in regions their axons normally innervate will not receive afferent synapses appropriate to the normal locations of their cell bodies.

Plasticity of Neural Connections

Although axonal regeneration in the central nervous system occurs only negligibly, considerable functional recovery commonly follows traumatic or pathological damage in many regions, especially when the lesion is not large. For example, destruction of a small area of cerebral cortex that had a well-defined motor or sensory function is followed by paralysis or loss of sensation, with recovery after several weeks. Similar recovery occurs after transection of tracts of fibers, provided the lesions are not too large. Recovery from paralysis caused by occlusion of blood vessels in the cerebral hemispheres (stroke) is commonly seen in clinical practice, and functional recovery may even follow partial transverse lesions of the spinal cord.

Functional recovery involves the taking over of the functions of the damaged region of the nervous system by other regions that remain intact. The reorganization of connections within the brain is known as **plasticity**. This may be an extension of a normally present adaptability used in the learning of often repeated tasks.

Structural changes accompany the functional plasticity that follows injury to the nervous system. Thus, when a group of neurons is deprived of part of its afferent input, the surviving preterminal axons, which may come from quite different places, commonly grow new branches that then form synapses at the sites denervated by the original lesion. This event, known as **axonal sprouting**, may occur over short distances within a small group of neurons or over greater distances, as when the axons of intact dorsal root ganglion cells extend their axons for three or four segments up and down the spinal cord after transection of neighboring dorsal roots. Axonal sprouting also occurs in the periphery; the anesthetic area of skin resulting from a peripheral nerve injury becomes smaller over several weeks, even if the severed nerve does not regenerate. The change is considered to be caused by sprouting of the axons of other cutaneous nerves within the skin. Comparable sprouting occurs in partially denervated skeletal muscles, with consequent enlargement of the motor units. Axonal sprouting involves intact axons and should not be confused with the regeneration of transected axons. It is probable that axonal sprouting accounts for functional plasticity and recovery after lesions in the central nervous system, but a causal relation has not yet been conclusively proved.

Methods for Investigating Neural Pathways and Functions

In histological material from normal animals, it is seldom possible to follow a tract of axons from its cell bodies of origin to the distant site in which it terminates. The small diameters and curved trajectories of axons, together with the fact that different pathways commonly occupy the same territory, make the direct tracing of connections impossible. It is, therefore, necessary to use experimental methods to determine the connections of the many groups of neurons in the brain and spinal cord. The results of investigations of neural connectivity in laboratory animals, especially the cat and monkey, may be applicable to the human brain. This transfer of data from animals to humans is usually justifiable when there are no major differences between the connections found in taxonomically diverse groups of animals; a pathway present in rats, dogs, and monkeys is likely to occur also in humans. When variation among species is found, it is hoped that neuroanatomical information gained from primates, such as monkeys, will be helpful with respect to the human brain. Sometimes injury and disease in the human nervous system can cause degeneration of particular tracts of axons. Postmortem examination of the degenerated fibers provides information, albeit of a limited accuracy, about normal human neural connections.

Neuroanatomical Methods Based on Degeneration

Until the introduction of methods based on axoplasmic transport, fiber tracts were traced by staining fibers undergoing wallerian degeneration after the placement of a destructive lesion at a selected site in the central nervous system of an animal. Although now largely of historical interest, such methods have contributed importantly to neuroanatomical knowledge.

The **Marchi technique**, which is still used on human postmortem material, depends on the staining of particles of degenerating myelin with osmium tetroxide in the presence of an oxidizing agent. The latter suppresses the staining of normal myelin, so that degenerating fibers appear as lines of black dots on a lighter background. The course of a tract can be followed in sections taken at appropriate intervals (Fig. 4-2). **Silver methods** for showing degenerating unmyelinated axons and synaptic terminals were rarely applicable to the human nervous system but were much used for laboratory animals.

Degenerating axonal terminals also can be recognized in **electron micrographs**. When the general area of projection of a group of neurons or of a tract is known from light microscopy, the exact mode of termination of the fibers on the dendrites, somata, or axons of the postsynaptic cells may be determined. As with silver degeneration methods, electron microscopy usually cannot be applied to human material because

the time of survival and the conditions of fixation of the tissue are critical.

Neuroanatomical Methods Based on Axoplasmic Transport

Research methods based on degenerating axons were replaced in the 1970s by much more sensitive techniques that reveal both the cells of origin and the sites of termination of axons. The results of the extensive use of methods based on axoplasmic transport have necessitated substantial revisions of earlier accounts of neuronal connections in the central nervous system.

In the **autoradiographic method**, a small volume of a radioactively labeled amino acid solution, commonly [^{3}H]leucine, is injected into the region that contains the cell bodies of the neurons being investigated. The amino acid is taken up by the neurons and is incorporated into proteins, which are transported distally along the axons to the presynaptic boutons. The animal is killed 24 to 48 hours later and the appropriate parts of the nervous system are chemically fixed to immobilize the labeled proteins. Sections are cut, and autoradiographs are prepared in the usual way. High concentrations of silver grains, indicating the presence of tritium in the tissue, are seen over the site of injection, over the terminal field of projection of the neurons, and often over the axons between these two regions.

With this technique, it has been possible to trace connections previously undetectable by the use of degeneration methods. It also has the important advantage that the labeled amino acid enters only the cell bodies and dendrites of neurons. Axons that happen to be passing through the site of injection do not take up the tracer, thus avoiding the confusion that often complicated the interpretation of areas of terminal degeneration.

Research methods using the axon reaction and staining degenerating fibers have been largely replaced by techniques that take advantage of the **uptake and axonal transport** of proteins and other substances. A histochemically detectable protein or a suitable fluorescent dye is injected into the region concerned. The foreign molecules are imbibed by presynaptic terminals in the region and transported retrogradely to their neuronal perikarya. The process takes 6 to 72 hours, according to the lengths of the axons and the substance used as a tracer.

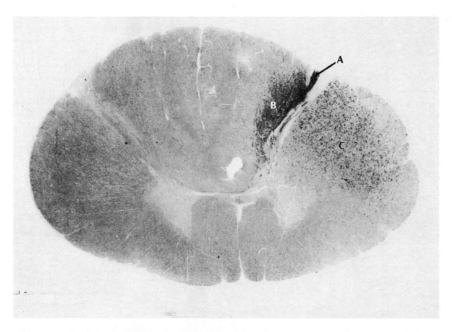

Figure 4-2. Section of the third cervical segment of a human spinal cord. The patient died 9 days after an injury that damaged the dorsal roots of the 2nd, 3rd, and 4th cervical nerves on the right side, together with the dorsal part of the right lateral funiculus of white matter in segment C2. The tissue was processed by the Marchi method, and degenerating myelin can be seen in (**A**) entering fibers of the 3rd right cervical dorsal root, (**B**) branches of fibers derived from dorsal roots C3 and C4, in the dorsal funiculus, and (**C**) descending corticospinal fibers in the lateral funiculus. (× 10)

The animal is then killed and the tissue is removed and appropriately fixed and sectioned. A protein tracer is localized by histochemical means, thus revealing the neuronal cell bodies that innervated the site of the injection (Fig. 4-3). A fluorescent tracer is observed directly by fluorescence microscopy.

The first protein to be used extensively as a tracer in this way was the enzyme peroxidase, extracted from the root of the horseradish plant. In recent years, the method has been made even more sensitive by the use of **lectins**, which are carbohydrate-binding proteins of plant origin. Lectins bind strongly to cell surfaces, including those of axonal terminals, and are then taken up into the cytoplasm and transported. The lectin is rendered histochemically detectable by its covalent conjugation with an enzyme, usually horseradish peroxidase. Other tracers, detectable by similar methods, include simple polysaccharides (Fig. 4-4) and some bacterial toxins.

Many neurons in the brain have axons that send branches to widely separated places. It is possible to demonstrate such branching by injecting a different tracer into each suspected terminal field. Dyes that fluoresce in different colors are commonly used for this purpose. If both tracers are present in a single cell body, that neuron has axonal branches that go to both sites of injection.

Proteins and dyes also are taken up and transported retrogradely by injured axons of passage, so care must be taken not to cause undue physical damage when injecting into an area that contains nerve endings whose cells of origin are to be identified. Uptake by injured axons may be deliberately studied by applying protein tracers at the sites of transection of tracts or to cut peripheral nerves.

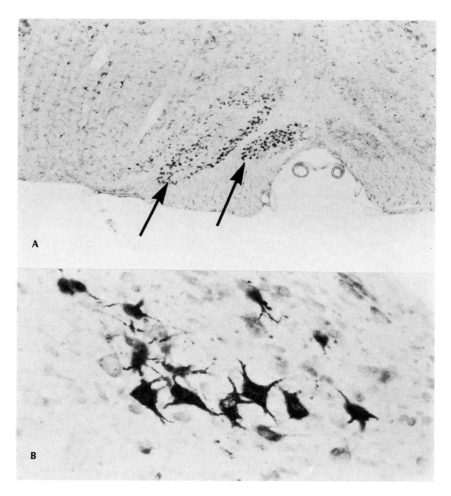

Figure 4-3. Transverse section through the ventral part of the medulla of a rat in which horseradish peroxidase was injected into the cortex of one cerebellar hemisphere 24 hours before the animal was killed. The section was treated for histochemical detection of peroxidase activity, revealed as a dark blue deposit that appears black in these photomicrographs. (**A**) Labeled cell bodies in the inferior olivary complex of nuclei (*arrows*), contralateral to the site of injection. (× 30) (**B**) Some of the labeled neurons at higher magnification. (× 150) Other cells appear gray because they were lightly counterstained with neutral red, a cationic dye. (*Courtesy of Dr. B. A. Flumerfelt*)

With the development of increased sensitivity in methods for the histochemical detection of peroxidase, it has become possible to study the anterograde as well as the retrograde transport of tracer proteins. The amount of protein taken up by cell bodies and dendrites is less than that absorbed by presynaptic terminals. However, an appreciable amount does enter the cell bodies and is transported orthogradely in the rapid component of the axoplasmic transport system. The protein is detected histochemically in the terminal and preterminal parts of axons, which have an appearance quite different from that of labeled perikarya. The method provides, for a smaller investment of time and effort, results comparable to those obtained by the autoradiographic method. Some lectins are especially suitable for anterograde tracing and provide remarkably clear delineation of the terminal branches of axons.

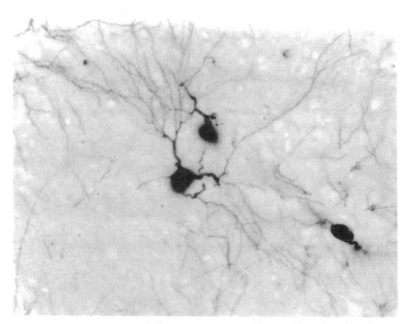

Figure 4-4. Parafascicular nucleus (one of the intralaminar nuclei of the thalamus) 48 hours after injection of biotinylated dextran into the striatum. Dextran is a bacterial carbohydrate that is taken up at synaptic terminals and retrogradely transported into the cell bodies and dendrites. The labeling compound, biotin, was made visible by virtue of its affinity for avidin, a protein extracted from egg white, which was itself labeled with the histochemically demonstrable enzyme peroxidase. The dark product of the histochemical reaction displays the dendrites of the thalamic neurons whose axons end in the striatum. The thalamostriate projection is discussed in Chapters 11 and 12. (*Courtesy of Dr. N. Rajakumar*)

Transsynaptic Tracing of Pathways

In some viral diseases, such as rabies, the infective agent spreads through the central nervous system by being passed from one neuron to another. Certain viruses are used for experimental neuronal tracing because they replicate within neurons, are transported within the axon, and are passed from one cell to another at synapses. The virus can be modified to make the cells that harbor it synthesize a histochemically detectable enzyme, or the viral protein may be stained immunohistochemically.

Metabolic Marking Methods

The sugar **2-deoxy-D-glucose** is an analogue of ordinary D-glucose. It enters cells in the same way as glucose but cannot be metabolized. When cells are active, their glucose uptake increases. Therefore, if an active cell is supplied with 2-deoxyglucose, this sugar will accumulate in the cytoplasm. A laboratory animal may be given an intravenous infusion of radioactively labeled 2-deoxyglucose while part of its nervous system is made highly active; for example, its visual system may be stimulated by light or its auditory system by sound. The radioactive sugar accumulates in all the neurons in the active system and may be detected there autoradiographically. In the visual system, for example, activity is detected in the retina, in certain layers of cells in the lateral geniculate body, and in the calcarine cortex (see Ch. 20 for an explanation of the significance of these regions).

The deoxyglucose method can reveal those structures in the brain that are active when a particular system of pathways is in use. It may thus be possible to determine which of a multitude of connections demonstrated by neuroanatomical tracing methods are the most important in relation to function.

Certain enzymes used in the metabolic activities of all cells can be demonstrated histochemically. **Cytochrome oxidase** is a notable example, and in regions that contain functionally active neurons, the activity of this enzyme is higher than in adjacent quiescent areas. Cytochrome oxidase histochemistry has been used with great success in the demonstration of columns of cells that respond to different visual stimuli in the cortex of the occipital lobe of the brain (see Ch. 14).

Regional Cerebral Blood Flow and Metabolism

In humans, it is possible to monitor blood flow in the cerebral cortex by computing regional variations in the gamma radiation detected around the head after injection of a suitable radioactive tracer. Sudden increases in blood flow are associated with activity in the underlying cortex. In clinical neurology, the technique is used to identify abnormally high or low blood flow caused by disease.

Similar information can be obtained by positron emission tomography (see Ch. 16), which provides pictorial and quantitative information about oxygen utilization or glucose uptake at sites deep within the brain.

Physiological and Pharmacological Methods

Anatomical studies of neuronal pathways are often supplemented by stimulating neurons and observing the destination of nerve impulses by recording the potentials evoked elsewhere. The accurate measurement of the time elapsed between stimulation and recording provides information that may help to determine the number of neurons, or synaptic delays, that are included in the pathway. This procedure is called "physiological neuronography."

Several **toxic substances** are used in laboratory animals as adjuncts to the study of neuroanatomy. For example, nicotine was first used a century ago by Langley to block synapses and thus establish their locations in autonomic ganglia.

Local injection of kainic acid or ibotenic acid kills many types of neurons without causing transection of passing fibers. These substances are analogues of glutamic acid, which is an excitatory transmitter. When kainic or ibotenic acid binds to glutamate receptors, the calcium channels of the postsynaptic cells are opened for unduly long times. Calcium ions that diffuse into the neurons activate proteolytic enzymes that destroy the cytoplasm. The result is a lesion more selective than one produced by physical methods. Cells that use monoamines as synaptic transmitters are selectively intoxicated by analogues of these substances. Thus neurons that make use of dopamine or norepinephrine are intoxicated by 6-hydroxydopamine, and serotonin cells are similarly sensitive to 5,6-dihydroxytryptamine.

Some poisonous lectins (notably ricin-60 from the castor bean) and other compounds (notably the antibiotic doxorubicin, which is used to treat some types of cancer) are taken up by axonal endings and by injured axons of passage and transported retrogradely to the neuronal cell bodies, where they inhibit nucleic acid and protein synthesis. This strategy, known as "suicide transport", is also useful for producing selective lesions to provide experimental models of diseases in which certain populations of neurons degenerate spontaneously.

SUGGESTED READING

Berry M: Regeneration of axons in the central nervous system. In Navaratnam V, Harrison RJ (eds): Progress in Anatomy, vol 3, pp 213–233. New York, Cambridge University Press, 1983

Cotman CW, Nieto-Sampedro M, Harris EW: Synapse replacement in the nervous system of adult vertebrates. Physiol Rev 61:684–784, 1981

Crutcher KA: Sympathetic sprouting in the central nervous system: A model for studies of axonal growth in the mammalian brain. Brain Res Rev 12:203–233, 1987

Fawcett JW, Keynes RJ: Peripheral nerve regeneration. Annu Rev Neurosci 13:43–60, 1990

Franklin RJM, Blakemore WF: The peripheral nervous system–central nervous system regeneration dichotomy: A role for glial cell transplantation. J Cell Sci 95:185–190, 1990

Hall SM: Regeneration in the peripheral nervous system. Neuropathol Exp Neurobiol 15:513–529, 1989

Kiernan JA: Hypotheses concerned with axonal regeneration in the mammalian nervous system. Biol Rev 54:155–197, 1979

Landau WM: Artificial intelligence: The brain transplant cure for parkinsonism. Neurology 40: 733–740, 1990

Lipton SA: Growth factors for neuronal survival and process regeneration. Arch Neurol 46:1241–1248, 1989

McLean JH, Shipley MT, Bernstein DI: Golgi-like transneuronal retrograde labelling with CNS injections of herpes simplex virus type 1. Brain Res Bull 22:867–881, 1989

Oorschot DE, Jones DG: Axonal regeneration in the mammalian central nervous system. Adv Anat Embryol Cell Biol 119:1–121, 1990

Purves D: Assessing some dynamic properties of the living nervous system. Quart J Exp Physiol 74:1089–1105, 1989

Schwab ME: Myelin-associated inhibitors of neurite growth. Exp Neurol 109:2–5, 1990

Sunderland S: Nerves and Nerve Injuries, 2nd ed. Edinburgh, Churchill-Livingstone, 1978

Regional Anatomy of the Central Nervous System

Five

The Human Nervous System: An Anatomical Viewpoint, Sixth Edition, Murray L. Barr and John A. Kiernan. J.B. Lippincott Company, Philadelphia, © 1993.

Spinal Cord

Important Facts

The spinal cord is shorter than the spinal canal in which it is suspended. Except in the neck, spinal cord segments are rostral to the corresponding vertebrae.

Cerebrospinal fluid can be sampled by inserting a needle into the subarachnoid space below the level of the conus medullaris.

The cross-sectional area of the central gray matter indicates the number of neurons: largest for segments supplying limbs.

The cross-sectional area of the white matter decreases caudally: fewer descending and ascending fibers.

Motor neurons are in the ventral horn; sensory axons enter the dorsal horn and the dorsal funiculi. Preganglionic autonomic neurons are laterally placed, in segments T1-L2 and S2-S4.

Ascending tracts include the uncrossed gracile and cuneate fasciculi (from sensory ganglia) and the crossed spinothalamic tract (from the dorsal horn). These are concerned with different types of sensation.

Descending motor tracts include the uncrossed vestibulospinal and the crossed lateral corticospinal tract. Hypothalamospinal and some reticulospinal fibers influence autonomic functions.

For most of the time, the stretch reflex, the gamma reflex loop, and the flexor or withdrawal reflex are suppressed by activity in the descending pathways.

Lesions in different parts of the spinal cord produce sensory and motor abnormalities appropriate to the functions of the tracts that have been transected. The segmental level of a lesion is indicated by the affected dermatomes and movements.

The spinal cord and dorsal root ganglia are directly responsible for innervation of the body, excluding most of the head. Afferent or sensory fibers enter the spinal cord through the dorsal roots of spinal nerves, and efferent or motor fibers leave by way of the ventral roots (the Bell-Magendie law). In addition to initiating spinal reflex responses, data originating in sensory endings are relayed to the brain stem and cerebellum, where they are used in various circuits, including those that influence motor performance. Sensory information is transmitted also to the brain stem, the thalamus, and the cerebral cortex, where it becomes part of conscious experience and may elicit immediate or delayed behavioral responses. Motor neurons in the spinal cord are excited or inhibited by impulses originating at various levels of the brain, from the medulla to the cerebral cortex.

As the tracts of the spinal cord are identified, references are made to components of the brain that are discussed in subsequent chapters. When the central nervous system is described by regions, it is necessary to probe ahead of the region under immediate consideration. An appreciation of the major systems is thus acquired step by step. The general sensory and motor systems are reviewed in Chapters 19 and 23, respectively.

Gross Features of the Spinal Cord and Nerve Roots

The spinal cord is a cylindrical structure, slightly flattened dorsoventrally, located in the spinal canal of the vertebral column. Protection for the cord is provided not only by the vertebrae and their ligaments, but also by the meninges and a cushion of cerebrospinal fluid.

Spinal Canal and Meninges

The innermost meningeal layer of **pia mater** adheres to the surface of the spinal cord. The outermost layer of thick dura mater forms a tube that extends from the level of the second sacral vertebra to the foramen magnum at the base of the skull, where it is continuous with the dura mater around the brain. The **arachnoid** lies against the inner surface of the dura mater, forming the outer boundary of the fluid-filled **subarachnoid space**. The spinal cord is suspended in the dural sheath by a **denticulate ligament** on each side. This ligament is in the form of a ribbon, which is attached along the lateral surface of the cord midway between the dorsal and ventral roots (Fig. 5-1). The lateral edge of the denticulate ligament is serrated. Twenty-one points or processes are attached to the dural sheath at intervals between the foramen magnum and the level at which the dura mater is pierced by the roots of the first lumbar spinal nerve. An

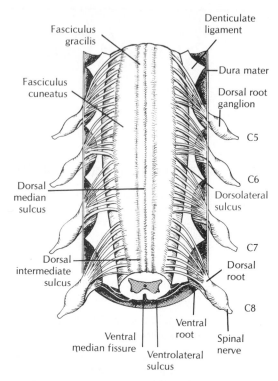

Figure 5-1. Dorsal view of the cervical enlargement of the spinal cord and the corresponding roots of spinal nerves.

epidural space, filled with fatty tissue that contains a venous plexus, intervenes between the dura and the wall of the spinal canal. The epidural space caudal to the second sacral vertebra also contains the roots of the most caudal spinal nerves.

Segments of the Cord, Roots, and Vertebral Column

The segmental nature of the spinal cord is demonstrated by the presence of 31 pairs of **spinal nerves**, but there is little indication of segmentation in its internal structure. Each dorsal root is broken up into a series of **rootlets** that are attached to the cord along the corresponding segment (see Fig. 5-1). The ventral root arises similarly as a series of rootlets. The spinal nerves are distributed as follows: cervical, 8; thoracic, 12; lumbar, 5; sacral, 5; coccygeal, 1. The first cervical nerves lack dorsal roots in 50% of people, and the coccygeal nerves may be absent.

EMBRYOLOGY AND GROWTH

Segments of the neural tube (neuromeres) correspond in position with segments of the vertebral column (scleromeres) until the 3rd month of fetal development. The vertebral column elongates more rapidly than the spinal cord during the remainder of fetal life. The cord, which is fixed at its rostral end, gradually advances; by the time of birth, the caudal end is opposite the disk between the second and third lumbar vertebrae. A slight difference in growth rate continues during childhood, bringing the caudal end of the cord in the adult opposite the disk between the first and second lumbar vertebrae (Fig. 5-2). This is an average level because the length of the spinal cord varies less than the length of the vertebral column. Thus the caudal end of the cord may be as high as the 12th thoracic vertebral body or as low as the 3rd lumbar vertebra. The subarachnoid space caudal to the end of the spinal cord is known as the **lumbar cistern**.

The rostral shift of the cord during development determines the direction of spinal nerve roots in the subarachnoid space. As shown in Figure 5-2, spinal nerves from C1 through C7 leave the spinal canal through the intervertebral foramina above the corresponding vertebrae. (The first and second cervical nerves lie on the vertebral arches of the atlas and axis, respectively.) The eighth cervical nerve passes through the foramen between the seventh cervical and first thoracic vertebrae because there are eight cervical cord segments and seven cervical vertebrae. From that point caudally, the spinal nerves leave the canal through foramina immediately below the pedicles of the corresponding vertebrae. All intervertebral foramina are slightly rostral to the levels of the intervertebral disks.

It is helpful when examining a patient with a possible spinal cord or nerve root lesion to determine the location of the cord segments in relation to vertebral spines or bodies; these are shown for reference in Figure 5-2.

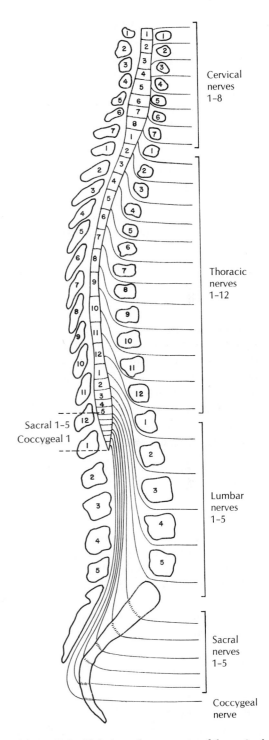

Figure 5-2. Relation of segments of the spinal cord and spinal nerves to the vertebral column. The vertebral bodies are on the right side, and the dorsal spines of the vertebrae on the left.

SPINAL AND VERTEBRAL LEVELS

The dorsal and ventral roots traverse the subarachnoid space and pierce the arachnoid and dura mater. At this point, the dura becomes continuous with the epineurium. After passing through the epidural space, the roots reach the intervertebral foramina, where the dorsal root ganglia are located. The dorsal and ventral roots join immediately distal to the ganglion to form the spinal nerve. The length and obliqueness of the roots increase progressively in a rostrocaudal direction because of the increasing distance between cord segments and the corresponding vertebral segments (see Fig. 5-2). The lumbosacral roots are, therefore, the longest and constitute the **cauda equina** in the lower part of the subarachnoid space. The cord ends as the **conus medullaris**, which tapers rather abruptly into a slender filament called the **filum terminale**, which lies in the middle of the cauda equina and has a distinctive bluish white color. The filum terminale picks up a dural investment opposite the second segment of the sacrum, and the resulting **coccygeal ligament** attaches to the dorsum of the coccyx. The filum terminale consists of pia mater and neuroglial elements; it is a vestige of the spinal cord of the embryonic tail, but in the adult, it has no functional significance.

LUMBAR PUNCTURE

It may be necessary to insert a needle into the subarachnoid space to obtain a sample of cerebrospinal fluid for analysis or for other reasons. A spinal lumbar puncture is the preferred method: the needle is inserted between the arches of the third and fourth lumbar vertebrae to enter the lumbar cistern without risk of damaging the spinal cord.

Limb Enlargements

The spinal cord is enlarged in two regions for innervation of the limbs. The **cervical enlargement** includes segments C4 to T1, with most of the corresponding spinal nerves forming the brachial plexuses for the nerve supply of the upper limbs. Segments L2 to S3 are included in the **lumbosacral enlargement**, and the corresponding nerves constitute most of the lumbosacral plexuses for the innervation of the lower limbs.

Segmental levels are most easily identified for anatomical or pathological study by labeling some of the nerve roots before removing the spinal cord. If this has not been done, the upper and lower levels of the limb enlargements are useful indicators. The sacral segments are short (2–3 mm, compared with 2–3 cm for cervical and thoracic segments), and at this level, the thicknesses of the ventral roots should be noted: ventral root S3 is conspicuously thinner than S2.

Internal Structure of the Spinal Cord

The surface of the spinal cord is marked by longitudinal furrows. The deep **ventral median fissure** contains connective tissue of the pia mater and branches of the anterior spinal artery. The **dorsal median sulcus** is a shallow midline furrow. The **dorsal septum**, composed of pial tissue, extends from the base of this sulcus almost to the gray matter.

Gray Matter and White Matter

As seen in transverse section, the gray matter has a roughly H-shaped or butterfly outline (Figs. 5-3, 5-4, and 5-5). The small **central canal** is lined by ependymal epithelium, and the lumen may be obliterated in places. The gray matter on each side consists of **dorsal** and **ventral horns** and an **intermediate zone**. A small **lateral horn**, containing sympathetic efferent neurons, is added in the thoracic and upper lumbar segments.

There are three main categories of neuron in the spinal gray matter. The smallest cells involved in local circuitry are the internuncial neurons, or **interneurons**. **Motor cells** of the ventral horn supply the skeletal musculature and consist of alpha and gamma motor neurons, whose functions were described in Chapter 3. (The somewhat similar cells of the lateral horn and the sacral autonomic nucleus

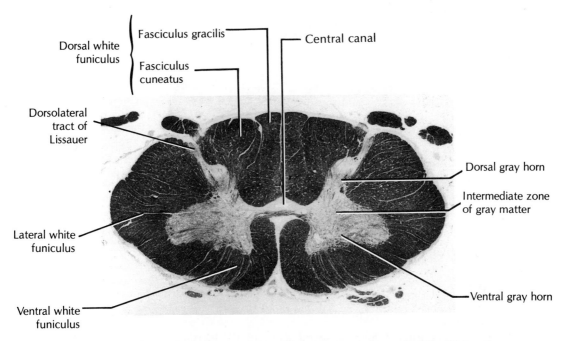

Figure 5-3. Seventh cervical segment. (Transverse section stained by Weigert's method for myelin, × 6)

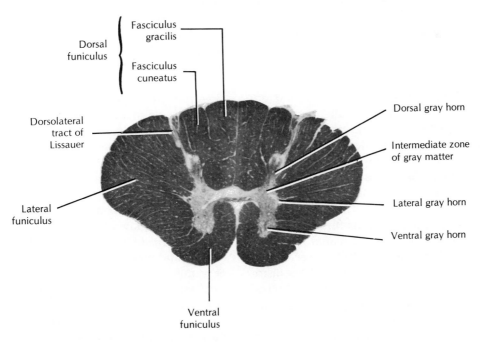

Figure 5-4. Second thoracic segment. (Weigert's stain, × 7)

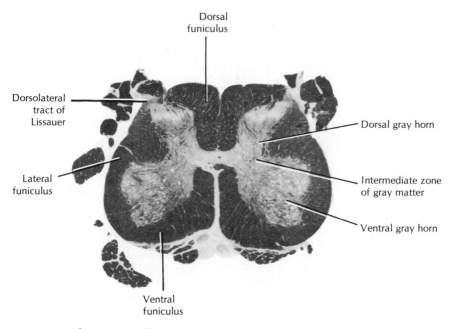

Dorsal funiculus

Dorsolateral tract of Lissauer

Lateral funiculus

Ventral funiculus

Dorsal gray horn

Intermediate zone of gray matter

Ventral gray horn

Figure 5-5. First sacral segment. (Weigert's stain, × 7)

are preganglionic neurons of the sympathetic and parasympathetic divisions of the autonomic system, respectively.) The cell bodies of **tract cells**, whose axons constitute the ascending fasciculi of the white matter, are located mainly in the dorsal horn.

The white matter consists of three funiculi (see Figs. 5-3, 5-4, and 5-5). (These are often called "columns," but this word is more appropriate for longitudinally aligned arrays of neuronal cell bodies in the gray matter.) The **dorsal funiculus**, bounded by the dorsal septum and the dorsal gray horn, consists of a medial **gracile fasciculus** and a lateral **cuneate fasciculus** above the midthoracic level. The former constitutes the entire dorsal funiculus caudal to the midthoracic region. The remainder of the white matter consists of **lateral** and **ventral funiculi**, between which there is no anatomical demarcation. The distribution of tracts in the lateral white matter justifies a more natural subdivision of the spinal white matter into dorsolateral and ventrolateral zones, separated by a plane that passes through the central canal and the denticulate ligament and a ventromedial area be-

tween the ventral horn and the ventral median fissure. Nerve fibers decussate in the **ventral white commissure**. The **dorsolateral tract** (of Lissauer) occupies the interval between the apex of the dorsal horn and the surface of the cord. The white matter consists of partially overlapping bundles (tracts or fasciculi) of fibers, as described later.

Although the general pattern of gray matter and white matter is the same throughout the spinal cord, regional differences are apparent in transverse sections (see Figs. 5-3, 5-4, and 5-5). For example, the amount of white matter increases in a caudal-to-rostral direction because fibers are added to ascending tracts and fibers leave descending tracts to terminate in the gray matter. The main variation in the gray matter is its increased volume in the cervical and lumbosacral enlargements for innervation of the upper and lower limbs. The small lateral horn of gray matter is characteristic of the thoracic and upper lumbar segments. Caudal to S2, the ventral fissure is shallow, so the left and right ventral horns blend together in a wide band of gray matter ventral to the central canal.

Neuronal Architecture of Spinal Gray Matter

As with other parts of the central nervous system, the spinal gray matter is composed of several neuronal populations. The cell types are classified according to their appearances under the microscope, and it has been found that cells of the same type are usually clustered together into groups. Because the architecture of the spinal gray matter is essentially the same along the length of the cord, the populations of similar neurons occur in long columns. When viewed in transverse sections of the spinal cord, many of the cell columns appear as layers, especially within the dorsal horn. Ten layers of neurons are recognized, known as the **laminae of Rexed**. Before the laminae were described in 1952, names were given to many of the cell columns, with all but a few of these names now having fallen into disuse. They were used differently by different authors, and confusing synonyms existed. The laminar scheme agrees well with the known sites of origin and termination of efferent and afferent fiber tracts, so it is possible to ascribe functions to at least some of the groups of neurons. The few unambiguous names still in use for cell columns are mentioned in association with the laminae in which they occur.

LAMINAR ORGANIZATION

The laminae of Rexed are numbered consecutively by Roman numerals, starting at the tip of the dorsal horn and moving ventrally into the ventral horn (Fig. 5-6).

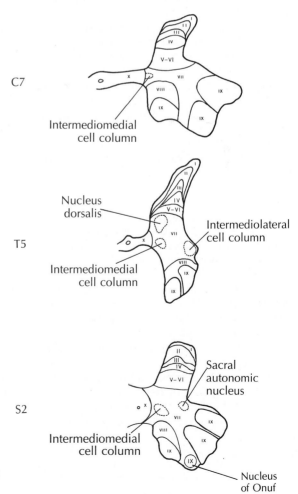

Figure 5-6. Positions of cytoarchitectonic laminae in the spinal gray matter.

Lamina I is a thin layer that caps the dorsal horn. It contains large, tangentially oriented neurons and smaller, stellate cells. Lamina I receives some of the incoming dorsal root fibers, and its large neurons contribute a small proportion of the axons of the contralateral spinothalamic tract.

Lamina II, also known as the **substantia gelatinosa** (of Rolando), consists of small, densely packed neurons (gelatinosa cells) that have numerous, richly branched dendrites. Its afferent fibers are collateral branches of incoming dorsal root axons, together with descending fibers, many of which come from the reticular formation of the medulla. The unmyelinated axons of the gelatinosa cells ascend or descend for up to four segments of the cord in the dorsolateral tract and in the adjacent white matter of the lateral funiculus. Their many branches make synaptic contacts in the other laminae of the dorsal horn at all these levels. The substantia gelatinosa is believed to be important for the editing of sensory input to the spinal cord, with the effect of determining which patterns of incoming impulses will produce sensations that will be interpreted by the brain as being painful. **Lamina III** also consists of interneurons and receives large numbers of fibers from the dorsal roots.

Lamina IV contains neurons with long dendrites that extend dorsally into laminae II and III. These are **tract cells**, with axons that cross the midline and enter the contralateral spinothalamic tract. Lamina IV is conspicuous in sections stained by Weigert's method (see Figs. 5-3, 5-4, and 5-5) because it contains more myelinated axons than any other part of the dorsal horn. Most of these are primary afferent fibers that come from the dorsal roots by way of the dorsal funiculus. Laminae I through VI all receive input from the dorsal roots, although this is densest in lamina IV. At the extreme rostral end of the spinal cord, laminae I, II, III, and IV become continuous with the caudal end of the spinal trigeminal nucleus.

Lamina V-VI is so named because the two laminae recognized by Rexed in the cat are indistinguishable from each other in the human spinal cord. This zone at the base of the dorsal horn contains tract cells that resemble those of lamina IV, mixed with interneurons of various shapes and sizes. It receives some primary afferent fibers and many descending fibers from

the brain, especially corticospinal fibers, most of which end in laminae V-VI, and VII. The tract cells in laminae IV and V-VI are collectively known as the **nucleus proprius**. Laterally, the gray matter at the base of the dorsal horn is mixed with longitudinal strands of white matter of the lateral funiculus. Sometimes the name "reticular formation" is applied to this region, which should not be confused with the reticular formation of the brain stem.[1]

Lamina VII is the largest cytoarchitectonic region of the spinal gray matter, occupying the intermediate zone between the dorsal and ventral horns as well as much of the space within the ventral horn. Its shape and position vary along the length of the cord, as do the shape and position of lamina VIII. Lamina VII contains many cells that function as interneurons, although most of these have long axons that run in the spinal white matter to the gray matter of other segments of the cord. The local circuitry is completed by collateral branches of the proximal parts of the axons of these cells.

There are some clearly delineated cell columns that do not fit well into the laminar scheme but usually are included in lamina VII. The **nucleus dorsalis** (nucleus thoracicus, or Clarke's column) is medial and ventral to the base of the dorsal horn in segments T1 to L3 or L4. This cell column is composed of large neurons with eccentric nuclei whose axons form the dorsal spinocerebellar tract. The ventral spinocerebellar tract originates from cells in laminae V-VI and VII as well as from neurons with cell bodies at the edge of the gray matter of the ventral horn in the lumbar segments. The latter are known as **spinal border cells**. The **inter-mediolateral cell column** occupies the lateral horn of the cord in segments T1 to L2 or L3. This column consists of the cell bodies of the preganglionic neurons of the sympathetic nervous system. The **sacral autonomic nucleus** is an equivalent column of cells in the lateral part of lamina VII in segments S2, S3, and S4. It consists of the cell bodies of the preganglionic neurons of the sacral division of the parasympathetic nervous system. The **intermedio-medial cell column** is present just lateral to lamina X throughout the length of the cord, but

---

[1] The reticular formation, described in Chapter 9, is a collection of groups of neurons that serve important functions in the medulla, pons, and midbrain.

it has a beaded structure and, therefore, cannot be seen in all transverse sections. It receives primary afferent fibers and may be involved in visceral reflexes.

Lamina VIII on the medial aspect of the ventral horn contains neurons with a variety of shapes and sizes. It is a site of termination of some descending fibers, including many of those of the vestibulospinal and reticulospinal tracts. The neurons project both ipsilaterally and contralaterally at the same and nearby segmental levels to laminae VII and IX.

Lamina IX takes the form of columns of neurons embedded in either lamina VII or lamina VIII. The cells in lamina IX include motor neurons, whose axons leave the spinal cord in the ventral roots to supply striated skeletal muscle fibers. The sizes of the cell bodies of motor neurons vary; those giving rise to long axons are among the largest of neurons, whereas those with shorter axons (and also those giving rise to the gamma efferent fibers to muscle spindles) are much smaller. In addition, lamina IX contains small neurons whose axons extend up and down the spinal cord in the fasciculus proprius adjacent to the gray matter. By virtue of collateral axonal branches that arise near the cell body, these cells also serve as local circuit neurons in the ventral horn.

Four columns of motor neurons (ventromedial, ventrolateral, central and dorsolateral), each with characteristic dendritic features visible in Golgi preparations, are recognized in the human ventral horn. The sizes and relative positions of the columns vary along the length of the spinal cord. In general, the ventrally and medially located neurons supply muscles in the neck and trunk, whereas cells in the dorsal and lateral parts of the ventral horn innervate the muscles of the limbs.

There are two additional motor nuclei in the cervical cord, one for the phrenic nerve and the other for the spinal root of the accessory nerve. The diaphragm develops from cervical myotomes and, although it migrates caudally during embryonic development, the origin of the diaphragm is reflected in its nerve supply. The **phrenic nucleus** is responsible for an enlargement of the ventromedial cell column in the ventral horn in segments C3 to C5, most prominently in C4. The **spinal accessory nucleus** consists of motor cells in the lateral region of the ventral horn in segments C1 to C5. The axons emerge in a series of rootlets along the lateral aspect of the spinal cord, just dorsal to the denticulate ligament. The rootlets converge to form the spinal root of the accessory nerve, which ascends along the side of the cord in the subarachnoid space and enters the posterior cranial fossa through the foramen magnum. The spinal root joins the cranial (medullary) root along the side of the medulla. The accessory nerve (see Ch. 8) then leaves the posterior cranial fossa through the jugular foramen, and the spinal component supplies the sternocleidomastoid and trapezius muscles.

In the second sacral segment, a prominent column of small neurons is embedded in a tract of unmyelinated fibers in the most ventral part of the ventral horn. This is the **nucleus of Onuf**. Its cells contribute axons to the pudendal nerve (roots S2–S4). The nucleus of Onuf supplies muscles in the pelvic floor, including the striated muscle sphincters that contribute to urinary and fecal continence. The nucleus also supplies the ischiocavernosus and bulbospongiosus muscles and contains more neurons in men than in women.

Lamina X surrounds the central canal. It contains neurons smaller than those in the adjacent laminae V-VI, VII, and VIII. A few dorsal root afferent fibers terminate in this area. There also are decussating axons and neuroglia. The ventral part of lamina X is one of the few places in which radial neuroglial cells (see Ch. 2) persist in the adult. Their cytoplasmic processes extend from the central canal to the pia mater of the ventral sulcus.

Outside the gray matter, an isolated group of neurons is present in the lateral funiculus, adjacent to the tip of the dorsal horn. This is the **lateral cervical nucleus**. It is found in segments C1 and C2, but is seldom conspicuous. This nucleus never contains more than half as many neurons as the equivalent cell column of the cat, and is absent in about 50% of people. It is possible that the human lateral cervical nucleus commonly merges into the nearby reflection of lamina I overlying the lateral aspect of the tip of the dorsal horn. Rostrally, the lateral cervical nucleus (in animals, and in humans when present) continues into the caudal third of the medulla. In cats and monkeys, the lateral cervical nucleus is an essential part of the spinocervicothalamic sensory pathway (see Ch. 19), but its importance in humans is not known.

In summary, the spinal gray matter is organized in the following way. Dorsal root afferents terminate predominantly in the dorsal horn. Impulses concerned with pain, temperature, and touch reach the tract cells, most with cell bodies in the deeper laminae of the dorsal horn, from which the spinothalamic tract originates. The sensory information transmitted to the brain, especially for pain, is subject to modification (editing) by interaction with other modalities of sensation and by impulses that reach the dorsal horn by way of various descending pathways. Lamina II (the substantia gelatinosa) is thought to have a prominent role in modifying the perception of pain. Motor neurons (lamina IX) supply the skeletal musculature. With the intervention of interneurons, the motor neurons usually come under the influence of dorsal root afferents for spinal reflexes and of several descending tracts for the control of motor activity by the brain. Of the neurons that constitute lamina IX, those supplying axial musculature are in the medial part of the ventral horn and those supplying the limbs are located more laterally. Distinctive columns of motor neurons include the phrenic and accessory nuclei in the cervical segments and the nucleus of Onuf in the sacral cord. Distinctive cell columns in the thoracic and upper lumbar segments (formally included with lamina VII) are the nucleus dorsalis, which gives rise to the dorsal spinocerebellar tract, and the intermediolateral cell column, which consists of preganglionic sympathetic neurons. The midsacral segments contain a less conspicuous intermediolateral column, the sacral autonomic nucleus. Spinal border cells in the lumbar segments contribute to the ventral spinocerebellar tracts.

Dorsal Root Entry Zone

Each dorsal root branches into six to eight rootlets as it approaches the spinal cord, and the axons become segregated into two divisions within each rootlet (Fig. 5-7). The lateral division contains most of the unmyelinated, or group C, axons and some thin group A myelinated axons. These axons enter the **dorso-lateral tract** (of Lissauer) where they divide into ascending and descending branches, each giving off collaterals that enter the dorsal horn. Some of these fibers extend as far as four segments rostral or caudal to the segment at which they entered the cord, but most terminate in their own or in immediately adjacent segments.

The medial division of dorsal root afferents, for modalities of sensation other than pain and temperature, consists largely of myelinated axons, including all the large-caliber, rapidly conducting sensory fibers. These enter the spinal white matter medial to the dorsal horn where, like those of the lateral division, they divide into ascending and descending branches. The descending branches run caudally within the dorsal funiculi for varying distances, some to nearby segments and others almost the whole length of the cord, to terminate eventually in the dorsal horn. Some of the long descending primary afferent fibers of the dorsal funiculi are collected into distinct bundles: the **fasciculus septomarginalis**, adjacent to the dorsal septum, and the **fasciculus interfascicularis**, between the gracile and cuneate fasciculi. The ascending branches of afferent fibers entering the dorsal funiculus are also of differing lengths, with many reaching the gracile and cuneate nuclei in the medulla. At the other extreme, many axons from the medial division of the dorsal root enter the gray matter at their own segmental levels. These fibers are conspicuous in lamina IV of the dorsal horn (Figs. 5-3 and 5-5). Primary afferent axons conveying signals from muscle spindles have some branches that terminate on motor neurons and are involved in the stretch reflex. Some of the synaptic arrangements in the dorsal gray horn are summarized in Figure 5-7.

Ventral Horn

The columns of cells constituting lamina IX contain motor neurons of two types, named after the diameters and, therefore, the conduction velocities of their axons. The alpha motor neurons supply the ordinary (extrafusal) fibers of striated skeletal muscles. The smaller gamma

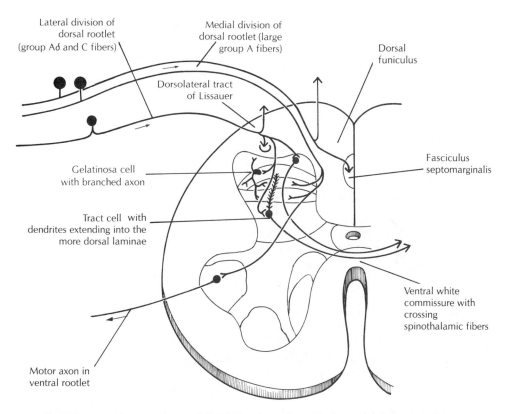

Figure 5-7. Neuronal circuitry of the dorsal horn of the spinal gray matter.

motor neurons are less numerous; they supply the intrafusal fibers of the neuromuscular spindles. The surfaces of both motor neuron types are densely covered with synaptic terminals, which release either excitatory or inhibitory transmitter substances. Each alpha motor neuron receives at least 20,000 synaptic contacts. The sources of the afferents are numerous; some are from descending tracts of the spinal cord, and others are branches of axons of primary afferent neurons. The greatest numbers, however, are from intrinsic cells of the spinal gray matter, which behave physiologically as interneurons. The interneurons are located mainly in lamina VII. They receive their afferents from one another, from descending tracts, and from primary afferent neurons concerned with all modalities of sensation.

A special type of interneuron, from the physiological standpoint, is the **Renshaw cell**, which receives excitatory synaptic input from branches of the axons of nearby motor neurons. The branched axon of a Renshaw cell forms inhibitory synaptic junctions on motor neurons, including the same ones that are presynaptic to the Renshaw cell itself. The Renshaw cells (which are in laminae VII and VIII) are also presynaptic and postsynaptic to other intraspinal neurons. The circuitry of the ventral horn is summarized in Figure 5-8.

Tracts of Ascending and Descending Fibers

The spinal white matter is divided into three longitudinally aligned **funiculi**, whose positions have already been described. Each funiculus contains tracts of ascending and descending fibers. The positions of the tracts have been approximately determined from clinical and pathological studies and from comparison

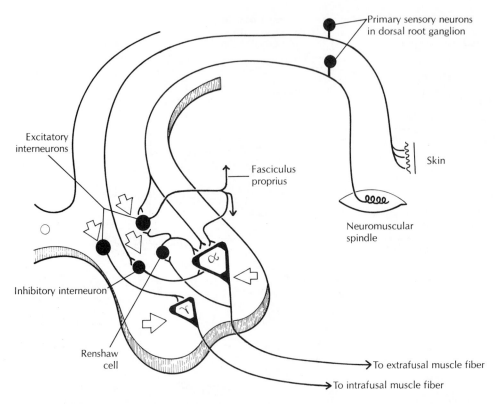

Figure 5-8. Neuronal circuitry of the ventral horn of the spinal gray matter, showing afferents to alpha (α) and gamma (γ) motor neurons. The interneurons also have long axonal branches that travel in the fasciculus proprius. Large red arrows point to the sites of termination of axons of descending tracts from the brain.

of these clinical data with the more exact information obtained from animal studies. Most neuroanatomy and clinical neurology textbooks contain diagrams such as Figure 5-9, showing the positions of the major tracts. It is important to realize that the precise positions of some tracts are not known with certainty and that the territories of the different tracts overlap one another considerably.

DORSAL FUNICULUS

The most important component of each dorsal funiculus is a large body of ascending axons derived from neurons located in the dorsal root ganglia. Other ascending fibers are axons of neurons in the dorsal horn. The ascending fibers are all ipsilateral. They are concerned especially with the discriminative qualities of sensation, including the ability to recognize changes in the positions of tactile stimuli applied to the skin. Conscious awareness of movement and of the positions of joints in the upper limb is also mediated by axons in the dorsal funiculi above the level of spinal segment T1. Fibers that carry the same proprioceptive modality from the lower limb travel in the dorsal funiculus only as far as the thoracic cord, where the axons end by synapsing in the nucleus dorsalis. The upward continuation of the pathway for position sense in the lower limb is located in the lateral funiculus (see Ch. 19). It was formerly thought that conscious appreciation of vibration required the integrity of the dorsal funiculi, but clinical observations indicate that this is not so. Both the dorsal and the lateral funiculi conduct impulses initiated by vibratory stimuli.

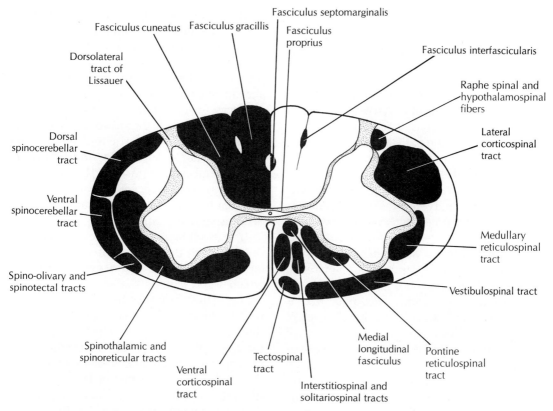

Figure 5-9. Major tracts of the spinal white matter at midcervical level. Ascending tracts are on the left; descending tracts are on the right.

As the spinal cord is ascended, axons are added to the lateral side of each dorsal funiculus. Consequently, in the upper cervical cord, the lowest levels of segmental innervation are represented in the most medial part of the gracile fasciculus and the uppermost levels, in the most lateral part of the cuneate fasciculus. These two fasciculi end, respectively, in the gracile and cuneate nuclei, which are located dorsally in the medulla. As a useful approximation, the gracile fasciculus and nucleus may be said to deal with sensations from the lower limb, and the cuneate fasciculus and nucleus may be said to deal with sensations from the upper limb. The orderly arrangement of different levels of the body in the dorsal funiculi is an example of **somatotopic lamination** in a tract. As will be seen, comparable lamination also exists in some other tracts of the spinal cord and brain.

The ascending sensory fibers are not the only axons in the dorsal funiculi. Descending axons arise from three sources: the neurons in the gracile and cuneate nuclei, the spinal gray matter, and the dorsal root ganglia. The gracilo- and cuneato-spinal pathways form part of a series of neural connections through which higher levels of the central nervous system are able to modify or edit the input of sensory messages from the cord. The spinospinal fibers, some of which run almost the full length of the cord in both directions, are probably involved in reflex coordination of the movements of the upper and lower limbs. The descending branches of incoming primary afferent axons provide a mechanism whereby the sensations arising in adjacent segmental levels of the body may be integrated so that meaningful patterns of impulses will ascend to the brain in the long ascending tracts.

LATERAL FUNICULUS

It is convenient to describe the dorsal and lateral halves of the lateral funiculus separately.

DORSOLATERAL FASCICULUS. The most conspicuous tract in the dorsal half of the lateral funiculus is the **lateral corticospinal tract**, which consists of axons of neurons in the cortex of the frontal and parietal lobes of the contralateral cerebral hemisphere. These fibers pass through the internal capsule, the basis pedunculi of the midbrain, the pons, and the medullary pyramid before decussating and entering the lateral funiculus of the cord. The corticospinal fibers from the frontal cortex terminate mainly in the intermediate gray matter and the ventral horn. Those from the parietal lobe end in the dorsal horn. The somatotopic lamination of the lateral corticospinal tract is such that fibers destined for the lowest levels of the spinal cord are the most laterally placed. In rodents and carnivores, a substantial **rubrospinal tract**, arising from the contralateral red nucleus, extends through most of the spinal cord immediately ventral to the lateral corticospinal tract. The rubrospinal tract is small in monkeys. In apes and humans, it is rudimentary and ends in the second cervical segment.

Experiments with animals indicate that the reticulospinal component of the dorsolateral funiculus arises in the nucleus raphe magnus in the reticular formation of the medulla and terminates in laminae I, II, and III. These unmyelinated fibers, constituting the **raphespinal tract** in the most dorsal part of the lateral funiculus, contain histochemically demonstrable quantities of serotonin, which they probably use as a neurotransmitter. The raphespinal tract modifies the transmission from the dorsal horn of impulses initiated by noxious stimuli, which produce painful sensations. Unmyelinated **hypothalamospinal fibers**, similarly located, arise from the paraventricular nucleus of the hypothalamus and end among the preganglionic autonomic neurons in segments T1 to L3 and S2 to S4. Some hypothalamospinal axons contain the peptide oxytocin.

Ascending fibers in the dorsal part of the lateral funiculus arise from cells in the dorsal horn. They convey impulses initiated by most modalities of cutaneous and deep sensation, probably including vibration, to the gracile and cuneate nuclei of the medulla. In cats and monkeys, the same region of white matter also contains the fibers of the **spinocervical tract**. The axons of this tract arise ipsilaterally from cells in the dorsal horn and terminate mainly in the lateral cervical nucleus. The spinocervical tract is concerned with cutaneous sensation, but its importance in the human central nervous system is uncertain.

The ascending fibers just described are located deep in the white matter. Superficially located is the **dorsal spinocerebellar tract**, which is present only above level L3. The axons of this tract arise from the cells of the nucleus dorsalis (Clarke's column) in the same side of the cord and terminate ipsilaterally in the cortex of the cerebellum, which they enter by way of the inferior cerebellar peduncle. In the lower medulla, axons of the dorsal spinocerebellar tract give off collateral branches that terminate in the nucleus Z of Brodal and Pompeiano. This nucleus is rostral to the gracile nucleus and forms part of the pathway for conscious proprioception (see Ch. 19) from the lower limb.

VENTROLATERAL FASCICULUS. Several tracts are present in the ventral half of the lateral funiculus. The largest is the **spinothalamic tract**, which consists of the ascending axons of neurons located in the gray matter of the opposite half of the cord. The cells of origin are mostly in the nucleus proprius of the dorsal horn (laminae IV and V-VI), although smaller numbers are present in laminae I, VII, VIII, and X. The axons cross the midline in the ventral white commissure close to the central canal and then traverse the ventral horn to enter the ventrolateral and ventral funiculi. The fibers of the spinothalamic tract end in thalamic nuclei. As they pass through the brain stem, some of these axons give off collateral branches to the reticular formation in the medulla and pons and to the periaqueductal gray matter in the midbrain. The spinothalamic tract conducts impulses concerned with tactile, thermal, and painful sensations. Its fibers are somatotopically arranged, with those for the lower limb lying most superficially and those for the upper limb lying closest to the gray matter. Distinct ventral and lateral spinothalamic tracts (respectively for touch and for pain and thermal sensation) were formerly recognized, but there seems to be little justification for such a subdivision. The functions of the spinothalamic fibers are discussed in more detail in Chapter 19.

The **ventral spinocerebellar tract** is located superficially in the ventrolateral funiculus. It arises from the base of the dorsal horn and from the spinal border cells of the ventral horn of the lumbosacral segments of the spinal cord and consists largely of crossed fibers. The tract ascends as far as the midbrain and then makes a sharp turn caudally into the superior cerebellar peduncle. The fibers cross the midline for a second time within the cerebellum before ending in the cerebellar cortex. Thus both spinocerebellar tracts convey sensory information (mainly proprioceptive) from one side of the body to the same side of the cerebellum. The other ascending components of the ventral half of the lateral funiculus are small. The **spinotectal tract** (also known, perhaps more accurately, as the spinomesencephalic tract) consists of fibers that originate in the same parts of the gray matter as the spinothalamic fibers, cross the midline, and then project rostrally to the periaqueductal gray matter, the superior colliculus, and various nuclei in the reticular formation of the midbrain. The **spinoreticular tract** also originates in laminae IV to VIII. It includes crossed fibers that terminate in the pontine reticular formation and uncrossed fibers that end in the medullary reticular formation. Many are collateral branches of spinothalamic fibers. They form part of the ascending reticular activating system (see Ch. 9), and may also be involved in the perception of pain and of various sensations that originate in internal organs. It is customary to indicate a small **spino-olivary tract** in the human spinal cord, but its existence in primates is uncertain. In the cat, this tract projects to the accessory olivary nuclei of the medulla contralateral to the cells of origin; the olivary nuclei, in turn, project across the midline to the cerebellar cortex.

A descending tract of the ventrolateral funiculus, the **medullary reticulospinal tract**, is derived largely from the gigantocellular reticular nucleus of the medulla. Most of its fibers are uncrossed, but a small proportion have crossed the midline in the medulla. This tract, together with the pontine reticulospinal tract (described below), is one of the descending pathways through which the brain directs and controls the activity of motor neurons. Whereas the corticospinal tract is concerned mainly with skilled volitional movements, the reticulospinal tracts control ordinary activities that do not require constant conscious effort.

VENTRAL FUNICULUS

The long tracts in this part of the spinal white matter are all descending ones. The **ventral corticospinal tract** comprises a small proportion of the corticospinal fibers, those that did not cross the midline in the lower part of the medulla. Most ventral corticospinal fibers probably decussate at segmental levels and terminate next to those of the larger lateral corticospinal tract. In a few people, most of the corticospinal fibers fail to decussate in the medulla and, therefore, descend ipsilaterally in the ventral funiculus or, rarely, in the ventrolateral fasciculus. The **vestibulospinal tract** is an uncrossed pathway that arises from the lateral vestibular nucleus (of Deiters) in the medulla. It is located in the lateral part of the ventral funiculus, and its axons terminate in lamina VIII and in the medial part of lamina VII. A few vestibulospinal fibers synapse directly with motor neurons in the cell columns of lamina IX. Although much is known about this tract in laboratory animals, human clinicopathological studies have yielded surprisingly little information. Its function is to mediate equilibratory reflexes, which are triggered by the activity of the vestibular apparatus of the internal ear and put into effect by the axial musculature and the extensors of the limbs.

The **pontine reticulospinal tract** originates in the ipsilateral pontine reticular formation and terminates bilaterally in the spinal gray matter, with some of the axons decussating in the ventral white commissure. The remaining tracts of the ventral funiculus are small. The descending component of the **medial longitudinal fasciculus** (also called the medial vestibulospinal tract, in which case the vestibulospinal tract previously described is designated as lateral) arises in the medial vestibular nucleus in the medulla. It is involved in movements of the head required for maintaining equilibrium and probably does not descend below the upper cervical levels of the spinal cord. Neither do the few fibers that constitute the **tectospinal tract** from the contralateral superior colliculus. The **interstitiospinal tract** is a small bundle that originates in the interstitial nucleus of Cajal and in the Edinger-Westphal nucleus, both of which are located in the rostral part of the midbrain. This tract is probably involved in visuomotor coordination. A small **solitariospinal tract**, from the solitary nucleus in the medulla and from certain nuclei of the medullary reticular formation, is present at all levels in animals. It is involved in rhythmic respiratory movements and may also mediate part of the higher control of autonomic functions.

FASCICULUS PROPRIUS

The fasciculus proprius, a zone containing both myelinated and unmyelinated fibers, is present in all the funiculi immediately adjacent to the gray matter (see Fig. 5-9). It contains **propriospinal (spinospinalis) fibers**, which connect different segmental levels of the gray matter. The shorter axons are closer to the gray matter than the longer fibers. Propriospinal fibers run both rostrally and caudally and have collateral branches that end in the gray matter near their own cell bodies, providing the functional equivalent of interneurons for reflexes within segments. Some neurons with axons in the fasciculus proprius extend for almost the whole length of the spinal cord and serve as necessary components of intersegmental spinal reflexes.

Spinal Reflexes

Certain neuronal connections in the spinal cord form the bases of spinal reflexes. The stretch reflex, gamma reflex loop, and flexor reflex are examples.

The **stretch reflex** has a two-neuron or monosynaptic reflex arc (Fig. 5-10). Slight

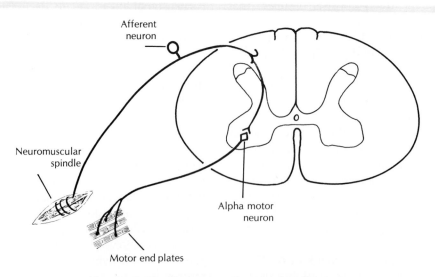

Figure 5-10. Monosynaptic stretch reflex arc.

stretching of a muscle stimulates the sensory endings in neuromuscular spindles, and the resultant excitation reaches the spinal cord by way of primary sensory neurons that have large group A axons. The proximal branches of these axons in the dorsal funiculus give off collateral branches that excite alpha motor neurons, causing the stretched muscle to contract. This is an important postural reflex. The neuromuscular spindles are delicate monitors of change in the length of the muscle, and the stretch reflex alters tension in such a way as to maintain a constant length. The stretch reflex forms the basis of the clinical **tendon jerks**, tests that are part of every physical examination. A sharp tap on the tendon causes synchronous discharges from the spindles in the muscle, with prompt reflex contraction. A diminished or absent tendon jerk indicates disease affecting either the afferent or the efferent neurons of the stretch reflex. Exaggerated jerks indicate a lack of inhibition of motor neurons by activity in descending tracts from the brain.

The reflex arc just described forms part of the **gamma reflex loop**, through which muscle tension comes under the control of descending motor pathways (Fig. 5-11). Fibers of these pathways (corticospinal, reticulospinal, vestibulospinal) excite gamma motor neurons, causing contraction of intrafusal muscle fibers and an increase in the rate of firing from sensory endings in the neuromuscular spindles (see Ch. 3). Through the monosynaptic reflex arc described for the stretch reflex, the sensory impulses are conveyed to alpha motor neurons that supply the main muscle mass.

In addition to the simple monosynaptic stretch reflex, there is a response with longer latency that occurs when a voluntarily contracting muscle is stretched. Physiological studies indicate that this slower reflex, which is most easily elicited in the hand, passes through the somatosensory and motor areas of the cerebral cortex.

The tension on a muscle is monitored by Golgi tendon organs. When the tension reaches a certain level, there is a distinct increase in the discharge from these receptors. The resulting nerve impulses reach interneurons in the spinal gray matter; these cells inhibit alpha motor neurons, and relaxation of the muscle follows. This reflex can prevent excessive tension on the muscle and tendon.

The **flexor reflex** also is protective. It consists of the withdrawal of a limb in response to a painful stimulus. At least three neurons are involved, so this is a polysynaptic reflex (Fig. 5-12). The cutaneous receptors are free nerve

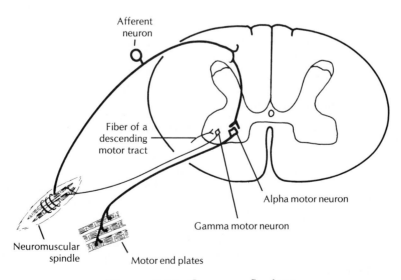

Figure 5-11. Gamma reflex loop.

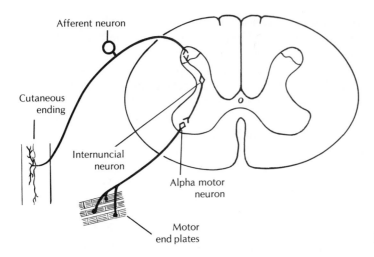

Figure 5-12. Flexor reflex arc.

endings that respond to potentially injurious stimuli, and the proximal branches of the afferent fibers synapse in the dorsal horn with interneurons. These end on alpha motor cells in several segments because a withdrawal response requires the action of muscle groups. Commissural neurons in the dorsal horn have axons that end in the contralateral ventral horn and, in a fully developed response, stimulate extension of the contralateral limb.

Anatomical and Clinical Correlations

Lesions of the spinal cord result from trauma, degenerative and demyelinating disorders, tumors, infections, and impairment of blood supply. The following notes on selected lesions show the necessity of understanding the intrinsic anatomy of the spinal cord to interpret signs and symptoms.

Clinical Examination

Testing for impairment or loss of cutaneous sensation is an important part of the neurological examination; it is particularly useful in detecting the site of a lesion that involves the spinal cord or nerve roots. The distribution of cutaneous areas (**dermatomes**) supplied by the spinal

nerves is shown in Figure 5-13.[2] Cutaneous areas supplied by adjacent spinal nerves overlap. For example, the upper half of the area supplied by T6 is also supplied by T5, and the lower half, by T7. There is, therefore, little or no sensory loss after interruption of a single dorsal root of a spinal nerve. The overlapping of dermatomes contrasts with the sharp delineation of the areas supplied by cutaneous nerves, which are formed in the limb plexuses by the mingling of fibers from various segmental nerve roots.

Reflex contraction of muscles also is used in testing for the integrity of segments of the cord and of the spinal nerves. The segments involved in four commonly tested **stretch or tendon reflexes** are as follows: biceps reflex, C5 and C6; triceps reflex, C6 to C8; quadriceps reflex (knee jerk), L2 to L4; gastrocnemius reflex (ankle jerk), S1 to S2.

Before specific pathological conditions are mentioned, it should be noted that a distinction is made between the effects of a lesion involving **lower motor neurons** as opposed to those involving **upper motor neurons**. Destruction or atrophy of lower motor neurons (in the present context, those of the ventral horn) results in flaccid paralysis of the affected muscles, diminished or absent tendon reflexes, and progressive

---

[2] Because different methods of investigation yield different results, a dermatomal map receiving general acceptance in all details has yet to be devised.

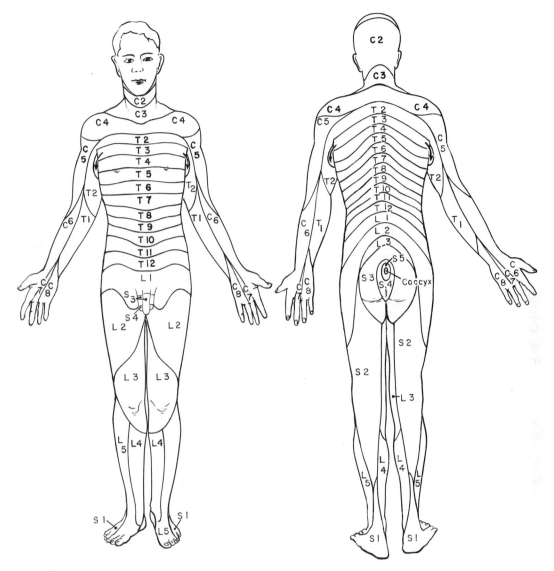

Figure 5-13. Cutaneous distribution of spinal nerves (dermatomes).

atrophy of the muscles deprived of motor fibers. The term "upper motor neuron lesion," although regularly used clinically, leaves much to be desired. The lesion may be in the cerebral cortex or in another part of the cerebral hemisphere, in the brain stem, or in the spinal cord. Thus the "upper motor neuron" is a collective term including all the descending pathways that control the activities of the neurons that supply the muscles. The following signs are associated with an upper motor neuron lesion after the acute effects have worn off: varying degrees of voluntary paralysis, which is severest in the upper limb; a positive Babinski's sign (upturning of the great toe and spreading of the toes on stroking of the sole); and spasticity with exaggerated tendon reflexes.

Spinal Transection

The cord may be damaged by penetrating wounds (caused by stabbing or gunfire) or by spinal fracture or dislocation (especially from road traffic accidents or diving into shallow water). Complete transection results in loss of all sensibility and voluntary movement below the lesion. The patient is **tetraplegic** (quadriplegic, with both arms and both legs paralyzed) if the upper cervical cord is transected and **paraplegic** (both legs paralyzed) if the transection is between the cervical and lumbosacral enlargements. During an initial period of **spinal shock**, lasting from a few days to several weeks, all somatic and visceral reflex activity is abolished. On return of reflex activity, there is spasticity of muscles and exaggerated tendon reflexes. Bladder and bowel functions are no longer under voluntary control.

The events following partial transection of the spinal cord depend on the size and location of the lesion. **Hemisection**, although unusual in the literal sense, is an instructive lesion anatomically. The neurological signs caudal to the hemisected region of the cord constitute the Brown-Séquard syndrome. Position sense, tactile discrimination, and the feeling of vibration are lost *on the side of the lesion* because of interruption of the dorsal and dorsolateral funiculi. There is anesthesia for pain and temperature *on the opposite side* because of interruption of the spinothalamic tract. Light touch is not much affected because of essentially bilateral conduction in the dorsal and lateral funiculi. The patient is **hemiplegic** (left or right upper and lower limbs paralyzed) if the lesion is in the upper cervical cord, whereas hemisection of the thoracic cord results in paralysis of the leg (**monoplegia**). The paralysis is *ipsilateral* to the lesion and of the upper motor neuron type.

Degenerative Diseases

The following degenerative diseases also illustrate the anatomical basis of neurological signs. In **subacute combined degeneration**, there is bilateral demyelination and loss of nerve fibers in the dorsal and dorsolateral funiculi. The principal causative factor is vitamin B_{12} deficiency, and the disorder is typically encountered in association with pernicious anemia. The lesion results in loss of the senses of position, discriminative touch, and vibration. The gait is ataxic (without coordination) because the patient is unaware of the position of the legs.

Amyotrophic lateral sclerosis is a bilateral degenerative disease. The degenerative process is largely restricted to the motor system, affecting the corticobulbar and corticospinal tracts (and perhaps other descending motor pathways) along with motor nuclei of cranial nerves and ventral horn motor cells. There is a combination of upper and lower motor neuron clinical signs, with the latter predominating in the terminal stages of the disease.

Syringomyelia is different from the disorders already mentioned, in that neuronal degeneration is not the primary pathological change. There is central cavitation of the spinal cord, usually beginning in the cervical region, with a glial reaction (gliosis) adjacent to the cavity. Decussating fibers for pain and temperature in the ventral white commissure are interrupted early in the disease. The cavitation and gliosis spread into the gray matter and white matter as well as longitudinally, leading to variable signs and symptoms, depending on the regions involved. The classical clinical picture is that of "yoke-like" anesthesia for pain and temperature over the shoulders and upper limbs accompanied by lower motor neuron weakness and consequent wasting of the muscles of the upper limbs. Spread of the cavitation and glial reaction into the lateral funiculi may result in voluntary paresis of the upper motor neuron type, affecting especially the lower limbs.

SUGGESTED READING

Abdel-Maguid TE, Bowsher D: The gray matter of the dorsal horn of the adult human spinal cord, including comparisons with general somatic and visceral afferent cranial nerve nuclei. J Anat 142:33–58, 1985

LaMotte C: Distribution of the tract of Lissauer and the dorsal root fibers in the primate spinal cord. J Comp Neurol 172:529–561, 1977

Matthews PBC: The human stretch reflex and the motor cortex. Trends Neurosci 14:87–91, 1991

Nathan PN, Smith MC: The rubrospinal and central tegmental tracts in man. Brain 105:223–269, 1982

Nathan PN, Smith MC, Deacon P: The corticospinal tracts in man. Course and location of fibres at different segmental levels. Brain 113:303–324, 1990

Nudo RJ, Masterton RB: Descending pathways to the spinal cord: A comparative study of 22 mammals. J Comp Neurol 277:53–79, 1988

Ralston DD, Ralston HJ: The terminations of corticospinal tract axons in the macaque monkey. J Comp Neurol 242:325–337, 1985

Renshaw B: Central effects of centripetal impulses in axons of spinal nerve roots. J Neurophysiol 9:191–204, 1946

Schoenen J, Faull RLM: Spinal cord: Cytoarchitectural, dendroarchitectural, and myeloarchitectural organization. In Paxinos G (ed): The Human Nervous System, ch. 2. San Diego: Academic Press, 1990

Smith MC, Deacon P: Topographical anatomy of the posterior columns of the spinal cord in man. The long ascending fibres. Brain 107:671–698, 1984

Swash M: Sphincter control systems in man. In Kenard C, Swash M (eds): Hierarchies in Neurology. A Reappraisal of a Jacksonian Concept, pp 169–180. London, Springer-Verlag, 1989

Truex RC, Taylor MJ, Smythe MQ, Gildenberg PL: The lateral cervical nucleus of the cat, dog and man. J Comp Neurol 139:93–104, 1970

Yezierski RP: Spinomesencephalic tract: Projections from the lumbosacral spinal cord of the rat, cat and monkey. J Comp Neurol 267:131–146, 1988

Six

The Human Nervous System: An Anatomical Viewpoint,
Sixth Edition, Murray L. Barr and John A. Kiernan. J.B.
Lippincott Company, Philadelphia. © 1993.

Brain Stem:
External Anatomy

Important Facts ▌

Proceeding laterally from the ventral midline, the anatomical landmarks at different levels are as follows. Each represents a functionally important nucleus or tract within the brain stem. The student must also know the sites of emergence of cranial nerves III to XII in relation to these landmarks.

Medulla: Pyramid, olive, inferior cerebellar peduncle; cuneate and gracile tubercles (below obex); floor of fourth ventricle (above obex).

Pons: Basal part of pons, middle cerebellar peduncle, superior cerebellar peduncle, floor of fourth ventricle.

Midbrain: Interpeduncular fossa, basis pedunculi, inferior or superior colliculus.

In the floor of the fourth ventricle motor nuclei of cranial nerves are typically medial and sensory nuclei lateral to the sulcus limitans. There are named areas for hypoglossal, vagal and vestibular nuclei. The facial colliculus overlies the abducens nucleus.

The superior and inferior medullary vela form the roof of the fourth ventricle, which narrows into the central canal caudally and the cerebral aqueduct rostrally.

Cerebrospinal fluid enters the fourth ventricle from the aqueduct and leaves by way of the median and lateral apertures.

The **brain stem** consists of the medulla oblongata, pons, and midbrain. Although each of the three regions has special features, they have certain fiber tracts in common, and each region includes nuclei of cranial nerves. The fourth ventricle is partly in the medulla and partly in the pons. It is advantageous therefore to describe the medulla, pons, and midbrain together. This chapter is concerned with the surface landmarks of the brain stem. For more details of the internal features of the brain stem (such as certain nuclei and tracts) that are mentioned in this chapter, see Chapter 7 or refer to the Index. The central connections and functions of the cranial nerves are explained in Chapter 8.

Medulla Oblongata

The medulla oblongata (or medulla) is about 3 cm long and widens gradually in a rostral direction. It rests on the basilar portion of the occipital bone and is concealed from above by the cerebellum. The junction of the spinal cord and medulla is at the upper rootlet of the first cervical nerve, level with the foramen magnum. The rostral limit of the medulla is clearly marked on the ventral surface by a prominent sulcus (Fig. 6-1 and 6-2). On the dorsal surface, the junction between the pons and medulla is an imaginary transverse line that passes between the caudal margins of the mid-

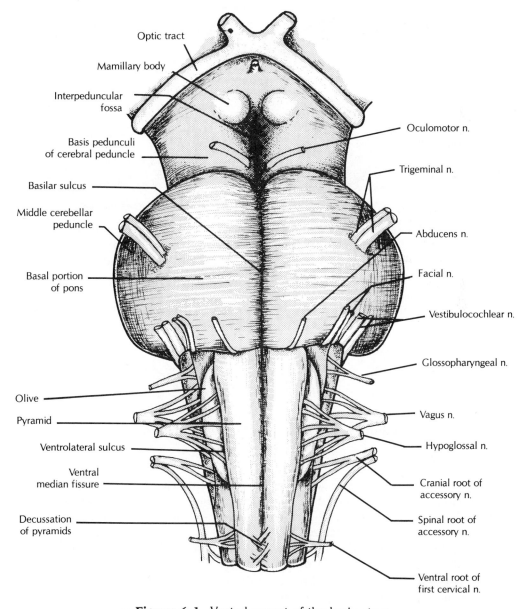

Figure 6-1. Ventral aspect of the brain stem.

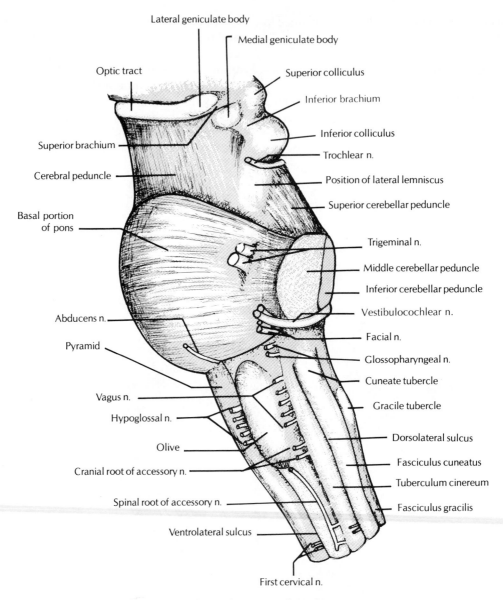

Figure 6-2. Lateral aspect of the brain stem.

dle cerebellar peduncles (Fig. 6-3). The dorsal surface, therefore, contains the caudal half of the fourth ventricle; this rostral end of the medulla is known as the **open portion**. That part of the medulla between the obex (see below) and the first cervical segment of the spinal cord is called the **closed portion**; it contains a continuation of the central canal of the spinal cord.

The ventricle results from a flexure of the embryonic brain with a dorsal concavity (the pontine flexure) and subsequent development of the large cerebellum with its thick peduncles. These events caused divergence of the dorsal halves of the maturing brain stem, so that its lumen widened out to form the fourth ventricle.

The longitudinal grooves previously de-

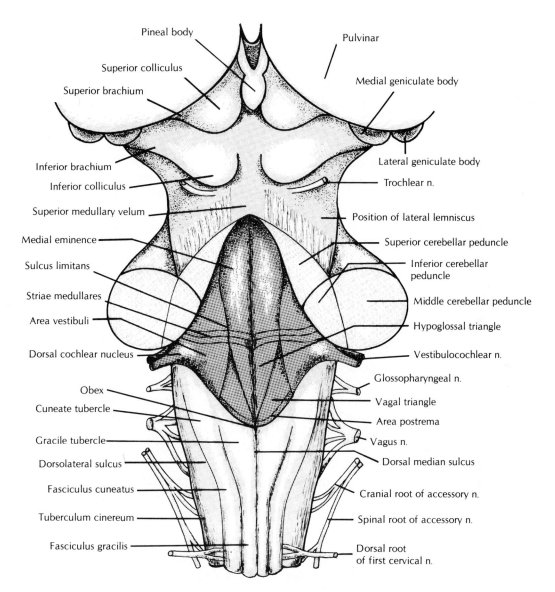

Figure 6-3. Dorsal aspect of the brain stem.

scribed for the spinal cord continue on the medulla. The ventral median fissure is interrupted at the spinomedullary junction by bundles of decussating fibers. These are corticospinal fibers that cross from the pyramid of the medulla to the opposite side of the cord, where they constitute the lateral corticospinal tract. The dorsal median, dorsolateral, and ventrolateral sulci also extend from the cord onto the surface of the medulla.

On each side, several bulges or eminences are outlined by the sulci. Ventrally, the **pyramid** (see Fig. 6-1) consists of corticospinal fibers. This is the origin of the term "pyramidal tract" as a synonym for corticospinal tract. Laterally (Fig. 6-2), the **olive** is a prominent oval swelling that marks the position of the inferior olivary nucleus. Rootlets of the glossopharyngeal, vagus, and accessory nerves are attached to the medulla just dorsal to the olive.

The **tuberculum cinereum**, immediately dorsal to these nerve rootlets, is a rather inconspicuous ridge that marks the position of the dorsal spinocerebellar tract and the more deeply situated spinal tract of the trigeminal nerve and its associated nucleus. The latter are comparable to the dorsolateral tract (of Lissauer) and the outer laminae of the dorsal horn in the spinal cord. The **gracile and cuneate fasciculi** continue from the spinal cord into the dorsal area of the medulla (see Fig. 6-2 and 6-3). The **gracile and cuneate tubercles** are slight elevations at the rostral ends of the corresponding fasciculi of the spinal cord. They contain the gracile and cuneate nuclei, in which the fibers of the fasciculi end. The apex of the V-shaped boundary of the inferior portion of the fourth ventricle, which is folded caudally over the most rostral 1 to 2 mm of the central canal, is known as the **obex**.

Seven cranial nerves are attached to the medulla or to the junction of the medulla and pons (see Figs. 6-1, 6-2, and 6-3). The **abducens nerve** emerges near the midline between the pons and the pyramid of the medulla. The nerve passes forward in the subarachnoid space beneath the pons, traverses the cavernous venous sinus (described in Chs. 25 and 26), and enters the orbit through the superior orbital fissure. The **facial** and **vestibulocochlear nerves** are attached to the brain stem at the caudal border of the pons well out laterally. The facial nerve, which is the more medial, has two roots, motor and sensory. The sensory root, which includes some efferent parasympathetic fibers, lies between the larger motor root and the vestibulocochlear nerve; it is therefore known as the **nervus intermedius** (of Wrisberg). The cochlear division of the vestibulocochlear nerve ends in the dorsal and ventral cochlear nuclei, which are situated on the base of the inferior cerebellar peduncle, whereas the vestibular division penetrates the brain stem deep to the root of the inferior cerebellar peduncle. The facial and vestibulocochlear nerves enter the internal acoustic meatus in the petrous temporal bone.

Roots of the **glossopharyngeal** and **vagus nerves** as well as those of the cranial division of the **accessory nerve** are attached to the medulla along a line between the olive and the tuberculum cinereum. The accessory nerve is motor, whereas the glossopharyngeal and vagus nerves are mixed, having sensory and motor components. The cranial root of the accessory nerve is joined by the spinal root, and the glossopharyngeal, vagus, and accessory nerves leave the posterior cranial fossa through the jugular foramen. Roots of the **hypoglossal nerve**, a motor nerve, emerge along the ventrolateral sulcus between the pyramid and the olive, and the nerve leaves the posterior fossa through the hypoglossal canal.

Pons

This part of the brain stem, which is about 2.5 cm long, owes its name to the appearance presented on its ventral surface (see Fig. 6-1), which is that of a bridge connecting the right and left cerebellar hemispheres. The appearance is deceptive as far as the constituent nerve fibers are concerned, as noted below.

The pons consists of quite different basal (ventral) and dorsal portions (see Figs. 7-9 and 7-10).

The **basal portion** is distinctive of this part of the brain stem. A shallow groove, the **basilar sulcus**, runs along its ventral surface in the midline. The pons merges laterally into the middle cerebellar peduncles, with the attachment of the **trigeminal nerve** marking the transition between the pons and the peduncle (see Figs. 6-1 and 6-2). The motor root of the trigeminal nerve is rostromedial to the larger sensory root. The trigeminal nerve enters the middle cranial fossa at the medial end of the petrous temporal bone, where the trigeminal ganglion is located. The three divisions of the nerve diverge from the ganglion, embedded in the dura mater. The ophthalmic division passes through the superior orbital fissure to reach the orbit. The maxillary division traverses the foramen rotundum, and the mandibular division traverses the foramen ovale.

Fibers from the cerebral cortex terminate ipsilaterally on nerve cells that compose the pontine nuclei, and axons of the latter cells cross the midline and then constitute the contralateral middle cerebellar peduncle. In effect, the basal pons is a large synaptic or relay station, providing a connection between the cortex of each cerebral hemisphere and the opposite cerebellar hemisphere as part of a circuit contributing to efficient voluntary movements. The cerebral cortex, basal pons, and cerebellum all increased in size during mammalian evolution and are best developed in the human brain. The corticospinal tracts traverse the basal portion of the pons before they enter the pyramids (see Fig. 7-9).

The dorsal portion or **tegmentum** of the pons is similar to much of the medulla and midbrain, in that it contains ascending and descending tracts and nuclei of cranial nerves. The dorsal surface of the pons is formed by the floor of the fourth ventricle.

The rostral part of the pons is known as the **isthmus of the brain stem**. A slight band-like elevation runs obliquely across the dorsolateral surface of the isthmus toward the inferior colliculus of the midbrain (see Fig. 6-2). This elevation is produced by the lateral lemniscus, which carries auditory fibers through the pons.

Fourth Ventricle

The **floor of the fourth ventricle** (rhomboid fossa) is broad in its midportion, narrowing toward the obex caudally and the aqueduct of the midbrain rostrally (see Fig. 6-3). The floor is divided into symmetrical halves by a median sulcus; the **sulcus limitans** further divides each half into medial and lateral areas. The vestibular nuclear complex lies beneath the floor of most of the lateral area. This area is therefore known as the **vestibular area** of the rhomboid fossa. Motor nuclei are located beneath the floor of the medial area. The caudal part of the rhomboid fossa is marked by two triangles or trigones. The rostral end of the **dorsal nucleus of the vagus nerve** lies beneath the vagal triangle (or ala cinerea), and the rostral end of the **hypoglossal nucleus** lies beneath the hypoglossal triangle. The **area**

postrema is a narrow strip between the vagal triangle and the most caudal part of the margin of the ventricle. Because the appearance of this part of the rhomboid fossa suggested the tip of a pen to early anatomists, the term **calamus scriptorius** was applied to it.

The **facial colliculus**, a slight swelling at the lower end of the **medial eminence** (see Fig. 6-3), is formed by fibers from the motor nucleus of the facial nerve looping over the abducens nucleus. There is a pigmented area, the **locus coeruleus**, at the rostral end of the sulcus limitans, indicating the site of a cluster of noradrenergic nerve cells that contain melanin pigment. In the middle of the floor of the fourth ventricle, delicate strands of nerve fibers emerge from the median sulcus, run laterally as the **striae medullares**, and enter the inferior cerebellar peduncle. The connections of these fibers are explained in Chapter 7.

The tent-shaped roof of the fourth ventricle protrudes toward the cerebellum. The rostral part of the roof is formed on each side by the **superior cerebellar peduncles**, which consist mainly of fibers proceeding from cerebellar nuclei into the midbrain. The V-shaped interval between the converging peduncles is bridged by the **superior medullary velum**, a sheet of tissue that consists of a layer of pia mater and one of ependyma with nerve fibers in between. The remainder of the roof consists of a thinner pial–ependymal membrane, the **inferior medullary velum**, which often adheres to the undersurface of the cerebellum. A deficiency of variable size in the inferior medullary velum constitutes the **median aperture** of the fourth ventricle, alternatively known as the **foramen of Magendie**. This hole provides the principal communication between the ventricular system and the subarachnoid space (Fig. 6-4).

The lateral walls of the fourth ventricle include the **inferior cerebellar peduncles**, which curve from the medulla into the cerebellum on the medial aspects of the middle peduncles (see Fig. 6-3). Lateral recesses of the ventricle extend around the sides of the medulla and open ventrally as the **lateral apertures** of the fourth ventricle (the **foramina**

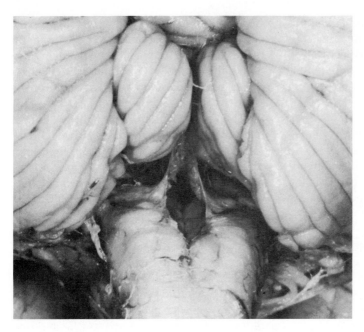

Figure 6-4. Median aperture of the fourth ventricle (foramen of Magendie), opening from the fourth ventricle into the cerebellomedullary cistern of the subarachnoid space. ($\times 2.5$)

of Luschka), which are two other channels through which cerebrospinal fluid enters the subarachnoid space (Fig. 6-5). These foramina are at the junction of the medulla, pons, and cerebellum (the cerebellopontine angles) near the attachment to the brain stem of the vestibulocochlear and glossopharyngeal nerves. The **choroid plexus** of the fourth ventricle is suspended from the inferior medullary velum; the plexus extends into the lateral recesses, and a small tuft usually protrudes through each foramen of Luschka.

Midbrain

The midbrain is about 1.5 cm long. Its ventral surface extends from the pons to the mamillary bodies of the diencephalon (see Fig. 6-1). The robust column of white matter on each side is the **basis pedunculi** (crus cerebri), which consists of fibers of the pyramidal motor system and corticopontine fibers. The deep depression between these two columns is the **interpeduncular fossa**. Many small blood vessels penetrate the midbrain in the floor of the interpeduncular fossa; this region is therefore known as the **posterior perforated substance**. The **oculomotor nerve** emerges

from the side of the interpeduncular fossa and passes forward through the cavernous venous sinus and then through the superior orbital fissure into the orbit.

The lateral surface of the midbrain (see Fig. 6-2) is formed mainly by the **cerebral peduncle**, which constitutes the major portion of this region of the brain stem on each side. The cerebral peduncle comprises the basis pedunculi and some internal structures, the substantia nigra and the tegmentum, which are described in Chapter 7.

The dorsal surface of the midbrain bears four rounded elevations, the paired **inferior** and **superior colliculi** (also called the corpora quadrigemina). These colliculi (see Figs. 6-2 and 6-3) make up the **tectum** and indicate the extent of the midbrain on the dorsal surface. The inferior colliculus is a relay nucleus on the auditory pathway. Fibers that connect the inferior colliculus with the specific thalamic nucleus for hearing (medial geniculate nucleus) form an elevation known as the **inferior brachium** (see Figs. 6-2 and 6-3). The superior colliculus is involved in the control of ocular movements and related movements of the head in response to visual and other stimuli. The **superior brachium** con-

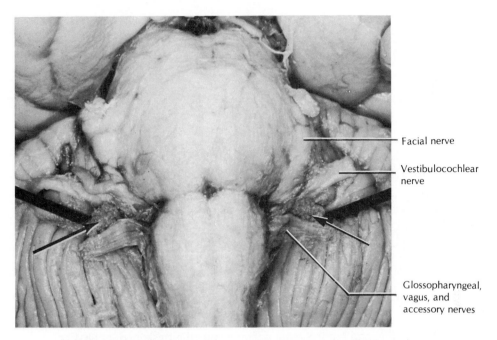

Facial nerve

Vestibulocochlear nerve

Glossopharyngeal, vagus, and accessory nerves

Figure 6-5. Lateral apertures of the fourth ventricle (foramina of Luschka). Tufts of choroid plexus (*arrows*) occupy the foramina, into which marker sticks (*black*) have been inserted. (× 1.5)

tains fibers proceeding from the cerebral cortex and the retina to the superior colliculus. Other fibers in the superior brachium terminate in the **pretectal area** ventral and just rostral to the superior colliculi; these fibers are part of a pathway from the retina for the pupillary light reflex. The **trochlear nerve** emerges from the brain stem immediately caudal to the inferior colliculus, curves around the midbrain, and enters the orbit after traversing the cavernous venous sinus.

The posterior part of the thalamus projects caudally beyond the plane of transition between the diencephalon and the midbrain (see Fig. 6-3). Consequently transverse sections at the level of the superior colliculi include thalamic nuclei, in particular those of the me-

dial and lateral geniculate bodies, and a prominent part of the thalamus known as the pulvinar (see Figs. 7-14 and 7-15).

SUGGESTED READING

Bertram EGM, Moore KL: An Atlas of the Human Brain and Spinal Cord. Baltimore, Williams & Wilkins, 1982

Montemurro DG, Bruni JE: The Human Brain in Dissection, 2nd ed. New York, Oxford University Press, 1988

Noback CR, Strominger NL, Demarest RJ: The Human Nervous System: Introduction and Review, 4th ed. Philadelphia, Lea & Febiger, 1991

Smith CG: Serial Dissections of the Human Brain. Baltimore, Urban & Schwarzenberg, 1981

Seven

The Human Nervous System: An Anatomical Viewpoint,
Sixth Edition, Murray L. Barr and John A. Kiernan. J.B.
Lippincott Company, Philadelphia, © 1993.

Brain Stem:
Nuclei and Tracts

Important Facts

The brain stem contains ascending and descending tracts, cranial nerve and other nuclei, and fibers connecting with the cerebellum.

The spinothalamic tract, which crossed in the spinal cord, is laterally located throughout the length of the brain stem.

The medial lemniscus is formed from axons that arise in the contralateral gracile and cuneate nuclei. The lemniscus is near the midline in the medulla, shifts laterally in the pons, and is laterally situated in the tegmentum of the midbrain.

Corticopontine and corticospinal fibers occupy the basis pedunculi. Corticopontine fibers end in the pontine nuclei. Corticospinal fibers continue caudally, forming the pyramid. Most pyramidal fibers decussate at the caudal end of the medulla.

The inferior olivary complex of nuclei and the pontine nuclei project across the midline to the cerebellum, in the inferior and middle cerebellar peduncles, respectively.

The superior cerebellar peduncles consist largely of fibers leaving the cerebellum. These decussate at the level of the inferior colliculi, and some end in the red nucleus, at the level of the superior colliculus.

The substantia nigra and the periaqueductal gray matter are present at all levels of the midbrain.

The seven motor nuclei of cranial nerves are the oculomotor and trochlear nuclei in the midbrain, the trigeminal motor nucleus in the pons, the facial motor and abducent nuclei at the pontomedullary junction, and the nucleus ambiguus and hypoglossal nucleus in the medulla.

Preganglionic parasympathetic nuclei include the Edinger-Westphal nucleus, the dorsal nucleus of the vagus, and some of the neurons in the nucleus ambiguus.

The only general somatic sensory nuclei are the three components (spinal, pontine, and mesencephalic) of the trigeminal nuclear complex. The only visceral sensory nucleus is the solitary nucleus, the most rostral part of which is the gustatory nucleus (for taste).

The two cochlear and the four vestibular nuclei receive special somatic sensory fibers. The lateral lemniscus extends for the length of the pons. The medial longitudinal fasciculus maintains its dorsomedial position throughout the brain stem.

The principal nuclei and fiber tracts of the brain stem are identified and discussed in this chapter. Long fiber tracts that traverse all or most of the brain stem are noted successively in the medulla, pons, and midbrain. A regional presentation of such tracts is not wholly desirable, and some pathways are reviewed as functional systems in Chapters 19 and 23. The nuclei of cranial nerves are included among the cell groups identified, but systematic descriptions of the functional components of the cranial nerves are reserved for Chapter 8.

Sections stained by the Weigert method are used as illustrations; the levels of the sections are shown in Figure 7-1. Some tracts are difficult to identify in such sections, although their location has been established from clinicopathological correlations in humans and from experimental work with laboratory animals. The sites of tracts are indicated in the illustrations, even though they cannot always be distinguished from adjacent white matter in sections of normal material.

The reticular formation is mentioned briefly here because the term is used in several contexts in the chapter. The reticular formation is a region in the dorsal parts of the medulla and pons and it extends rostrally into the tegmentum of the midbrain. It is traversed by small bundles of myelinated axons that course in all directions, and it contains overlapping populations of neurons that are not easily classified into groups, although numerous nuclei are recognized. The reticular formation has several functions of primary importance, including the following: an influence on levels of consciousness and degrees of alertness (ascending reticular activating system); a role in the control of movement through efferents to the spinal cord and to motor nuclei of cranial nerves; and a contribution to visceral and other involuntary activities through groups of neurons that function as cardiovascular and respiratory "centers." In view of its special histological characteristics and functional importance, the reticular formation is discussed separately in Chapter 9, as are several smaller nuclei of the brain stem.

Medulla

At the level of the pyramidal decussation there is an extensive rearrangement of gray matter and white matter in the transitional zone between the spinal cord and the medulla. The ventral gray horns continue into the region of the decussation where they include motor cells for the first cervical nerve and the spinal root of the accessory nerve. Here the gray matter is traversed obliquely by bundles of fibers that pass from the pyramids to the lateral corticospinal tracts (Figs. 7-2 and 7-3). Dorsal expansions of the gray matter at the level of the pyramidal decussation form the gracile and cuneate nuclei. The dorsal gray horns of the spinal cord are replaced by the spinal trigeminal nuclei. Above the decussation, the medulla has a complex structure that is entirely different from that of the spinal cord (Figs. 7-4 to 7-7). The inferior olivary nucleus, which is dorsal and lateral to the pyramid, is the most prominent feature of the rostral half of the

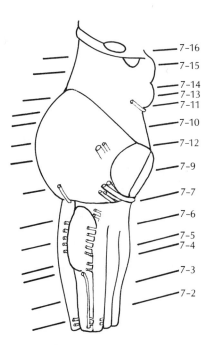

Figure 7-1. Key to levels of the series of Weigert-stained sections of the brain stem that illustrate this chapter.

7-16
7-15
7-14
7-13
7-11
7-10
7-12
7-9
7-7
7-6
7-5
7-4
7-3
7-2

(text continues on page 101)

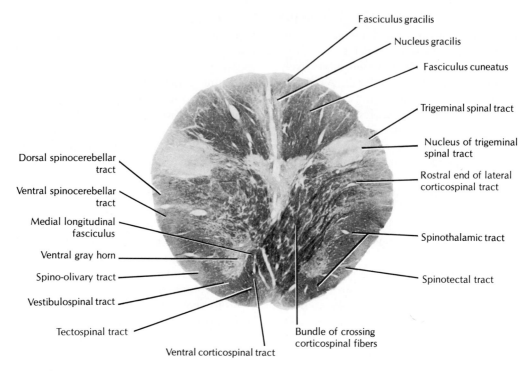

Figure 7-2. Junction of the medulla and spinal cord. (Weigert stain, × 5)

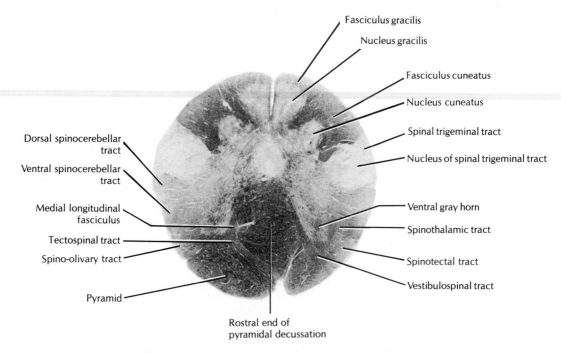

Figure 7-3. Medulla at the rostral end of the pyramidal decussation. (Weigert stain, × 4.5)

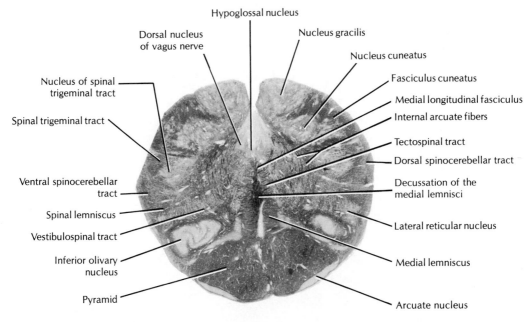

Figure 7-4. Medulla at the caudal end of the inferior olivary nucleus. (Weigert stain, × 4)

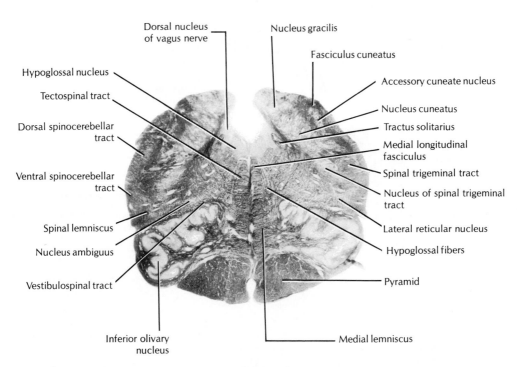

Figure 7-5. Medulla at the level of transition between its closed and open portions. (Weigert stain, × 3)

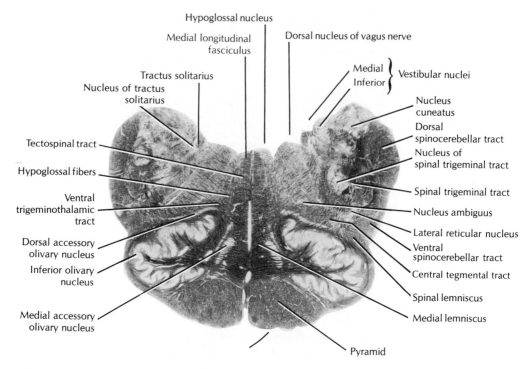

Figure 7-6. Medulla at the midolivary level. (Weigert stain, × 3.25)

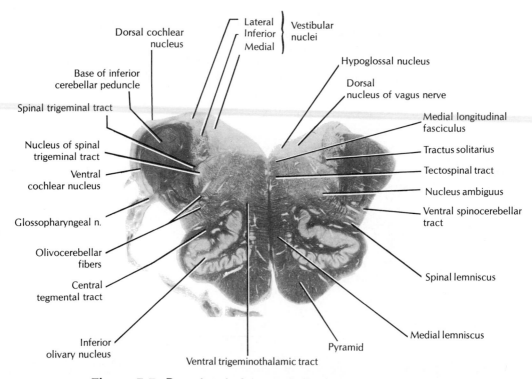

Figure 7-7. Rostral end of the medulla. (Weigert stain, × 2.5)

medulla. Near the pons, the base of the inferior cerebellar peduncle appears as a distinctive area of white matter in the dorsolateral part of the medulla (see Fig. 7-7).

Ascending Pathways

MEDIAL LEMNISCUS SYSTEM

It will be recalled (see Ch. 5) that long dorsal funiculus fibers reaching the medulla from the spinal cord transmit impulses for discriminative touch, proprioception, and vibration as an ipsilateral pathway. The **gracile fasciculus** is concerned with tactile sensations for the leg and lower trunk, whereas impulses that mediate touch and proprioception from the upper trunk, arm, and neck are transmitted in the **cuneate fasciculus**. Proprioceptive sensation from the lower limb is relayed to the medulla by collateral branches of some of the axons that constitute the dorsal spinocerebellar tract. These branches terminate in the **nucleus Z** (of Brodal and Pompeiano), which is just rostral to the gracile nucleus. Conduction for the vibratory sense was once thought to be confined to the dorsal funiculus. It is now known that a supplementary pathway exists in the lateral funiculus of the spinal cord.

The **gracile nucleus**, in which fibers of the corresponding fasciculus terminate, is present throughout the closed portion of the medulla. The fibers of the cuneate fasciculus end in the **cuneate nucleus**, which first appears slightly rostral to the beginning of the gracile nucleus and continues beyond the latter nucleus. There is a somatotopic representation in these nuclei. Thus fibers that enter the spinal cord in a specific segment synapse with a specific group of cells in the nuclei. Such a point-to-point projection of fibers in sensory pathways forms an anatomical basis for recognition of the source of a stimulus.

The myelinated axons of the cells in the gracile nucleus (and nearby nucleus Z) and the cuneate nucleus pursue a curved course to the midline as **internal arcuate fibers**, which are clearly shown in Figure 7-4. After crossing the midline in the **decussation of the medial lemnisci**, these fibers turn rostrally in the **medial lemniscus**. This is one of the most conspicuous tracts of the brain stem, occupying the interval between the midline and the inferior olivary nucleus in the medulla (see Figs. 7-6 and 7-7). Fibers that conduct sensory signals from the contralateral foot are most ventral (ie, adjacent to the pyramid). The opposite side of the body is then represented sequentially, so that fibers for the neck are in the most dorsal part of the medial lemniscus. After traversing the pons and midbrain, the tract ends in the thalamic nucleus for general sensation, which is the lateral division of the ventral posterior (VPL) nucleus of the thalamus. (Cervicothalamic fibers from the opposite lateral cervical nucleus [commonly absent in humans; see Ch. 5] reach the same thalamic nucleus by joining the medial lemniscus).

SPINOTHALAMIC AND SPINOTECTAL TRACTS

The spinothalamic tract for pain, temperature, and touch on the opposite side of the body continues into the medulla without appreciable change in position. This is also true of the spinotectal (or spinomesencephalic) tract, which conveys somesthetic data to the superior colliculus and the reticular formation of the midbrain. The two tracts soon merge to form the **spinal lemniscus**, which traverses the lateral area of the medulla dorsal to the inferior olivary nucleus (see Figs. 7-4 to 7-7). The spinotectal fibers leave the spinal lemniscus in the rostral midbrain, and the spinothalamic fibers continue to the ventral posterior nucleus of the thalamus. Collateral branches of the same fibers go to the intralaminar and posterior groups of nuclei of the thalamus. (The thalamic nuclei are described in Ch. 11.)

SPINORETICULAR FIBERS

The spinoreticular tracts in the ventral and lateral white matter of the cord continue into the brain stem where their constituent axons synapse with cells of the reticular formation. They transmit sensory data, especially from the skin and internal organs. Many spinoreticular fibers are collateral branches of fibers of the spinothalamic tract. Axons of cells in the reticular formation project caudally to the spinal cord and rostrally to the thalamus, and impulses transmitted by the ascending fibers influence neuronal activity throughout much of the cerebral cortex through thalamic relays.

There are at least three routes from the spinal cord to the thalamus and cerebral cortex. The **medial lemniscus system** proceeds without interruption, mainly to the ventral posterior thalamic nucleus, which in turn projects to the primary somatosensory area of the cerebral cortex. The **neospinothalamic system** consists of the axons of those tract cells that do not have collateral branches to the reticular formation. These are phylogenetically recent (ie, mammalian) pathways, which became increasingly important as the thalamus and cerebral cortex increased in size and functional significance during evolution. Sensory data also reach the intralaminar group of thalamic nuclei through the **paleospinothalamic system**, which exists in all vertebrate animals. This is a less direct pathway, consisting of spinoreticular fibers (ones that are not collaterals of the spinothalamic tract) and reticulothalamic fibers, which are the rostrally projecting axons of neurons of the reticular formation. These ascending fibers from the reticular formation end in the intralaminar nuclei, which project to the cerebral cortex generally. This diffuse pathway influences levels of consciousness and degrees of alertness, and it also is involved in the awareness (but not the localization) of pain.

The **lateral reticular nucleus**, whose afferents include spinoreticular fibers and which is related functionally to the cerebellum, is an exceptionally distinct group of cells of the reticular formation situated dorsal to the inferior olivary nucleus and near the surface of the medulla (see Figs. 7-4, 7-5, and 7-6).

SPINOCEREBELLAR TRACTS

The **dorsal** and **ventral spinocerebellar tracts**, which relay proprioceptive signals mainly from the lower limb, traverse the medulla in the periphery of the lateral area (see Figs. 7-2 to 7-6). The dorsal tract, which is uncrossed, originates in the nucleus dorsalis (nucleus thoracicus or Clarke's column) of the thoracic and upper lumbar segments of the spinal cord. The ventral tract, on the other hand, is largely crossed, and many of its cells of origin are in the lumbosacral enlargement of the cord. The dorsal spinocerebellar fibers enter the inferior cerebellar peduncle (Figs. 7-7 and 7-8), whereas the ventral spinocerebellar tract continues through the pons and enters the cerebellum by way of the superior cerebellar peduncle. For the upper limb, pathways equivalent to the spinocerebellar tracts involve the accessory cuneate nucleus.

Medullary Nuclei Connected with the Cerebellum

ACCESSORY CUNEATE NUCLEUS

The accessory or external cuneate nucleus is lateral to the cuneate nucleus (see Fig. 7-5). The afferents to the accessory cuneate nucleus are fibers that entered the spinal cord in cervical dorsal roots; many such afferents are in fact collateral branches of fibers that end in the cuneate nucleus. Efferents from the accessory cuneate nucleus, accompanied by a few fibers from the cuneate nucleus, enter the cerebellum by way of the inferior peduncle. These **cuneocerebellar fibers** supplement the dorsal spinocerebellar tract by providing a pathway from proprioceptive and other sensory endings in the neck and upper limb. The functions of the accessory cuneate nucleus and cuneocerebellar tract (for the upper limb) are equivalent to those of the nucleus thoracicus and the dorsal spinocerebellar tract (for the lower limb): both transmit proprioceptive signals along rapidly conducting axons to the cerebellum.

INFERIOR OLIVARY COMPLEX OF NUCLEI

Several groups of neurons in the medulla and pons are known as **precerebellar nuclei**. They receive afferents from various sources and project to the cerebellum. These nuclei include the components of the inferior olivary complex. The largest component is the **inferior olivary nucleus**, which is shaped like a

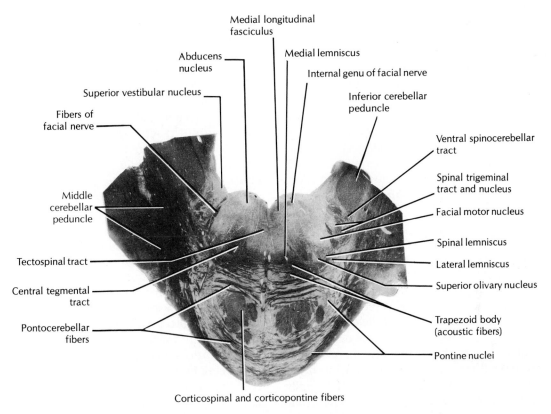

Figure 7-8. Caudal region of the pons. (Weigert stain, × 2.4)

crumpled bag or purse with the hilus facing medially (see Figs. 7-5, 7-6, and 7-7). The **medial accessory olivary nucleus** lies between the medial lemniscus and the inferior olivary nucleus, and the **dorsal accessory olivary nucleus** is immediately dorsal to the inferior olivary nucleus (see Fig. 7-6). The inferior olivary complex receives afferents from the contralateral dorsal horn of all levels of the spinal cord and from the ipsilateral red nucleus (in the midbrain) and cerebral cortex. Spino-olivary projections are predominantly to the accessory olivary nuclei, whereas cortico-olivary and rubro-olivary projections are mainly to the principal inferior olivary nucleus.

The **central tegmental tract** is in part a pathway from the red nucleus and the periaqueductal gray matter of the midbrain to the inferior olivary complex. These sources relay signals from the spinal cord, the cerebral cortex, the cerebellum, and (in laboratory animals) many other parts of the central nervous system. The terminal portion of the central tegmental tract forms a dense layer on the dorsal surface of the inferior olivary nucleus, best seen in Figure 7-7. The tract also contains numerous ascending fibers from the reticular formation of the brain stem and from the solitary nucleus (of the medulla). The ascending fibers proceed to the diencephalon.

Olivocerebellar fibers constitute the projection from the inferior olivary complex. Fibers from the principal nucleus occupy its interior and leave through the hilus. After decussating in the midline, the strands of myelinated olivocerebellar fibers curve in a dorsolateral direction through the reticular formation and enter the inferior cerebellar peduncle, of which they are the largest single component (see Fig. 7-7). The accessory olivary nuclei project to regions of the cerebellum concerned with the maintenance of equilibrium and the stereotyped movements of postural changes and locomotion. The inferior olivary nucleus projects to the part of the cerebellum that ensures efficiency and precision of voluntary movements. The inferior olivary complex is the main source of a type of afferent to the cerebellar cortex called climbing fibers, which terminate on and excite the Purkinje cells. Physiological studies indicate that the inferior olivary complex of nuclei channels into the cerebellum programs of instructions for subsequent use in the coordination of learned patterns of movement.

ARCUATE NUCLEUS

The arcuate nucleus on the surface of the pyramid (see Fig. 7-4) receives collateral branches of corticospinal fibers. The axons of cells in the arcuate nucleus enter the cerebellum by way of the inferior cerebellar peduncle, which they reach by two routes. Some travel over the lateral surface of the medulla as the **external arcuate fibers**; the remainder run dorsally in the midline of the medulla and then laterally in the **striae medullares** in the floor of the fourth ventricle. The connections of the arcuate nucleus are similar to those of the cell groups in the basal portion of the pons (see Ch. 10). Both receive afferents from the ipsilateral cerebral cortex and project across the midline to the cerebellum.

Descending Tracts

CORTICOSPINAL TRACT

The parent cell bodies of the corticospinal (pyramidal) tract are in an area of cerebral cortex that occupies adjoining regions of the frontal and parietal lobes. The corticospinal fibers traverse the medullary center of the cerebral hemisphere and the internal capsule to reach the brain stem. The fibers continue as a compact bundle in the basis pedunculi of the midbrain, but the tract is broken up into small strands on entering the basal portion of the pons. These strands coalesce in the caudal pons, and the corticospinal tract is again a compact body of white matter in the pyramid of the medulla (see Figs. 7-4 to 7-7).

The proportion of fibers that cross over in the **decussation of the pyramids** varies among people, but on the average, about 85% enter the decussation. The rostral limit of the pyramidal decussation appears in Figure 7-3, and a bundle of fibers passing through the gray matter from a pyramid to the opposite **lateral corticospinal tract** is shown in Figure 7-2. The 15% of non-decussating fibers continue into the ventral funiculus of the cord as the **ventral corticospinal tract**. The corticospinal fibers terminate in the base of the dorsal horn, the intermediate gray matter, and the ventral horn, and a few synapse directly with motor neurons. Each pyramid contains about 1 million fibers of varying size. The thickest and most rapidly conducting fibers come from the giant pyramidal cells of Betz in the primary motor area. These are the ones believed to end in synaptic contact with the cell bodies of motor neurons in the spinal cord.

The corticospinal tracts are often thought of as being exclusively motor, and this is indeed their major functional aspect. However, axons of cortical origin also modulate the transmission of somatic sensory information to the brain by synapsing with neurons in the gracile and cuneate nuclei and in the dorsal horn that form parts of major sensory pathways.

TRACTS THAT ORIGINATE IN THE MIDBRAIN

The **central tegmental tract** has already been mentioned as arising from the ipsilateral red nucleus and other gray areas of the midbrain. It terminates in the inferior olivary complex. A bundle of axons from the contralateral red nucleus continues caudally as the **rubrospinal tract**, which comes to occupy a position ventral to the lateral corticospinal tract in the spinal cord. Rubrospinal fibers are numerous in most mammals, but in humans the tract is a tiny bundle that ends in the upper two cervical segments of the spinal cord.

The **tectospinal tract** originates in the superior colliculus of the midbrain, and the fibers cross at that level to the opposite side of the brain stem. The tract (see Figs. 5-9, 7-5 and

7-14) is probably insignificantly small in humans. **Tectobulbar fibers** go from the superior colliculus to the reticular formation of the pons and upper medulla. They are involved in the control of eye movements (see Ch. 8).

Nuclei of Cranial Nerves and Associated Tracts

HYPOGLOSSAL, ACCESSORY, VAGUS, AND GLOSSOPHARYNGEAL NERVES

The **hypoglossal nucleus** gives rise to axons that innervate the tongue muscles. This nucleus is a column of motor cells near the midline throughout most of the medulla. The nucleus is in the central gray matter of the closed part of the medulla (see Fig. 7-4) and beneath the hypoglossal triangle of the rhomboid fossa (see Figs. 7-5, 7-6, and 7-7). The myelinated axons leaving the nucleus are directed ventrally between the medial lemniscus and the inferior olivary nucleus (see Figs. 7-5 and 7-6); they continue lateral to the pyramid and emerge as the rootlets of the hypoglossal nerve along the ventrolateral sulcus (between the pyramid and the olive). The **nucleus ambiguus** lies within the reticular formation, dorsal to the inferior olivary nucleus (Figures 7-5, 7-6, and 7-7). This important cell column supplies the muscles of the soft palate, pharynx, larynx, and upper esophagus through the cranial root of the accessory nerve and the vagus and glossopharyngeal nerves. It also contains parasympathetic neurons whose axons end in the cardiac ganglia and control the heart rate. The **dorsal nucleus of the vagus nerve** is the largest parasympathetic nucleus in the brain stem; it contains the cell bodies of preganglionic neurons for smooth muscle and glandular elements of the thoracic and abdominal viscera. The nucleus lies lateral to the hypoglossal nucleus in the gray matter that surrounds the central canal (see Fig. 7-4) and extends rostrally beneath the vagal triangle of the rhomboid fossa (see Figs. 7-5, 7-6, and 7-7).

A bundle of visceral afferent fibers known as the **solitary tract** lies along the lateral side of the dorsal nucleus of the vagus nerve (see Figs. 7-5, 7-6, and 7-7). This tract consists of caudally directed fibers whose cell bodies are in the inferior ganglia of the vagus and glossopharyngeal nerves and in the geniculate ganglion of the facial nerve. The fibers terminate in the **solitary nucleus** (nucleus of the solitary tract), a column of cells that lies adjacent to and partly surrounds the tract. Some vagal and glossopharyngeal afferents have important roles in visceral reflexes, and others transmit impulses for taste from the epiglottis and posterior one-third of the tongue. The fibers contributed by the facial nerve are for taste in the anterior two-thirds of the tongue and in the palate.

VESTIBULOCOCHLEAR NERVE

Nuclei in the rostral part of the medulla receive the fibers of the cochlear and vestibular divisions of the eighth cranial nerve. The **dorsal cochlear nucleus**, lying on the base of the inferior cerebellar peduncle, is shown in Figure 7-7, and parts of the **ventral cochlear nucleus** appears lateral to the peduncle in the same figure. Fibers leaving the cochlear nuclei are noted later, in the description of the pons.

The **vestibular nuclei**, beneath the vestibular area of the rhomboid fossa, comprise the **superior, lateral, medial**, and **inferior vestibular nuclei**, which differ in their cytoarchitecture and connections. The superior nucleus is in the pons (see Fig. 7-8), whereas the remaining nuclei are in the medulla (see Figs. 7-6 and 7-7). The vestibular nerve penetrates the brain stem ventral to the inferior cerebellar peduncle and medial and slightly rostral to the attachment of the cochlear nerve. Most vestibular nerve fibers end in the vestibular nuclei, and a few enter the cerebellum through the inferior peduncle. Descending branches of vestibular nerve fibers that terminate in the inferior vestibular nucleus, together with vestibulospinal fibers from the lateral vestibular nucleus, give the inferior nucleus a stippled appearance in transverse sections (see Fig. 7-7). In addition to the primary vestibulocerebellar fibers, numerous secondary fibers proceed from the vestibular nuclei into the cerebellum through the inferior peduncle.

Vestibular nuclei project to the spinal cord by way of two tracts. The larger of these is the **vestibulospinal tract**, for which the cells of origin are in the lateral vestibular (Deiters') nucleus. Vestibulospinal fibers run caudally, dorsal to the inferior olivary nucleus, in the position indicated in Figures 7-4 and 7-5. The tract is deflected ventrally at the level of the pyramidal decussation (see Figs. 7-2 and 7-3) and continues into the ipsilateral ventral funiculus of the spinal cord.

Fibers from the vestibular nuclei account for most of those in the **medial longitudinal fasciculus**, which extends rostrally and caudally adjacent to the midline (see Figs. 7-2 to 7-7). The ascending fibers will be identified later in the pons and midbrain. The parent cell bodies of the descending fibers are in the medial vestibular nucleus and are mainly ipsilateral. Below the pyramidal decussation they are joined by the nearby tectospinal and ventral corticospinal tracts, and there is considerable intermingling of the three categories of fibers in the ventral funiculus of the cervical cord.

TRIGEMINAL NERVE

The trigeminal nerve contributes a tract and associated nucleus to the internal structure of the medulla. Many fibers of the trigeminal sensory root turn caudally on entering the pons. They constitute the **spinal trigeminal tract**, so named because some of the fibers extend as far as the third cervical segment of the spinal cord. The spinal tract transmits data for pain, temperature, and touch from the extensive area of distribution of the trigeminal nerve. The fibers terminate in the subjacent **spinal trigeminal nucleus** (nucleus of the spinal trigeminal tract). The tract and nucleus lie deep to the root of the inferior cerebellar peduncle and the dorsal spinocerebellar tract in the rostral part of the medulla (see Figs. 7-4 through 7-7). More caudally, they lie under the surface area of the medulla known as the tuberculum cinereum (see Figs. 7-2 and 7-3). Many of the descending fibers are unmyelinated or thinly myelinated, and the nucleus consists principally of small neurons. The spi-

nal trigeminal tract and its nucleus share, therefore, some structural and functional characteristics with the dorsolateral tract of Lissauer and the outermost four laminae of the dorsal horn of the spinal gray matter. The **ventral trigeminothalamic tract** (see Fig. 7-6) is a crossed fasciculus that arises from neurons in the nucleus of the spinal tract (and the pontine trigeminal nucleus) and in the adjacent part of the reticular formation, and ends in the ventral posterior nucleus of the thalamus. Conducting sensory signals from the opposite side of the head, the ventral trigeminothalamic tract is comparable functionally to the spinothalamic tract for the body generally.

Pons

The main features in Weigert-stained sections through the pons are its division into basal (ventral) and dorsal (tegmental) regions and the prominent cerebellar peduncles (Figs. 7-8 and 7-9). The basal portion consists of longitudinal fiber bundles, transverse fibers, and collections of nerve cells in the intervals between longitudinal and transverse fasciculi. The longitudinal bundles are numerous and small at rostral levels (Figs. 7-9 and 7-10), but many coalesce as they approach the medulla (see Fig. 7-8).

Dorsal Portion (Tegmentum)

The pontine tegmentum is structurally similar to the medulla and midbrain. There are, therefore, tracts that were encountered in the medulla, together with components of several cranial nerves.

TRACTS AND CEREBELLAR PEDUNCLES

The **medial lemniscus** "rotates" in passing from the medulla into the pons, where it takes up a position in the most ventral part of the tegmentum. The lemniscus has a roughly oval outline at the level shown in Figure 7-8; it moves laterally farther forward and becomes flatter (see Figs. 7-9 and 7-10). The medial lemniscus rotates in such a way that fibers from the cuneate nucleus are medial to those

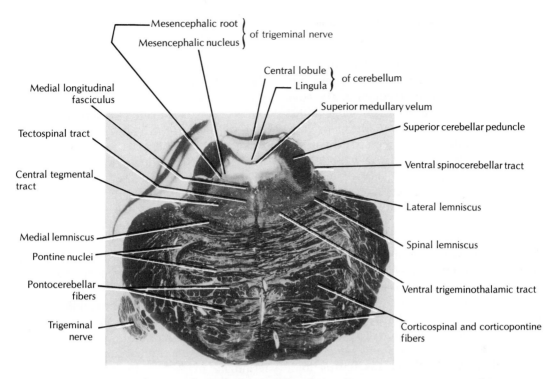

Figure 7-9. Section through the middle of the pons. (Weigert stain, × 2.3)

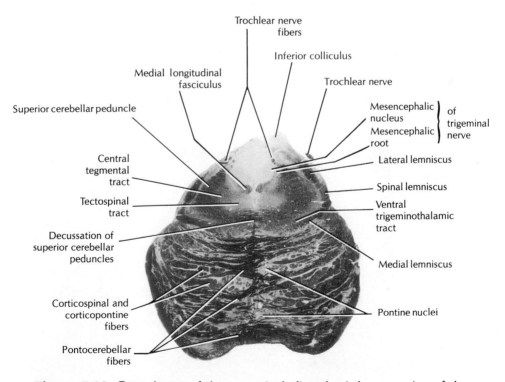

Figure 7-10. Rostral part of the pons, including the isthmus region of the pontine tegmentum. (Weigert stain, × 2.2)

from the gracile nucleus. The somatotopic representation is therefore neck, arm, trunk, and leg, in a medial-to-lateral sequence. The **spinal lemniscus** is near the lateral edge of the medial lemniscus throughout the pons (see Figs. 7-8, 7-9, and 7-10). The **ventral spinocerebellar tract** traverses the most lateral part of the tegmentum (see Fig. 7-8) and then curves dorsally and enters the cerebellum through the superior peduncle (Figs. 7-9 and 7-11).

With respect to descending tracts, the **central tegmental tract** is medial to the fibers of the superior cerebellar peduncle at the level of the pontine isthmus (see Fig. 7-10), in the central area of the tegmentum at midpontine levels (see Fig. 7-9) and dorsal to the medial lemniscus in the caudal region of the pons (see Fig. 7-8). As in the medulla and spinal cord, the **medial longitudinal fasciculus** and **tectospinal tract** are near the midline in the pontine tegmentum (see Figs. 7-8 through 7-10),

The **inferior cerebellar peduncles** enter the cerebellum from the caudal part of the pons. In this location, they lie medial to the middle cerebellar peduncles, forming the lateral walls of the fourth ventricle (see Fig. 7-8). Olivocerebellar fibers are the most numerous in the inferior peduncle, followed by fibers of the dorsal spinocerebellar tract. Smaller components are cuneocerebellar fibers from the accessory cuneate nucleus, fibers from the arcuate nucleus and the reticular formation of the medulla, and fibers from the pontine and spinal trigeminal nuclei. The region of the inferior cerebellar peduncle immediately adjoining the fourth ventricle consists of fibers that enter the cerebellum from the vestibular nerve and vestibular nuclei, together with fibers that arise in the parts of the cerebellum concerned with maintaining equilibrium. The latter fibers terminate in vestibular nuclei and in the reticular formation.

The **superior cerebellar peduncles** (see Fig. 7-9) consist mainly of cerebellar efferent

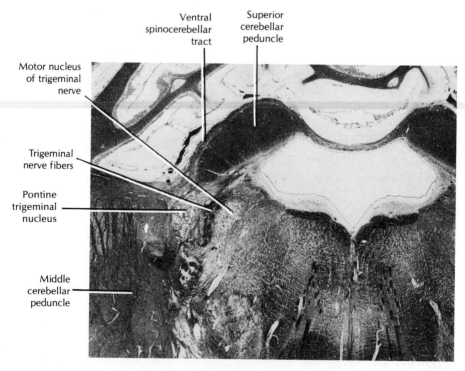

Figure 7-11. Part of a section through the middle of the pons, at the level of the pontine and motor trigeminal nuclei. (Weigert stain, × 5.5)

fibers that originate in cerebellar nuclei and enter the brain stem immediately caudal to the inferior colliculi of the midbrain. The fibers cross the midline at the level of the inferior colliculi in the **decussation of the superior cerebellar peduncles** (Figs. 7-10, 7-12, and 7-13). Most continue rostrally to the ventral lateral nucleus of the thalamus, from which fibers project to motor areas of cortex in the frontal lobe, and the remainder end in the red nucleus and in the reticular formation. The superior cerebellar peduncle also contains fibers that enter the cerebellum: the ventral spinocerebellar tract as well as fibers from the red nucleus and the mesencephalic trigeminal nucleus.

NUCLEI OF CRANIAL NERVES AND ASSOCIATED TRACTS

VESTIBULOCOCHLEAR NERVE. Fibers from the dorsal and ventral cochlear nuclei cross the pons to ascend in the lateral lemniscus of the opposite side. Most of the decussating fibers constitute the **trapezoid body** (see Fig. 7-8), which intersects the medial lemnisci. It is difficult to distinguish these slender bundles of acoustic fibers from nearby bundles of pontocerebellar fibers. Some fibers from the ventral cochlear nuclei end in the **superior olivary nucleus** (see Fig. 7-8), from which more ascending fibers are added to the auditory pathway. Fibers from the cochlear and superior olivary nuclei turn rostrally in the lateral

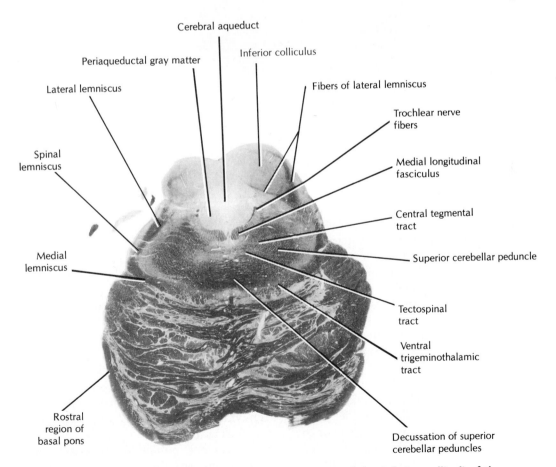

Figure 7-12. Section through the basal pons and the inferior colliculi of the midbrain. (Weigert stain, × 3)

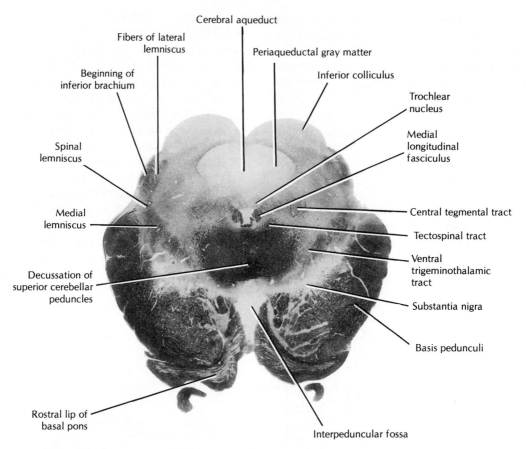

Cerebral aqueduct

Fibers of lateral lemniscus

Periaqueductal gray matter

Beginning of inferior brachium

Inferior colliculus

Trochlear nucleus

Medial longitudinal fasciculus

Spinal lemniscus

Medial lemniscus

Central tegmental tract

Tectospinal tract

Decussation of superior cerebellar peduncles

Ventral trigeminothalamic tract

Substantia nigra

Basis pedunculi

Rostral lip of basal pons

Interpeduncular fossa

Figure 7-13. Midbrain at the level of the rostral ends of the inferior colliculi. (Weigert stain, × 3)

part of the tegmentum to form the **lateral lemniscus** (see Fig. 7-8). This tract is lateral to the medial lemniscus in the first part of its course (see Fig. 7-9) and then moves dorsally to end in the inferior colliculus of the midbrain (see Fig. 7-10). The auditory pathway continues through the inferior brachium to the medial geniculate body of the thalamus and then to the auditory area of cortex in the temporal lobe. The auditory system is more fully described in Chapter 21.

Of the four vestibular nuclei, only the **superior vestibular nucleus** is (Figure 7-8). Fibers from all the vestibular nuclei, some crossed and some uncrossed, ascend in the **medial longitudinal fasciculus**, which runs near the midline and close to the floor of the fourth ventricle throughout the pons (see

Figs. 7-8 to 7-10). The fibers terminate mainly in the abducens, trochlear, and oculomotor nuclei; the connections thereby established coordinate movements of the eyes with movements of the head. The medial longitudinal fasciculus also contains other groups of fibers concerned with movement of the eyes. These are discussed in Chapter 8.

FACIAL AND ABDUCENS NERVES. The **facial motor nucleus**, which supplies the muscles of expression, is a prominent group of typical motor neurons in the ventrolateral part of the tegmentum (see Fig. 7-8). Axons arising from the nucleus course dorsomedially and then form a compact bundle, the **internal genu**, which loops over the caudal end of the abducens nucleus beneath the facial colliculus of the rhomboid fossa. The bundle of fibers that forms the genu then runs forward along the medial side of the abducens nucleus and curves again over its rostral end (see right side of Fig. 7-8). After leaving the genu, the fibers pass between the nucleus of origin and the spinal trigeminal nucleus, emerging as the motor root of the facial nerve at the junction of the pons and medulla.

The **abducens nucleus** innervates the lateral rectus muscle of the eye. It is located beneath the facial colliculus, as noted above (see Fig. 7-8). The efferent fibers of the nucleus proceed in a ventral direction with a caudal inclination and leave the brain stem as the abducens nerve between the pons and the pyramid of the medulla (see Fig. 6-1).

TRIGEMINAL NERVE. The **spinal trigeminal tract** and **nucleus** are in the lateral part of the tegmentum of the caudal half of the pons (see Fig. 7-8), lateral to the fibers of the facial nerve. The pontine tegmentum also contains two other trigeminal nuclei (see Fig. 7-11). The **pontine trigeminal nucleus** (also known as the chief or principal nucleus) is at the rostral end of the spinal trigeminal nucleus. It receives fibers for touch, especially discriminative touch. Fibers from the pontine trigeminal nucleus project to the thalamus, along with fibers from the spinal nucleus, in the **ventral trigeminothalamic tract** (see Figs. 7-9 and 7-10). A **dorsal trigeminothalamic tract**, consisting of crossed and uncrossed fibers, originates in the pontine trigeminal nuclei exclusively. (Alternatively, all the trigeminothalamic fibers are said to compose the **trigeminal lemniscus**.) The **motor nucleus**, which is medial to the pontine trigeminal nucleus (see Fig. 7-11), contains the motor neurons that supply the muscles of mastication and a few other muscles.

The **mesencephalic nucleus of the trigeminal nerve** is a slender column of cells beneath the lateral edge of the rostral part of the fourth ventricle (see Figs. 7-9 and 7-10), extending into the midbrain. These unipolar cells are unusual because they are cell bodies of primary sensory neurons and the only such cells in the central nervous system. Fibers from the nucleus form the **mesencephalic root of the trigeminal nerve** (see Figs. 7-9 and 7-10); most are distributed through the mandibular division of the nerve to proprioceptive endings in the muscles of mastication.

Basal Portion

The basal or ventral portion of the pons (see Figs. 7-8 through 7-10) is especially large in humans because of its connections with those parts of the cortex of the cerebral and cerebellar hemispheres that increased in size during mammalian evolution. The basal pons contains longitudinal and transverse bundles of fibers and the pontine nuclei.

The longitudinal fasciculi are descending fibers that entered the pons from the basis pedunculi of the midbrain. Many are **corticospinal fibers** that pass through the pons to reassemble as the pyramids of the medulla. There also are numerous **corticopontine fibers**, which originate in widespread areas of cerebral cortex and establish synaptic contact with cells of the **pontine nuclei** of the same side. Except in the caudal one-third of the pons, in which there are large regions of pontine gray matter (see Fig. 7-8), the pontine nuclei are small groups of cells scattered among the longitudinal and transverse fasciculi (see Figs. 7-9 and 7-10). The nuclei consist of small and medium-size polygonal cells. Their axons cross the midline, forming the conspicuous transverse bundles of **pontocerebellar fibers**, and enter the cerebellum through the **middle cerebellar peduncle**. The activities of the cerebral cortex, which include neural events that underlie volitional movements, are made available to the cerebellar cortex through the relay in the pontine nuclei. The cerebellar cortex influences motor areas in the frontal lobe of the cerebral hemisphere through a pathway that includes the dentate nucleus of the cerebellum and the ventral lateral nucleus of the thalamus. The well-developed circuit linking the cerebral and cerebellar cortices contributes to the precision and efficiency of voluntary movements.

Midbrain

The internal structure of the midbrain is shown in Figures 7-12 to 7-15. The sections shown in Figures 7-12 and 7-13 are through the inferior colliculi. The planes of the sections are such that Figure 7-12 includes the basal pons and Figure 7-13 shows the extreme rostral lip of the basal pons (see Fig. 7-1). Figures 7-14 and 7-15 show more rostral levels that include the superior colliculi and certain thalamic nuclei that are in the same transverse plane.

For descriptive purposes, the midbrain is divided into the following regions (see Fig. 7-14): the **tectum**, which consists of the paired inferior and superior **colliculi** (corpora quadrigemina); the **basis pedunculi**, which

is a dense mass of descending fibers; and the **substantia nigra**, which is a prominent zone of gray matter immediately dorsal to the basis pedunculi. The remainder of the midbrain comprises the **tegmentum**, which contains fiber tracts, the prominent red nuclei, and the periaqueductal gray matter surrounding the cerebral aqueduct (aqueduct of Sylvius). The term **cerebral peduncle** refers to all of the midbrain on each side, exclusive of the tectum.

Tectum and Associated Tracts

INFERIOR COLLICULUS

The inferior colliculus is a large nucleus incorporated into the auditory pathway to the cerebral cortex. Fibers of the lateral lemniscus en-

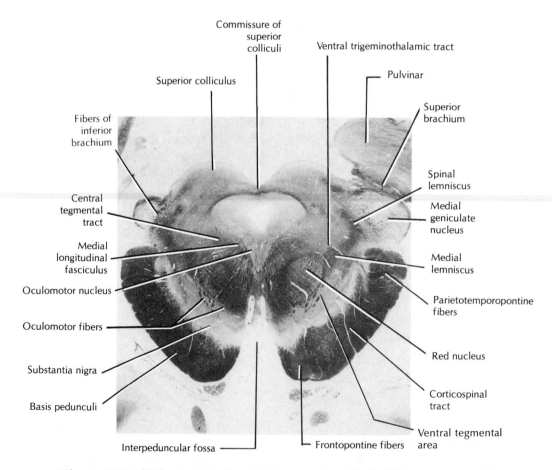

Figure 7-14. Midbrain at the level of the superior colliculi. (Weigert stain, × 3)

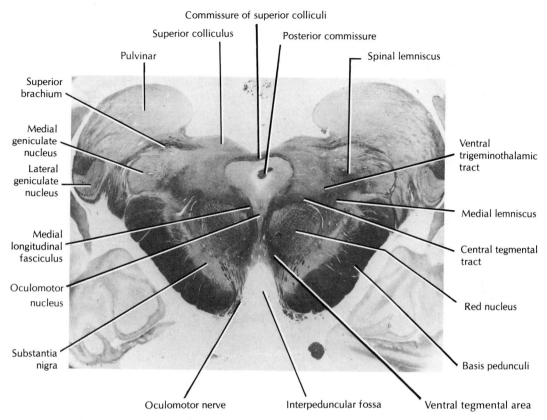

Figure 7-15. Midbrain at the level of the rostral ends of the superior colliculi. The section also includes parts of the thalamus and some cortex of the temporal lobes. (Weigert stain, × 2)

velop the nucleus and enter it from superficial and deep aspects (see Fig. 7-12). Fibers from the inferior colliculus traverse the inferior brachium to reach the medial geniculate body of the thalamus (see Figs. 7-13 to 7-15), which in turn projects to the auditory cortex in the temporal lobe. There are commissural fibers between the inferior colliculi, accounting in part for the bilateral cortical projection from each ear.

Some fibers from the inferior colliculus pass forward into the superior colliculus. From the latter site, through a polysynaptic pathway described in Chapter 8, nerve impulses reach cranial nerve nuclei that supply the extraocular muscles, and a few tectospinal fibers influence spinal motor neurons in the cervical region. A pathway is thereby established for reflex turning of the eyes and head toward the source of an unexpected sound.

SUPERIOR COLLICULUS

The superior colliculi (see Figs. 7-14 and 7-15) differ from the inferior colliculi both in phylogenetic background and in function. The optic tectum of the midbrain in lower vertebrates is the homologue of the superior colliculi. The optic tectum constitutes an important integrating center for visual and somesthetic data, especially in fish and amphibia, in which it is larger than the telencephalon. In some of the lower mammals, such as rodents, most of the axons of the optic tract terminate in the superior colliculus. In higher mammals, including humans, most of the fibers from the retina go instead to the lateral geniculate body of the thalamus. The importance of the optic tectum has left an imprint in the mammalian superior colliculus in the form of a complex structure consisting of seven alternating layers of white matter and gray matter.

The cortex of the occipital lobe is the largest source of afferent fibers to the human superior colliculus. Corticotectal fibers come from the visual cortex in the occipital lobe. Other corticotectal afferents are derived from an area of the frontal lobe called the frontal eye field. Corticotectal fibers (which are ipsilateral) make up most of the **superior brachium**, which reaches the superior colliculus by passing between the pulvinar and the medial geniculate body of the thalamus (see Figs. 7-14 and 7-15). Through collicular efferents (to be described), this connection between the cortex and the superior colliculus is responsible for both voluntary and involuntary movements of the eyes and head, as when rapidly shifting the direction of gaze (saccadic movements) or when following objects passing across the visual field (smooth pursuit movements). Corticotectal fibers that originate in the occipital cortex also participate in the ocular response of accommodation (ie, thickening of the lens and constriction of the pupil), which accompanies convergence of the eyes when viewing a near object.

Some fibers of the optic tract reach the superior colliculus by way of the superior brachium and constitute the afferent limb of a reflex pathway that assists in turning the eyes and head to follow an object moving across the field of vision. In addition, spinotectal fibers terminate in the superior colliculus and transmit data from general sensory endings, of which those in the skin are the most important. The connections thereby established presumably serve to direct the eyes and head toward the source of cutaneous stimuli. Another source of afferents to the superior colliculus is the pars reticulata of the substantia nigra, which thereby connects the corpus striatum (see Ch. 12) with the parts of the midbrain that control movements of the eyes and head.

Efferents from the superior colliculus are distributed to the spinal cord and nuclei of the brain stem. The few fibers destined for the spinal cord curve around the periaqueductal gray matter, cross to the opposite side in the **dorsal tegmental decussation** (of Meynert), and continue caudally near the midline as the tectospinal tract (see Figs. 7-12 and 7-13). Efferents to the brain stem, known as **tectobulbar fibers**, are, for the most part, directed bilaterally. They go to the pretectal area, to the accessory oculomotor nuclei, and to the paramedian pontine reticular formation. These regions project to the nuclei of the oculomotor, trochlear, and abducens nerves, which supply the eye muscles. (Neural control of these muscles is discussed in Ch. 8.) Other efferent fibers from the superior colliculus terminate in the reticular formation near the motor nucleus of the facial nerve, providing a reflex pathway for protective closure of the eyelids when there is a sudden visual stimulus.

The superior colliculi are interconnected by the **commissure of the superior colliculi** (see Figs. 7-14 and 7-15). The **posterior commissure** is a robust bundle that runs transversely, just dorsal to the transition between the cerebral aqueduct and the third ventricle. A small piece of the commissure in the midline is included in the section shown in Figure 7-15. Despite the substantial size of the posterior commissure, the connections of its fibers are not all known. Some have been identified as coming from the superior colliculus and the following smaller nuclei nearby: pretectal area, habenular nuclei (in the epithalamus of the diencephalon), and the accessory oculomotor nuclei.

PRETECTAL AREA

The pretectal area consists of four small nuclei rostral to the lateral edge of the superior colliculus. The pretectal area receives fibers from the retina by way of the optic tract and the superior brachium. These fibers are probably all collateral branches of axons destined for the lateral geniculate body of the thalamus. Efferent fibers travel to the Edinger-Westphal nucleus (origin of preganglionic parasympathetic fibers in the oculomotor nerve) of each side. The pretectal area is thereby included in a reflex pathway for the pupillary response to light, with the pupils becoming smaller as the intensity of light increases. Other afferents to the pretectal area come from the superior colliculus, the visual cortex, and the frontal eye fields, and other efferent fibers go from the pretectal area to the accessory oculomotor nuclei. Through these connections, the pretectal area is included in the pathways for the cortical control of eye movement (see Ch. 8).

Tegmentum

FASCICULI PROCEEDING TO THE THALAMUS

The **medial lemniscus** continues to be a readily identifiable fasciculus as it traverses the midbrain in the lateral area of the tegmentum to its termination in the ventral posterior nucleus of the thalamus (see Figs. 7-13 to 7-15). The **spinal lemniscus** is dorsolateral to the medial lemniscus, this spatial relation being continued from the pontine tegmentum. Spinotectal fibers leave the spinal lemniscus to enter the superior colliculus, and some end in the periaqueductal gray matter. The spinothalamic fibers continue into the diencephalon, where they end in the ventral posterior and other thalamic nuclei. Some spinothalamic fibers send branches into the periaqueductal gray matter of the midbrain.

RED NUCLEUS AND ASSOCIATED TRACTS

The red nucleus is a prominent component of the tegmentum. The nucleus is egg-shaped (round in transverse section) and extends from the caudal limit of the superior colliculus into the subthalamic region of the diencephalon. The nucleus is more vascular than the surrounding tissue and is named from its pinkish hue in a fresh specimen. Myelinated nerve fibers that pass through the red nucleus give it a punctate appearance in Weigert-stained sections (see Figs. 7-14 and 7-15).

Afferent fibers from the contralateral cerebellum reach the red nucleus by way of the superior cerebellar peduncle and its decussation (see Fig. 7-13). Corticorubral fibers come from the motor areas of the ipsilateral cerebral hemisphere. Many other afferents to the red nucleus have been detected in animals, but their significance in the human brain is not known.

The red nucleus gives rise to a small number of axons that cross the midline in the **ventral tegmental decussation** (of Forel) and continue through the brain stem into the lateral funiculus of the spinal cord as the rubrospinal tract. This is a minor pathway in the human brain, and its few fibers terminate in the first two segments of the cervical spinal gray matter. Some descending fibers accompany the rubrospinal fibers initially and then end in the facial motor nucleus and in those nuclei of the reticular formation that project to the cerebellum. In addition to these crossed projections, large numbers of **rubro-olivary fibers** travel in the ipsilateral central tegmental tract to terminate in the inferior olivary complex, which projects across the midline to the cerebellum. There are probably also some direct rubrocerebellar fibers that traverse the superior cerebellar peduncles and end in certain central nuclei of the cerebellum (globose and emboliform nuclei).

Nuclei of Cranial Nerves and Associated Tracts

VESTIBULOCOCHLEAR NERVE

Certain tracts that originate in the sensory nuclei of cranial nerves continue into the midbrain; two are associated with the vestibulocochlear nerve. The **lateral lemniscus** was identified in the discussion of the inferior colliculus. The **medial longitudinal fasciculus** is adjacent to the midline (see Figs. 7-12 to 7-15), in the same general position as at lower brain stem levels. Most of its fibers originate in vestibular nuclei, and those that reach the midbrain end in the trochlear, oculomotor, and accessory oculomotor nuclei. The fasciculus also contains association fibers connecting the abducens, trochlear, and oculomotor nuclei.

TRIGEMINAL NERVE

The **ventral trigeminothalamic tract**, which arises from the spinal and pontine trigeminal nuclei, continues through the midbrain near the medial lemniscus (see Figs. 7-12 to 7-15). **Dorsal trigeminothalamic fibers** from the pontine trigeminal nuclei of both sides traverse the midbrain tegmentum some distance dorsal to the ventral tract. The **mesencephalic nucleus** of the trigeminal nerve continues from the pons into the lateral region of the periaqueductal gray matter throughout most of the midbrain.

TROCHLEAR AND OCULOMOTOR NERVES

The **trochlear nucleus** is in the periaqueductal gray matter at the level of the inferior colliculus, where it lies just dorsal to the medial longitudinal fasciculus (see Fig. 7-13). Fibers from the nucleus curve dorsally around the periaqueductal gray matter, with a caudal slope (see Figs. 7-10 and 7-12). On reaching the dorsal surface of the brain stem, the fibers decussate in the superior medullary velum and emerge as the trochlear nerves just behind the inferior colliculi. The trochlear nerve supplies the superior oblique muscle of the eye.

The **oculomotor nucleus** is in reality a group of subnuclei in and adjacent to the midline in the ventral part of the periaqueductal gray matter at the level of the superior colliculus. The paired nuclei have a V-shaped outline in sections (see Figs. 7-14 and 7-15). Bundles of fibers from the nucleus pursue a curved course through the tegmentum, with many of them passing through the red nucleus (see Fig. 7-14), and then emerge along the side of the interpeduncular fossa to form the oculomotor nerve (see Fig. 7-15). The oculomotor nerve supplies the extraocular muscles, with the exception of the lateral rectus and superior oblique. It also supplies the striated fibers of the levator palpebrae superioris muscle, which opens the eye. Distinct subnuclei supply the individual muscles. The oculomotor nucleus includes a parasympathetic component, the **Edinger-Westphal nucleus**, concerned with the ciliary and sphincter pupillae muscles of the eye.

Substantia Nigra

The substantia nigra is a large nucleus that is situated between the tegmentum and the basis pedunculi throughout the midbrain (see Figs. 7-13 through 7-15) and extends into the subthalamic region of the diencephalon. The nucleus is rudimentary in lower vertebrates, makes its first definitive appearance in mammals, and is largest in the human brain. The black color is due to the dopaminergic neurons of the **pars compacta**, adjacent to the tegmentum. These cells contain cytoplasmic inclusion granules of melanin pigment. The number of melanin granules is few at birth and increases rapidly during childhood and then more slowly throughout life. The pigment, which is probably a by-product of dopamine metabolism, is present in albinos. Functionally, the substantia nigra is associated with the corpus striatum, a large body of gray matter in the forebrain.

The major source of fibers afferent to the pars compacta is the striatum (caudate nucleus plus the outer part, known as the putamen, of the lentiform nucleus). The efferent fibers from the pars compacta go to the striatum. These connections form part of a larger piece of neuronal circuitry and are discussed in Chapters 12 and 23.

The region of the substantia nigra bordering the basis pedunculi consists of cells that lack pigment and is called the **pars reticulata**. Its cellular architecture and the afferent and efferent connections indicate that it is probably a detached part of the internal segment of the globus pallidus, which is the inner part of the lentiform nucleus (see Ch. 12). The pars reticulata contains neurons that project to the superior colliculus, providing a pathway whereby the corpus striatum can participate in the control of eye movements.

Parkinson's Disease

The importance of the substantia nigra is apparent when the disturbances of motor function in **Parkinson's disease** (paralysis agitans) are considered. The clinical features of this crippling disorder are muscular rigidity, a slow tremor, and bradykinesia or poverty of movement. The last is manifest as a mask-like face, difficulty in initiating movements, and loss of all unnecessary involuntary movements such as swinging the arms when walking. All three features combine to cause a typical shuffling gait, with a tendency to fall forward and difficulty in stopping. The most consistent pathological finding in Parkinson's disease is degeneration of the melanin-containing cells in the pars compacta of the substantia nigra. Most cases of Parkinson's disease have no known cause, but a few are due to poisons, including manganese compounds (industrial exposure in some mines) and MPTP (1-methyl-4-phenyl-1,2,4,6-tetrahydropyridine), present in illegally manufactured heroin. Some drugs (see below) can cause transient parkinsonian symptoms by blocking the normal actions of dopamine on neurons.

Biochemical and histochemical research have provided the basis for therapy. Dopamine, normally present in the substantia nigra and in the striatum, is virtually absent from these sites in Parkinson's disease. Administration of dopamine might replace the regulatory action of the substantia nigra on the striatum, but this amine does not cross the blood–brain barrier. A metabolic precursor that does gain access to brain tissue has been used instead. This precursor is L-DOPA (L-dihydroxyphenylalanine), and its conversion to dopamine occurs in the surviving neurons of the pars compacta. The administration of L-DOPA (levodopa) does not stop the loss of neurons, but it relieves the motor abnormalities in Parkinson's disease until there are not enough nigral neurons left to deliver dopamine to the striatum. Other drugs used to treat Parkinsonism include inhibitors of an enzyme that degrades dopamine and anticholinergic agents, which work indirectly by suppressing the actions of the cholinergic interneurons of the striatum. Surgical treatment of Parkinson's disease consists of destroying parts of the brain that are overactive when there is not enough

dopaminergic modulation of the striatum. The ventral lateral nucleus of the thalamus is the site most often chosen for such lesions, but some relief of symptoms follows either surgical or spontaneous pathological damage almost anywhere in the base of the cerebral hemisphere. In the late 1980s, many attempts were made to treat patients with Parkinson's disease by transplanting cells potentially capable of secreting dopamine (taken from the patient's adrenal gland or from aborted human fetuses) into either the caudate nucleus or the striatum. Not surprisingly (see Ch. 2), these operations provided only transient relief of the symptoms.

VENTRAL TEGMENTAL AREA

The ventral tegmental area (of Tsai) is another population of dopaminergic neurons, on the medial aspect of the cerebral peduncle, between the substantia nigra and the red nucleus. The axons of these cells end in the hypothalamus, the hippocampal formation, and other parts of the limbic system. These projections, sometimes called the **mesolimbic dopaminergic system**, have been intensively studied in animals because their actions are blocked by drugs that are useful in the clinical management of schizophrenia and other mental disorders. The drugs antagonize dopamine at its postsynaptic receptors, and their most serious adverse effect is a syndrome that resembles Parkinson's disease.

Basis Pedunculi

The basis pedunculi (crus cerebri) consists of fibers of the pyramidal and corticopontine systems (see Figs. 7-13 through 7-15 and Ch. 23).

Corticospinal fibers constitute the middle three-fifths of the basis pedunculi; the somatotopic arrangement is that of fibers for the neck, arm, trunk, and leg in a medial to lateral direction. **Corticobulbar (corticonuclear) fibers** are located between the corticospinal and frontopontine tracts, but many leave the basis pedunculi and continue to their destinations through the tegmentum of the midbrain and pons. The majority of the corticobulbar fibers end in the reticular formation near the motor nuclei of cranial nerves (the trigeminal and facial motor nuclei, the nucleus ambiguus, and the hypoglossal nucleus). A few make direct synaptic contacts with the motor neurons in these nuclei. In addition to these pathways, which have obvious motor functions, there are corticobulbar fibers to the pontine and spinal trigeminal nuclei and to the solitary nucleus. Axons of cortical origin that end in the gracile and cuneate nuclei also are classified as corticobulbar. Thus corticobulbar connections are involved in modulating the transmission of sensory information rostrally from the brain stem as well as in the control of movement.

Corticopontine fibers are divided into two large bundles. The **frontopontine tract** occupies the medial one-fifth of the basis pedunculi. The lateral one-fifth consists of the **parietotemporopontine tract**, most of whose fibers originate in the parietal lobe. Corticopontine fibers end in the basal pons, synapsing with the cells of the pontine nuclei.

Visceral Pathways in the Brain Stem

The **ascending visceral pathways** in the spinal cord are in the ventral and ventrolateral funiculi. They may be considered to be parts of the spinothalamic and spinoreticular tracts. Data of visceral origin reach the reticular formation, the thalamus, and the hypothalamus.

Physiologically important visceral afferents reach the **solitary nucleus** in the medulla by way of the vagus and glossopharyngeal nerves (see Ch. 8). The solitary nucleus also receives afferents for taste through the vagus, glossopharyngeal, and facial nerves. Ascending fibers from the solitary nucleus travel ipsilaterally in the central tegmental tract and terminate in the hypothalamus and in the most medial part of the ventral posterior medial nucleus of the thalamus. From the latter site, information with respect to taste is relayed to a cortical taste area in the parietal and insular lobes. A small **solitariospinal tract** that originates in the solitary nucleus terminates on preganglionic autonomic neurons in the spinal cord.

There are two descending pathways whose cells of origin are located in the hypothalamus. **Mamillotegmental fibers** originate in the mamillary body of the hypothalamus; they terminate in the reticular formation of the midbrain, which projects to autonomic nuclei in the brain stem and spinal cord. Fibers from other hypothalamic nuclei, notably the paraventricular nucleus, run caudally in the **dorsal longitudinal fasciculus** (of Schütz), a bundle of unmyelinated fibers in the periaqueductal gray matter of the midbrain. Some terminate in the reticular formation of the brain stem and the dorsal nucleus of the vagus nerve, and the hypothalamospinal fibers proceed to autonomic nuclei in the spinal cord. Thus impulses of hypothalamic origin reach the preganglionic sympathetic and sacral parasympathetic neurons both directly and through relays in the reticular formation. Clinical evidence indicates that fibers influencing the sympathetic nervous system descend ipsilaterally through the lateral part of the medulla.

Anatomical and Clinical Correlations

Vascular lesions are among the more important causes of damage to the brain. **Hemorrhage** into the brain stem usually has serious consequences because the escaping blood destroys regions of the reticular formation that control the vital functions of respiration and circulation. **Vascular occlusion** results in neurological signs that depend on the location and size of the affected region. The following examples are presented to show the correlation between clinical signs and the location of the lesion.

The **medial medullary syndrome** results from occlusion of a medullary branch of the vertebral artery; the size of the infarction depends on the distribution of the particular artery involved. In

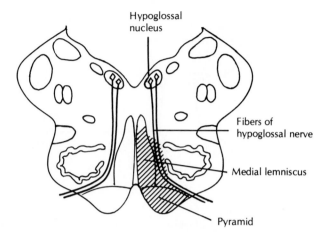

Figure 7-16. Site of a lesion producing the medial medullary syndrome.

the example shown in Figure 7-16, the affected area includes the pyramid and most of the medial lemniscus on one side. The lesion extends far enough laterally to include fibers of the hypoglossal nerve as they pass between the medial lemniscus and the inferior olivary nucleus. A patient with this lesion has contralateral hemiparesis as well as impairment of the sensations of position and movement and of discriminative touch on the opposite side of the body. Paralysis of the tongue muscles is ipsilateral. This is an example of "crossed" or "alternating" paralysis, in which the body below the neck is affected on the side opposite the lesion, whereas muscles supplied by a cranial nerve are affected on the same side as the lesion.

Occlusion of a vessel supplying the lateral area of the medulla results in the **lateral medul-** lary (**Wallenberg's**) syndrome. Typically, the occluded vessel is a medullary branch of the posterior inferior cerebellar artery. The infarcted area (Fig. 7-17) includes the spinal trigeminal tract and its nucleus, causing ipsilateral loss of pain and temperature sensibility in the area of distribution of the trigeminal nerve. Below the neck there is contralateral loss of pain and temperature sensation because of interruption of fibers of the spinothalamic tract in the spinal lemniscus. Because the medial lemniscus is intact, touch sensation is diminished rather than abolished. Destruction of the nucleus ambiguus causes paralysis of the muscles of the soft palate, pharynx, and larynx on the side of the lesion, with difficulty in swallowing and phonation. The descending pathway to the intermediolateral cell column of the spinal cord is usually in-

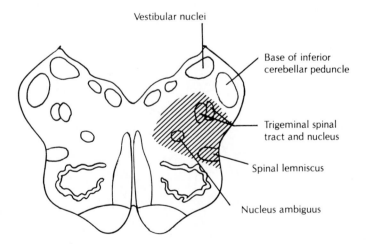

Figure 7-17. Site of a lesion producing the lateral medullary syndrome.

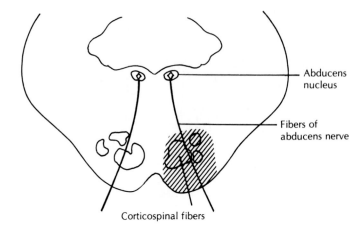

Figure 7-18. Site of a lesion in the basal pons involving descending motor fibers and the abducens nerve.

cluded in the area of degeneration, thereby causing **Horner's syndrome** (small pupil, drooping of the upper eyelid [ptosis] and slight enophthalmos) and warm, dry skin of the face, all on the side of the lesion. The infarcted region may extend dorsally to include the base of the inferior cerebellar peduncle and vestibular nuclei, causing dizziness, cerebellar ataxia, and nystagmus. Cerebellar signs are more pronounced if infarction of part of the cerebellum is added to that of the medulla (posterior inferior cerebellar artery thrombosis).

Lesions in the basal region of the pons or the midbrain may produce alternating paralysis, similar to that described for the medial medullary syndrome. Figure 7-18 shows an area of infarction in one side of the caudal region of the pons, resulting from occlusion of a pontine branch of the basilar artery. Interruption of corticospinal and other descending motor fibers causes contralateral hemiparesis. Inclusion of abducens nerve fibers in the lesion causes paralysis of the lateral rectus muscle on the ipsilateral side, resulting in a medial strabismus or squint.

The position of a vascular lesion in the basal region of a cerebral peduncle, which can follow occlusion of a branch of the posterior cerebral artery, is shown in Figure 7-19. This causes **Weber's syndrome**, consisting of contralateral hemiparesis due to interruption of corticospinal and other descending motor fibers and ipsilateral paralysis of ocular muscles because of inclusion of oculomotor nerve fibers in the infarcted area. There is paralysis of all the extraocular muscles except the lateral rectus and superior oblique. The most obvious signs are loss of ability to raise the upper eyelid and lateral strabismus, together with dilation of the pupil because of interruption of parasympathetic fibers that control the sphincter pupillae muscle.

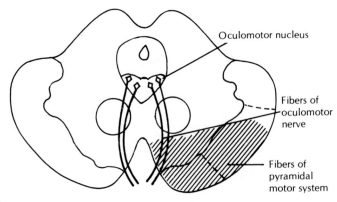

Figure 7-19. Site of a lesion in the midbrain involving descending motor fibers and the oculomotor nerve.

SUGGESTED READING ⸺

Hirsch WL, Kemp SS, Martinez AJ, Curfin H, Latchaw RE, Wolf G: Anatomy of the brainstem: correlation of in vitro MR images with histologic sections. Am J Neuroradiol 10:923–928, 1989

Nathan PW, Smith MC: The rubrospinal and central tegmental tracts in man. Brain 105:223–269, 1982

Nathan PW, Smith MC: The location of descending fibres to sympathetic neurons supplying the head and neck. J Neurol Neurosurg Psychiat 49:187–194, 1986

Nieuwenhuys R, Voogd J, van Huijzen C: The Human Central Nervous System. A Synopsis and Atlas, 3rd ed. Berlin, Springer-Verlag, 1988

Olszewski J, Baxter D: Cytoarchitecture of the Human Brain Stem, 2nd ed. Basel, S Karger, 1954; reprint, 1982

Riley HA: An Atlas of the Basal Ganglia, Brain Stem and Spinal Cord. New York, Hafner, 1960

Sadjadpour K, Brodal A: The vestibular nuclei in man: A morphological study in the light of experimental findings in the cat. J Hirnforsch 10:299–323, 1968

Saper CB: Anatomical substrates for the hypothalamic control of the autonomic nervous system. In Brooks CMcC, Koizumi K, Sato A (eds): Integrative Actions of the Autonomic Nervous System, ch. 24. Amsterdam, Elsevier-North Holland, 1979

Eight

The Human Nervous System: An Anatomical Viewpoint, Sixth Edition, Murray L. Barr and John A. Kiernan. J.B. Lippincott Company, Philadelphia, © 1993.

Cranial Nerves

Important Facts

The cranial nerves (I–XII) have motor, parasympathetic, and sensory functions.

Eye Movements

III, IV, and VI supply extraocular muscles.

Voluntary saccadic eye movements are controlled by the frontal eye field and smooth pursuit movements by the occipital cortex.

The descending pathways for conjugate horizontal gaze include the paramedian pontine reticular formation and the medial longitudinal fasciculus (MLF). Internuclear ophthalmoplegia is caused by interruption of the MLF.

Nuclei in the rostral midbrain are involved in vertical eye movements.

Other Motor Functions

The trigeminal motor nucleus supplies masticatory and a few other muscles through the mandibular division of V.

The facial motor nucleus supplies the facial muscles and the stapedius. The lower half of the face is controlled by the contralateral cerebral hemisphere. The upper half is bilaterally controlled, and therefore not paralyzed by an "upper motor neuron" lesion.

The muscles of the larynx and pharynx are supplied by neurons in the nucleus ambiguus, mostly by way of X.

XI consists largely of motor fibers for the trapezius and sternocleidomastoid muscles, from segments C1 to C5.

The protruded tongue deviates toward the abnormal side if there is weakness of the muscles supplied by XII.

Preganglionic Parasympathetic Fibers

III contains preganglionic fibers from the Edinger-Westphal nucleus. They end in the ciliary ganglion, which supplies the sphincter pupillae and ciliary smooth muscles. Loss of the light reflex is the first sign of compression of III.

Salivary and lacrimal glands are supplied by parasympathetic ganglia, which receive preganglionic innervation from VII and IX. Preganglionic axons in X are from two nuclei in the medulla.

General Sensory Functions

All general somatic sensory fibers from cranial nerve ganglia (V, IX; some from VII, X) end in trigeminal nuclei.

Touch sensation is relayed through the pontine trigeminal nucleus and the rostral part of the spinal trigeminal nucleus.

Pain and temperature fibers descend ipsilaterally in the spinal trigeminal tract and end in the caudal part of its nucleus.

Trigeminothalamic fibers cross the midline in the brain stem and ascend to the contralateral thalamus (VPm nucleus).

The caudal part of the solitary nucleus receives visceral afferent fibers (IX and X) for cardiovascular and respiratory reflexes.

Special Senses

I, II, and VIII are discussed in Chapters 17, 20, 21, and 22.

Taste fibers (VII, IX, and a few from X) go in the solitary tract to the rostral end of the solitary nucleus. Solitariothalamic fibers go to the most medial part of the VPm.

The cranial nerves, listed in the order in which numbers are assigned to them, are as follows. These numbers were introduced by von Sömmering in 1798.

1. (or I) Olfactory
2. (or II) Optic
3. (or III) Oculomotor
4. (or IV) Trochlear
5. (or V) Trigeminal
6. (or VI) Abducens
7. (or VII) Facial
8. (or VIII) Vestibulocochlear
9. (or IX) Glossopharyngeal
10. (or X) Vagus
11. (or IX) Accessory
12. (or XII) Hypoglossal

In addition to motor and general sensory functions, five special senses are served by various cranial nerves. Of the special senses, the olfactory system is an integral part of the forebrain (see Ch. 17). The optic and vestibulocochlear nerves are discussed in the section on systemic neuroanatomy, in which the visual, auditory, and vestibular systems are described (see Chs. 20, 21, and 22). The special sense of taste (gustatory system) is dealt with in this chapter because the primary sensory neurons for taste are in the same ganglia as sensory neurons that have other functions in the facial, glossopharyngeal, and vagus nerves.

Oculomotor, Trochlear, and Abducens Nerves

The third, fourth, and sixth cranial nerves supply the extraocular muscles with motor fibers; their nuclei, therefore, consist of multipolar motor neurons and receive afferents from the same sources. The oculomotor nucleus includes in addition a parasympathetic component.

OCULOMOTOR NERVE

The **oculomotor nucleus** is situated in the periaqueductal gray matter of the midbrain, ventral to the aqueduct at the level of the supe-

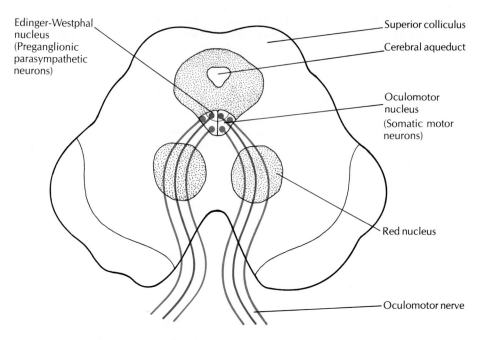

Figure 8-1. Origin of the oculomotor nerve in the midbrain. (Motor neurons are red; preganglionic parasympathetic neurons are blue.)

rior colliculus (Fig. 8-1). The paired nuclei have a triangular outline in transverse section and are bounded laterally by the medial longitudinal fasciculi. The cells for individual extraocular muscles (including the levator palpebrae superioris) are localized in longitudinal groups; these subnuclei are represented bilaterally, except for one, which is situated dorsocaudally in the midline. According to Warwick's schema for the oculomotor nucleus of the monkey, there are three laterally disposed cell groups, which supply the inferior rectus, inferior oblique, and medial rectus muscles. On the medial side of these, there is a subnucleus for the superior rectus muscle. The unpaired cell group supplies the levator palpebrae superioris muscle on each side. Myelinated axons from each oculomotor nucleus curve ventrally through the tegmentum, with many of them passing through the red nucleus. The fibers emerge as rootlets along the side of the interpeduncular fossa, and these rootlets converge immediately to form the oculomotor nerve.

Oculomotor fibers are partly crossed and partly uncrossed. Although full details are lacking for humans, it appears that only uncrossed fibers supply the inferior rectus, inferior oblique, and medial rectus muscles. The superior rectus muscle receives crossed fibers only, and the levator palpebrae superioris muscles of both sides are supplied by the unpaired subnucleus.[1] The small sizes of the motor units, in which about six muscle fibers are supplied by a nerve fiber, attest to the delicate neuromuscular mechanisms required for coordinated movement of the eyes in binocular vision.

Mixed with the motor neurons of the oculomotor nucleus are neurons whose axons pass in the medial longitudinal fasciculus to the trochlear and, especially, the abducens nuclei of the same and the opposite sides. These **internuclear neurons** mediate inhibition of antagonistic muscles whenever the eyes are moved.

The **Edinger-Westphal nucleus** is dorsal

---

[1] This statement refers to the striated skeletal fibers of this muscle. The levator also contains smooth-muscle fibers, which are innervated by sympathetic nerve fibers with cell bodies in the superior cervical ganglion (see Ch. 24).

to the rostral two-thirds of the main oculomotor nucleus, and its smaller cells are similar to those of other preganglionic parasympathetic neurons. Fibers from the Edinger-Westphal nucleus accompany other oculomotor fibers into the orbit, where they terminate in the **ciliary ganglion**. Postganglionic fibers (the axons of the neurons in the ganglion) pass through the **short ciliary nerves** to the eyeball, in which they supply the sphincter pupillae muscle of the iris and the ciliary muscle. The Edinger-Westphal nucleus also contributes fibers to the small interstitiospinal tract, which is probably concerned with visuomotor coordination.

A lesion that interrupts fibers of the oculomotor nerve causes paralysis of all extraocular muscles except the superior oblique and lateral rectus muscles. The sphincter pupillae muscle in the iris and the ciliary muscle in the ciliary body are functionally paralyzed, although they are not denervated. The consequences of such a lesion are lateral strabismus caused by unopposed action of the lateral rectus muscle, inability to direct the eye medially or vertically, and drooping of the upper eyelid (ptosis). Interruption of the parasympathetic fibers causes dilation of the pupil, enhanced by unopposed action of the dilator pupillae muscle in the iris, which has a sympathetic innervation. There is no longer pupillary constriction in response to an increase of light intensity or in accommodation for near objects, nor does the ciliary muscle contract to allow the lens to increase in thickness for focusing on a near object. The preganglionic parasympathetic fibers run superficially in the nerve and are therefore the first axons to suffer when the nerve is affected by external pressure. Consequently *the first sign of compression of the oculomotor nerve is ipsilateral slowness of the pupillary response to light.*

TROCHLEAR NERVE

The **trochlear nucleus** for the superior oblique muscle is immediately caudal to the oculomotor nucleus, at the level of the inferior colliculus (Fig. 8-2). Trochlear nerve fibers have an unusual course and is the only nerve to emerge from the dorsum of the brain stem.

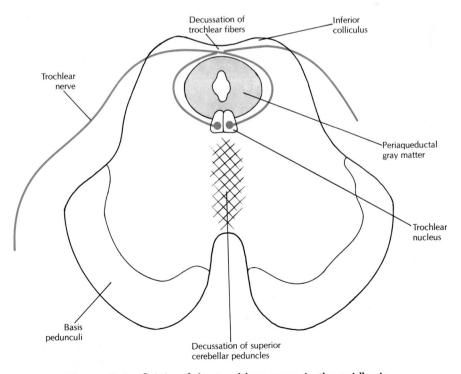

Figure 8-2. Origin of the trochlear nerve in the midbrain.

Small bundles of fibers curve around the periaqueductal gray matter with a caudal slope and decussate in the superior medullary velum with fibers from the companion nucleus; the slender nerve emerges immediately caudal to the inferior colliculus. The superior oblique muscle, like the superior rectus, is therefore supplied by crossed fibers. The function of the superior oblique muscle is to rotate and depress the eyeball. Paralysis of the muscle, as in the rare occurrence of an isolated lesion of the trochlear nerve, causes vertical diplopia (double vision). The diplopia is maximal when the eye is directed downward and inward, and a person so affected experiences difficulty in walking downstairs.

ABDUCENS NERVE

The **abducens nucleus** for the lateral rectus muscle is situated beneath the facial colliculus in the floor of the fourth ventricle (Fig. 8-3). A bundle of facial nerve fibers curves over the nucleus, contributing to the facial colliculus. The motor neurons in the abducens nucleus give rise to axons that pass through the pons in a ventrocaudal direction, emerging from the brain stem at the junction of the pons and the pyramid. The abducens nucleus also contains internuclear neurons whose axons travel to the part of the oculomotor nucleus concerned with supplying the medial rectus muscle.

Interruption of the abducens nerve causes medial strabismus and inability to direct the affected eye laterally. Functional impairment of any of the extraocular muscles causes diplopia. The separation between the two images is greatest when the patient attempts to look in the direction of action of the weak or paralyzed muscle.

An understanding of the neuroanatomical basis of ocular movements, discussed below, is essential for the clinical analysis of impairment of these movements.

AFFERENTS TO NUCLEI THAT SUPPLY EXTRAOCULAR MUSCLES

The main part of the oculomotor nucleus (ie, all but the parasympathetic component) and the trochlear and abducens nuclei receive fibers from the same sources, as is to be expected. These afferents are concerned with the control of both voluntary and involuntary eye movements. Voluntarily initiated conjugate movements of the eyes include those that occur when scanning a landscape or reading a printed page. These movements, known as **saccadic eye movements**, are rapid, with each being completed in 20 to 50 msec. Slower

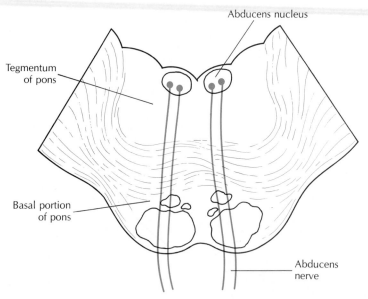

Figure 8-3. Origin of the abducens nerve in the midbrain.

Abducens nucleus

Tegmentum of pons

Basal portion of pons

Abducens nerve

movements of the eyes are possible only when tracking a moving object in the visual field. These largely involuntary **smooth pursuit movements** are mentioned later in connection with visual fixation. **Vergence movements**, in which both eyes move medially to look at a near object or laterally to look into the distance, can also occur slowly.

VOLUNTARY EYE MOVEMENTS

The area of the cerebral cortex that controls voluntary eye movements is the **frontal eye field**, located anterior to the motor cortex. Electrical stimulation of the frontal eye field results in conjugate deviation of the eyes to the opposite side. A destructive lesion there causes both eyes to deviate to the same side—looking away from the paralyzed side of the body if the motor cortex has been damaged by the same lesion. There are probably no direct corticobulbar fibers from any part of the cerebral cortex to the nuclei of cranial nerves III, IV, and VI. Instead, the voluntary control of eye movements is mediated by a polysynaptic pathway that involves the frontal cortex, superior colliculus, pretectal area, accessory oculomotor nuclei, and, finally, oculomotor, trochlear, and abducens nuclei (Fig. 8-4). (The four pairs of accessory oculomotor nuclei, in the rostral midbrain, are shown in Fig. 9-8.) The internuclear neurons, whose axons travel in the medial longitudinal fasciculus to interconnect the three motor nuclei, inhibit all motor neurons supplying muscles that are

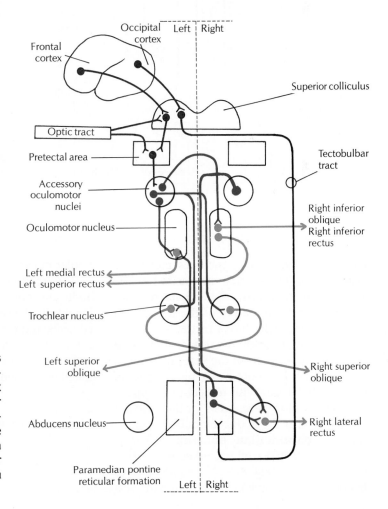

Figure 8-4. Some pathways for the control of eye movements by the cerebral cortex and superior colliculus. (Motor neurons are red; neurons ending in the motor nuclei are blue; neurons originating in the cerebral cortex, superior colliculus, and pretectal area are black.)

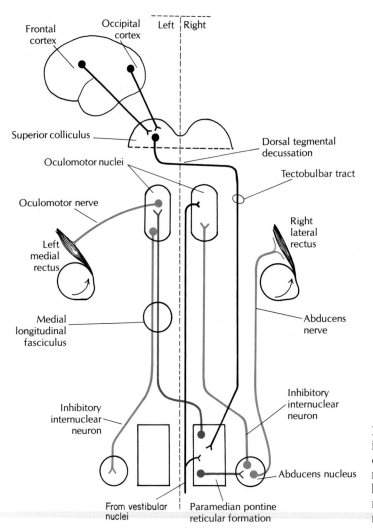

Figure 8-5. Pathways involved in conjugate lateral movements of the eyes. (Motor neurons are red; projections of the PPRF are blue; inhibitory internuclear neurons are green; other neurons are black.)

passively lengthened as the eyes move. For example, the coordinated contraction of the left lateral rectus and the right medial rectus is associated with inhibition of the left medial rectus and the right lateral rectus.

The medial longitudinal fasciculus also transmits impulses from the vestibular nuclei and provides for coordinated movements of the eyes and head. With respect to conjugate movements of the eyes, cells in the reticular formation near the abducens nucleus constitute the **paramedian pontine reticular formation (PPRF),** which serves as a "center for lateral gaze" (Fig. 8-5). The PPRF receives fibers from the superior colliculus and the ves-

tibular nuclei and from other parts of the reticular formation. It sends fibers to the ipsilateral abducens nucleus and, through the medial longitudinal fasciculus, to those cells of the contralateral oculomotor nucleus that supply the medial rectus muscle. The actions of the medial and lateral recti are thereby coordinated in horizontal movements of the eyes.[2] A

---

[2] This coordination is a function of both the PPRF and the internuclear neurons contained in the abducens nucleus. Formerly both populations of cells were thought to reside in a region named the parabducens nucleus, but this term is now obsolete, because it does not refer to any real anatomical entity.

lesion in the PPRF causes paralysis of conjugate gaze to the ipsilateral side.

A small lesion in the medial longitudinal fasciculus in the upper part of the pons is most often due to multiple sclerosis, a disease in which there are scattered plaques of demyelination in the central nervous system. This lesion causes **internuclear ophthalmoplegia**, in which the ipsilateral eye cannot adduct when the contralateral eye abducts and also exhibits nystagmus. These abnormalities are evident only when the patient is asked to gaze to the side opposite that of the lesion; contraction of the medial rectus occurs normally with convergence of the eyes for looking at a near object. The paralysis of adduction of the ipsilateral eye is attributed to transection of fibers from the contralateral PPRF to the ipsilateral oculomotor nucleus. The associated nystagmus in the abducting (contralateral) eye is a useful diagnostic sign, thought to be due to interruption of inhibitory internuclear fibers.

Comparable "centers" for conjugate movement of the eyes in the vertical plane are present in the upper midbrain bilaterally. A lesion that involves the rostral interstitial nucleus of the medial longitudinal fasciculus (one of the accessory oculomotor nuclei) causes paralysis of downward gaze. A lesion located a little farther caudally or, alternatively, one that transects the posterior commissure causes paralysis of upward gaze. These disorders of vertical eye movements can result from pressure by a tumor of the pineal gland.

FIXATION AND CONVERGENCE

The eyes are normally directed toward some object in the center of the field of vision. If the object moves, both eyes will execute smooth-pursuit movements to maintain visual fixation, which contributes importantly to awareness of the position of the head and, integrated with other sensory information, helps in the maintenance of the body's equilibrium. These slow eye movements are largely involuntary. They are controlled principally by the cortex of the occipital lobe, including both the primary visual area and the surrounding visual association cortex, although there is experimental evidence for simultaneous involvement of the frontal eye fields. Electrical stimulation of these areas results in conjugate movement of the eyes to the opposite side. The descending connections of the occipital cortex are essentially the same as those of the frontal eye field (see Fig. 8-4). The direct visual input from the retina to the superior colliculus may also be involved in reflex eye movements for visual fixation.

Convergence occurs when both eyes are focused on a near object. The neuroanatomical substrates of convergence are poorly understood but are presumed to be similar to those just described for visual fixation. Convergence requires the integrity of the occipital cortex but not that of the frontal eye field or of the PPRF. The descending pathway probably includes synaptic relays in the superior colliculus and in the accessory oculomotor nuclei.

LIGHT AND ACCOMMODATION REFLEXES

The Edinger-Westphal nucleus is a parasympathetic autonomic nucleus concerned mainly with reflex responses to light and accommodation. An increase in the intensity of light falling on the retina causes constriction of the pupil. The afferent limb of the reflex arc involves fibers in the optic nerve and optic tract that reach the pretectal area by way of the superior brachium (Fig. 8-6). The pretectal area projects to the Edinger-Westphal nucleus, from which fibers traverse the oculomotor nerve to the ciliary ganglion in the orbital cavity. Postganglionic fibers travel through the short ciliary nerves to the sphincter pupillae muscle of the iris. Some neurons in the pretectal area send their axons across the midline in the posterior commissure to the contralateral Edinger-Westphal nucleus. Consequently both pupils constrict when a light is shone into only one eye. This response of the contralateral iris is known as the consensual light reflex.

The accommodation of the lens accompanies ocular convergence produced by visual fixation on a near object. Impulses that originate in the occipital cortex and are relayed to the Edinger-Westphal nucleus through the superior colliculus appear to initiate the accom-

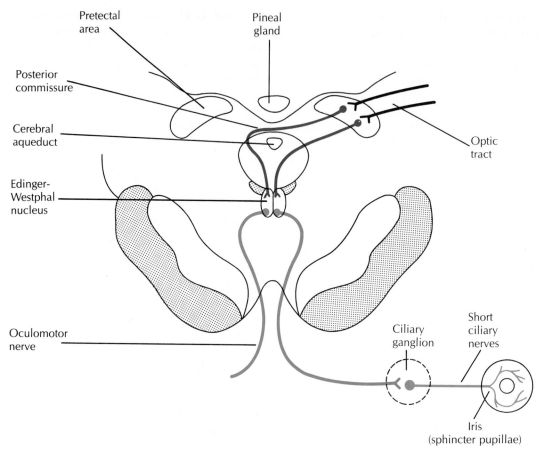

Figure 8-6. The pupillary light reflex. (Sensory fibers are black; central inter-neurons are blue; preganglionic parasympathetic neurons are red; post-ganglionic neurons are green.)

modation response. The efferent part of the pathway consists of preganglionic and post-ganglionic fibers from the Edinger-Westphal nucleus and the ciliary ganglion, respectively. The postganglionic fibers supply the ciliary muscle, which, on contraction, allows the lens to increase in thickness and thereby increases refractive power for focusing on a near object. The sphincter pupillae muscle contracts at the same time, sharpening the image by decreasing the diameter of the pupil and reducing spherical aberration in the refractive media.

The different pathways for pupillary responses to light and accommodation are differently affected by disease. For example, in the **Argyll Robertson pupil**, there is constric-

tion when attention is directed to a near object, but pupillary constriction in response to light is absent. The Argyll Robertson pupil is characteristically seen in patients with tabes dorsalis, a syphilitic disease of the central nervous system. Loss of the pupillary light reflex alone should be the result of a small lesion in the pretectal or periaqueductal region, but pathological changes cannot always be found in these sites. The Argyll Robertson pupil is irregular and smaller than normal, probably because of disease of the iris itself. The **Holmes-Adie pupil** responds more slowly than the other to both light and accommodation. It is attributed to death of some neurons in the ciliary ganglion, for no known reason, and may be associated (also for no known reason) with sluggish stretch reflexes throughout the body. The pupillary abnormality of **Horner's syndrome** is explained in Chapter 24.

Trigeminal Nerve

The trigeminal nerve is the principal sensory nerve for the head and is the motor nerve for the muscles of mastication and several small muscles.

Sensory Components

The cell bodies of most of the primary sensory neurons are in the **trigeminal** (semilunar or gasserian) **ganglion**, with the remainder being in the mesencephalic trigeminal nucleus.

The peripheral processes of trigeminal ganglion cells constitute the ophthalmic and maxillary nerves and the sensory component of the mandibular nerve. The cell bodies of sensory neurons for the three divisions of the nerve occupy anatomically discrete regions within the ganglion. The mandibular nerve also includes proprioceptive fibers from the mesencephalic nucleus. The trigeminal nerve is responsible for sensation from the skin of the face and forehead, the scalp as far back as the vertex of the head, the mucosa of the oral and nasal cavities and the paranasal sinuses, and the teeth (Fig. 8-7). The trigeminal nerve also contributes sensory fibers to most of the dura mater (see Ch. 26) and to the cerebral arteries. The scalp of the back of the head and an area of skin at the angle of the jaw are supplied by the

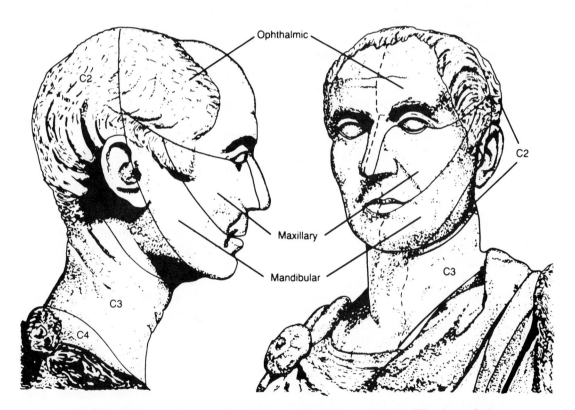

Figure 8-7. Cutaneous innervation of the head and neck. The boundaries between the territories of the three divisions of the trigeminal nerve do not overlap appreciably, as do the boundaries between spinal dermatomes. (*With permission, from Kiernan JA: Introduction to Human Neuroscience, p. 148. Philadelphia, JB Lippincott, 1987*)

second and third cervical nerves. The external ear has a complicated and overlapping innervation. The anterior border of the auricle, the anterior wall of the external acoustic meatus, and the anterior part of the tympanic membrane receive trigeminal fibers. The concha of the auricle, much of the acoustic meatus and tympanic membrane, and a cutaneous area behind the ear are supplied by the facial and vagus nerves. The helix and the posterior surface are supplied by the second and third cervical nerves.

PONTINE TRIGEMINAL NUCLEUS

The central processes of trigeminal ganglion cells make up the large sensory root of the trigeminal nerve; these fibers enter the pons and terminate in the pontine and spinal trigeminal nuclei. The pontine trigeminal nucleus, also called the chief, principal, or superior sensory nucleus, is in the dorsolateral area of the pontine tegmentum at the level of entry of the sensory fibers (Fig. 8-8). Large-diameter fibers for discriminative touch terminate in the pontine trigeminal nucleus. Other fibers divide on nearing the nucleus; one branch enters it and the other branch turns caudally in the spinal tract and ends in the nucleus of the spinal tract. These afferents are mainly for light touch, and both nuclei must therefore participate in this sensory modality.

SPINAL TRIGEMINAL TRACT AND ITS NUCLEUS

Large numbers of sensory root fibers of intermediate size and many fine, unmyelinated fibers turn caudally on entering the pons. These fibers for pain, temperature, and light touch combine with descending branches of the afferents mentioned above to form the spinal trigeminal tract (see Fig. 8-8). The tract includes a small complement of fibers from the facial, glossopharyngeal, and vagus nerves. The latter fibers are for general somatic sensation from part of the external ear, the mucosa of the posterior part of the tongue, the pharynx, and the larynx. Some fibers of the spinal tract descend as far as the upper three segments of the cord, where they intermingle

with fibers of the dorsolateral tract of Lissauer. There is a spatial arrangement of fibers in the sensory root and spinal tract, corresponding to the three divisions of the trigeminal nerve. In the sensory root, ophthalmic fibers are dorsal, mandibular fibers are ventral, and maxillary fibers are in between. There is a rotation of the fibers as they enter the brain stem, with the result that in the trigeminal spinal tract, the mandibular fibers are dorsal and the ophthalmic fibers are ventral. Fibers from the facial, glossopharyngeal, and vagus nerves are dorsal to the mandibular fibers.

Fibers of the spinal tract terminate in the subjacent spinal trigeminal nucleus (see Fig. 8-8) and also in the reticular formation medial to the nucleus. The spinal nucleus extends from the pontine trigeminal nucleus to the caudal limit of the medulla; the nucleus of the spinal tract and the dorsal portion (laminae I–IV) of the dorsal gray horn are indistinguishable from each other in the upper three cervical segments of the spinal cord. The nearby reticular formation corresponds to laminae V-VI and VII of the spinal gray matter. Trigeminothalamic fibers arise from cells in this region as well as from those of the spinal and pontine trigeminal nuclei.

Based on cytoarchitecture, the spinal nucleus divided into three subnuclei. The **pars caudalis**, which extends from the level of the pyramidal decussation to spinal segment C3, receives fibers for pain and temperature. The integrity of the pars caudalis and of the caudal end of the spinal trigeminal tract are essential for the perception of pain that originates in the same side of the head. In the first three cervical segments, laminae I through IV of the dorsal gray horn are concerned with pain and temperature in both the trigeminal area of distribution and in that of the most rostral cervical nerves (neck and back of the head).

Of the remaining two regions of the spinal trigeminal nucleus (see Fig. 8-8), the **pars interpolaris** extends from the level of the rostral third of the inferior olivary nucleus to that of the pyramidal decussation. The **pars oralis** extends from the pars interpolaris rostrally to the pontine trigeminal nucleus, which

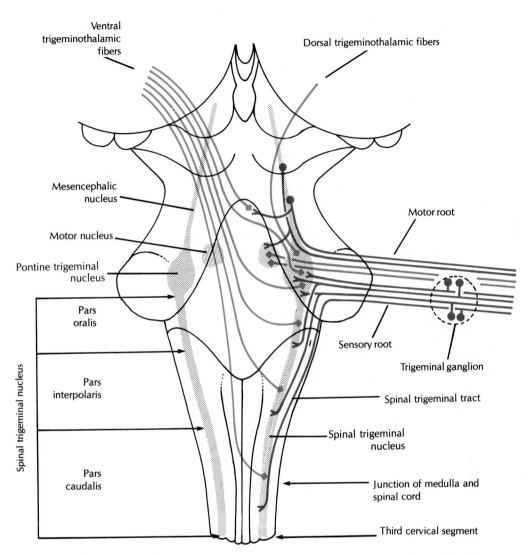

Figure 8-8. Nuclei of the trigeminal nerve and their connections. (Primary sensory neurons are blue; trigeminothalamic neurons are green; motor neurons are red.)

it resembles in its cellular architecture. Fibers of the spinal tract terminating in these regions appear to be mainly concerned with touch, including some discriminative touch in the case of the pars oralis, although there is evidence that the pars interpolaris receives some pain afferents from the teeth.

Some efferent fibers from the sensory trigeminal nuclei terminate in motor nuclei of the trigeminal and facial nerves, the nucleus ambiguus, and the hypoglossal nucleus. These mediate reflex responses to stimuli applied to the area of distribution of the trigeminal nerve. An example is the **corneal reflex**: touching the cornea causes the eyelids to close; the afferent fibers are in the ophthalmic nerve and the efferent fibers of the reflex arc are in the facial nerve. As a further example, irritation of the nasal mucosa causes **sneezing**. For this reflex, afferent impulses in the maxillary nerve are relayed to motor nuclei of the trigeminal and facial nerves, the nucleus ambiguus, the hypoglossal nucleus, and (through a reticulospinal relay) the phrenic nucleus and motor cells in the spinal cord that supply the intercostal and other respiratory muscles.

Projections from the spinal trigeminal nuclei to the reticular formation may provide a source of cutaneous stimuli for the parts of the reticular formation concerned with consciousness and arousal. Other fibers enter the cerebellum through the inferior peduncle. The principal pathway from the pontine and spinal trigeminal nuclei to the thalamus is the crossed **ventral trigeminothalamic tract** (see Fig. 8-8), which ascends close to the medial lemniscus. Smaller numbers of fibers, crossed and uncrossed, proceed from the pontine trigeminal nucleus to the thalamus in the **dorsal trigeminothalamic tract**. The combined tracts are commonly called the **trigeminal lemniscus**. The fibers end in the medial division of the ventral posterior nucleus (VPm) of the thalamus, which projects to the inferior end of the first somatosensory area of the cerebral cortex.

MESENCEPHALIC TRIGEMINAL NUCLEUS

The mesencephalic nucleus is a slender strand of cells extending from the pontine trigeminal nucleus into the midbrain (see Fig. 8-8). The nucleus is located beneath the lateral edge of the floor of the fourth ventricle in the pons and in the lateral region of the periaqueductal gray matter in the midbrain. The unipolar cells are primary sensory neurons in an unusual location; they are the only such cells that are incorporated into the central nervous system, rather than being in cerebrospinal ganglia. The axons of these cells constitute the slender **mesencephalic root** of the trigeminal nerve, which runs alongside the mesencephalic nucleus. Each axon divides into a peripheral and a central branch. Most of the peripheral branches enter the motor root of the trigeminal nerve and are distributed within the mandibular division (see Fig. 8-8). These fibers end in deep proprioceptive-type receptors adjacent to the

teeth of the lower jaw and in neuromuscular spindles in the muscles of mastication. Some fibers from the mesencephalic nucleus traverse the sensory root and the trigeminal ganglion for distribution by way of the maxillary division to endings in the hard palate, adjacent to the teeth of the upper jaw. Central branches of the axons of some cells of the mesencephalic nucleus terminate in the motor nuclei of the trigeminal nerve. This connection establishes the stretch reflex that originates in neuromuscular spindles in the masticatory muscles, together with a reflex for control of the force of the bite. Other central branches synapse with cells of the reticular formation, from which fibers proceed to the thalamus along with other trigeminothalamic fibers. In addition, a few fibers from the mesencephalic nucleus enter the cerebellum through the superior peduncle.

Motor Component

The **trigeminal motor nucleus**, consisting of typical multipolar neurons, is situated medial to the chief sensory nucleus (see Figs. 7-11 and 8-8). Fibers from the motor nucleus constitute the bulk of the motor root, which joins sensory fibers of the mandibular nerve just distal to the trigeminal ganglion. This nerve supplies the muscles of mastication (masseter, temporalis, and lateral and medial pterygoid muscles) and several smaller muscles—the tensor tympani, tensor veli palatini, digastric (anterior belly), and mylohyoid muscles. The motor nucleus receives afferents from the corticobulbar tract; most of these are crossed, but there is a significant proportion of uncrossed fibers. Some of the corticobulbar neurons contact the motor neurons directly, but the majority end in the nearby reticular formation and influence the trigeminal motor nucleus through interneurons.

Afferents for reflexes come mainly from the sensory trigeminal nuclei, including the mesencephalic nucleus. In addition to the stretch reflex, there is a **jaw-opening reflex**, in which the contractions of the masseter, temporalis, and medial pterygoid muscles are inhibited as a result of painful pressure applied to the teeth. Cells that supply the tensor tympani muscle receive acoustic fibers from the superior olivary nucleus. The tensor tympani, by reflex contraction, checks excessive movement of the tympanic membrane caused by loud sounds.

Clinical Considerations

Of the diseases that affect the trigeminal nerve, **trigeminal neuralgia**, or **tic douloureux**, is of special importance. In this disorder there are paroxysms of excruciating pain in the area of distribution of one of the trigeminal divisions, usually with periods of remission and exacerbation. The maxillary nerve is most frequently involved, then the mandibular nerve, and least frequently the ophthalmic nerve. The paroxysm, which is of sudden onset, is often set off by touching an especially sensitive area of skin. In most patients, the symptoms are relieved by carbamazepine, a drug otherwise used to treat epilepsy. If medical treatment fails, major surgery is warranted because of the severity of the pain. Many cases of trigeminal neuralgia are cured if a small aberrant artery is moved away from the sensory root of the nerve. Other surgical procedures aim to interrupt the pain pathway from the affected cutaneous area to the spinal trigeminal nucleus. Lesions may be placed in the trigeminal ganglion or in the sensory root of the nerve, but these can impair corneal sensitivity, which affords protection from damage that might lead to corneal ulceration. Transection of the spinal trigeminal tract in the lower medulla abolishes the ability to feel pain in the face. The somatotopic lamination of the tract permits placement of a small lesion that restricts the analgesic area to the territory of a single division of the trigeminal nerve.

Another painful disorder that commonly affects the trigeminal nerve is **herpes zoster** (see Ch. 19).

The sensory and motor nuclei and the intracranial fibers of the trigeminal nerve may be included in areas damaged by vascular occlusion, trauma, tumor growth, or other lesions in or near the brain stem. Interruption of the motor fibers causes paralysis and eventual atrophy of the muscles of mastication. The mandible deviates to the affected side because of the unopposed action of the contralateral lateral pterygoid muscle, which protrudes the jaw. Interruption of corticobulbar fibers does not cause complete paralysis of the masticatory muscles on the side opposite the lesion because the motor nucleus also receives some uncrossed fibers from the motor cortex.

Facial Nerve

The facial nerve has two sensory components: one supplies taste buds and the other contributes cutaneous fibers to part of the external ear. There are also two efferent components: one for the facial muscles of expression and one for the submandibular and sublingual salivary glands and the lacrimal gland.

Sensory Components

The cell bodies of primary sensory neurons are in the **geniculate ganglion** (Fig. 8-9), situated at the bend of the nerve as it traverses the facial canal in the petrous temporal bone.

GUSTATORY FIBERS

The peripheral processes of cells for taste, which compose most of the ganglion, enter the chorda tympani branch of the facial nerve, which joins the lingual branch of the mandibular nerve. The fibers are distributed to taste buds in the anterior two-thirds of the tongue, most of which are along its lateral border. The fibers for palatal taste buds follow a complicated route, and, as is also true of parasympathetic fibers in the facial and glossopharyngeal nerves, an understanding of the gross anatomy of the head is necessary to visualize their course (Fig. 8-10). In brief, these sensory fibers leave the facial nerve in the greater petrosal branch at the level of the geniculate ganglion; this branch proceeds into the pterygopalatine fossa above the palate, where

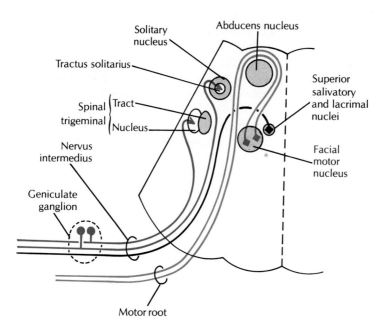

Figure 8-9. Components of the facial nerve in the brain stem. (Primary sensory neurons are blue; motor neurons are red; preganglionic parasympathetic neurons are black.)

the fibers join palatine branches of the maxillary division of the trigeminal nerve. The trigeminal fibers of the palatine nerves provide for general sensation in the palate and on the inner surface of the gums, whereas the fibers from the facial nerve terminate in taste buds in the hard and soft palates.

The central processes of geniculate ganglion cells that subserve taste enter the brain stem in the **nervus intermedius** (which is the sensory and parasympathetic root of the facial nerve) and turn caudally in the solitary tract (see Fig. 8-9). The facial nerve fibers in this fasciculus are joined more caudally by gustatory fibers from the glossopharyngeal and vagus nerves. Fibers from these three sources terminate in the **solitary nucleus**, a column of cells adjacent to and partly surrounding the tract. Only the large-celled rostral part of the nucleus receives taste fibers; it is sometimes called the **gustatory nucleus**. The caudal part, whose cells are small, receives general visceral afferents. Fibers from the gustatory nucleus run rostrally in the ipsilateral central tegmental tract, through the midbrain and subthalamic region, to their site of termination in the most medial part of the **ventral posterior nucleus of the thala-**

mus.[3] This thalamic nucleus projects to the cortical area for taste, which is adjacent to the general sensory area for the tongue and extends onto the insula and forward to the frontal operculum. Physiological evidence has shown that in animals, gustatory stimuli influence the hypothalamus, amygdala, and cortex of the limbic system but probably not through specific ascending projections from the brain stem. Like the functionally related olfactory system (see Ch. 17), the pathway for taste does not cross the midline.

CUTANEOUS FIBERS

The cutaneous sensory fibers leave the facial nerve just after it leaves the facial canal at the stylomastoid foramen (see Fig. 8-10). These fibers are distributed to the skin of the concha of the auricle, a small area behind the ear, the wall of the external acoustic meatus, and the external surface of the tympanic membrane.

---

[3] This is also known as the ventromedial basal thalamic nucleus. In mammals other than primates, a relay in the parabrachial nucleus, in the rostral pons, is interposed between the gustatory nucleus and the thalamus. Possible gustatory connections of the parabrachial nucleus are few or absent in monkeys, and there is no evidence for their existence in the human brain.

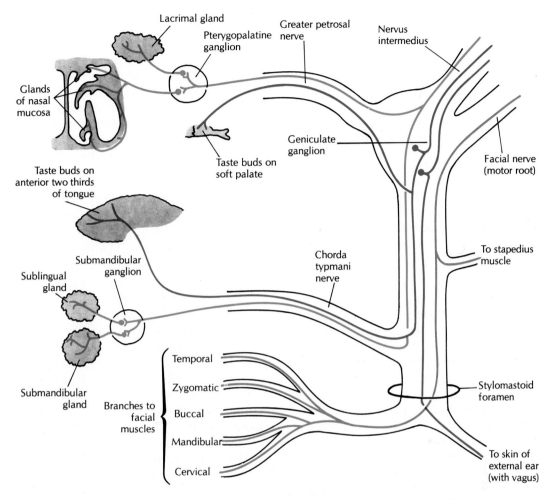

Figure 8-10. Components of the peripheral parts of the facial nerve. (Primary sensory neurons are blue; motor neurons are red; preganglionic and postganglionic parasympathetic neurons are green.)

The central processes of the geniculate ganglion cells for cutaneous sensation enter the brain stem in the nervus intermedius. They continue into the spinal tract of the trigeminal nerve (see Fig. 8-9) and terminate in the subjacent nucleus of the spinal tract.

Efferent Components

FOR SUPPLY OF STRIATED MUSCLES

The motor component is the most important part of the nerve from the clinical viewpoint. The **facial motor nucleus** is situated in the caudal one-third of the ventrolateral part of the pontine tegmentum (see Fig. 8-9). Efferent fibers of the nucleus pursue an unexpected course. Directed initially toward the floor of the fourth ventricle, the fibers form a compact bundle that loops over the caudal end of the abducens nucleus, runs forward along its medial side, and loops again over the rostral end of the nucleus. The fibers then proceed to the point of emergence of the motor root of the facial nerve by passing between the nucleus of origin and the spinal trigeminal nucleus. The configuration of the fiber bundle around the abducens nucleus is called the **internal genu**. (The external genu of the facial nerve is in the facial canal at the level of the geniculate ganglion.)

The explanation for the course of facial motor fibers in the pons is based on a migration of cells in the embryo. It has been suggested that neurons destined to form the abducens and facial nuclei are intermingled at an early embryonic stage. The facial neurons subsequently move in a ventrolateral direction under the influence of the spinal trigeminal tract and its nucleus. Concurrently the abducens neurons move dorsomedially toward the medial longitudinal fasciculus. The fibers extending from the facial nucleus to the region of the abducens nucleus indicate the direction and extent of the change in position of the nuclei during embryonic development. Such shifts in position of groups of nerve cells during development are said to be the result of **neurobiotaxis**, a term introduced by Ariëns Kappers in 1914 to indicate the tendency of neurons to migrate toward major sources of stimuli.

The motor root of the facial nerve consists entirely of fibers from the motor nucleus. They supply the muscles of expression (mimetic muscles), the platysma and stylohyoid muscles, and the posterior belly of the digastric muscle. The facial nerve also supplies the stapedius muscle of the middle ear; by reflex contraction in response to loud sounds, this small muscle prevents excessive movement of the stapes.

The facial motor nucleus receives afferents from several sources, including important connections for reflexes. Tectobulbar fibers from the superior colliculus complete a reflex pathway that provides for closure of the eyelids in response to intense light or a rapidly approaching object. Fibers from trigeminal sensory nuclei function in the corneal reflex and in chewing or sucking responses on placing food in the mouth. Fibers from the superior olivary nucleus on the auditory pathway permit reflex contraction of the stapedius muscle.

Corticobulbar afferents are crossed, except for those that terminate on cells supplying the frontalis and orbicularis oculi muscles, which receive both crossed and uncrossed fibers. *Contralateral voluntary paralysis of only the lower facial muscles is therefore a feature of upper motor neuron lesions.* Under such circumstances, however, the facial muscles continue to respond involuntarily, and often excessively, to changing moods and emotions. Emotional changes of facial expression are typically lost in Parkinson's disease (mask-like face), although voluntary use of the facial muscles is retained. The neuroanatomical basis for the two types of control of facial movement is not known.

PARASYMPATHETIC NUCLEI

The **superior salivatory** and **lacrimal nuclei** consist of indefinite clusters of small cells, partly intermingled, that are medial to the facial motor nucleus (see Fig. 8-9). The positions of these nuclei in the human brain are not known with certainty. They contain the cell bodies of preganglionic neurons for the submandibular and sublingual salivary glands and for the lacrimal gland. Fibers from the nuclei leave the brain stem in the nervus intermedius and continue in the facial nerve until branches are given off in the facial canal in the petrous temporal bone. The fibers follow devious routes to their destinations, running part of the way in branches of the trigeminal nerve (see Fig. 8-10). Briefly stated, fibers from the superior salivatory nucleus leave the facial nerve in the chorda tympani branch and join the lingual branch of the mandibular nerve to reach the floor of the oral cavity. There they terminate in the **submandibular ganglion** and on scattered neurons within the submandibular gland. Short postganglionic fibers are distributed to the parenchyma of the submandibular and sublingual glands, where they stimulate secretion and cause vasodilation.

Fibers from the lacrimal nucleus leave the facial nerve in the greater petrosal branch and terminate in the **pterygopalatine ganglion** (also called the sphenopalatine ganglion) located in the pterygopalatine fossa. Postganglionic fibers for the stimulation of secretion and vasodilation reach the lacrimal gland through the zygomatic branch of the maxillary nerve. Other secretomotor postganglionic fibers are distributed to mucous glands in the mucosa that lines the nasal cavity and the paranasal sinuses.

The superior salivatory nucleus comes under the influence of the hypothalamus, perhaps through the dorsal longitudinal fasciculus, and of the olfactory system through relays in the reticular formation. Data from taste buds and from the mucosa of the oral cavity are received by way of the solitary nucleus and sensory trigeminal nuclei, respectively. The chief sources of impulses to the lacrimal nucleus are presumed to be the hypothalamus for emotional responses and the spinal trigeminal nucleus for lacrimation caused by irritation of the cornea and conjunctiva.

Clinical Considerations

A facial paralysis commonly accompanies hemiplegia caused by occlusion of an artery supplying the contralateral internal capsule or motor cortex. For reasons already stated, only the lower half of the face is affected. When a unilateral facial paralysis involves the musculature around the eyes and in the forehead in addition to that around the mouth, the lesion must involve either the cell bodies in the facial nucleus or their axons. In a common condition known as **Bell's palsy**, the facial nerve is affected as it traverses the facial canal in the petrous temporal bone, with rapid onset of weakness (paresis) or paralysis of the facial muscles on the affected side. The cause is edema (perhaps due to a viral infection) of the facial nerve and adjacent tissue in the facial canal. The signs of Bell's palsy depend not only on the severity of the axonal compression, but also on where the nerve is affected in its passage through the facial canal (see Fig. 8-10). All functions of the nerve are lost if the damage is proximal to the geniculate ganglion. In addition to the paralysis of facial muscles, there is a loss of taste in the anterior two-thirds of the tongue and in the palate of the affected side, together with impairment of secretion by the submandibular, sublingual, and lacrimal glands. Also, sounds seem abnormally loud (hyperacusis) because of paralysis of the stapedius muscle.

In mild cases, the nerve fibers are not damaged severely enough to result in wallerian degeneration, and the prognosis is favorable. Recovery is slow and frequently incomplete when it must rely on nerve fiber regeneration. There is no regeneration into the brain stem of sensory fibers that have been interrupted on the central side of the geniculate ganglion. In the case of such a lesion in the proximal part of the nerve, some regenerating salivatory fibers may find their way into the greater petrosal nerve and reach the pterygopalatine ganglion. This results in lacrimation (crocodile tears) when aromas and taste sensations cause stimulation of cells in the superior salivatory nucleus. When the nerve is affected in the distal part of the facial canal after the greater petrosal and chorda tympani branches are given off, the condition is limited to paresis or paralysis of both the upper and the lower facial muscles on the side of the lesion.

Glossopharyngeal, Vagus, and Accessory Nerves

The ninth, tenth, and eleventh cranial nerves have much in common functionally and share certain nuclei in the medulla. To avoid repetition, it is convenient to consider them together.

Afferent Components

The glossopharyngeal and vagus nerves include sensory fibers for the special visceral sense of taste from the posterior one-third of the tongue, pharynx, and epiglottis, together with general visceral afferents from the carotid sinus, carotid body, and viscera of the thorax and abdomen. There are also general sensory fibers for pain, temperature, and touch from the mucosa of the back of the tongue, from the pharynx and nearby regions, from the skin of part of the ear, and from parts of the dura mater. The cell bodies of primary sensory neurons are in the superior and inferior ganglia[4] of the ninth and tenth cranial nerves.

---

[4] Commonly used alternative names for the vagal sensory ganglia are the **nodose ganglion** (= inferior ganglion) and the **jugular ganglion** (superior ganglion). The old name **petrosal ganglion** applied strictly to the inferior glossopharyngeal ganglion, but sometimes it is used to include both the ganglia of the ninth cranial nerve, which do not differ in their functional connections.

VISCERAL AFFERENTS

The cell bodies for the **gustatory fibers** are in the glossopharyngeal ganglia and in the inferior ganglion of the vagus nerve. The fibers are distributed through the glossopharyngeal nerve to taste buds on the back of the tongue as well as to the few that occur in the pharyngeal mucosa. Vagal fibers supply taste buds on the epiglottis; these are unimportant because few persist into adult life. Central processes of the ganglion cells join the solitary tract and terminate in the rostral portion of the solitary nucleus—the gustatory nucleus (Fig. 8-11).

General visceral afferent neurons receive signals used for reflex regulation of cardiovascular, respiratory, and alimentary function. Their cell bodies are in the glossopharyngeal and inferior vagal ganglia, together with the neurons for taste. These fibers in the glossopharyngeal nerve supply the carotid sinus at the bifurcation of the common carotid artery, and the adjacent carotid body. Nerve endings in the wall of the carotid sinus function as baroreceptors, which monitor arterial blood pressure. The carotid body contains chemoreceptors, which monitor the concentration of oxygen in the circulating blood. Vagal fibers similarly supply baroreceptors in the aortic arch and chemoreceptors in the small aortic bodies adjacent to the arch. The vagus nerve contains many afferent fibers that are distributed to the viscera of the thorax and abdomen; impulses conveyed centrally are important in reflex control of cardiovascular, respiratory, and alimentary functions. The central processes of the primary sensory neurons for these reflexes descend in the solitary tract and end in the more caudal part of its nucleus (see Fig. 8-12). Connections from the latter site are established bilaterally with several regions of the reticular formation. Reticulobulbar and reticulospinal connections provide pathways for reflex responses mediated by parasympathetic and sympathetic efferents.

Some axons from the solitary nucleus proceed rostrally to the hypothalamus. Others probably go to the ventral posteromedial nucleus of the thalamus for conscious sensations

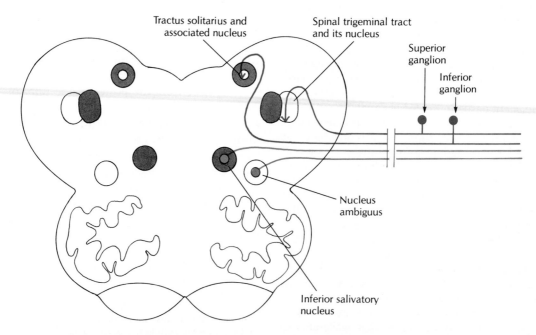

Figure 8-11. Components of the glossopharyngeal nerve in the medulla. (Primary sensory neurons are blue; motor neurons are red; preganglionic parasympathetic neurons are green.)

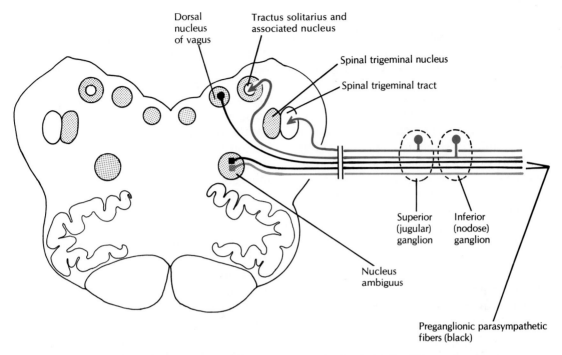

Figure 8-12. Components of the vagus nerve in the medulla. (Primary sensory neurons are blue; motor neurons are red; preganglionic parasympathetic neurons are black.)

other than pain, such as fullness or emptiness of the stomach. Still others constitute the small solitariospinal tract, which terminates on preganglionic autonomic neurons in the spinal cord.

OTHER AFFERENT FIBERS

The glossopharyngeal nerve includes fibers for the general sensations of pain, temperature, and touch in the mucosa of the posterior one-third of the tongue, upper part of the pharynx (including the tonsillar area), auditory or eustachian tube, and middle ear. The vagus nerve carries fibers with the same functions to the lower part of the pharynx, the larynx, and the esophagus. The cell bodies of these sensory neurons are in the glossopharyngeal ganglia and the superior ganglion of the vagus nerve. Their central processes enter the spinal trigeminal tract and terminate in its nucleus (see Figs. 8-11 and 8-12). The afferents for touch from the pharynx are important in the **gag reflex**, through a pathway that includes the

nucleus ambiguus and the hypoglossal nucleus.

The vagus nerve sends general sensory (pain) fibers to the dura mater that lines the posterior fossa of the cranial cavity. Through its auricular branch, it contributes sensory fibers to the concha of the external ear, a small area behind the ear, the wall of the external acoustic meatus, and the tympanic membrane. The cell bodies are in the superior ganglion of the nerve, and the central processes join the spinal trigeminal tract. The area of skin and tympanic membrane supplied by the auricular branch of the vagus nerve is coextensive with that supplied by the facial nerve.

Efferent Components

The ninth, tenth, and eleventh cranial nerves include motor fibers for striated muscles, and the ninth and tenth nerves contain parasympathetic efferents.

FOR SUPPLY OF STRIATED MUSCLES

The **nucleus ambiguus** is a slender column of motor neurons situated dorsal to the inferior olivary nucleus (Fig. 8-13; see also Figs. 8-11 and 8-12). Fibers from the nucleus are directed dorsally at first. They then turn sharply to mingle with other fibers in the glossopharyngeal and vagus nerves, and some of them constitute the entire cranial root of the accessory nerve. The nucleus ambiguus supplies muscles of the soft palate, pharynx, and larynx, together with striated muscle fibers in the upper part of the esophagus. (The only muscle in these regions not supplied by this nucleus is the tensor veli palatini muscle, which is innervated by the trigeminal nerve.)

A small group of cells in the rostral end of the nucleus ambiguus supplies the stylopharyngeus muscle through the glossopharyngeal nerve (see Fig. 8-11). A large region of the nucleus supplies the remaining pharyngeal muscles, the cricothyroid muscle (an external muscle of the larynx), and the striated muscle of the esophagus through the vagus nerve (see Fig. 8-12). Fibers from the caudal part of the nucleus leave the brain stem in the **cranial root of the accessory nerve** (see Fig. 8-13). They join the spinal root of the accessory nerve temporarily and then constitute the internal ramus of the nerve, which passes over to the vagus nerve in the region of the jugular foramen (Fig. 8-14). These fibers supply muscles of the soft palate and the intrinsic muscles of the larynx. (It would be simpler, although contrary to convention, to consider the cranial root of the accessory nerve as part of the vagus nerve, leaving the spinal root as the definitive accessory nerve.)

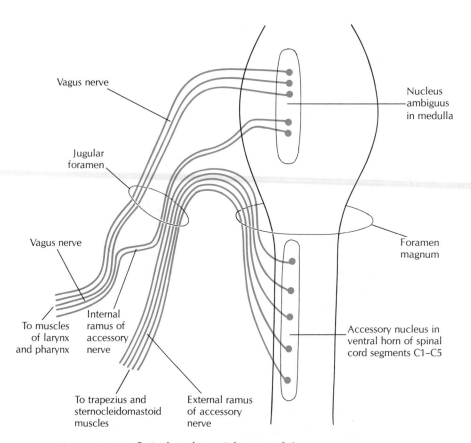

Figure 8-13. Spinal and cranial roots of the accessory nerve.

The nucleus ambiguus receives afferents from sensory nuclei of the brain stem, most importantly from the spinal trigeminal nucleus and from the solitary nucleus. These connections establish reflexes for coughing, gagging, and vomiting, with the stimuli arising in the mucosa of the respiratory and alimentary passages. Corticobulbar afferents are both crossed and uncrossed; muscles supplied by the nucleus ambiguus are, therefore, not paralyzed in the event of a unilateral lesion of the upper motor neuron type.

The nucleus ambiguus is not composed solely of motor neurons. As described further on, some of its cells are preganglionic parasympathetic neurons for control of the heart rate.

Motor neurons for the sternocleidomastoid and trapezius muscles differentiate in the embryo near cells that are destined to form the nucleus ambiguus. The former cells migrate into the spinal cord (segments C1 to C5) and become the **accessory nucleus** in the lateral part of the ventral gray horn. Arising as a series of rootlets along the side of the cord, just dorsal to the denticulate ligament, the **spinal root of the accessory nerve** ascends next to the spinal cord, thus retracing the migration of its cells of origin (see Fig. 8-13). On reaching the side of the medulla by passing through the foramen magnum, the spinal and cranial roots unite and continue as the accessory nerve as far as the jugular foramen. Fibers from the nucleus ambiguus then join the vagus nerve, as already noted, and those of spinal origin proceed to the sternocleidomastoid and trapezius muscles. Corticospinal fibers that control the spinal accessory neurons are almost all crossed. There is, therefore, contralateral weakness (paresis) of the sternocleidomastoid and trapezius muscles if an upper motor neuron lesion is present.

PARASYMPATHETIC NUCLEI

There are parasympathetic fibers in the glossopharyngeal and vagus nerves. The **inferior salivatory nucleus** is a small collection of cells caudal to the superior salivatory nucleus and probably near the rostral tip of the nucleus ambiguus (see Fig. 8-11). (Its exact location in the human brain is uncertain.) Fibers from the inferior salivatory nucleus are included in the glossopharyngeal nerve, enter its tympanic branch, and reach the **otic ganglion** by way of the tympanic plexus and the lesser petrosal nerve. Postganglionic fibers join the auriculotemporal branch of the mandibular nerve and thus reach the parotid gland. The parasympathetic supply to the parotid gland is secretomotor and vasodilatory. The inferior salivatory nucleus is influenced by stimuli from the hypothalamus, olfactory system, solitary nucleus, and sensory trigeminal nuclei.

The largest parasympathetic nucleus is the **dorsal nucleus of the vagus nerve** (also called "dorsal motor nucleus," but it does not directly innervate muscles). This column of cells is in the gray matter around the central canal and beneath the vagal triangle in the floor of the fourth ventricle. The axons of the cells in the dorsal nucleus constitute the majority of the preganglionic parasympathetic fibers of the vagus nerve. They end in the pulmonary plexus and in abdominal viscera, mostly in the myenteric and submucous plexuses of the alimentary canal (see Ch. 24).

Other vagal parasympathetic neurons have their cell bodies in the **nucleus ambiguus**. The axons of these neurons terminate in small ganglia associated with the heart. In some laboratory animals, about 10% of the cardioinhibitory neurons are in the dorsal nucleus of the vagus. In others, the cardiac ganglia receive all their afferent fibers from the nucleus ambiguus and none from the dorsal nucleus. It seems likely that the nucleus ambiguus contains most or all of the vagal neurons that control the human heart.

The dorsal nucleus of the vagus nerve and the visceral efferent neurons of the nucleus ambiguus are influenced, directly or indirectly, by the hypothalamus, the olfactory system, autonomic "centers" in the reticular formation, and the solitary nucleus.

Isolated lesions that involve the ninth, tenth, or eleventh cranial nerves separately are uncommon. Vascular occlusions, however,

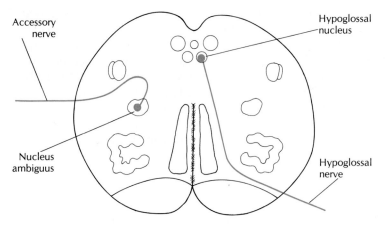

Figure 8-14. Hypoglossal nerve and origin of the cranial root of the accessory nerve in the medulla.

can destroy the central nuclei. A unilateral lesion of the nucleus ambiguus, for example, results in ipsilateral paralysis of the soft palate, pharynx, and larynx, with the expected signs of hoarseness and difficulty in breathing and swallowing. Medullary lesions typically involve long sensory or motor pathways as well as cranial nerve nuclei (see Ch. 7).

Hypoglossal Nerve

The **hypoglossal nucleus** lies between the dorsal nucleus of the vagus nerve and the midline of the medulla (Fig. 8-14). The hypoglossal triangle in the floor of the fourth ventricle marks the position of the rostral part of the nucleus. Fibers from the hypoglossal nucleus course ventrally on the lateral side of the medial lemniscus and emerge along the sulcus between the pyramid and the olive. The hypoglossal nerve supplies the intrinsic muscles of the tongue and the three extrinsic muscles (genioglossus, styloglossus, and hyoglossus). The nucleus receives afferents from the solitary nucleus and the sensory trigeminal nuclei for reflex movements of the tongue in swallowing, chewing, and sucking in response to gustatory and other stimuli from the oral and pharyngeal mucosae.

Corticobulbar afferents are predominantly crossed; a unilateral upper motor neuron lesion, therefore, causes paresis of the opposite side of the tongue.[5] Paralysis and eventual atrophy of the affected muscles follow destruction of the hypoglossal nucleus or interruption of the nerve. The tongue *deviates to the weak side* on protrusion because of the unopposed action of the contralateral genioglossus muscle.

Sensory Nerve Supply of Neuromuscular Spindles

The striated skeletal muscles supplied by cranial nerves all execute movements that are delicately controlled. Proprioceptive input is therefore physiologically important. The following account is based on the results of animal experimentation; there is no reliable information relating to humans.

Extraocular Muscles

The extraocular muscles contain spindles of a special type. Their sensory fibers in the ophthalmic nerve come from neurons in the trigeminal ganglion with axons that terminate in the pars interpolaris of the spinal trigeminal nucleus. Although eye movements are guided principally

[5] Usually, only corticobulbar fibers are mentioned when discussing upper motor neuron lesions and their effects on muscles supplied by cranial nerves. In fact, voluntary control of the musculature is mediated also through pathways from the cortex that include the reticular formation. Corticoreticular as well as corticobulbar fibers are interrupted in a typical upper motor neuron lesion.

by visual stimuli, experiments with human volunteers have shown that passive movement of one eye causes misjudgment of direction by the other eye, indicating that proprioception is necessary for accurate binocular vision.

Masticatory and Facial Muscles

Sensory fibers that originate in the mesencephalic nucleus of the trigeminal nerve supply neuromuscular spindles in muscles innervated by the mandibular division, together with other proprioceptors associated with the muscles of mastication and pressure-sensitive endings adjacent to the teeth and in the hard palate. However, cell bodies for afferents from the temporomandibular joint have been traced to the trigeminal ganglion.

The presence of spindles in the facial muscles has not been conclusively established.

Muscles Supplied by Cranial
Nerves IX, X and XI

Sensory fibers in laryngeal muscles have been identified in the vagus nerve; the cell bodies must be in a ganglion of the vagus nerve because innervated spindles persist after section of the nerve proximal to the ganglia. Proprioceptors in the sternocleidomastoid and trapezius muscles receive sensory fibers through the second, third, and fourth cervical nerves, which provide the muscles with innervation additional to that from the accessory nerve.

The Tongue

Some of the cell bodies of sensory neurons that supply spindles in the tongue are in the inferior ganglion of the vagus nerve, with the fibers passing over to the hypoglossal nerve through an anastomotic connection. The muscles of the tongue also receive proprioceptive fibers from cells in dorsal root ganglia of the second and third cervical nerves. They enter the hypoglossal nerve through the ansa hypoglossi in the anterior triangle of the neck.

Classification of Cranial and Spinal Nerve Components

The components, including associated sensory, motor, and autonomic nuclei, of the cranial and spinal nerves can be classified under seven headings. Four components are present in spinal nerves; three more are added to include the special senses and to recognize the different embryonic origins of the muscles of the head. Cranial nerve nuclei in the brain stem are shown in Figure 8-15 according to the following classification, which is based on the classic embryological and comparative anatomical studies of C. J. Herrick.

Afferent Components

The **special somatic afferent** group consists of those special senses that relate the body to the external environment. This group consists of the optic nerve (included by convention) and the cochlear and vestibular nuclei.

General somatic afferent nuclei receive impulses from general sensory endings and are, therefore, concerned with pain, temperature, touch, and proprioception. The cells are in the dorsal gray horn of the spinal cord, the gracile and cuneate nuclei, and the sensory trigeminal nuclei.

Special visceral afferents are for taste, with second-order neurons in the rostral part of the solitary nucleus (gustatory nucleus). The olfactory nerves are conventionally considered as special visceral afferent because of the influence of smell on visceral functions.

General visceral afferent components are for visceral reflexes and for sensations such as fullness of hollow organs and pain of visceral origin. The second-order neurons are in the dorsal gray horn of the spinal cord and the caudal portion of the solitary nucleus.

Efferent Components

Motor neurons included under the heading of **general somatic efferents** supply muscles derived from myotomes of the embryonic somites. They are in the ventral horn of the spinal cord and in the oculomotor, trochlear, abducens, and hypoglossal nuclei.

Special visceral efferents supply muscles derived from the branchial arches of the embryo. They are classified as "visceral" because of the respiratory function of the analogous gill arches in aquatic forms. There are three special visceral efferent nuclei: the trigeminal motor nucleus for the muscles of mastication, which develop from the first branchial arch; the facial

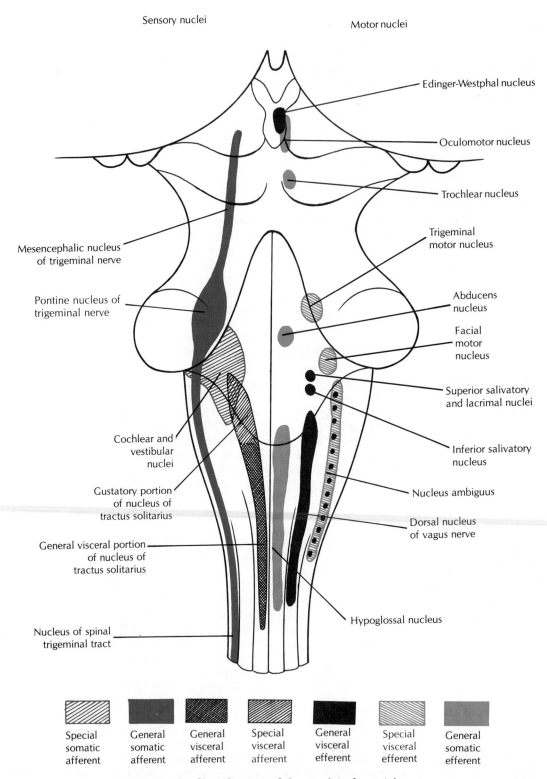

Sensory nuclei

Motor nuclei

Edinger-Westphal nucleus

Oculomotor nucleus

Trochlear nucleus

Mesencephalic nucleus
of trigeminal nerve

Trigeminal
motor nucleus

Pontine nucleus of
trigeminal nerve

Abducens
nucleus

Facial
motor
nucleus

Superior salivatory
and lacrimal nuclei

Cochlear and
vestibular
nuclei

Inferior salivatory
nucleus

Gustatory portion
of nucleus of
tractus solitarius

Nucleus ambiguus

Dorsal nucleus
of vagus nerve

General visceral portion
of nucleus of
tractus solitarius

Hypoglossal nucleus

Nucleus of spinal
trigeminal tract

| Special somatic afferent | General somatic afferent | General visceral afferent | Special visceral afferent | General visceral efferent | Special visceral efferent | General somatic efferent |

Figure 8-15. Classification of the nuclei of cranial nerves.

motor nucleus for the muscles of expression, of second branchial arch derivation; and the nucleus ambiguus for muscles of the palate, pharynx, larynx, and upper esophagus, with these muscles being derived from the third, fourth, and fifth branchial arches. The spinal accessory nucleus, because of its embryonic origin mentioned earlier in this chapter, is also usually included in the special visceral efferent category.

General visceral efferents are the preganglionic neurons of the autonomic nervous system. In the spinal cord, they include the intermediolateral cell column in the thoracic and upper lumbar segments and the parasympathetic cells in the sacral cord. In the brain stem, this category consists of the Edinger-Westphal nucleus, lacrimal nucleus, superior and inferior salivatory nuclei, dorsal nucleus of the vagus nerve, and some of the cells in the nucleus ambiguus.

Centrifugal fibers in the vestibulocochlear nerve (see Chs. 21 and 22) and in the optic nerves of some animals are not included in the classical list of components because they were not known at the time the classification was devised. The name **special somatic efferent** is appropriate for efferent axons that modify the activities of the special sensory receptors.

SUGGESTED READING

Bender MB: Brain control of conjugate horizontal and vertical eye movements. A survey of the structural and functional correlates. Brain 103: 23–69, 1980

Büttner-Ennever JA (ed): Neuroanatomy of the Oculomotor System. Reviews of Oculomotor Research, vol 2. Amsterdam, Elsevier, 1988

Cruccu G, Berardelli A, Inghilleri M, Manfredi M: Corticobulbar projections to upper and lower facial motoneurons. A study by magnetic transcranial stimulation in man. Neurosci Lett 117: 68–73, 1990

Davies AM, Lumsden A: Ontogeny of the somatosensory system: Origins and early development of primary sensory neurons. Annu Rev Neurosci 13:61–73, 1990

FitzGerald MJT, Sachithanandan SR: The structure and source of lingual proprioceptors in the monkey. J Anat 128:523–552, 1979

Gauthier GM, Nommay D, Vercher JL: Ocular muscle proprioception and visual localization of targets in man. Brain 113:1857–1871, 1990

Hamilton RB, Pritchard TC, Norgren R: Central distribution of the cervical vagus nerve in Old and New World primates. J Auton Nerv Syst 19: 153–169, 1987

Ito S, Ogawa H: Cytochrome oxidase staining facilitates unequivocal visualization of the primary gustatory area in the fronto-operculo-insular cortex of macaque monkeys. Neurosci Lett 130: 61–64, 1991

Jenny A, Smith A, Decker J: Motor organization of the spinal accessory nerve in the monkey. Brain Res 441:352–356, 1988

Keller EL, Heinen SJ: Generation of smooth pursuit eye movements: Neuronal mechanisms and pathways. Neurosci Res 11:79–107, 1991

MacAvoy MG, Gottlieb JP, Bruce CJ: Smooth pursuit eye movement representation in the primate frontal eye field. Cerebral Cortex 1:95–102, 1991

May M (ed): The Facial Nerve. New York, Thieme, 1986

Norgren R: Gustatory system. In Paxinos G (ed): The Human Nervous System, pp 845–861. San Diego, Academic Press, 1990

O'Rahilly R: On counting cranial nerves. Acta Anat 133:3–4, 1988

Plecha DM, Randall WC, Geis GS, Wurster RD: Localization of vagal preganglionic somata controlling sinoatrial and atrioventricular nodes. Am J Physiol 255:R703–R708, 1988

Porter JD: Brainstem terminations of extraocular muscle primary afferent neurons in the monkey. J Comp Neurol 247:133–143, 1986

Ruskell GL, Simons T: Trigeminal nerve pathways to the cerebral arteries in monkeys. J Anat 155:23–37, 1987

Wilson-Pauwels L, Akesson EJ, Stewart PA: Cranial Nerves. Anatomy and Clinical Comments. Toronto, BC Dekker, 1988

Nine

The Human Nervous System: An Anatomical Viewpoint, Sixth Edition, Murray L. Barr and John A. Kiernan. J.B. Lippincott Company, Philadelphia, © 1993.

Reticular Formation

Important Facts

The reticular formation of the brain stem contains several populations of neurons with long dendrites surrounded by interlacing bundles of nerve fibers.

The precerebellar reticular nuclei are probably concerned with coordination of muscle contractions.

The raphe nuclei include many serotonergic neurons, with extensively distributed axons. Rostrally projecting serotonergic neurons are active in sleep. Caudally projecting neurons, which receive afferents from the periaqueductal gray matter, modulate pain sensation.

The central group of nuclei includes the cells of origin of motor reticulospinal fibers. Rostral projections are concerned with eye movements and, possibly, with the conscious state.

Cholinergic reticular nuclei influence stereotyped movements through connections with the central group and the basal ganglia of the forebrain.

Catecholaminergic neurons in the locus coeruleus and elsewhere have axons that go to most parts of the brain and spinal cord, probably to increase the speed of reflex responses and the general level of alertness.

Through connections with appropriate sensory, motor, and autonomic neurons, the laterally located parvocellular, parabrachial, and superficial medullary reticular areas are concerned with the regulation of feeding and of the respiratory and circulatory systems.

The area postrema, which contains permeable blood vessels, is a chemoreceptor that mediates some physiological responses to blood-borne stimuli, including drug-induced vomiting.

The paramedian pontine reticular formation, the perihypoglossal nuclei, and the accessory oculomotor nuclei are involved in the control of eye movements.

This chapter describes the anatomy and connections of the groups of neurons that constitute the reticular formation of the brain stem and reviews the involvement of the reticular formation in sleep and consciousness as well as in sensory and motor functions. There are also descriptions of a few other nuclei in the brain stem that were not discussed in Chapters 7 and 8.

Broadly defined, the **reticular formation** consists of a substantial portion of the dorsal part of the brain stem in which the groups of neurons and intersecting bundles of fibers present a netlike (reticular) appearance in transverse sections. It excludes nuclei of cranial nerves, long tracts that pass through the brain stem, and the more conspicuous masses of gray matter. Some "excluded" structures, however, such as the medial lemniscus and the nucleus ambiguus, are located within the territory of the reticular formation. The neurons of the reticular nuclei all have unusually long dendrites that extend into parts of the brain stem remote from the cell bodies. Their architecture enables them to receive and integrate synaptic inputs from most or all of the axons that project to or through the brain stem.

Through its direct and indirect connections with all levels of the central nervous system, the reticular formation contributes to several functions, including the sleep–arousal cycle, perception of pain, control of movement, and regulation of visceral activity. Although such adjectives as "primitive" and "diffuse" have been applied to the reticular formation, it is not a mass of randomly interconnected neurons. The parts of the reticular formation differ from one another in their cytoarchitecture, connections, and physiological functions. Aggregations of neurons are thereby recognized, and are called nuclei even though not all are as clearly circumscribed as nuclei elsewhere. As in every part of the nervous system, information obtained through research continues to reveal higher and higher degrees of orderly structural organization than were previously thought to exist.

Nuclei of the Reticular Formation

The nuclei of the reticular formation (Figs. 9-1 and 9-2) can be classified as follows: the precerebellar nuclei, the raphe nuclei, the central group of nuclei, cholinergic and catecholamine cell groups, the lateral parvocellular reticular area, the parabrachial area, and the superficial medullary neurons. There are also functionally designated "centers," recognized mainly from experiments in animals, that do not always correspond to anatomically defined populations of neuronal cell bodies.

PRECEREBELLAR RETICULAR NUCLEI

The lateral reticular nucleus (see Figs. 9-1 and 9-2A), the paramedian reticular nucleus (see Fig. 9-2A), and the pontine reticulotegmental nucleus (see Fig. 9-1) project to the cerebellum. These, the precerebellar reticular nuclei are functionally quite separate from the rest of the reticular formation; they are, therefore, considered in Chapter 10, which deals with the cerebellum.

RAPHE NUCLEI

The raphe nuclei are in the midline of the brain stem. The cells are interspersed among bundles of decussating axons, which are the most conspicuous feature of the raphe in sections stained for myelin. The raphe nuclei form a contiguous column, but individual nuclei with different cytoarchitecture and efferent projections are recognized at different levels. Some of these are named in Figures 9-1 and 9-2. Many of the raphe neurons have been shown by histochemical methods to synthesize and secrete serotonin (5-hydroxytryptamine), and this amine is believed to be their principal synaptic transmitter. Hardly anything is known of the connections of those raphe neurons that do not synthesize serotonin. The axons of the serotonergic raphe neurons are fine, unmyelinated, and greatly branched. They are distributed to gray matter throughout the central nervous system. The projections mentioned below are the most prominent (Fig. 9-3).

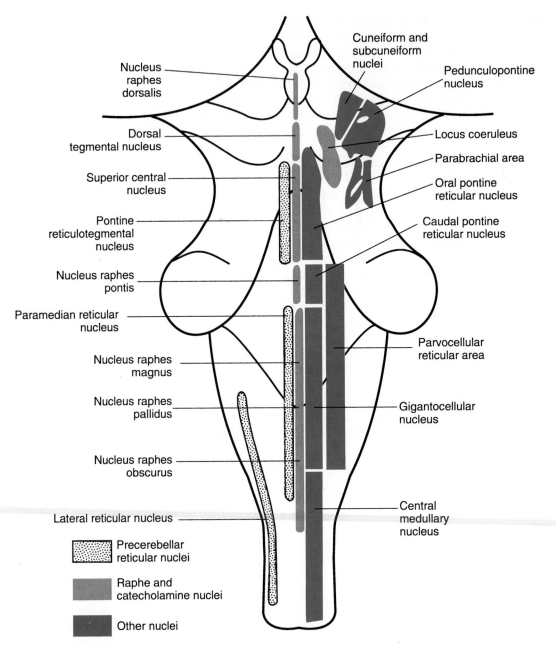

Figure 9-1. Diagram showing the positions of the larger nuclei of the reticular formation of the brain stem.

The **medullary raphe nuclei** (nucleus raphes magnus, nucleus raphes pallidus, and nucleus raphes obscurus)[1] receive afferents from the spinal cord, the gracile and cuneate nuclei, the trigeminal sensory nuclei, and the periaqueductal gray matter. They project to the cerebellum, to the dorsal and ventral horns of the spinal gray matter, to the trigeminal nuclei, and to the preganglionic autonomic neurons

---

[1] For a note on the terminology of nuclei of the raphe, look up **raphe** in the Glossary.

of the brain stem and cord. The input from the periaqueductal gray matter and the projection to the spinal dorsal horn are important from a clinical standpoint because activity of this pathway can suppress the conscious awareness of pain.

Afferents to the **raphe nuclei of the midbrain and rostral pons** (nucleus raphes pontis, superior central nucleus, nucleus raphes dorsalis, and dorsal tegmental nucleus) include fibers from the prefrontal cortex and from several components of the limbic system (see Ch. 18), including the hippocampal formation, the hypothalamus, the interpeduncular nucleus, and the ventral tegmental area. The axons of the neurons in the rostral raphe nuclei extend to all parts of the forebrain, to the cerebellum, and to the noradrenergic nuclei of the brain stem.

The best understood functions of the raphe nuclei are those related to pain and sleep. They are discussed later in this chapter.

CENTRAL GROUP OF RETICULAR NUCLEI

The central group of reticular nuclei includes the central medullary nucleus and the gigantocellular nucleus[2] in the medulla, the caudal and oral pontine reticular nuclei, and the cuneiform and subcuneiform nuclei in the midbrain (see Figs. 9-1 and 9-2). The latter two are laterally located but are included in the central

(text continues on page 154)

---

[2] The nuclei of the reticular formation have been given many names. We use those that seem to be in current use. The central medullary nucleus (formally known as the nucleus centralis medullae oblongatae) also is called the ventral reticular nucleus. The gigantocellular nucleus also is known as the gigantocellular reticular nucleus and as the magnocellular reticular nucleus.

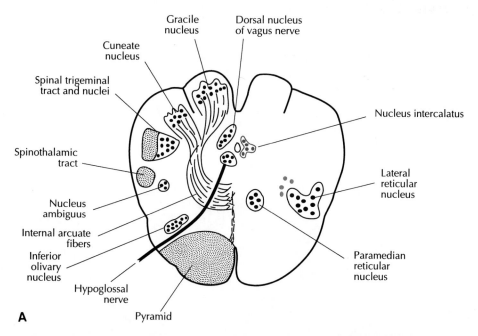

Figure 9-2. Diagrammatic transverse sections of the brain stem. The left side of each figure shows nuclei and tracts that are major anatomical landmarks. The right side shows the positions of reticular and other nuclei discussed in this chapter. *Black dots* (•) indicate precerebellar nuclei; *red dots* indicate groups of serotonin- (raphe nuclei) and catecholamine-containing nuclei; *blue dots* are for other nuclei. (**A**) Nuclei at the level of the caudal pole of the inferior olivary nucleus. (The unlabeled red dots indicate scattered adrenergic neurons.)

(continued)

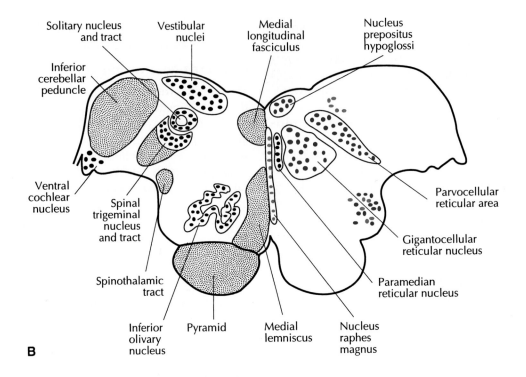

B

Labels in panel B:
- Solitary nucleus and tract
- Vestibular nuclei
- Medial longitudinal fasciculus
- Nucleus prepositus hypoglossi
- Inferior cerebellar peduncle
- Ventral cochlear nucleus
- Spinal trigeminal nucleus and tract
- Spinothalamic tract
- Inferior olivary nucleus
- Pyramid
- Medial lemniscus
- Nucleus raphes magnus
- Paramedian reticular nucleus
- Gigantocellular reticular nucleus
- Parvocellular reticular area

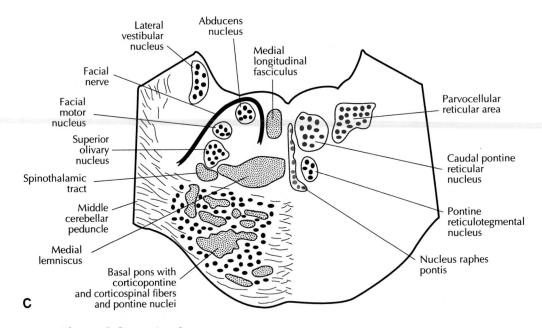

C

Labels in panel C:
- Lateral vestibular nucleus
- Abducens nucleus
- Medial longitudinal fasciculus
- Facial nerve
- Facial motor nucleus
- Superior olivary nucleus
- Spinothalamic tract
- Middle cerebellar peduncle
- Medial lemniscus
- Basal pons with corticopontine and corticospinal fibers and pontine nuclei
- Parvocellular reticular area
- Caudal pontine reticular nucleus
- Pontine reticulotegmental nucleus
- Nucleus raphes pontis

Figure 9-2. *(continued)*
(B) Nuclei at the level of the rostral pole of the inferior olivary nucleus. (The unlabeled red dots indicate groups of noradrenergic and adrenergic neurons. The blue dots dorsolateral to the inferior olivary nucleus indicate the probable position of the ventral superficial reticular area of the medulla.) **(C)** Nuclei in the pontine tegmentum at the level of the internal genu of the facial nerve.

(continued)

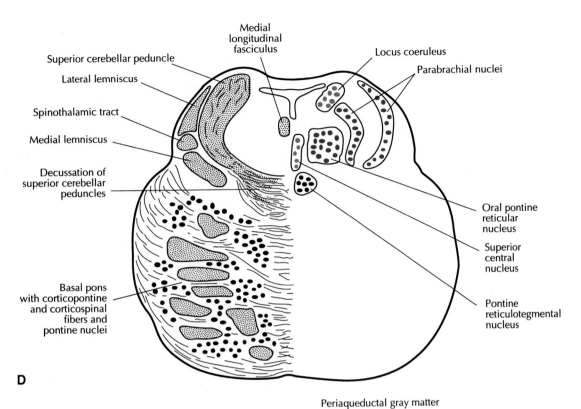

D

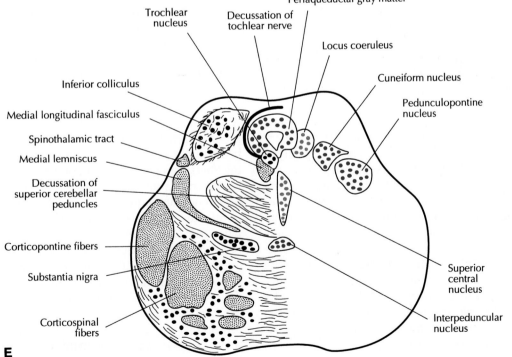

E

Figure 9-2. (*continued*)
(D) Pontine tegmentum at a level rostral to the motor trigeminal nucleus.
(E) Nuclei at the level of the caudal pole of the inferior colliculus.

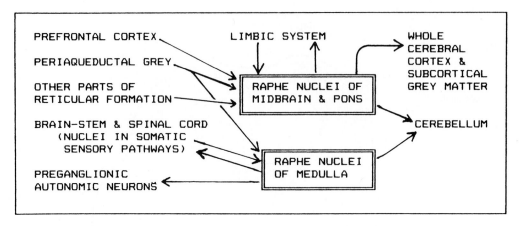

Figure 9-3. Major connections of the serotonergic raphe nuclei. (*With permission from Kiernan JA: Some functional pathways in the central nervous system. In Kelley WN (ed): Textbook of Internal Medicine, 2nd ed, pp 2138–2145. Philadelphia, JB Lippincott, 1992.*)

group because of their similar connections and functions. The paramedian pontine reticular formation (PPRF), which is importantly involved in conjugate lateral movements of the eyes (see Ch. 8), includes neurons of both pontine reticular nuclei.

The central nuclei receive **afferents from sensory systems**: these include the spinoreticular tracts, collateral branches from the spinothalamic and trigeminothalamic tracts, and collateral branches of ascending axons of the gustatory and auditory systems. Tectoreticular fibers from the superior colliculus provide input from the visual system. Olfactory stimulation has been shown by physiological methods to evoke activity in the reticular formation, possibly mediated by fibers that descend from olfactory areas of the cerebral cortex. Thus all the general and special sensory pathways contribute synaptic inputs to the neurons of the central group of reticular nuclei. **Other afferent fibers** come from the fastigial nucleus of the vestibulocerebellum, the reticular formation of the midbrain, the cholinergic reticular nuclei (see below), the hypothalamus, and the premotor area of the cerebral cortex (Fig. 9-4).

Neurons of the central reticular nuclei typically have axons with long ascending and de-scending branches. In the brain stem, these axons also have numerous horizontally directed collateral branches, which synapse with the long dendrites of other reticular neurons (Fig. 9-5), including those of the raphe and catecholamine neurons. The long **descending fibers** constitute the medial (or pontine) and lateral (or medullary) reticulospinal tracts located, respectively, in the ventral and lateral funiculi of the spinal white matter. The reticulospinal tracts are important motor pathways (discussed later in this chapter and Ch. 23). **Ascending axons** from the central group of reticular nuclei travel in the central tegmental tract (which also contains descending fibers going to the inferior olivary nucleus) to the intralaminar thalamic nuclei and the basal cholinergic nuclei of the substantia innominata in the base of the forebrain. The latter (see Ch. 12) include the nucleus basalis of Meynert, the nucleus of the diagonal band, and certain nuclei of the septal area. The intralaminar nuclei and the basal forebrain cholinergic nuclei project diffusely to the whole cerebral cortex. The possible involvement of these ascending projections in maintaining consciousness is reviewed later in this chapter. The intralaminar thalamic nuclei also provide a major input to the corpus striatum, a large

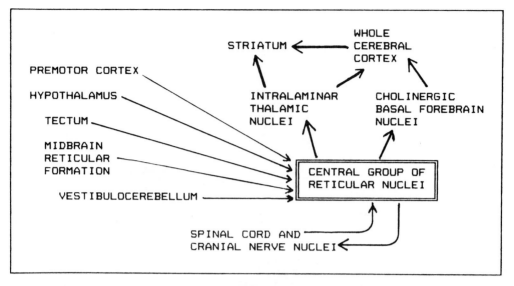

Figure 9-4. Major connections of the central group of reticular nuclei. (*With permission from Kiernan JA: Some functional pathways in the central nervous system. In Kelley WN (ed): Textbook of Internal Medicine, 2nd ed, pp 2138–2145. Philadelphia, JB Lippincott, 1992.*)

component of the forebrain best known for its involvement in motor control (see Chs. 12 and 24).

CHOLINERGIC NEURONS

The reticular formation contains at least two groups of neurons that contain choline acetyltransferase, the enzyme that catalyzes the synthesis of acetylcholine. The larger of these is in the **pedunculopontine nucleus** (see Figs. 9-1 and 9-2), in the rostral pons and caudal midbrain. The smaller is nearby, in the pontine periventricular gray matter. These nuclei receive descending afferent fibers from the pallidum (see Ch. 12) and the substantia nigra pars reticulata. They project caudally to the central group of reticular nuclei and rostrally to the subthalamic nucleus in the diencephalon and to the pallidum in the telencephalon. The cholinergic nuclei in the reticular formation have been suspected of involvement in stereotyped motor functions, such as locomotion, and in consciousness and arousal. These functions are similar to those proposed for the nuclei of the central group.

CATECHOLAMINE NUCLEI

The catecholamines are noradrenaline (norepinephrine), adrenaline (epinephrine), and dopamine. Neurons believed to use these substances as synaptic transmitters are identified by histochemical methods for the amines and for enzymes involved in their synthesis. The largest group of central noradrenergic neurons, and the only one easily recognized in ordinary anatomical preparations, is the **locus coeruleus** or nucleus pigmentosus (see Figs. 9-2C and 9-2D). This collection of pigmented neurons is found at the pontomesencephalic junction, rostral and lateral to the facial and trigeminal motor nuclei. Six smaller groups of noradrenergic neurons are present in the lateral part of the reticular formation in the medulla, pons, and midbrain. There also are two groups of adrenergic neurons in the medulla, one in the ventrolateral reticular formation and the other within the solitary nucleus (see Figs. 9-2A and 9-2B).

The noradrenergic cells resemble other neurons of the reticular formation in having long dendrites and in receiving **afferent fi-**

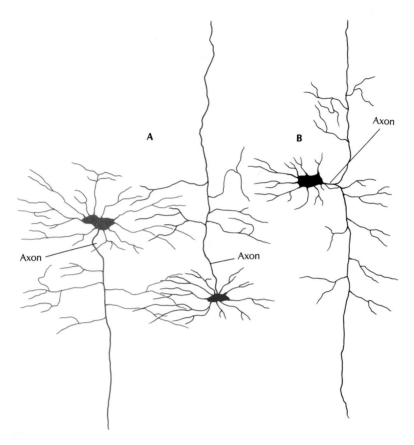

Figure 9-5. Neurons of the reticular formation. **(A)** Interaction between dendrites and collateral axonal branches of neurons with ascending (*blue*) and descending (*red*) projections. **(B)** A neuron whose axon divides into long ascending and descending branches.

bers from many parts of the central nervous system (Fig. 9-6). Those to the locus coeruleus come from the central group of reticular nuclei and from the nucleus prepositus hypoglossi. (The latter group of cells, mentioned at the end of this chapter is also involved in the control of eye movements.) The laterally located noradrenergic neurons probably receive descending afferents from the periaqueductal gray and other components of the reticular formation and from the hypothalamus, amygdala, and prefrontal cortex.

Each noradrenergic neuron has an unmyelinated axon with numerous long branches. These branches go to many regions of the central nervous system, though they are not as extensively distributed as the axons of the serotonergic raphe nuclei. Most of the **efferent fibers** of the locus coeruleus travel rostrally in the central tegmental tract, the medial forebrain bundle, and a smaller bundle that lies ventrolateral to the periaqueductal gray matter. The fibers ascending from the locus coeruleus in the central tegmental tract and medial forebrain bundle terminate in the hypothalamus, the basal cholinergic nuclei of the forebrain, and the amygdala. Of those in the more dorsally located bundle, some go to the cerebellar nuclei and cortex. Others ascend in the walls of the third ventricle and eventually end in the thalamus, habenular nuclei, basal cholinergic nuclei of the forebrain, amygdala, ol-

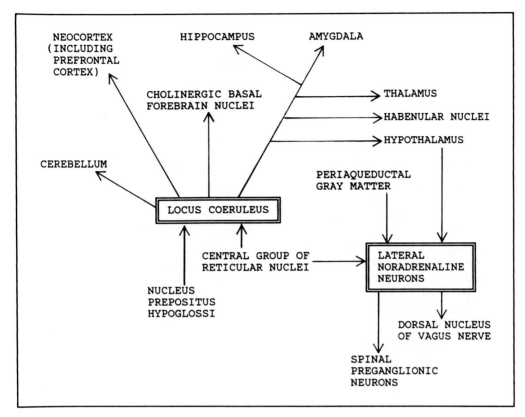

Figure 9-6. Major connections of the noradrenergic nuclei of the brain stem.

factory bulb, hippocampal formation, and most of the neocortex. The projections to the amygdala and hippocampus are particularly prominent (see Fig. 9-6).

Descending noradrenergic axons, which are predominantly from the lateral medullary catecholamine nuclei, end in contact with preganglionic autonomic neurons in the medulla (dorsal nucleus of the vagus) and spinal cord (thoracolumbar sympathetic and sacral parasympathetic nuclei). Dopaminergic neurons in the ventral tegmental area, which is not part of the reticular formation, have similar connections with the limbic forebrain (see Ch. 18).

The noradrenaline released by axons from the locus coeruleus and related cell groups probably acts mainly as a modulator of synapses between other neurons. The effects on spinal reflexes and on alertness are generally excitatory. Although the actions of the noradrenergic reticular neurons seem to be rather nonspecific, the anatomical distribution of the axons to the neocortex is topographically organized.

PARVOCELLULAR RETICULAR AREA

The parvocellular reticular area is in the medulla and pons, lateral to the gigantocellular and pontine reticular nuclei and medial to the spinal and pontine trigeminal nuclei (see Figs. 9-1 and 9-2). Afferent fibers probably come from these sensory nuclei and from the cerebral cortex. The neurons in the parvocellular reticular area project to the motor nuclei of the hypoglossal, facial, and trigeminal nerves. These connections indicate involvement in reflexes concerned with feeding, rather than in consciousness and arousal as was once thought. An "expiratory center" identified by electrical stimulation in animals is located within the medullary parvocellular reticular area. Stimulation in this region also can cause acceleration of the heart and increased arterial blood pressure.

PARABRACHIAL AREA

Rostral to the parvocellular reticular area, the medial and lateral **parabrachial nuclei** and the nearby **Kolliker-Fuse nucleus** are in the lateral part of the reticular formation of the caudal midbrain, close to the fibers of the superior cerebellar peduncle. This area has many connections. Afferent fibers come from the solitary nucleus and from the cortex of the insula and adjoining parts of the parietal lobe. The axons of parabrachial neurons project rostrally to the hypothalamus, preoptic area, intralaminar thalamic nuclei, and amygdala. In many mammals, though probably not in primates, the parabrachial nuclei also form part of the sensory pathway for taste. Thus the parabrachial area serves as a relay station in ascending pathways for visceral sensations. The Kolliker-Fuse nucleus is coextensive with the "pneumotaxic center" recognized by physiologists as a region concerned with the regulation of respiratory rhythm.

SUPERFICIAL MEDULLARY RETICULAR NEURONS

The ventral superficial reticular area in the medulla is another region concerned with cardiovascular and respiratory regulation. Afferents are from the spinal cord and solitary nucleus. They include fibers activated by the baroreceptors of the carotid and aortic sinuses and by the oxygen-sensitive chemoreceptors of the carotid and aortic bodies. Some of these medullary neurons respond directly to changes in the pH or carbon dioxide concentration in the nearby cerebrospinal fluid. The ventral superficial reticular area projects to the hypothalamus and to preganglionic autonomic neurons in the medulla and spinal cord. There are functional connections also with the motor neurons that supply the muscles of respiration.

Functions of the Reticular Formation

Sleep and Arousal

PHYSIOLOGICAL ASPECTS OF CONSCIOUSNESS

The sleeping and awake states normally follow a rhythm with the same periodicity as the alternation of night and day. Within the nocturnal phase, sleep may be light (easily awakened) or deep (requiring a strong sensory stimulus for arousal). In addition, there are episodes of sleep in which there are rapid eye movements (**REM sleep**). At such times, a substantial sensory stimulus is needed for arousal, but the brain is very active. A person suddenly awakened during REM sleep usually reports dreaming.

The varying level of consciousness is paralleled by changes in the **electroencephalogram (EEG)**, which is a crude indicator of the activity of the cerebral cortex. The fluctuations in voltage recorded from a point on the scalp are the sum of the variations in the membrane potentials of the dendrites of neurons in the underlying cerebral cortex (see also Ch. 14). Dendritic potentials are responses to activity of afferent axons, most of which come from neurons in the thalamus. Large potentials are recorded when thalamic neurons are firing synchronously, whereas low-voltage activity indicates that each cortical neuron is responding differently to its thalamic afferents. The EEG waves of a fully alert person are of low voltage and high frequency, indicating *desynchronization* of thalamocortical circuits. With progressive deepening of sleep, the waves become taller (*synchronization*) and longer ("slow wave sleep"). In REM sleep, the EEG is desynchronized despite the fact that such sleep is deep in the sense of being resistant to sensory stimulation.

NEUROANATOMICAL CORRELATES

The central group of reticular nuclei was once thought to be the major part of the **ascending reticular activating system**, receiving convergent synaptic input from pathways for all types of sensation and sending signals rostrally to the thalamus and then to the whole cerebral cortex (see Fig. 9-4). Thus any increase in the general level of sensory stimulation would lead to increased neuronal activity in the cerebral cortex and a more alert or wakeful condition. Such a view accords with many experimental and clinical observations, including the irreversible coma that follows bilateral destruction of the medial part of the reticular formation at or above upper pontine levels. However, there also is evidence for the involvement of at least two other pathways. The **noradrenergic neurons** of the reticular formation may provide another ascending projection that excites neurons throughout the cerebral cortex. The cells of the locus coeruleus are active only in awake, attentive animals; they are quiescent in sleep (including REM sleep). The hypothalamus (see Ch. 11) contains **histamine-secreting neurons** with axons that end in all parts of the central nervous system. Pharmacological studies indicate that histamine of neuronal origin participates in arousal.

It has been known for many years that there are systems of neurons that actively induce sleep. These include the **serotonergic neurons** of the raphe nuclei, with axons distributed to all parts of the central nervous system. The raphe neurons are active in deep sleep, which may be due in part to a widespread inhibitory action of serotonin in the thalamus and cerebral cortex. Dreaming may be due to occasional release of the telencephalic neurons from serotonergic inhibition. A simultaneous reduction of inhibition of the PPRF could account for the accompanying movements of the eyes.

Pain

Through spinal afferents and projections to the thalamus, the central group of reticular nuclei forms part of an **ascending pathway** for the poorly localized perception of pain. Such sensation persists after transection of the spinothalamic tracts (see Ch. 19).

A **descending inhibitory pathway** consists of the axons of serotonergic raphe neurons that project to the dorsal horn and spinal trigeminal nucleus. This system inhibits the transmission rostrally of impulses that report pain. Electrical stimulation of the periaqueductal gray matter (which projects to the nucleus raphes magnus in the medulla) results in loss of the ability to experience pain from sites of injury or disease. Curiously, the analgesic action of a few minutes' stimulation can last for several hours.

Peptide neurotransmitters or neuromodulators known as enkephalins are released at synapses in the periaqueductal gray matter, raphe nuclei, and substantia gelatinosa of the dorsal horn of spinal gray matter. The enkephalins have analgesic actions similar to those of morphine and related opiate drugs, which bind to the same postsynaptic receptor molecules. The analgesic effects of stimulation of the periaqueductal gray matter and those of the medicinally used opiates require the integrity of the raphespinal tract in the dorsolateral funiculus of the spinal cord. Drugs that antagonize morphine, such as naloxone, are able to prevent the analgesia brought about by electrical stimulation of the nucleus raphes magnus or the periaqueductal gray matter. Other opiate-like peptides, the endorphins, have been found in several parts of the brain and in the pituitary gland. It is believed that the opiates produce their pharmacological effects by mimicking the actions of enkephalins and endorphins. Thus the principal anatomical sites of the relief of pain by morphine are thought to be the periaqueductal gray matter, medullary raphe nuclei, and dorsal horn.

Somatic Motor Functions

The reticulospinal tracts constitute one of the major descending pathways involved in the control of movement. The others are the corticospinal and vestibulospinal tracts. Equivalent reticulobulbar connections supply the motor nuclei of cranial nerves. The **pontine reticulospinal tract**, which originates in the caudal and oral pontine reticular nuclei, descends in the ventral funiculus of the same side of the spinal cord. The **medullary retic-**

ulospinal tract arises from the gigantocellular nuclei of both sides and descends in the ventrolateral funiculus. Some of the uncrossed fibers of both these tracts decussate in the ventral white commissure of the cord before terminating. The reticulospinal tracts consequently project both ipsilaterally and bilaterally to the spinal gray matter. They end on interneurons and influence the motor neurons indirectly through synaptic relays within the spinal cord.

Research with animals indicates that regions of the central group of reticular nuclei that give rise to most of the reticulospinal fibers are located slightly rostral to the levels that send the most profuse ascending projections to the thalamus (see Fig. 9-5). Because of the extensive interaction of collateral axonal branches with dendrites in the reticular formation, activity in the reticulospinal neurons is affected by activity in the rostrally projecting reticulothalamic neurons. With respect to motor functions, important afferents to the central group of reticular nuclei come from the motor cortex of the cerebral hemispheres, the cholinergic pedunculopontine nucleus (see Figs. 9-2D and 9-4), the cerebellar nuclei, and the spinal cord. It is noteworthy that corticoreticular fibers from the motor cortex terminate principally in the parts of the central nuclear group that give rise to the greatest numbers of reticulospinal axons.

The **raphespinal tract** is a reticulospinal pathway, best known for the involvement of its serotonergic neurons in the modulation of pain sensation. There is evidence, however, that raphespinal projections may also modulate the activities of motor neurons, which are made more excitable by serotonin. Drugs that block the action of serotonin have been used clinically to alleviate the spasticity that follows damage to the major descending motor pathways.

Visceral Activities

Certain regions in the reticular formation regulate **visceral functions and breathing** through connections rostrally with the amygdala and hypothalamus, and caudally with nuclei of the autonomic outflow and with respiratory motor neurons in the phrenic nucleus and thoracic cord. The functions of the superficial medullary reticular neurons in mediating reflex responses to the systemic blood pressure and the degree of oxygenation of the blood were mentioned earlier in this chapter. Other cardiovascular and respiratory regions, commonly referred to as "centers," have been identified by electrical stimulation within the brain stem in laboratory animals. Some of these centers are fields within the network of dendrites in the reticular formation rather than compact collections of cell bodies. Maximal inspiratory and expiratory responses are obtained from the gigantocellular nucleus and the parvocellular reticular area, respectively, in the medulla. A pneumotaxic center in the parabrachial area of the pons corresponds to the Kolliker-Fuse nucleus, and influences respiratory rhythm.

Stimulation in the medial part of the reticular formation of the medulla has a depressor effect on the circulatory system, with slowing of the heart rate and lowering of blood pressure. The opposite effects are produced by stimulation in laterally located sites. Damage to the brain stem is life-threatening because of the presence of these regions involved in the control of vital functions.

Miscellaneous Nuclei of the Brain Stem

The **area postrema** is a narrow strip of neural tissue in the caudal part of the floor of the fourth ventricle between the vagal triangle and the margin of the ventricle (see Fig. 6-3). It is richly vascular, with capillaries of large diameter (sinusoids). The blood–brain barrier, which elsewhere prevents certain substances from entering nervous tissue from the blood, is lacking. Among other possible connections, the area postrema receives visceral afferents from the spinal cord, and there are reciprocal connections with the solitary nucleus. The area has been shown experimentally to be a chemoreceptor region for emetic drugs such as apomorphine and digoxin. It may, therefore, function in the physiology of vomiting.

The **perihypoglossal nuclei** are three quite conspicuous groups of neurons in the caudal medulla: the nucleus intercalatus (between the hypoglossal nucleus and the dorsal nucleus of the vagus; see Fig. 9-2A), the nucleus of Roller (ventrolateral to the hypoglossal nucleus), and the nucleus prepositus hypoglossi (rostral to the hypoglossal nucleus; see Fig. 9-2B), which is the largest and is continuous at its rostral end with the PPRF (see Fig. 8-5).

These nuclei receive afferents from several sources, including the cerebral cortex, vestibular nuclei, accessory oculomotor nuclei, and PPRF. Efferent fibers proceed mainly to the nuclei of cranial nerves III, IV, and VI, which they reach by passing in the medial longitudinal fasciculus. The perihypoglossal nuclei form part of the complex circuitry for movements of the eyes. Lesions in the nucleus prepositus hypoglossi impair the ability to keep the eyes fixed on a visual target, although conjugate movements are still performed accurately. The projection of this nucleus to the locus coeruleus, mentioned earlier (see Fig. 9-6), has no obvious relation to ocular movements.

The **accessory oculomotor nuclei** are the interstitial nucleus of Cajal, the nucleus of Darkschewitsch, the nucleus of the posterior commissure, and the rostral interstitial nucleus of the medial longitudinal fasciculus. They are situated at the junction of the mid-

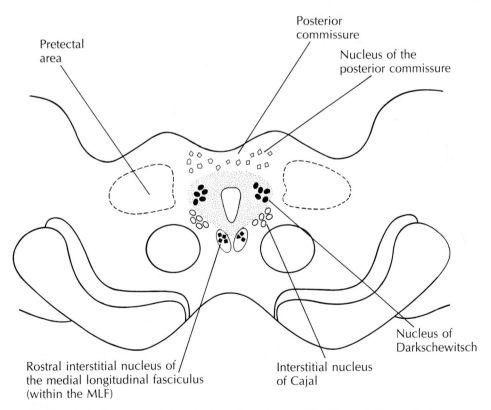

Figure 9-7. Some nuclei at the junction of the midbrain and diencephalon, at the level of the posterior commissure. (Stippling shows the extent of the periaqueductal gray matter. The red nucleus, substantia nigra and basis pedunculi are outlined but not labeled.)

brain and the diencephalon, near the rostral end of the cerebral aqueduct, and are concerned with movements of the eyes. Their positions are shown in Figure 9-7. The specific connections and functions of the individual nuclei are poorly understood, so they are treated as a group in the discussion of ocular movements in Chapter 8. The interstitial nucleus of Cajal is notable in that, together with the Edinger-Westphal nucleus, it sends some axons caudally as the interstitiospinal tract. This minor pathway probably contributes to visuomotor coordination. The rostral interstitial nucleus of the medial longitudinal fasciculus is part of the circuitry necessary for vertical eye movements.

The **periaqueductal gray matter** surrounds the cerebral aqueduct of the midbrain. Although afferent and efferent connections have been traced in laboratory animals with regions ranging from the spinal cord to parts of the telencephalon, its physiological role is largely obscure. As mentioned earlier, electrical stimulation of the periaqueductal gray matter causes analgesia, and this effect is mediated by way of the descending projection of the nucleus raphes magnus in the medulla. The nucleus of Darkschewitsch is within the territory of the periaqueductal gray matter, but its connections indicate that it is one of the accessory oculomotor nuclei.

The **interpeduncular nucleus** is in the midline, ventral to the periaqueductal gray matter and near the roof of the most rostral part of the interpeduncular fossa. This nucleus lies on a pathway through which the limbic system projects to autonomic nuclei in the brain stem and spinal cord. Lateral to the interpeduncular nucleus, in the medial part of the cerebral peduncle, is a population of dopamine-secreting neurons known as the **ventral tegmental area**. This, too, has connections with the limbic system and is discussed in Chapter 18.

SUGGESTED READING

Decker MW, McGaugh JL: The role of interactions between the cholinergic system and other neuromodulatory systems in learning and memory. Synapse 7:151–168, 1991

Foote SL, Morrison JH: Extrathalamic modulation of cortical function. Annu Rev Neurosci 10: 67–95, 1987

Kelly DD: Sleep and dreaming. In Kandel ER, Schwartz JH, Jessell TM (eds): Principles of Neural Science, 3rd ed, pp 792–804. New York, Elsevier-North Holland, 1991

Mantyh PW: Connections of the periaqueductal gray in the monkey. J Neurophysiol 49:567–594, 1983

Martin GF, Holstege G, Mehler WR: Reticular formation of the pons and medulla. In Paxinos G (ed): The Human Nervous System, pp 203–220. San Diego, Academic Press, 1990

Moruzzi G, Magoun HW: Brain stem reticular formation and activation of the EEG. Electroenceph Clin Neurophysiol 1:455–473, 1949

Nieuwenhuys R, Voogd J, van Huijzen C: The Human Central Nervous System. A Synopsis and Atlas, 3rd ed. Berlin, Springer-Verlag, 1988

Noback CR, Strominger NL, Demarest RJ: The Human Nervous System, 4th ed. Philadelphia, Lea & Febiger, 1991

Olszewski J, Baxter D: Cytoarchitecture of the Human Brain Stem, 2nd ed. Basel, Karger, 1982

Parnavelas JG, Papadopoulos GC: The monoaminergic innervation of the cerebral cortex is not diffuse and nonspecific. Trends Neurosci 12:315–319, 1989

Posner MI, Peterson SE: The attention system of the human brain. Annu Rev Neurosci 13:25–42, 1990

Saper CB: Function of the locus coeruleus. Trends Neurosci 10:343–344, 1987

Wada H, Inagaki N, Yamatodani A, Watanabe T: Is the histaminergic neuron system a regulatory center for whole-brain activity? Trends Neurosci 14:415–418, 1991

Wainberg M, Barbeau H, Gauthier S: The effects of cyproheptadine on locomotion and on spasticity in patients with spinal cord injuries. J Neurol Neurosurg Psychiatry 53:754–763, 1990

Ten

The Human Nervous System: An Anatomical Viewpoint, Sixth Edition, Murray L. Barr and John A. Kiernan. J.B. Lippincott Company, Philadelphia, © 1993.

Cerebellum

Important Facts

The hemispheres, vermis, flocculus, nodule, and tonsil are major landmarks of the cerebellar cortex.

Afferent fibers end in the three-layered cerebellar cortex. The Purkinje cells have axons that end in the cerebellar nuclei.

The fastigial, interposed, and dentate nuclei receive branches of all cerebellar afferent fibers and the output of the cortex. These nuclei contain the cerebellar efferent neurons.

The superior cerebellar peduncle contains cerebellar efferent fibers and the ventral spinocerebellar tract. The middle cerebellar peduncle consists of fibers from the contralateral pontine nuclei, and the inferior cerebellar peduncle contains olivocerebellar and dorsal spinocerebellar fibers and the vestibulocerebellar and fastigiobulbar connections.

The vestibular system is connected ipsilaterally with the vestibulocerebellum, which comprises the flocculonodular lobe and the fastigial nucleus. This nucleus projects to the ipsilateral vestibular nuclei and to the reticular formation.

Proprioceptive signals are carried ipsilaterally to the spinocerebellum, which consists of vermis, paravermal zones, and interposed nuclei. These nuclei project to the contralateral ventrolateral (VL) thalamic nucleus. The VL projects to the primary motor cortex.

The cerebral cortex influences the contralateral cerebellar hemisphere and dentate nucleus (pontocerebellum) by way of a relay in the pontine nuclei. The dentate nucleus projects to the contralateral VL thalamic nucleus.

These connections determine that each side of the body is represented ipsilaterally in the cerebellum and that postural functions are localized in and near the midline.

The cerebellum learns and executes instructions for movements, ensuring coordination of the force, extent, and duration of the contractions of muscles.

A lesion in or near the midline cause disorders of posture and gait, whereas a lesion in a hemisphere causes defective control of movements of the ipsilateral limbs.

Although the cerebellum has an abundant input from sensory receptors, it is essentially a motor part of the brain, functioning in the maintenance of equilibrium and in the coordination of muscle contractions. The cerebellum makes a special contribution to synergy of muscle action (ie, to the synchronized contractions and relaxations of different muscles that make up a useful movement). The cerebellum ensures that there is contraction of the proper muscles at the appropriate time, each with the correct force. There is reason to believe that the cerebellum participates in the learning of patterns of neuronal activity needed for carrying out movements and also in the execution of these encoded instructions. The cerebellum increased in size in the course of vertebrate evolution. The large size in the human brain coincides with the need for synergy of muscles, especially for maintenance of the erect posture and in learned activities that require precisely orchestrated hand movements.

Despite their complexity, the activities of the cerebellum have long been thought to occur without any conscious awareness. This traditional viewpoint may not be entirely correct: imagined movements are accompanied by an increase in cerebellar blood flow that is larger than the increase detected in the motor areas of the cerebral cortex. Damage to the cerebellum causes disturbances of motor function without voluntary paralysis.

The cerebellum consists of a **cortex**, or surface layer, of gray matter contained in transverse folds or folia, a medullary center of white matter, and four pairs of **central nuclei** embedded in the medullary center. Three pairs of **cerebellar peduncles**, composed of nerve fibers, connect the cerebellum with the brain stem.

Gross Anatomy

The superior cerebellar surface is elevated in the midline, conforming to the dural reflection or tentorium that forms a roof for the posterior cranial fossa. The inferior surface is deeply grooved in the midline; the remainder of this surface is convex on each side and rests on the floor of the posterior cranial fossa (Fig. 10-1).

Certain terms are useful to identify regions of the cerebellar surface. The region in and near the midline is known as the **vermis** and the remainder, as the **hemispheres**. The superior vermis is not demarcated from the hemispheres, but the inferior vermis lies in a deep depression (the vallecula) and is well delineated. The term **paravermal zone** is used for the medial parts of the hemispheres for 1 to 2 cm on either side of the vermis.

Three major regions, the flocculonodular, anterior, and posterior lobes, are recognized in the horizontal plane (see Fig. 10-1). The **flocculonodular lobe** (or lobule) is a small component, the oldest phylogenetically, that lies at the rostral edge of the inferior surface. The nodule is the rostral portion of the inferior vermis, and the flocculi are irregularly shaped masses on each side. The cerebellum is deeply indented by several transverse fissures. The **dorsolateral fissure** (also called the posterolateral fissure) along the caudal border of the flocculonodular lobe is the first of these to appear during embryonic development. The main mass of the cerebellum (all but the flocculonodular lobe) consists of anterior and posterior lobes. The **anterior lobe** is that part of the superior surface rostral to the **primary fissure**.[1] The remainder of the cerebellum on both surfaces constitutes the **posterior lobe**.

The roof of the rostral part of the fourth ventricle is formed by the superior cerebellar peduncles and by the superior medullary velum that bridges the interval between them (Fig. 10-2; see also Fig. 7-10). The remainder of the roof consists of the thin inferior medullary velum, formed by pia mater and ependyma. This membrane, in which a deficiency constitutes the median aperture of the fourth ventricle or foramen of Magendie (see Fig.

---

[1] This, despite its name, is the second fissure to appear during embryonic development.

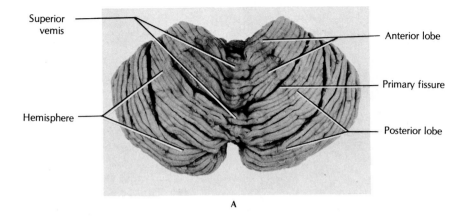

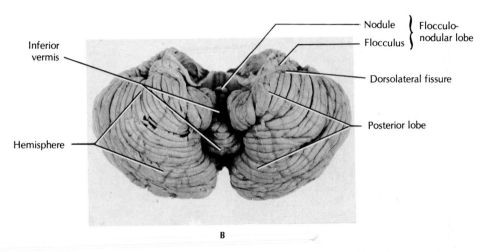

Figure 10-1. The cerebellum. **(A)** Superior surface. **(B)** Inferior surface. (× 0.66)

6-4), commonly adheres to the inferior vermis. The three pairs of peduncles are attached to the cerebellum in the interval between the flocculonodular and anterior lobes.

Other fissures outline further subdivisions or lobules, especially in the posterior lobe. The names given to these lobules by early anatomists have no functional significance; neither is there uniform acceptance of a single system of nomenclature. Figure 10-3 is provided for reference, if smaller subdivisions of the cerebellum need to be identified. The position of the **tonsils** is clinically significant because

these parts of the cerebellar hemispheres are close to the medulla and can compress this vital part of the brain stem if the contents of the posterior fossa of the skull are displaced downward into the foramen magnum. The tonsil is also an angiographic landmark, imparting a characteristic curve to the course of the posterior inferior cerebellar artery.

Three functional divisions of the cerebellum are recognized, based on the destinations of different categories of afferent fibers. Cortical histology is uniform throughout the cerebellum, unlike the cerebral cortex, in

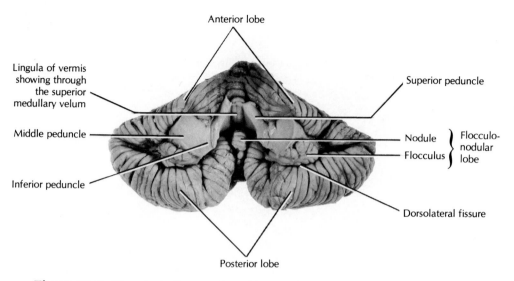

Figure 10-2. The cerebellum as viewed from in front and below, showing the cut surfaces of the cerebellar peduncles. (× 0.66)

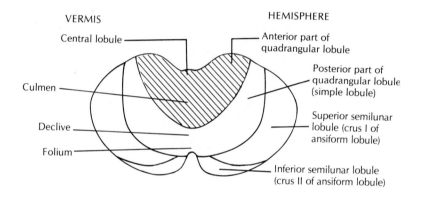

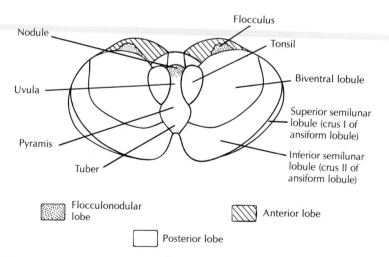

Figure 10-3. Anatomical names of parts of the cerebellum. (The *lingula*, not seen in these drawings, is a small, flattened portion of the superior vermis beneath the central lobule and adherent to the superior medullary velum; see Fig. 10-2).

which there are histologically different areas. The four central nuclei are likewise similar at the cellular level. The cortex and nuclei are, therefore, described at this point, after which the functional divisions and their individual connections are discussed.

Cerebellar Cortex

Because of the extensive folding of the cerebellar surface in the form of thin transverse **folia**, 85% of the cortical surface is concealed. There is, therefore, a large cortical area. It is about three-quarters as extensive as that of the cerebral cortex.

Cortical Layers

Three layers are seen in histological sections. From the surface to the white matter of the folium, these are the molecular layer, the layer of Purkinje cells, and the granule cell layer (Fig. 10-4). The **Purkinje cell layer** consists of a single row (in sections) of bodies of Purkinje cells, which are the principal cells of the cerebellar cortex. The **molecular layer** contains some interneurons but is largely a synaptic zone, made up of profusely branching dendrites of Purkinje cells and the axons of the granule cells. The term *molecular* is derived from the punctate appearance of this layer in sections stained for nerve fibers. The **granule cell layer** consists of closely packed interneurons, of which the most abundant are the granule cells. The axons of these small interneurons extend into the molecular layer.

Of the afferent fibers to the cortex, **mossy fibers** terminate in synaptic contact with granule cells of the innermost layer, whereas **climbing fibers** enter the molecular layer and wind among the dendrites of Purkinje cells. The only fibers that leave the cortex are axons of Purkinje cells. These fibers terminate in central nuclei of the cerebellum, with the exception of some fibers from the cortex of the floc-

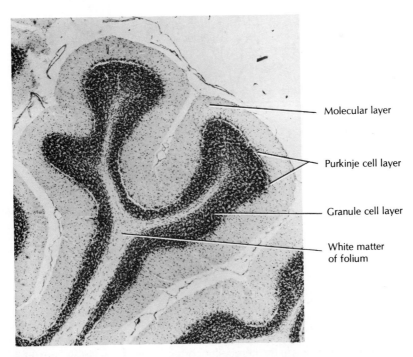

Molecular layer

Purkinje cell layer

Granule cell layer

White matter of folium

Figure 10-4. Transverse section of cerebellar folia showing the three layers of the cortex and the underlying white matter. (Stained with cresyl violet, × 35)

culonodular lobe that proceed to the brain stem.

Cytoarchitecture

The five neuron types in the cerebellar cortex establish a complex but remarkably regular pattern of intracortical circuits. The precise three-dimensional orientation of dendrites and axons, as shown by the Golgi staining method and by electron microscopy, has encouraged the study of cortical physiology at the cellular level by means of recording microelectrodes. The basic pattern of the neurons is indicated in Figure 10-5.

Granule Cells and Mossy Fibers

The granule cells are small and closely packed together in the deepest cortical layer. Each cell has a spherical nucleus with a coarse chromatin pattern, and the scanty cytoplasm lacks clumps of Nissl substance. The short dendrites have

claw-like endings that are contacted by mossy fibers. The unmyelinated axon enters the molecular layer, where it bifurcates and runs parallel with the folium. Because of the density of the granule cell population, the whole molecular layer contains closely arranged parallel fibers. Each granule cell axon traverses the dendritic trees of some 450 Purkinje cells, making synaptic contacts with their dendritic spines. These axons also synapse with dendrites of stellate, basket, and Golgi cells in the molecular layer.

A large proportion of the afferent fibers to the cerebellum are mossy fibers that terminate in synaptic relation with dendrites of granule cells. While still in the white matter, a mossy fiber divides into several branches, which may enter the cortex of adjacent folia. On entering the granule cell layer, the fiber loses its myelin sheath and there is further terminal branching. Along the terminal portion of the fiber and at its end, there are swellings known as rosettes, with which the dendrites of several granule cells make synaptic contact. The synaptic configuration that includes the rosette of a mossy fiber, dendrites of granule cells, and the axon of a Golgi cell (see Stellate and Golgi Cells) is known

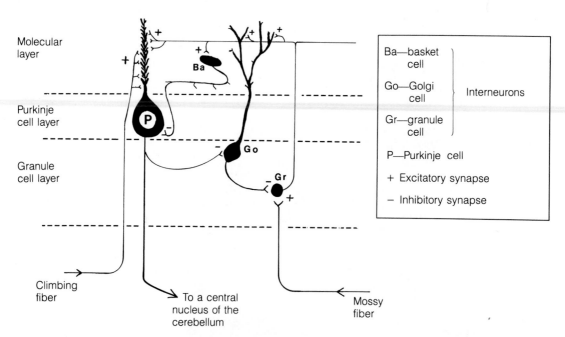

Figure 10-5. Neurons in the cerebellar cortex, showing excitatory and inhibitory synapses. (*With permission, from Kiernan JA: Introduction to Human Neuroscience. Philadelphia, JB Lippincott, 1987*)

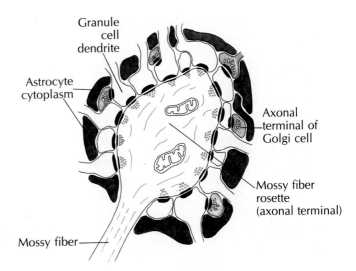

Figure 10-6. Ultrastructure of a synaptic glomerulus in the granule cell layer.

as a **glomerulus** (Fig. 10-6). The whole synaptic complex is invested by cytoplasmic processes of protoplasmic astrocytes. These take up and metabolize the amino acid neurotransmitters released by the presynaptic boutons, thereby preventing diffusion to nearby glomeruli.

Purkinje Cells and Climbing Fibers

There are about 15 million Purkinje cells. They are easily recognized by their flask-shaped cell bodies. Their most remarkable characteristic is profuse dendritic branching in the molecular layer, in a plane transverse to the folium. The primary and secondary branches are smooth, whereas the finer branches bear regularly spaced spines. Electron micrographs show synaptic junctions where the spines indent parallel fibers. The parallel arrangement of axons of granule cells and the transverse orientation of dendrites of Purkinje cells, with respect to a folium, provide maximal opportunity for a Purkinje cell to receive stimuli from a large number of granule cells and also allow a granule cell to contact many Purkinje cells. The molecular layer is, therefore, a rich synaptic field to which stellate, basket, and Golgi cells also contribute.

Axons of Purkinje cells traverse the granule cell layer, acquire myelin sheaths, and terminate mainly in central cerebellar nuclei. Collateral branches given off by the axons synapse with adjacent Purkinje cells and with Golgi cells in the outer part of the granule cell layer (see Fig. 10-5).

As the mossy fibers have a special relation-ship with granule cells, so the climbing fibers have a special relationship with Purkinje cells. Climbing fibers enter the cortex from the medullary center, traverse the granule cell layer, and wind among the dendritic branches of Purkinje cells like a vine growing on a tree. Each climbing fiber makes synaptic contact with the smooth surface of the larger branches of a Purkinje cell dendrite. The climbing fibers probably all originate in the inferior olivary complex of nuclei.

Basket Cells

The basket cells are scattered in the molecular layer near the bodies of Purkinje cells. The dendrite of a basket cell branches in the transverse plane of the folium, receiving synaptic contacts from many granule cell axons. The axon of a basket cell is directed across the folium, and collateral branches form characteristic synapses with about 250 Purkinje cells. Each collateral forms a basket-like arrangement around the cell body of a Purkinje cell, with the fibers concentrating around the axon hillock, where synaptic contacts are made (Fig. 10-7). Because of an overlapping arrangement, collateral branches of several basket cell axons synapse with a single Purkinje cell.

Stellate and Golgi Cells

Granule, Purkinje, and basket cells have special features, whereas stellate and Golgi cells are similar to small neurons elsewhere in the nervous system.

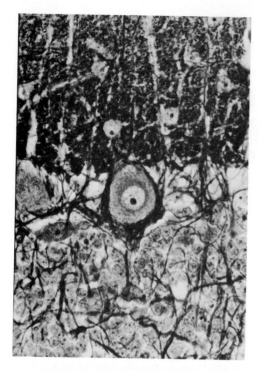

Figure 10-7. Cell body of a Purkinje cell situated between the molecular layer (*above*) and the granule cell layer of the cerebellar cortex. Most of the fibers surrounding the Purkinje cell body are preterminal branches of basket cell axons. (Cajal's silver nitrate method, × 450)

There are scattered stellate cells in the superficial part of the molecular layer whose dendrites are contacted by axons of granule cells. Axons of stellate cells synapse mainly with Purkinje cell dendrites; a few enter the innermost cortical layer and establish a feedback circuit by synapsing with granule cells. The Golgi cells are situated in the outer portion of the granule cell layer, and their dendrites extend into the molecular layer, where they are contacted by parallel fibers. Other afferents to Golgi cells are collateral branches of Purkinje cell axons. Axons of Golgi cells enter glomeruli, where they synapse with the dendrites of granule cells (see Fig. 10-6).

Intracortical Circuits

Recordings from microelectrodes inserted into the cerebellar cortex have yielded information about whether synapses between specific types of neuron produce an excitatory postsynaptic potential (EPSP) or an inhibitory postsynaptic potential (IPSP). These observations, supplemented by immunohistochemical and pharmacological studies of neurotransmitters and their receptors, show that the synapses made by axons afferent to the cerebellum (ie, by the mossy and climbing fibers) are all excitatory. The granule cells also make excitatory synapses with the Purkinje cells (see Fig. 10-5). The excitatory transmitter is probably glutamate. All the other cerebellar interneurons make inhibitory synapses, with gamma-aminobutyric acid (GABA) as the probable transmitter. The excitatory input to the cortex is thereby modified by intracortical circuits that inhibit Purkinje cells, and therefore suppress transmission from cortex to central nuclei. For example, parallel fibers produce an EPSP in stellate and basket cells, but synapses between these and Purkinje cells produce an IPSP. Parallel fibers also excite Golgi cells, which inhibit granule cells. The inhibitory circuits include more synapses than do the excitatory relays. Therefore, an afferent volley to the cortex first produces an EPSP in a Purkinje cell, followed after 1 to 2 msec by an IPSP. The inhibitory circuits limit the area of cortex excited and the degree of excitation resulting from an incoming volley.

Aminergic Fibers

Large numbers of noradrenergic axons enter the cerebellum through its superior peduncle. These unmyelinated fibers, which come from the locus coeruleus, end by branching profusely in the molecular layer (see Fig. 10-5). The noradrenaline released from these afferent fibers may have a modulatory action at the synapses between parallel fibers and Purkinje cells. The cerebellar cortex also contains some serotonergic axons from the raphe nuclei of the reticular formation (see Ch. 9). It has been suggested that noradrenaline and serotonin may have opposing actions, the former amine enhancing and the latter reducing the excitatory action of glutamate on the dendrites of Purkinje cells.

Central Nuclei

Four pairs of nuclei are embedded deep in the medullary center; in a medial to lateral direction, they are the fastigial, globose, emboliform, and dentate nuclei (Fig. 10-8).

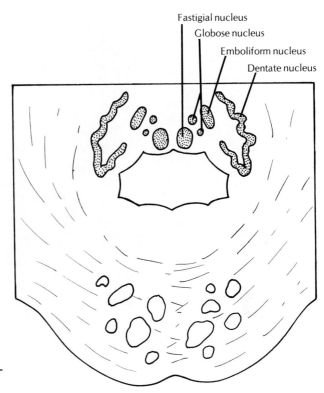

Fastigial nucleus
Globose nucleus
Emboliform nucleus
Dentate nucleus

Figure 10-8. Central nuclei of the cerebellum.

The **fastigial nucleus** is nearly spherical, close to the midline, and almost in contact with the roof of the fourth ventricle. The **globose nucleus** consists of two or three small cellular masses, and the larger **emboliform nucleus** is oval or plug-shaped. In mammals as high in the phylogenetic scale as the monkey, a single nucleus (the nucleus interpositus or **interposed nucleus**) is situated between the fastigial and dentate nuclei. In apes and humans, the interposed nucleus is represented by the globose and emboliform nuclei. The **dentate nucleus** is the most prominent of the central nuclei; this mammalian nucleus is largest in primates, especially in humans. The dentate nucleus has the irregular shape of a crumpled purse, similar to that of the inferior olivary nucleus, with the hilus facing medially. Its efferent fibers occupy the interior of the nucleus and leave through the hilus.

The input to the cerebellar nuclei is from (a) sources outside the cerebellum and (b) the Purkinje cells of the cortex. The extrinsic input consists of pontocerebellar, spinocerebellar, and olivocerebellar fibers, together with fibers from the precerebellar reticular nuclei. *Most of these afferents are collateral branches of fibers proceeding to the cerebellar cortex.* A few rubrocerebellar fibers end in the globose and emboliform nuclei, and the fastigial nucleus receives afferents from the vestibular nerve and nuclei. The fastigial nucleus discharges to the brain stem through the inferior cerebellar peduncle, whereas efferents from the other nuclei leave the cerebellum through the superior peduncle and end in the brain stem and in the thalamus.

Results of physiological studies have indicated that the input to the central nuclei from outside the cerebellum is excitatory, whereas the input from Purkinje cells, which use GABA as their transmitter substance, is inhibitory. Crudely processed information in the central nuclei is refined by impulses received from the cortex. The combination of the two inputs maintains a tonic discharge from the central nuclei to the brain stem and thalamus. This

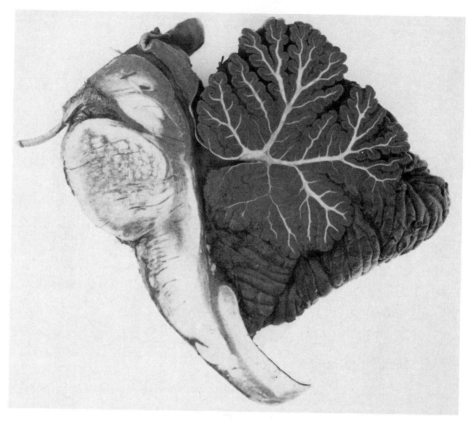

Figure 10-9. Midline structures of the brain stem and cerebellum, showing the *arbor vitae cerebelli* in the vermis. The cut surface of the specimen has been stained by a method that differentiates gray matter (*dark*) and white matter (*light*). ($\times$ 1.5)

discharge changes constantly according to the afferent input to the cerebellum at any given time.

Cerebellar Peduncles

The white matter is scanty in the region of the vermis, where it produces a branching tree-like pattern (the *arbor vitae cerebelli*) in a sagittal section (Fig. 10-9). Each hemisphere contains a large medullary center in which the dentate nucleus is embedded (Fig. 10-10). This white matter consists of afferent fibers to the cortex, axons of Purkinje cells proceeding to the central nuclei, and efferent fibers of the nuclei. The afferent and efferent systems are discussed in connection with the functional divisions of the cerebellum. They are identified

at this point only as components of the cerebellar peduncles.

The **inferior cerebellar peduncle** consists mainly of fibers entering the cerebellum, with the largest contingent being of those that originate in the contralateral inferior olivary complex of nuclei. The other components are the dorsal spinocerebellar tract, cuneocerebellar fibers, fibers from the vestibular nerve and nuclei, the arcuate nucleus,[2] the nucleus of the spinal trigeminal tract, the pontine trigeminal nucleus, and the raphe and precerebellar retic-

---

[2] The arcuate nucleus in the ventral part of the medulla was briefly discussed in Chapter 7. It has afferent and efferent connections similar to those of the pontine nuclei and is probably a caudally displaced part of this neuronal population.

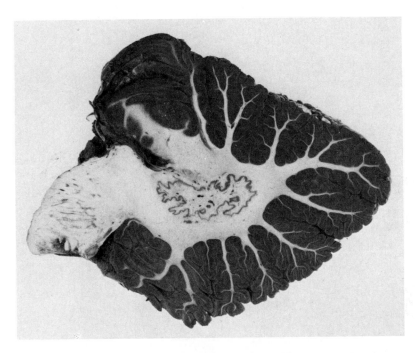

Figure 10-10. Cerebellar surface in a sagittal plane through a hemisphere, stained to differentiate gray matter (*dark*) and white matter (*light*). The dentate nucleus is shown, embedded in the white matter of the hemisphere. ($\times$ 1.5)

ular nuclei. The inferior cerebellar peduncle also contains efferent fibers that proceed from the flocculonodular lobe and fastigial nucleus to the vestibular nuclei and to the central group of reticular nuclei of the medulla and pons.

The **middle cerebellar peduncle** consists of pontocerebellar fibers that originate in the pontine nuclei. The **superior cerebellar peduncle** consists mainly of efferent fibers from the globose, emboliform, and dentate nuclei. The other fibers in the superior peduncles are afferent to the cerebellum. They include the ventral spinocerebellar tract on the dorsolateral surface of the peduncle, fibers that originate in the locus coeruleus, a few fibers from the red nucleus, and fibers from the mesencephalic nucleus of the trigeminal nerve.

Functional Anatomy

Three divisions of the cerebellum are recognized on the basis of phylogeny (Fig. 10-11).

The **archicerebellum**, which is the only component of the cerebellum in fishes and in lower amphibians, consists of the flocculonodular lobe, together with a region of the inferior vermis known as the uvula (see Fig. 10-3). The **paleocerebellum** makes its first appearance in higher amphibians and is larger in reptiles and birds. In humans, it is represented by the superior vermis in the anterior lobe and by part of the inferior vermis in the posterior lobe. The cerebellar hemispheres, together with the superior vermis in the posterior lobe, constitute the **neocerebellum**, which is found only in mammals and is largest in humans.

These phylogenetic divisions of the cerebellum correspond in large part with divisions based on the major sources of afferent fibers (Fig. 10-12). Thus the archicerebellum is identical to the **vestibulocerebellum**, which receives input from the vestibular nerve and nuclei. Those parts of the vermis that constitute the paleocerebellum, together with the ad-

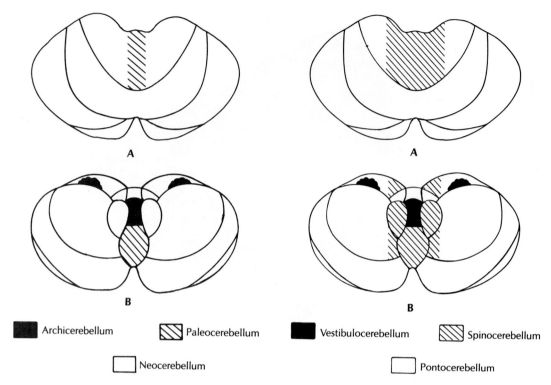

Figure 10-11. Phylogenetic regions of the cerebellum. **(A)** Superior surface. **(B)** Inferior surface.

Figure 10-12. Functional regions of the cerebellum. **(A)** Superior surface. **(B)** Inferior surface.

jacent (neocerebellar) medial or paravermal zones of the hemispheres, make up the **spinocerebellum**. This is the site of termination of the spinocerebellar tracts and cuneocerebellar fibers, which convey proprioceptive and other sensory information. The remainder of the neocerebellum (ie, the large lateral parts of the hemispheres and the superior vermis in the posterior lobe) constitutes the **pontocerebellum**. The contralateral pontine nuclei send afferent fibers to this area. There is some overlapping of the three divisions; for example, some pontocerebellar fibers terminate in the cortex of the spinocerebellum.

VESTIBULOCEREBELLUM

The vestibulocerebellum receives afferent fibers from the vestibular ganglion and from the vestibular nuclei of the same side (Fig. 10-13). These enter the cerebellum in the medial part of the inferior cerebellar peduncle. Some of the

afferent fibers from these sources terminate in the fastigial nucleus, which also receives collateral branches of the axons destined for the cortex of the vestibulocerebellum. The cortex and nucleus also receive afferents from the accessory olivary nuclei.

Some Purkinje cell axons from the vestibulocerebellar cortex proceed to the brain stem (an exception to the general rule that such fibers end in central nuclei), but most terminate in the fastigial nucleus. Fibers from the cortex and the **fastigial nucleus** traverse the medial portion of the inferior cerebellar peduncle to their termination in the vestibular nuclear complex and in the central group of reticular nuclei. (One bundle of fastigiobulbar fibers, known as the **uncinate fasciculus** [of Russell], has an aberrant course. The fasciculus crosses the midline, passes through the other fastigial nucleus, and then curves over the root of the superior cerebellar peduncle to

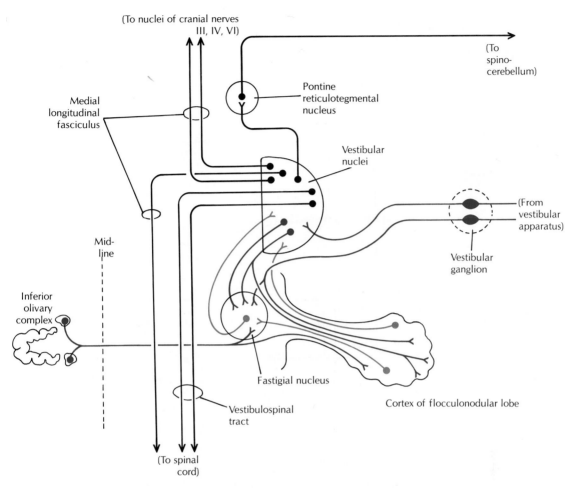

Figure 10-13. Connections of the vestibulocerebellum and vestibular nuclei.

join other efferent fibers of the vestibulocerebellum in the contralateral inferior peduncle.)

In summary, the vestibulocerebellum influences motor neurons through the vestibulospinal tract, the medial longitudinal fasciculus, and reticulospinal fibers. It is concerned with adjustment of muscle tone in response to vestibular stimuli. It coordinates the actions of muscles that maintain equilibrium and participates in other motor responses to vestibular stimulation (see Ch. 22).

SPINOCEREBELLUM

The following afferent systems project to the spinocerebellar cortex. (a) The dorsal and ventral **spinocerebellar tracts** convey data from proprioceptive endings and from touch and pressure receptors (Fig. 10-14). The dorsal tract, consisting of the axons of the neurons constituting the **nucleus thoracicus** in spinal segments T1 to L3 or L4, conveys information from the trunk and leg. The ventral tract, which arises in various parts of the lumbosacral gray matter (see Ch. 5), is involved mainly in conduction from the leg. (b) **Cuneocerebellar fibers** from the **accessory cuneate nucleus** (see Ch. 7) are equivalent, for the arm and neck, to those of the dorsal spinocerebellar tract. Most of the fibers afferent to the cells of origin of the spinocerebellar and cuneocerebellar tracts have ascended in the dorsal funiculi of the spinal cord.

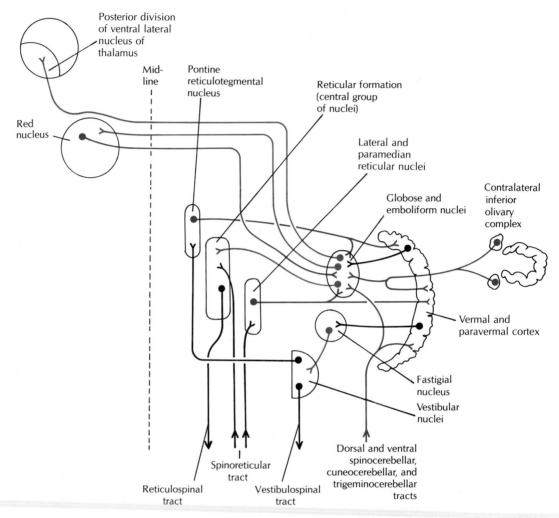

Figure 10-14. Connections of the spinocerebellum.

Data from cutaneous receptors are carried by spinoreticular fibers to the **lateral** and **paramedian reticular nuclei** (see Figs. 9-1 and 9-2), from which fibers project to the cerebellum. These two nuclei also receive afferent fibers from primary motor and sensory areas of the cerebral cortex. Another precerebellar reticular nucleus that projects to the vermis and medial parts of the hemispheres is the **reticulotegmental nucleus** in the pons (see Fig. 9-1). This nucleus receives afferents from the cerebral cortex and from the vestibular nuclei. Finally, the spinocerebellum receives

fibers from all three **trigeminal sensory nerve** and from the accessory olivary nuclei (in which spino-olivary tracts terminate). Collateral branches of the axons from the various afferent sources terminate in the globose and emboliform nuclei, which also receive a small contingent of fibers from the red nucleus.

Each half of the body is represented in the ipsilateral cerebellar cortex; if afferent fibers have crossed the midline from cells of origin at lower levels, they cross again in the medullary center of the cerebellum. In the monkey, and probably also in humans, the limbs are represented in two areas: one in and alongside the vermis in the anterior lobe, and the other in the medial part of the hemisphere on the inferior surface of the posterior lobe. The "head area" is in the superior vermis and the immediately adjacent cortex of the posterior lobe. Somatotopic representation in the spinocerebellum is less clearly defined than in some areas of the cerebral cortex; there is overlap of different inputs, so that trains of impulses from various sources may reach the same Purkinje cell.

The spinocerebellar cortex projects to the **fastigial nucleus** (from the vermis) and to the **globose and emboliform nuclei** (from the paravermal zones of the hemispheres). Synergy of muscle action and control of muscle tonus are effected in part through fastigiobulbar connections, as described for the vestibulocerebellum. Fibers from the globose and emboliform nuclei traverse the superior cerebellar peduncle and terminate in the central group of reticular nuclei. Thus the spinocerebellum may influence motor neurons through reticulospinal fibers and a similar projection to motor nuclei of cranial nerves. Alpha and gamma motor neurons are involved in cerebellar control of muscle action, and the influence of the spinocerebellum on the skeletal musculature is ipsilateral.

Some fibers from the globose and emboliform nuclei traverse the superior cerebellar peduncle and end in the red nucleus. Others pass through or around the **red nucleus** and continue to the **ventral lateral nucleus of the thalamus**, from which fibers project to the primary motor area of the cerebral cortex. The main projection of the red nucleus is through the central tegmental tract to the inferior olivary complex of nuclei.

In summary, the spinocerebellum receives information from proprioceptive and exteroceptive endings and from the cerebral cortex. These data are processed in the circuitry of the cerebellar cortex, which modifies and refines the discharge of nerve impulses from the central nuclei. Motor neurons are influenced mainly through relays in the vestibular nuclei, the reticular formation, and the primary motor

area of the cerebral cortex. The end result is control of muscle tone and synergy of collaborating muscles, as appropriate at any moment for the adjustment of posture and in many types of movement, including those of locomotion.

PONTOCEREBELLUM

Pontocerebellar fibers constitute the whole of the middle cerebellar peduncle. These fibers, which originate in the **pontine nuclei** (nuclei pontis) of the opposite side, are distributed to the vermis of the anterior and posterior lobes and throughout the cortex of the cerebellar hemispheres. The large lateral regions of the hemispheres constitute the pontocerebellum. Through **corticopontine tracts** that originate in widespread areas of the contralateral cerebral cortex (especially that of the frontal and parietal lobes) and the pontocerebellar projection, the cortex of a cerebellar hemisphere receives information concerning volitional movements that are about to take place or are in progress. Some of the pontine nuclei receive afferents from the superior colliculus and relay data used by the cerebellum in the control of visually guided movements.

Purkinje cell axons from the pontocerebellar cortex terminate in the **dentate nucleus**, the efferent fibers of which compose most of the superior cerebellar peduncle. After traversing the decussation of the peduncles, some dentatothalamic fibers give off collateral branches that go to the red nucleus and the inferior olivary complex, but the great majority pass through or around the red nucleus and end in the **ventral lateral nucleus of the thalamus**. This thalamic nucleus projects in turn to the primary motor area of cortex in the frontal lobe. Through these connections, the pontocerebellum can modify activity in corticospinal, corticoreticular, and reticulospinal pathways (see Fig. 10-15).

The output of the dentate nucleus, like that of the other cerebellar nuclei, fluctuates according to the excitatory input from extracerebellar sources and the refinement of discharge by the inhibitory action of Purkinje cells. Mainly through its influence on the cere-

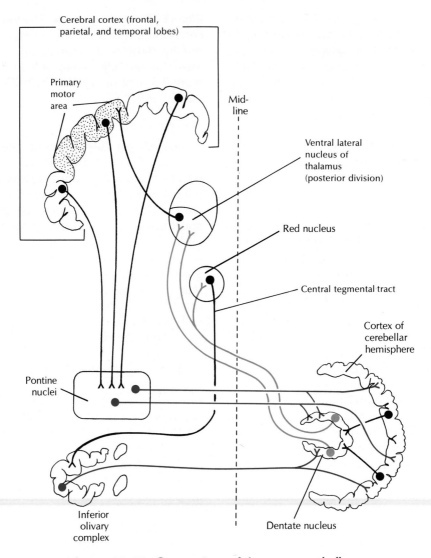

Figure 10-15. Connections of the pontocerebellum.

bral motor cortex, the pontocerebellum ensures a smooth and orderly sequence of muscle contractions and the intended precision in the force, direction, and extent of volitional movements. These functions are particularly important for the upper limb. A cerebellar hemisphere influences the musculature of the same side of the body because of the compensating decussations of the superior cerebellar peduncles and of the corticospinal tracts and other descending pathways.

ADDITIONAL CEREBELLAR CONNECTIONS AND FUNCTIONS

There is a large contingent of **olivocerebellar fibers** from the inferior olivary nucleus and from the dorsal and medial accessory olivary nuclei in the medulla. These cross the midline and enter the contralateral inferior cerebellar peduncle to be distributed to all parts of the cerebellar cortex. Olivocerebellar fibers also end in cerebellar nuclei. The principal inferior olivary nucleus projects to the cortex of the pontocerebellum and to the dentate nucleus, whereas the accessory olivary nuclei project to the spinocerebellar and vestibulocerebellar cortex and to the emboliform, globose, and fastigial nuclei. In addition to the rubro-olivary fibers indicated in Figure 10-15, the main afferents to the inferior olivary nucleus are from the sensorimotor strip of cortex of the ipsilateral cerebral hemisphere (see Ch. 7).

The climbing fibers from the inferior olivary complex are believed to carry instructions relating to movements that have not yet been performed. The patterns or programs concerned are stored in the cerebellum, probably as structural or functional modifications of synapses. It has been suggested that transmitters or other substances released from climbing fibers induce changes in the numbers and positions of the nearby synapses between parallel fibers and the dendrites of Purkinje cells. The execution and coordination of learned movements are mediated by the mossy fiber afferents, of which those from the pontine nuclei are the most numerous in primates. When a monkey makes an intended movement, the neurons in the dentate nucleus (which receives its excitatory afferents from the pontine nuclei) are active several milliseconds before those in the primary motor area.

The movements coordinated by the pontocerebellum are usually guided by input from the **special senses**, especially vision. In monkeys, impulses of visual and acoustic origin reach the superior vermis of the posterior lobe through relays in the pontine nuclei. Tectopontine fibers from the superior colliculus to the dorsal region of the pontine nuclei convey acoustic data as well as visual data because of a connection from the inferior to the superior colliculus. Stimuli perceived by the eyes and ears are also able to influence the cerebellum through corticopontine fibers that originate in visual and auditory areas of the cerebral cortex.

Results of animal experiments have shown that the cerebellum also has a role in **visceral functions**. Under certain conditions, electrical stimulation of the spinocerebellar cortex produces respiratory, cardiovascular, pupil- lary, and urinary bladder responses. They are sympathetic in nature when the anterior lobe is stimulated and parasympathetic when the tonsils (see Fig. 10-3) of the posterior lobe are stimulated. The postulated pathway includes the interposed nuclei, reticular formation and hypothalamus.

Cerebellar Disorders

Pathological conditions are classified broadly into those that affect the vermis and flocculonodular lobe (the vestibulocerebellum and spinocerebellum) and those that affect the hemispheres (pontocerebellum).

MIDLINE LESIONS

The midline portions of the cerebellum may be invaded by a tumor, typically a "medulloblastoma" that occurs in childhood. In adults, a similar syndrome may be seen in chronic alcoholism, which causes degeneration of the vermis. The patient has an unsteady, staggering **ataxic gait**, walks on a wide base, and sways from side to side. **Cerebellar nystagmus** is "pendular," with eye movements of equal speed in both directions, usually in the horizontal plane. It is attributed to interruption of connections of the vermis with the ocular motor nuclei by way of the vestibular nuclei and the reticular formation. The signs are at first limited to a disturbance of equilibrium; however, additional cerebellar signs appear when a tumor invades other parts of the cerebellum.

NEOCEREBELLAR SYNDROME

With respect to the cerebellar hemispheres, signs of dysfunction accompany lesions that interrupt afferent pathways, cause destruction of the cortex and medullary center, or involve the central nuclei or the efferent pathways in the superior cerebellar peduncle. The motor disorder is severer and more enduring when a lesion involves the central nuclei or the superior cerebellar peduncle. When the lesion is unilateral, the signs of motor dysfunction are on the same side of the body.

The following signs, in varying degrees of severity, are those of a neocerebellar syndrome. Movements are **ataxic** (intermittent or jerky). There is **dysmetria**; for example, when the patient reaches out with the finger to an object, the finger overshoots the mark or deviates from it (**past-pointing**). Rapidly alternating movements, such as flexion and extension of the fingers or pronation and supination of the forearm, are performed in a clumsy manner (**adiadochokinesis**). **Asynergy** is separation of smoothly flowing voluntary movements into successions of mechanical or puppet-like movements (**decomposition of movement**). There may be **hypotonia** of muscles, which also tire easily. Cerebellar **tremor**, which occurs most frequently with demyelinating lesions in the cerebellar peduncles, usually occurs at the end of a particular movement (**intention tremor**). **Dysarthria** is evident if asynergy involves muscles used in speech, which is then thick and monotonous (slurring; scanning speech). There may be nystagmus, if the lesion encroaches on the vermis. The deficits noted are superimposed on volitional movements that are themselves basically intact.

SUGGESTED READING

Brooks VB: The Neural Basis of Motor Control. New York, Oxford University Press, 1986

Decety J, Sjöholm H, Ryding E, Stenberg G, Ingvar DH: The cerebellum participates in mental activity: Tomographic measurements of regional cerebral blood flow. Brain Res 535:313–317, 1990

FitzGerald MJT: Neuroanatomy Basic and Clinical. 2nd ed. London, Ballière Tindall, 1992

Lalonder R, Botez MI: The cerebellum and learning processes in animals. Brain Res Rev 15:325–332, 1990

Llinás RR, Walton KD: Cerebellum. In Shepherd GM (ed): The Synaptic Organization of the Brain, 3rd ed., pp. 214–245. New York, Oxford University Press, 1990

Tredici G, Barajon I, Pizzini G, Sanguineti I: The organization of corticopontine fibres in man. Acta Anat 137:320–323, 1990

Walton J: Introduction to Clinical Neuroscience, 2nd ed. London, Ballière Tindall, 1987

Eleven

The Human Nervous System: An Anatomical Viewpoint, Sixth Edition, Murray L. Barr and John A. Kiernan. J.B. Lippincott Company, Philadelphia, © 1993.

Diencephalon

Important Facts

The thalamus, epithalamus, and hypothalamus form the walls and floor of the third ventricle. The thalamus also forms the floor of the lateral ventricle.

The reticular nucleus of the thalamus modulates the exchange of signals between other thalamic nuclei and the cerebral cortex.

Neurons in the thalamus are reciprocally connected with the cerebral cortex. Most thalamic nuclei also receive subcortical afferents.

The ventral group of thalamic nuclei includes the medial and lateral geniculate bodies, the ventral posterior nucleus (VPm and VPl), and the ventral lateral nucleus (VLp and VLa). These are parts of major sensory and motor pathways.

The intralaminar nuclei of the thalamus receive afferents from the spinal cord, brain stem reticular formation, and globus pallidus. They project to the whole neocortex and the striatum. Involvement in arousal, awareness, and motor control is suspected.

The anterior and lateral dorsal nuclei of the thalamus are parts of the limbic system.

The mediodorsal thalamic nucleus receives afferents from the amygdala and entorhinal area and projects to the prefrontal cortex. The lateral posterior nucleus and the pulvinar are connected with the parietal and occipital association cortex.

The subthalamus contains various bundles of fibers connected with the thalamus, the rostral parts of some midbrain nuclei, and the subthalamic nucleus. The last-named is connected with the pallidum; a destructive lesion causes hemiballismus.

The epithalamus consists of the stria medullaris thalami, habenular nuclei, posterior commissure, and pineal gland.

The hypothalamus contains several nuclei. Afferents include fibers from the limbic forebrain and the brain stem. Some hypothalamic neurons directly sense changes in hormone concentrations, osmotic pressure, and temperature of the blood.

Hypothalamic efferent fibers go to the brain stem and spinal cord for control of autonomic and other involuntary functions.

Some hypothalamic neurons secrete hormones, including those of the posterior lobe of the pituitary gland. Releasing factors enter the hypophysial portal vessels and control the secretion of anterior pituitary hormones.

The diencephalon and telencephalon together constitute the cerebrum, of which the diencephalon forms the central core and the telencephalon, the cerebral hemispheres. Because it is almost entirely surrounded by the hemispheres, only the ventral surface of the diencephalon is exposed to view, in an area that contains hypothalamic structures (Fig. 11-1). This area is bounded in front by the optic chiasma and on each side by the optic tract and the region where the internal capsule becomes the basis pedunculi of the midbrain. The diencephalon is divided into symmetrical halves by the slit-like third ventricle. As seen in a median section (Fig. 11-2), the junction of the midbrain and diencephalon is represented by a line that passes through the posterior commissure and is immediately caudal to the mamillary body. The boundary between the diencephalon and the telencephalon is represented by a line that traverses the interventricular foramen (foramen of Monro) and the optic chiasma.

Gross Features

SURFACES

Each half of the diencephalon has the following landmarks and relations. The **medial surface** of the diencephalon forms the wall of the third ventricle (see Fig. 11-2). In about 70% of brains, a bridge of gray matter, the **interthalamic adhesion** or massa intermedia, joins the left and right thalami. A bundle of nerve fibers called the **stria medullaris thalami** forms a prominent ridge along the junction of the medial and dorsal surfaces. The ependymal lining of the third ventricle is reflected from one side to the other along the striae medullares, forming the roof of the ventricle from which a small choroid plexus is suspended.

The **dorsal surface** is largely concealed by the fornix (Fig. 11-3), which is a robust bundle of fibers that originates in the hippocampal formation of the temporal lobe, curves over the thalamus, and ends mainly in the mamillary

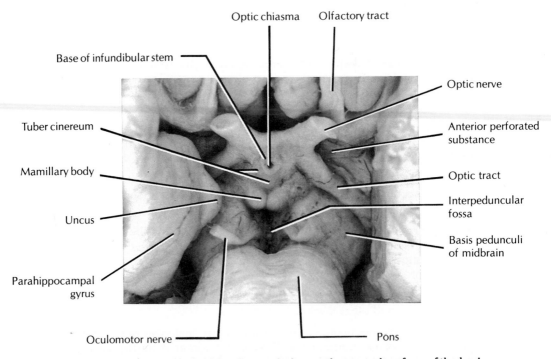

Figure 11-1. Landmarks of the diencephalon on the ventral surface of the brain. Part of the left temporal lobe (right-hand side of picture) has been cut away. (× 1.5)

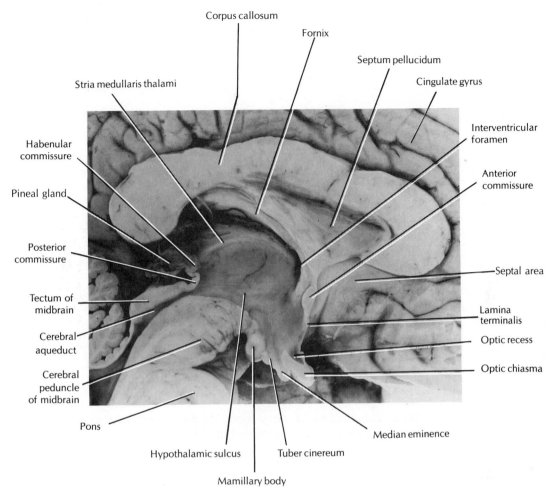

Figure 11-2. Central region of the brain in median section. (× 1.25)

body. Between the left and right fornices, vascular connective tissue known as the **tela choroidea** is continuous with the vascular core of the choroid plexuses of the lateral and third ventricles. Lateral to the fornix, the dorsal surface of the thalamus forms the floor of the central part of the lateral ventricle, much of which is concealed by the choroid plexus (see Fig. 11-3).

The **lateral surface** is bounded by the **internal capsule**, which is a thick band of fibers connecting the cerebral cortex with the thalamus and other parts of the central nervous system. The **ventral surface** of the diencephalon presents to the surface of the brain, as previously noted.

MAJOR COMPONENTS

The diencephalon consists of four components, or regions, on each side. These are the thalamus, subthalamus, epithalamus, and hypothalamus. The **thalamus**, by far the largest component, is subdivided into nuclei that have different afferent and efferent connections. Certain thalamic nuclei receive sensory input for the general and special senses (except smell); these nuclei project to corresponding sensory areas of the cerebral cortex. Other thalamic nuclei are connected with motor and association areas of the cortex, and yet others participate in emotional expression, memory, and sleep. The **subthalamus** is a complex

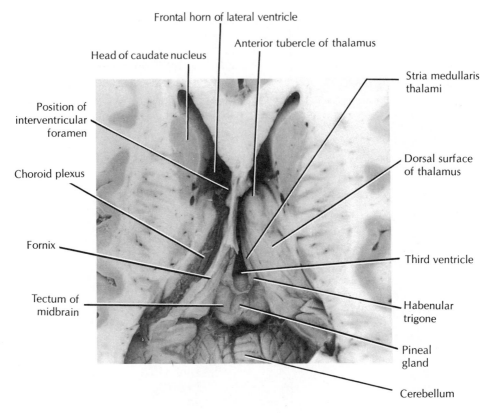

Figure 11-3. Dorsal aspect of the diencephalon. The fornix and the choroid plexus of the lateral ventricle have been removed on the right side. ($\times$ 1)

region ventral to the thalamus; it includes a nucleus with motor functions (the subthalamic nucleus), ascending tracts that terminate in the thalamus, and bundles of fibers proceeding from the cerebellum and corpus striatum to the thalamus. The reticular formation, red nucleus, and substantia nigra extend from the midbrain part way into the subthalamus. The **epithalamus**, situated dorsomedial to the thalamus and adjacent to the roof of the third ventricle, is a particularly old part of the diencephalon phylogenetically. It includes the pineal gland (also called the pineal body or epiphysis cerebri) as well as nuclei and tracts concerned with autonomic and behavioral responses to emotional changes. The **hypothalamus** occupies the region between the third ventricle and the subthalamus; it is the part of the forebrain that integrates and controls the

activities of the autonomic nervous system and of several endocrine glands. The neurohypophysis, which includes part of the pituitary gland, is an outgrowth of the hypothalamus.

Thalamus

The thalamus, which is about 3 cm anteroposteriorly and 1.5 cm in the other two directions, makes up four-fifths of the diencephalon. Thin laminae of white matter partially outline the thalamus; the **stratum zonale** on the dorsal surface, best developed anteriorly (see Fig. 11-12), is one such sheet of nerve fibers. The **external medullary lamina** is a thin layer of nerve fibers that covers the lateral surface of the thalamus (see Fig. 11-9). It consists of thalamocortical and corticothalamic fibers that run along the surface of the thalamus briefly before entering or leaving the internal capsule. The external medullary lamina and internal capsule are separated by an attenuated layer of nerve cells that compose the reticular nucleus of the thalamus. The **internal medullary lamina** (Fig. 11-4*B*; see also Fig. 11-9), consisting of fibers that enter and leave the various thalamic nuclei, divides the thalamus into three gray masses. These are a lateral nuclear mass, the medial nuclei, and the anterior nuclei, with the latter enclosed by a bifurcation of the lamina.

Scheme of Thalamic Organization

Knowledge of the nuclei of the thalamus has come from comparative anatomy, experimental tracing of connections, and physiological study of the effects of stimulation and ablation. Notable investigators of the thalamus include Clark and Walker[1] in the 1920s and 1930s. Their recognition of groups of ''specific'' and ''nonspecific'' nuclei is no longer tenable, but their terminology is still in use. The modern view of thalamic organization comes from numerous investigators in the 1970s and 1980s and is derived from animal experimentation, using electron microscopy, microelectrodes, and tracing methods based on axoplasmic transport.

Every nucleus of the thalamus except the reticular nucleus sends axons to the cerebral cortex, either to a sharply defined area or diffusely to a large area. Every part of the cortex receives fibers from the thalamus, probably from at least two nuclei. Every thalamocortical projection is faithfully copied, with great anatomical precision, by a reciprocal corticothalamic connection. Thalamic nuclei receive other afferent fibers from subcortical regions. There is probably only one noncortical structure, the neostriatum (see Ch. 12), that receives fibers from the thalamus.

Both the thalamocortical and the corticothalamic axons give collateral branches to neurons in the reticular nucleus, whose neurons project to the other nuclei of the thalamus (Fig. 11-5). Contrary to earlier beliefs, there are no connections between the various nuclei of the main mass of the thalamus, although each individual nucleus contains interneurons. The synapses of the interneurons are inhibitory, and most are dendrodendritic. Other synapses in the thalamus are excitatory. The general plan of thalamic connections is shown in Figure 11-5.

Reticular Nucleus

As noted, the reticular nucleus is a thin sheet of nerve cells between the external medullary lamina and the internal capsule (see Fig. 11-9). Despite its name, it is not connected with the reticular formation of the brain stem. The nucleus receives collateral branches of corticothalamic and thalamocortical fibers. The axons of cells in the reticular nucleus project into the deeper parts of the thalamus to end in the same nuclei that gave rise to afferents to those cells (see Fig. 11-5). All the other thalamic nuclei and all areas of the cerebral cortex are associated with corresponding regions in the reticular nucleus. The modulation by the reticular nucleus of the exchange of signals between the thalamus and cortex has been studied electrophysiologically, but a simple function cannot yet be assigned to these connections.

Intralaminar Nuclei

The intralaminar nuclei are partly surrounded by the fibers of the internal medullary lamina. The **centromedian nucleus**,[2] in the posterior part of the thalamus, is the largest member of the group (Figs. 11-6 to 11-8; see also Fig. 11-4*C*). A smaller **parafascicular nucleus** is medial to the centromedian nucleus and adjacent to the habenulointerpeduncular fas-

(*text continues on page 188*)

---

[1] Biographical summaries can be found in the list of ''Investigators Mentioned in the Text'' at the end of the book.

[2] This nucleus, also called the *centrum medianum* and the *centre médian de Luys*, should not be confused with the small central medial nucleus, which is in the massa intermedia.

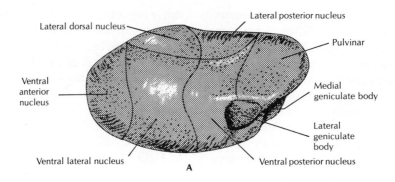

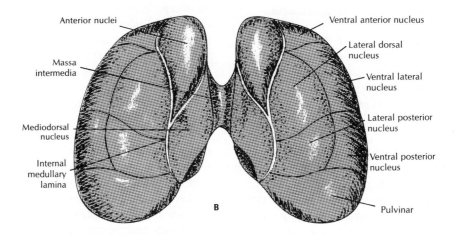

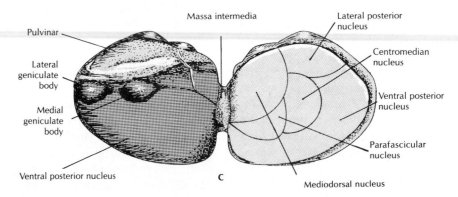

Figure 11-4. Model of the thalami, showing the positions of the larger nuclei. **(A)** Lateral view. **(B)** Dorsal view. **(C)** Posterior view, with the posterior part of the right thalamus cut away. *(Model made by Dr. D. G. Montemurro)*

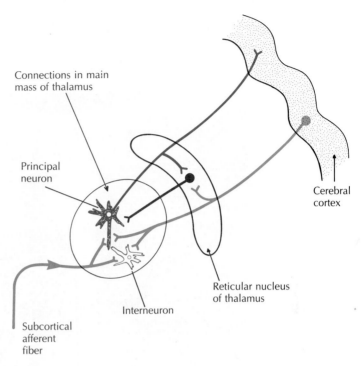

Figure 11-5. Scheme of neuronal connections of the thalamus.

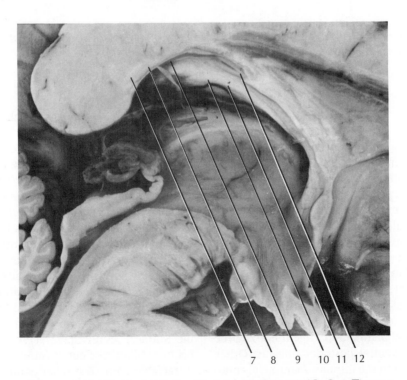

Figure 11-6. Key to levels for Figures 11-7 to 11-12. See Figures 11-2 and 11-3 for names of gross anatomical landmarks.

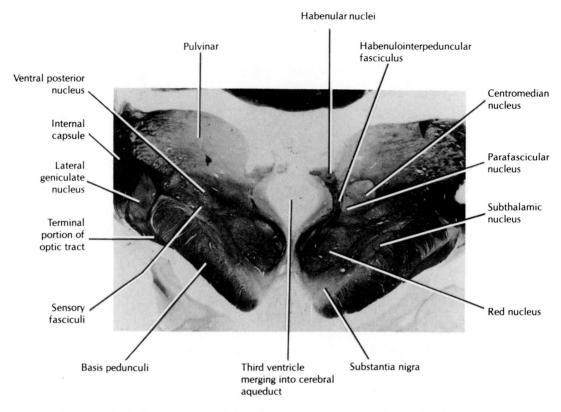

Figure 11-7. Transverse section at the transition between the midbrain and the diencephalon, immediately caudal to the mamillary bodies. (Weigert stain, × 1.8)

ciculus (see Fig. 11-7). The **central lateral nucleus**, in the more anterior part of the internal medullary lamina, is too small to be seen as a pale area in Figures 11-9 and 11-10. The other two intralaminar nuclei (central lateral and paracentral) are too small in humans to merit consideration here.

The intralaminar nuclei receive afferents from the central group of nuclei of the reticular formation of the brain stem (mainly to the centromedian and parafascicular nuclei) and the collateral branches of spinothalamic and trigeminothalamic fibers (mainly to the central lateral nucleus). The principal destination of the spinothalamic and trigeminothalamic fibers is the ventral posterior nucleus. Other fibers afferent to the intralaminar nuclei come from the locus coeruleus, the parabrachial

nuclei, the cerebellum, and the globus pallidus (which is part of the corpus striatum).

The two-way cortical connections of the intralaminar nuclei are with extensive areas of the frontal and parietal lobes. The pathway from the reticular formation through the intralaminar nuclei to the cerebral cortex is thought to provide the anatomical basis for the influence of sensory input to the brain stem and spinal cord on levels of consciousness and degrees of alertness. It also provides for vague awareness of sensory stimulation without specificity or discriminative qualities, but with emotional responses, especially to painful stimuli. Surgical lesions have been placed in the centromedian nucleus in attempts to relieve intractable pain. The relief obtained in some patients was probably attributable to the tran-

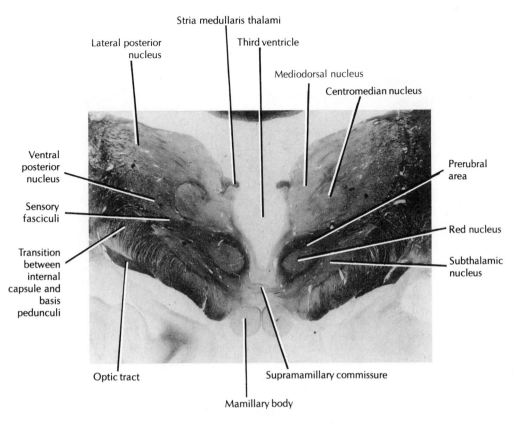

Figure 11-8. Diencephalon at the level of the mamillary bodies. (Weigert stain, × 1.8)

section of spinothalamic fibers that pass through this nucleus and the surrounding parts of the internal medullary lamina before terminating in the central lateral and ventral posterior nuclei.

The intralaminar nuclei also project to the caudate nucleus and putamen, which compose the striatum (see Chs. 12 and 23). These connections may form part of the neuronal circuitry that controls movements, or they may indicate that the corpus striatum is involved in consciousness and arousal.

Ventral Group of Nuclei

The ventral tier of thalamic nuclei includes groups of neurons that form relays in the major sensory and motor pathways. The medial and lateral geniculate bodies (see Fig. 11-4), which contain some of the nuclei of the ventral tier, are sometimes said to compose the **meta-thalamus**.

MEDIAL GENICULATE BODY

The medial geniculate body, located on the auditory pathway, consists of four subnuclei, which are not discussed separately here. It forms a swelling on the posterior surface of the thalamus beneath the pulvinar (see Figs. 7-15, 7-16, and 11-4). Afferent fibers to the medial geniculate body constitute the **inferior brachium** coming from the inferior colliculus, which is the terminus of the lateral lemniscus. The nucleus receives data from the spiral organ (organ of Corti) of both sides, but predominantly from the opposite ear. This bilateral

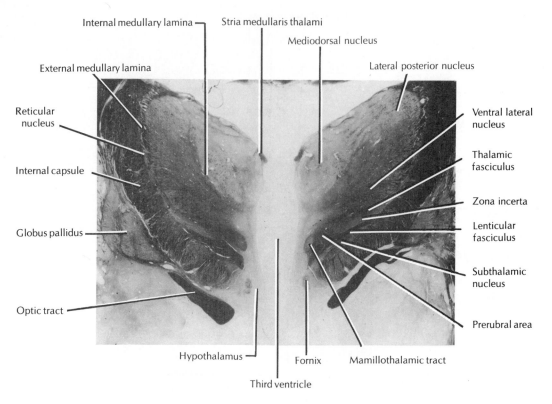

Internal medullary lamina — Stria medullaris thalami

Mediodorsal nucleus

External medullary lamina Lateral posterior nucleus

Reticular nucleus Ventral lateral nucleus

Thalamic fasciculus

Internal capsule Zona incerta

Lenticular fasciculus

Globus pallidus Subthalamic nucleus

Optic tract Prerubral area

Hypothalamus Fornix Mamillothalamic tract

Third ventricle

Figure 11-9. Diencephalon at the level of the middle of the tuber cinereum. (Weigert stain, × 1.8)

projection stems from the presence of some ipsilateral fibers in the lateral lemniscus, and from commissural fibers that pass between the inferior colliculi and between the nuclei of the lateral lemnisci (see Ch. 21). There is a topographical pattern in the ventral portion of the medial geniculate body with respect to pitch; the pattern simulates a spiral, corresponding to the configuration of the organ of Corti.

Fibers emerging from the medial geniculate body constitute the auditory radiation, which terminates in the auditory area of the temporal lobe (see Fig. 11-13). Awareness of sounds is a function of the auditory cortex, and the adjacent association cortex provides for discriminative aspects of hearing and recognition on the basis of past experience.

LATERAL GENICULATE BODY

The lateral geniculate body beneath the pulvinar marks the position of the **dorsal lat-** **eral geniculate nucleus**[3] on the visual pathway to the cerebral cortex (see Figs. 11-4 and 11-7). The nucleus consists of six layers of neurons, numbered consecutively from the ventral surface. The lateral geniculate body is the terminus of most of the fibers of the optic tract, and it projects to the visual area of the cortex. The fibers afferent to the lateral geniculate body originate in the ganglion cell layer of the retina; they are divided equally between those from the lateral half of the ipsilateral eye and those from the medial half of the contralateral eye, with the latter fibers having crossed the midline in the optic chiasma. Each nucleus, therefore, receives signals from the opposite field of vision. The crossed fibers termi-

[3] The ventral nucleus of the lateral geniculate body (or pregeniculate nucleus) is small in the human brain. It is a continuation of the reticular nucleus of the thalamus and probably has similar connections.

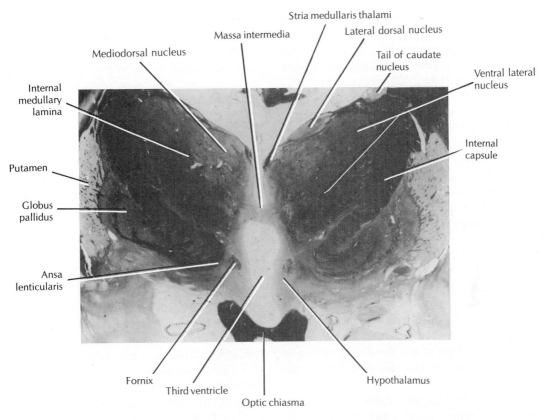

Internal medullary lamina

Mediodorsal nucleus

Massa intermedia

Stria medullaris thalami

Lateral dorsal nucleus

Tail of caudate nucleus

Ventral lateral nucleus

Internal capsule

Putamen

Globus pallidus

Ansa lenticularis

Fornix

Third ventricle

Optic chiasma

Hypothalamus

Figure 11-10. Diencephalon at the level of the optic chiasma. (Weigert stain, × 1.8)

nate in layers 1, 4, and 6, and the uncrossed fibers end in layers 2, 3, and 5.

There is a detailed point-to-point projection of the retina on the dorsal lateral geniculate nucleus. The superior retinal quadrants project to the medial part of the nucleus, the inferior quadrants to the lateral part, and the macular region for central vision to the posterior part of the nucleus. Axons of cells in the nucleus constitute the **geniculocalcarine tract**, which terminates in the visual area of the occipital lobe adjacent to the calcarine sulcus (see Fig. 11-13). At this site and in the surrounding association cortex, there is awareness of visual stimuli accompanied by discriminative and mnemonic aspects of vision.

VENTRAL POSTERIOR NUCLEUS

The ventral posterior nucleus (see Figs. 11-4, 11-7, and 11-8) is part of the pathway for

conscious appreciation of **somatic sensations** arising from skin, muscles, and internal parts of the body. This sensory system is discussed in Chapter 19. All the fibers of the medial lemniscus and most of those of the spinothalamic and trigeminothalamic tracts terminate in the ventral posterior nucleus.[4] This large thalamic nucleus is also involved in two of the special senses. It receives fibers concerned with **awareness of position and movement** (from the vestibular nuclear complex) and ascending fibers concerned with **taste** (from the gustatory nucleus, which is the rostral end of the solitary nucleus).

There is a detailed topographical projection

---

[4] Fibers from the contralateral lateral cervical nucleus go to the ventral posterior nucleus in the cat and monkey, but this pathway is probably small and unimportant in humans (see Ch. 5).

of the opposite half of the body on the ventral posterior nucleus. The lower limb is represented in its dorsolateral part, with the upper limb in an intermediate position and the head most medially. The medial region that receives sensory data from the head is usually referred to as the **ventral posteromedial division** of the nucleus (**VPm**), and the larger lateral portion for the remainder of the body is the **ventral posterolateral division** (**VPl**). The image of the body is distorted, in that the more important parts with respect to sensory function, such as the hand and face, are disproportionately large. The topographical projection of the body on the ventral posterior nucleus (and on the somesthetic area of cortex) is the basis for precise recognition of the sources of stimuli. Fibers from the vestibular nuclei terminate in or close to the region that receives the trigeminothalamic tract. The gustatory fibers end in the most medial part of the ventral posterior nucleus of the thalamus, which is also called the **ventral medial basal nucleus**.

Nerve fibers leave the lateral aspect of the ventral posterior nucleus in large numbers, traverse the internal capsule and medullary center of the cerebral hemisphere, and end in the first somesthetic area of cortex in the parietal lobe (see Fig. 11-13). The opposite side of the body has an inverted representation in the somesthetic cortex, with the portions assigned to the head and hand being disproportionately large. The location of the vestibular cortical area is uncertain. It may be in the superior temporal gyrus, posterior to the auditory area.

VENTRAL LATERAL NUCLEUS

The ventral lateral nucleus (**VL**) has posterior (**VLp**) and anterior (**VLa**) divisions (see Figs. 11-4, 11-10 and 11-11). The VLp receives fibers from cerebellar nuclei, mainly the dentate nucleus, and the VLa receives fibers from the globus pallidus of the corpus striatum. Axons of neurons in both divisions of VL enter the internal capsule and proceed to cortical areas of the frontal lobe. The VLp is connected with the primary motor area on the precentral gyrus, whereas the VLa communicates with the more

anteriorly situated premotor area (see Fig. 11-13). Some symptoms of paralysis agitans (Parkinson's disease) can be ameliorated by a surgically placed lesion in the VL nucleus, but modern drugs have largely replaced this form of therapy (see Ch. 7).

VENTRAL ANTERIOR NUCLEUS

The large ventral anterior nucleus[5] (Fig. 11-12; see also Fig. 11-4) projects to extensive areas of the frontal lobe of the cerebral cortex. Little is known of its subcortical connections or functions.

Posterior Group of Nuclei

In the most caudal region of the thalamus, there is a group of nuclei known as the posterior group or complex. It consists of part of the pulvinar, part of the medial geniculate body, and two small nuclei, the suprageniculate nucleus and the nucleus limitans. Some of the spinothalamic and trigeminothalamic fibers terminate in the nuclei of the posterior group, from which axons project to the cortex of the insula and to nearby parts of the parietal and temporal lobes, including the second somesthetic area. For the perception of pain, the posterior and intralaminar nuclei are probably as important as the ventral posterior nucleus of the thalamus. The pathway through the ventral posterior nucleus to the primary somesthetic area of the cortex is necessary, however, for the conscious appreciation of the precise sites from which pain and all other somatic sensations originate.

Lateral Group of Nuclei

The lateral dorsal nucleus, the lateral posterior nucleus, and the four nuclei of the pulvinar are in the dorsal part of the lateral nuclear mass (see Figs. 11-4 and 11-7 to 11-10).

The **lateral dorsal nucleus** is a poorly understood part of the limbic system; it re-

---

[5] The name "ventral anterior" has often been applied to the VLa nucleus, but current usage favors VLp and VLa for the parts of the thalamus that receive cerebellar and pallidal afferents.

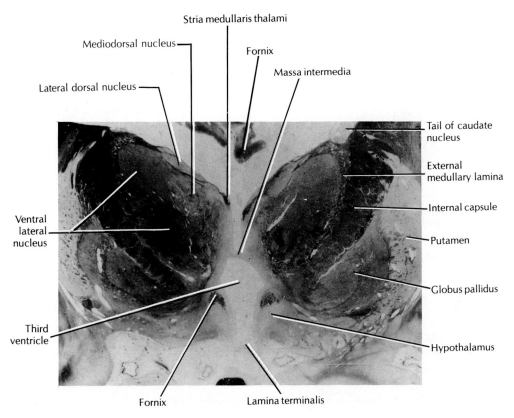

Figure 11-11. Diencephalon rostral to the level of the optic chiasma. (Weigert stain, × 1.8)

ceives afferent fibers from the hippocampus, and it projects to the cingulate gyrus in the cerebral hemisphere. The connections of this nucleus, therefore, have much in common with those of the nearby anterior group of thalamic nuclei.

The **lateral posterior nucleus** is connected reciprocally with the somatosensory association cortex of the parietal lobe, but its subcortical afferent connections have yet to be determined. The nuclei of the **pulvinar** also project to sensory association areas in the parietal, temporal, and occipital lobes. Some nuclei of the pulvinar receive input from the superior colliculus and the pretectal area, and a few fibers from the retina also end there. A projection of the pulvinar on the visual cortex of the occipital lobe forms the terminal link of a series of neurons that runs in parallel with the main visual pathway. It is probably not very important in humans, and it cannot take over visual functions if the pathway through the lateral geniculate body is disrupted.

Medial Group of Nuclei

The medial group consists of the large mediodorsal nucleus[6] (see Figs. 11-4 and 11-10) and the smaller medioventral nucleus. The latter, which also has been called the "midline" group, includes cell groups known as the nucleus reuniens and the paratenial nucleus.

---

[6] The mediodorsal nucleus also is known as the medial nucleus and as the dorsomedial nucleus. Subnuclei with different connections are recognized by some authorities. Connections of the mediodorsal nucleus with the hypothalamus, formerly thought to form an important part of the circuitry of the prefrontal area, probably do not exist.

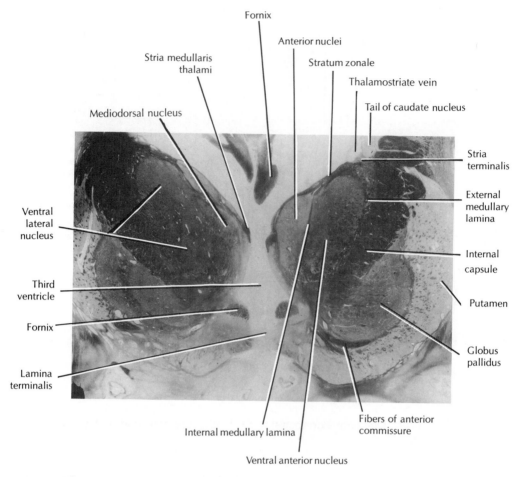

Figure 11-12. Rostral end of the diencephalon. (Weigert stain, × 2)

MEDIODORSAL NUCLEUS

The connections of the mediodorsal nucleus are with the limbic system and with the cortex of the frontal lobe. Afferent fibers come from the entorhinal cortex (at the anterior end of the parahippocampal gyrus, on the inferior surface of the temporal lobe) and from the nearby amygdaloid body. There is a large reciprocal connection between the mediodorsal nucleus and the prefrontal cortex, which is the association cortex of the frontal lobe (Fig. 11-13). A bundle of fibers known as the **inferior thalamic peduncle** passes ventrally to the base of the hemisphere and provides connections between the mediodorsal thalamic nucleus and the orbital cortex of the frontal lobe. Collateral branches of fibers of the spin-othalamic tract have been traced to the mediodorsal nucleus in monkeys; they may be involved in emotional responses to pain (see Ch. 19).

The functions of the mediodorsal nucleus are inferred from the effects of destructive lesions. Severe anxiety states have been ameliorated by placing lesions bilaterally in the mediodorsal nuclei or, more commonly, by severing the connections between these nuclei and the prefrontal cortices (**leukotomy**, or prefrontal lobotomy). Sometimes the procedure has been followed by inappropriate social behavior and impairment of judgment and foresight, so this form of psychosurgery has largely been abandoned in favor of medical therapy. In patients with intractable pain, relief has been

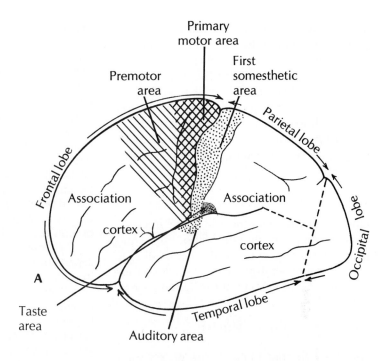

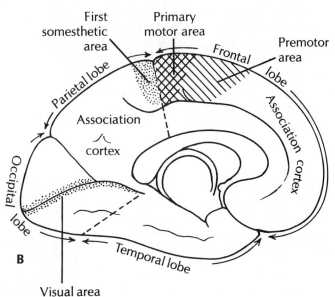

Figure 11-13. Cortical areas connected with thalamic nuclei. **(A)** Lateral surface of left cerebral hemisphere. **(B)** Medial surface of left cerebral hemisphere.

provided by bilateral prefrontal leukotomy. This operation does not cause analgesia or any other definable sensory deficit. The presence of the pain is no longer distressing, however, and the patient will say that the pain is still there but that it does not hurt.

The mediodorsal thalamic nucleus appears also to play a role in memory. In Korsakoff's syndrome, in which amnesia is a characteristic symptom, the degenerative changes in the brain follow a variable pattern. The lesions are typically in regions that surround the third ventricle, and the mediodorsal nucleus is reported as being most consistently affected.

Memory deficits have been reported after surgical destruction of the mediodorsal thalamic nuclei. These changes are difficult to interpret because the pathological and surgical damage affect passing fibers in addition to neuronal cell bodies. Fibers that pass through this region include those of the mamillothalamic tract, which forms part of a circuit believed to be used in the acquisition of new memories (see Ch. 18).

MEDIOVENTRAL NUCLEUS

Little is known about the role of this nucleus. Its connections are with the hippocampus and parahippocampal gyrus in the temporal lobe of the cerebral hemisphere, so that it is considered to be a component of the limbic system.

Anterior Group of Nuclei

The three anterior thalamic nuclei (see Figs. 11-4B and 11-12) are responsible for the anterior tubercle of the thalamus, which forms the posterior or caudal boundary of the interventricular foramen (of Monro; see Figs. 11-2 and 11-3). These nuclei are included in the limbic system of the brain, which is concerned with memory and other behavioral functions (see Ch. 18). The anterior thalamic nuclei receive afferent fibers from the mamillary bodies of the posterior hypothalamus through the mamillothalamic fasciculus (bundle of Vicq d'Azyr) and have reciprocal connections with the cortex of the cingulate gyrus. The lateral dorsal thalamic nucleus, considered earlier, has similar cortical connections but receives its afferents from the hippocampus.

Thalamic Syndrome and Central Neurogenic Pain

The thalamic syndrome is a disturbance of the somatosensory aspects of thalamic function subsequent to a lesion (usually vascular in origin) that involves the ventral posterior parts of the thalamus. Adjacent structures, including the internal capsule, are also involved in these lesions. The symptoms vary according to the lo-

cation and extent of the damage. Proprioception and the sensations of touch, pain, and temperature are typically impaired on the opposite side of the body. When the threshold is reached, the sensation is exaggerated, painful, perverted, and exceptionally disagreeable. For example, the prick of a pin may be felt as a severe burning sensation, and even music that is ordinarily pleasing may be disagreeable. There is spontaneous pain in some instances, which may become intractable to analgesics. There may also be emotional instability, with spontaneous or forced laughing and crying. It is impossible to attribute any of these symptoms to destruction of individual thalamic nuclei.

Pain may also result from destructive lesions in parts of the central nervous system other than the thalamus, including the spinal cord, brain stem, and the cortex and white matter of the parietal lobe. In all these conditions, there is impairment of the perception of real sensory stimuli, attributable to damage to the somatosensory pathways (see Ch. 19). The physiology of pain of the central origin is poorly understood, but it has been hypothesized that the condition is due to abnormal activity in thalamic and cortical neurons that have been deprived of their normal afferents.

Subthalamus

The subthalamus contains sensory fasciculi, rostral extensions of midbrain nuclei, fiber bundles from the cerebellum and the globus pallidus, and the subthalamic nucleus. Fibers in the supramamillary commissure (see Fig. 11-8) interconnect subthalamic structures.

The **sensory fasciculi** are the medial lemniscus, spinothalamic tract, and trigeminothalamic tracts. They are spread out immediately beneath the ventral posterior nucleus of the thalamus, in which the fibers terminate (see Figs. 11-7 and 11-8).

The **substantia nigra** and **red nucleus** extend from the midbrain part way into the subthalamus (see Figs. 11-7 and 11-8). Dentatothalamic fibers, which have crossed the midline in the decussation of the superior cerebellar peduncles, both surround and traverse the red nucleus and then continue forward in the **prerubral area**, or **field H of Forel** (H from the German *Haube*, a cap; see Figs. 11-8 and 11-9). The dentatothalamic fibers, accompanied by some from the globose and emboliform nuclei, contribute to the thalamic fasciculus (see below) and end in the posterior division (VLp) of the ventral lateral nucleus of the thalamus.

Efferent fibers of the globus pallidus are contained in two bundles, the lenticular fasciculus and the ansa lenticularis (see Figs. 11-9, 11-10, and 12-5). The **lenticular fasciculus** consists of fibers that cut across the internal capsule to reach the subthalamus, where they form a band of white matter known as **field H₂ of Forel**. The fibers reverse direction in the prerubral area, enter the **thalamic fasciculus (field H₁ of Forel)**, and terminate in the anterior division (VLa) of the ventral lateral thalamic nucleus. At a more rostral level, the **ansa lenticularis** makes a sharp bend around the medial edge of the internal capsule, continues in the thalamic fasciculus, and also ends in the VLa nucleus of the thalamus. A few fibers from the globus pallidus turn caudally into the midbrain, where they terminate in the pedunculopontine nucleus, which is one of the cholinergic nuclei in the reticular formation of the brain stem (see also Chs. 9 and 23).

The mesencephalic reticular formation extends into the subthalamus, where it appears as the **zona incerta** between the lenticular and thalamic fasciculi (see Fig. 11-9). The connections and functions of the zona incerta are similar to those of the nearby lateral hypothalamic area. Through connections with the subfornical organ (a chemosensitive nucleus, described later in this chapter) and the hypothalamus, the zona incerta is involved in the regulation of drinking behavior.

The **subthalamic nucleus** (body of Luys) is biconvex and lies against the medial side of the internal capsule (see Figs. 11-7 to 11-9). The subthalamic nucleus has reciprocal connections with the globus pallidus, which are described in more detail in Chapters 12 and 23. These fibers constitute the **subthalamic fasciculus**, which cuts across the internal capsule. The subthalamic nucleus also receives some afferent fibers from the pedunculopontine nucleus and sends some efferents to the substantia nigra.

A lesion in the subthalamic nucleus causes a motor disturbance on the opposite side of the body known as **hemiballismus**. The condition is characterized by involuntary movements that come on suddenly with great force and rapidity. The movements are purposeless and of a throwing or flailing type, although they may be choreiform or jerky. The spontaneous movements occur most severely at proximal joints of the limbs, especially the arms. The muscles of the face and neck are sometimes also involved.

Epithalamus

The epithalamus consists of the habenular nuclei and their connections and the pineal gland.

HABENULAR NUCLEI

A slight swelling in the habenular trigone marks the position of the medial and lateral habenular nuclei (see Figs. 11-3 and 11-7). Afferent fibers are received through the **stria medullaris thalami**, which runs along the dorsomedial border of the thalamus (see Figs. 11-2, 11-3, and 11-9) and also is considered part of the epithalamus. Most of the cells of origin of the stria are situated in the septal area. This area is on the medial surface of the frontal lobe beneath the rostral end of the corpus callosum (see Fig. 11-2) and is part of the limbic system of the brain, considered in Chapter 18.

The habenular nuclei give rise to a well-defined bundle of fibers known as the **habenulointerpeduncular fasciculus** (fasciculus retroflexus of Meynert; see Fig. 11-7). The main destination of the fasciculus is the interpeduncular nucleus in the roof of the interpeduncular fossa of the midbrain. Through relays in the reticular formation, the interpeduncular nucleus influences neurons in the hypothalamus and preganglionic autonomic neurons.

PINEAL GLAND

The pineal gland or body, also called the epiphysis, has the shape of a pine cone. It is attached to the diencephalon by the pineal stalk, into which the third ventricle extends as the pineal recess (see Figs. 11-2 and 11-3). The **habenular commissure** in the dorsal wall of the stalk includes fibers of the stria medullaris thalami that terminate in the opposite habenular nuclei. The ventral wall of the pineal stalk is attached to the **posterior commissure**. The pineal gland and its stalk develop as an outgrowth from the ependymal roof of the third ventricle.

The pineal organ has undergone remarkable evolutionary changes. In some types of fish and amphibian, the distal part of the epiphysis contains light-sensitive cells beneath a thin cranial vault. The axons of associated neurons enter the habenular commissure and then pass into the diencephalon. In birds and mammals, the pineal gland has the structural organization of an endocrine gland, although in some species, it contains a small nucleus of neurons that are reciprocally connected with the habenular nuclei. The mammalian pineal gland receives most of its afferent nerve supply from the superior cervical ganglion of the sympathetic trunk through the nervus conarii, which runs subendothelially in the straight sinus (within the tentorium cerebelli) before penetrating the dura and distributing its branches to the pineal parenchyma.

Histologically, the parenchymatous cells (pinealocytes) are arranged as cords separated by connective tissue. These cells have granular cytoplasm and processes that end in bulbous expansions close to blood vessels at the surface of the cellular cords or in the intervening connective tissue septa. The cords also contain neuroglial cells that resemble astrocytes. After about age 16, granules of calcium and magnesium salts appear and later coalesce to form larger particles (brain sand). The deposits are a useful radiographic landmark for determining whether or not the pineal gland is displaced by a space-occupying lesion.

Clinical observations have suggested an antigonadotrophic function for the human pineal gland because a pineal tumor developing around the time of puberty may alter the age of onset of pubertal changes. Puberty may be precocious if the tumor is of a type that destroys parenchymatous cells, or delayed if the tumor is derived from them. Experimental work has placed these observations on a more sound basis.

Pinealectomy in young animals stimulates growth of the reproductive organs, with genital hypertrophy, precocious opening of the vagina in females, and changes in the estrous cycle. Administration of pineal extracts has the contrary effect through inhibition of the gonads. Chemical extraction of bovine pineal glands has produced several possible active principles, including melatonin, an indoleamine related to serotonin. In lower vertebrates, melatonin causes clumping of melanin granules in the pigment-bearing cells of the skin, with concomitant lightening of overall color. In humans, the circulating level of melatonin falls sharply with the onset of puberty. In women of reproductive age, there are cyclic variations, with the melatonin levels reaching minimum values at the time of ovulation.

In mammals, as in lower vertebrates, the activity of the pineal organ is influenced by light; its antigonadotrophic activity is highest when the animal is in the dark and lowest when the animal is in a light environment. The pathway is known to originate in the retina; it also is known that the sympathetic innervation has an inhibitory effect on the gland. A connection between the retina and the intermediolateral cell column in the upper thoracic segments of the spinal cord is, therefore, required. This connection has been shown in animals to begin as fibers leaving the optic tract near the optic chiasma, with these fibers terminating in the suprachiasmatic nucleus of the hypothalamus. Hypothalamospinal fibers traveling in the dorsal longitudinal fasciculus and terminating in the lateral horn of the upper thoracic segments of the spinal cord presumably complete the pathway.

The sites of action of the pineal hormone(s) are still being investigated. The target cells may be in the gonads or in the pars distalis of the pituitary gland. Alternatively, they may be neurosecretory cells in the hypothalamus that produce releasing factors for the gonadotrophin-producing cells of the pituitary, or neurons that project to the hypothalamus. Results of some studies have implicated cells of the central nervous system, either hypothalamic cells or neurons in the reticular formation of the midbrain projecting to the hypothalamus. In addition to the antigonadotrophic function, there is some evidence that pineal hormones influence pituitary cells that produce the growth (somatotrophic) hormone (STH), the thyroid-stimulating hormone (TSH), and the adrenocorticotrophic hormone (ACTH).

Hypothalamus

The hypothalamus, which occupies only a small part of the brain and weighs about 4 g, has a functional importance that is quite out of proportion to its size. Input from the limbic system has a special behavioral significance, and afferents from the brain stem convey information that is largely of visceral origin. However, the hypothalamus, is not influenced solely by neuronal systems; some of the constituent nerve cells respond to properties of the circulating blood, including temperature, osmotic pressure, and the levels of various hormones. Hypothalamic function becomes manifest through efferent pathways to autonomic nuclei in the brain stem and spinal cord and through an intimate relation with the hypophysis or pituitary gland by means of **neurosecretory cells**. These cells elaborate the hormones of the neurohypophysis and produce releasing factors that control the hormonal output of the adenohypophysis. By these means, the hypothalamus has a major role in producing responses to emotional changes and to needs signaled by hunger and thirst and is instrumental in maintaining a constant internal environment (homeostasis).

Anatomy and Terminology

The hypothalamus surrounds the third ventricle ventral to the hypothalamic sulci (see Fig. 11-2). The mamillary bodies are distinct swellings on the ventral surface (see Fig. 11-1). The region bounded by the mamillary bodies, optic chiasma, and beginning of the optic tracts is known as the **tuber cinereum**. The **infundibular stem** arises from the **median eminence** just behind the optic chiasma and expands to form the **infundibular process** or pars nervosa of the pituitary gland. The median eminence, infundibular stem, and infundibular process have similar cytological and functional characteristics; together they constitute the **neurohypophysis**. For reference, these and some other names applied to the hypothalamo-hypophysial system are summarized in Table 11-1.

The columns of the fornix traverse the hypothalamus to reach the mamillary bodies and serve as points of reference for sagittal planes that divide each half of the hypothalamus into **medial and lateral zones**. The medial zone is subdivided into **suprachiasmatic, tuberal, and mamillary regions**, with ventral structures as landmarks. The medial zone consists of gray matter in which several nuclei are recognized on the basis of cellular characteristics and connections. It also includes a thin layer of fine myelinated and unmyelinated fibers beneath the ependymal lining of the third ventricle. The lateral zone or area contains fewer nerve cells, but there are many fibers, with most of them running in a longitudinal direction.

Hypothalamic Nuclei

The lamina terminalis represents the rostral end of the embryonic neural tube and limits the third ventricle anteriorly (Fig. 11-14). The lamina extends from the optic chiasma to the anterior commissure. The lamina terminalis and anterior commissure are telencephalic structures. So is the gray matter immediately behind the lamina terminalis (the **preoptic area**), although its connections and functions are inseparable from those of the anterior (rostral) part of the medial zone of the hypothalamus.[7]

---

[7] The essential unity of the preoptic area and hypothalamus emphasizes the artificiality of naming and delineating parts of the body. The primary and secondary brain vesicles (see Fig. 1-2) are recognized for purposes of embryological and anatomical description, but they are not really defined by lines that separate functionally different regions of the brain.

TABLE 11-1

Hypothalamo-hypophysial Nomenclature (See also Fig. 11-16.)

Name	Definition
Adenohypophysis	Derivatives of Rathke's pouch, an outgrowth from the entoderm of the embryonic pharynx, comprising the pars distalis, pars intermedia, and pars tuberalis
Anterior lobe	Largest part of the adenohypophysis (= pars distalis)
Hypophysis cerebri	Pituitary gland, with its stalk and the median eminence
Hypothalamo-hypophysial tract	Collective name for neurosecretory axons arising in the supraoptic and paraventricular nuclei
Infundibular process	Another name for the neural lobe of the pituitary gland
Infundibular stem	Neural tissue of the pituitary stalk
Median eminence	Part of the neurohypophysis that also is part of the tuber cinereum (see Figs. 11-16 and 11-17)
Neural lobe	Neural tissue of the posterior lobe of the pituitary gland (= infundibular process or pars nervosa)
Neurohypophysis	Diencephalic parts of the hypophysis: median eminence, infundibular stem, and neural lobe
Pars distalis	Anterior lobe of the pituitary gland
Pars intermedia	Adenohypophysial cells in the anterior part of the posterior lobe of the pituitary gland
Pars nervosa	Another name for the neural lobe of the pituitary gland
Pars tuberalis	Layer of adenohypophysial cells on the surface of the median eminence and pituitary stalk
Pituicytes	Atypical astrocytes of the neurohypophysis
Pituitary gland	Adenohypophysis and neurohypophysis
Pituitary stalk	Infundibular stem, together with part of the pars tuberalis, and pituitary portal veins
Posterior lobe	Collective name for the pars nervosa and pars intermedia
Tanycytes	Special ependymal cells (see Ch. 2) with long basal processes that end in the median eminence
Tubero-hypohypophysial tract	Collective name for neurosecretory axons ending in the median eminence

MEDIAL ZONE

Within the medial zone (see Fig. 11-14), the suprachiasmatic region contains the supraoptic, paraventricular, suprachiasmatic, and anterior nuclei. The **supraoptic nucleus** consists of large cells and is best developed above the junction of the optic chiasma and optic tract. The **paraventricular nucleus** contains large cells in a matrix of smaller neurons. These two nuclei are conspicuous in Nissl-stained sections and have a plentiful supply of capillaries. The cells of the supraoptic and paraventricular nuclei elaborate neurohypophysial hormones, and secretory granules in the cytoplasm are evidence of neurosecretory activity. Axons from the nuclei constitute the hypothalamo-hypophysial tract, whose fibers terminate throughout the neurohypophysis where the hormones are released into capillary blood. The **suprachiasmatic nucleus** is a small cluster of neurons on each side of the midline immediately dorsal to the optic chiasma. Axons of retinal origin leave the chiasma to terminate in this nucleus.

The **anterior nucleus** is similar to the preoptic area cytologically, and they are not clearly demarcated from each other. One group of intensely staining cells in this region is notable for containing more than twice as many neurons in men as in women. The difference is due to neuronal death, which begins at age 4 years, in the female brain.

The tuberal region contains the **ventro-**

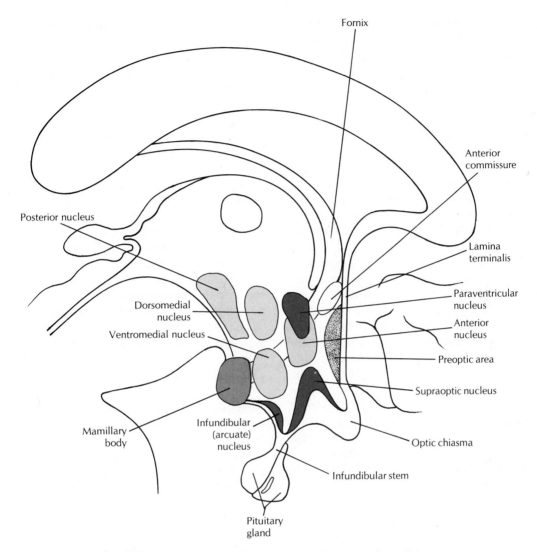

Figure 11-14. Nuclei in the medial zone of the hypothalamus.

medial, **dorsomedial**, and **infundibular (arcuate) nuclei**, with each nucleus consisting of small neurons. The mamillary region includes the **mamillary body** and the **posterior nucleus**. In humans, the mamillary body is occupied almost entirely by a medial mamillary nucleus, and the remainder consists of an intermediate and a lateral nucleus. The cells of the lateral nucleus are large, whereas the bulk of the mamillary body is made up of small neurons. The posterior hypothalamic nucleus consists of large neurons in a background of small ones.

LATERAL ZONE

The large nerve cells throughout the lateral zone are relatively sparse and collectively constitute the **lateral nucleus** of the hypothalamus. The cells are interspersed with longitudinally running nerve fibers that pass to or from hypothalamic nuclei or through the area. This zone includes the **lateral tuberal nucleus**, which consists of several groups of nerve cells near the surface of the tuber cinereum. The human hypothalamus is characterized by the large size of the medial mamillary nucleus, the well-defined lateral tuberal nucleus, and the presence of large neurons in the posterior and lateral nuclei. The lateral zone of the hypothalamus merges caudally with the ventral tegmental area of the midbrain.

Afferent Connections

As mentioned previously, the hypothalamus receives information from diverse sources in order to serve as the main integrator of the autonomic and endocrine systems.

Ascending afferents convey data of visceral origin, including the special visceral sense of taste. The pathways are not well defined, compared with somatic sensory tracts leading to the thalamus. Most of the fibers that ascend to the hypothalamus arise from nuclei in the reticular formation of the brain stem, including the catecholamine, serotonin, and cholinergic cell-groups and the parabrachial nuclei. Some of the ascending fibers are included in the dorsal longitudinal fasciculus, and others are in the medial forebrain bundle. Both these fasciculi also contain efferent fibers of the hypothalamus. Somatic sensory information, especially from erotogenic zones such as the nipples and genitalia, also reaches the hypothalamus.

The cells of origin of the **medial forebrain bundle** are chiefly in the septal area, with other fibers coming from the intermediate and lateral olfactory areas (see Ch. 17). The bundle, therefore, conducts data related to basic emotional drives and the sense of smell. It runs caudally in the lateral zone of the hypothalamus, giving off fibers to various hypothalamic nuclei. Other fibers of the bundle continue through the hypothalamus to the raphe nuclei of the reticular formation of the midbrain and pons. It also contains ascending fibers that originate in the locus coeruleus and the ventral tegmental area of the brain stem and terminate in the hypothalamus. The medial forebrain bundle is smaller in the human brain than in the brains of animals that rely heavily on the sense of smell.

A second input related to smell and emotional drives comes from the amygdaloid body. This nuclear complex is situated in the temporal lobe in the region of the uncus (see Fig. 11-1). A slender strand of fibers known as the **stria terminalis** arises from the amygdaloid body, arches over the thalamus along the medial side of the caudate nucleus (see Figs. 11-12 and 16-9), and ends in the preoptic area, the anterior nucleus of the hypothalamus and the septal area (see Ch. 18).

The **fornix**, which originates in the hippocampal formation of the temporal lobe, is the largest of the fiber bundles that end in the hypothalamus. As mentioned earlier, the fornix arches over the thalamus and into the hypothalamus, where most of its fibers end in the mamillary body (Fig. 11-15). There also are direct **corticohypothalamic fibers**, especially from the orbital surface of the frontal lobe. These reach the hypothalamus by way of the anterior limb of the internal capsule (see Ch. 16).

Efferent Connections

There are two principal descending pathways from the hypothalamus. The first of these begins as thinly myelinated and unmyelinated **periventricular fibers** beneath the ependyma of the third ventricle, continuing into the **dorsal longitudinal fasciculus** in the periaqueductal gray matter of the midbrain. Many of these descending fibers originate from the small cells of the paraventricular nucleus. Some end in the dorsal nucleus of the vagus nerve and, it may be presumed, in the salivatory and lacrimal nuclei. Other fibers continue into the spinal cord to terminate in the intermediolateral cell column and sacral autonomic nucleus. Thus the hypothalamus can directly influence the preganglionic neurons of the sympathetic and parasympathetic nervous systems. Through relays in the reticular formation, and reticulobulbar and reticulospinal fibers, the hypothalamus also influences the activity of certain motor neurons that supply striated muscles used in feeding and drinking. These include cells in the motor nuclei of the trigeminal and facial nerves, the nucleus ambiguus, and the hypoglossal nucleus. Motor neurons of the spinal cord are influenced by the

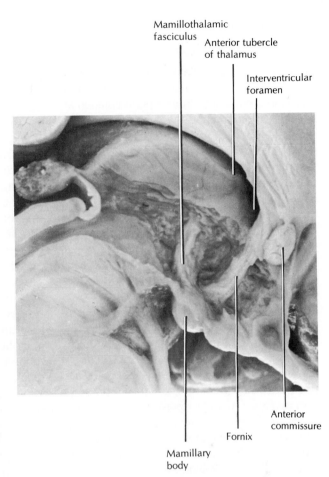

Mamillothalamic fasciculus

Anterior tubercle of thalamus

Interventricular foramen

Anterior commissure

Fornix

Mamillary body

Figure 11-15. Dissection showing the fornix and mamillothalamic fasciculus on the left side. Gray matter has been removed piecemeal from the wall of the third ventricle to display the bundles of myelinated fibers. ($\times$ 2)

hypothalamus for temperature regulation, as in shivering to raise the body temperature.

The fibers of a second descending pathway, the **mamillotegmental fasciculus**, are collateral branches of fibers of the mamillothalamic fasciculus that turn caudally and end in nuclei of the reticular formation of the midbrain and pons. Thus impulses originating in the mamillary body reach autonomic nuclei in the brain stem and spinal cord through synaptic relays in the reticular formation. Finally, axons of some hypothalamic neurons reach the reticular formation by way of the medial forebrain bundle as well as through an indirect pathway that includes the stria medullaris thalami and habenular nuclei.

Activity within the hypothalamus is transmitted rostrally to thalamic and cortical components of the limbic system (see Ch. 18). The large **mamillothalamic fasciculus** (bundle of Vicq d'Azyr) projects to the anterior nuclei of the thalamus, which in turn have reciprocal connections with the cortex of the cingulate gyrus (see Fig. 11-15). Through these connections, the hypothalamus is thought to participate in the acquisition of new memories, the subjective experience of emotions, and the visceral manifestations of emotions through the autonomic nervous system.

The hypothalamus also sends fibers to a region lateral to it called the substantia innominata, which contains the large neurons of the basal cholinergic nuclei of the forebrain (see Ch. 12). These nuclei project to the whole of the cerebral cortex, and their involvement in higher mental functions has been suggested.

Functional Considerations

AUTONOMIC AND RELATED ASPECTS

Knowledge of hypothalamic function has been derived partly from human clinicopathological correlations but largely from experimentation in animals. In interpreting the effects of electrical stimulation or of destructive lesions, it is necessary to appreciate that the axons of neurons in the anterior parts of the medial zone of the hypothalamus pass through the posterior parts of the medial zone and through the lateral zone on their way to the brain stem. It is, therefore, difficult to attribute functions to individual hypothalamic nuclei.

The responses most regularly elicited by stimulation of the anterior hypothalamus (preoptic area and anterior nucleus) include slowing of the heart rate, vasodilation, lowering of blood pressure, salivation, increased peristalsis in the gastrointestinal tract, contraction of the urinary bladder, and sweating. These effects are mediated peripherally by cholinergic neurons, including those of the parasympathetic system (see Ch. 24). Noradrenergic sympathetic responses are most readily elicited by stimulation in the region of the posterior and lateral nuclei, and they include cardiac acceleration, elevation of blood pressure, cessation of peristalsis in the gastrointestinal tract, dilation of the pupils, and hyperglycemia.

Regulation of body temperature is an instructive example of the role of the hypothalamus in maintaining homeostasis. Certain hypothalamic cells monitor the temperature of blood and initiate physiological changes necessary to maintain a normal body temperature. Thermosensitive neurons in the anterior hypothalamus respond to an increase in temperature of the blood and activate mechanisms that promote heat loss, such as cutaneous vasodilation and sweating. A lesion in the anterior hypothalamus may, therefore, result in hyperthermia. Cells in the posterior hypothalamic nucleus respond to lowering of blood temperature, triggering such responses as cutaneous vasoconstriction and shivering, for conservation and production of heat. A lesion in the posterior part of the hypothalamus destroys cells involved in conservation and production of heat, and it also interrupts fibers running caudally from the heat-dissipating region. This results in a serious impairment of temperature regulation in either a cold or a hot environment.

Hypothalamic regulation of food and water intake also has been demonstrated by electrical stimulation and by placing small electrolytic lesions in the hypothalamus. A hunger or feeding "center" has been located in the lateral zone, and a "satiety center" (inhibiting food intake) has been demonstrated in the region of the ventromedial nucleus. The neurons in these parts of the hypothalamus are influenced by the glucose level of the blood, by visceral afferent fibers, and by the olfactory and limbic systems. Destruction of the ventromedial nucleus (satiety center) in a laboratory animal results in excessive food intake and obesity. Naturally occurring lesions in humans also result in obesity, and the cell bodies or axons of cells that regulate the output of gonadotrophic hormones by the adenohypophysis may be destroyed at the same time. The combination of obesity and deficiency of secondary sex characteristics is known as the adiposogenital, or Fröhlich's, syndrome. The zona incerta of the subthalamus, the lateral and ventromedial hypothalamic nuclei, and the subfornical organ are interconnected to control water intake.

RELATIONS OF THE HYPOTHALAMUS TO THE PITUITARY GLAND (HYPOPHYSIS)

Neurohypophysial hormones are synthesized in the hypothalamus; hormone production by the adenohypophysis is also controlled by hypothalamic hormones. The nervous system, through the neurosecretory function of hypothalamic cells, has, therefore, an intimate relation with the endocrine system. Only the major features of the hypothalamo-hypophysial system are discussed here; the subject is a large one, constituting much of the science of **neuroendocrinology**. The anatomical nomenclature special to this system is explained in Table 11-1 and illustrated in Figure 11-16. Some of the clinical and endocrinologi-

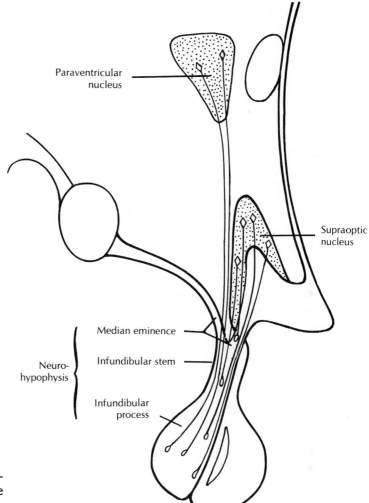

Figure 11-16. Hypothalamo-hypophysial tract and the three parts of the neurohypophysis.

cal terminology is explained in the Glossary at the end of the book.

NEUROHYPOPHYSIS. As noted previously, the neurohypophysis consists of the median eminence, infundibular stem, and infundibular process, all of which are of diencephalic origin in the embryo (see Fig. 11-16). Histologically, it is made up of axonal endings, blood vessels, and atypical astrocytes known as **pituicytes**. Although hormones enter the blood from the neurohypophysis, they are synthesized in the cell bodies of the large neurosecretory cells of the supraoptic and paraventricular nuclei. The hormones are **vasopressin** (also called anti-diuretic hormone or ADH) and **oxytocin**. Vasopressin has two properties, vasoconstrictor and antidiuretic, the former of which is probably of little physiological importance. Oxytocin causes contraction of myoepithelial cells that surround the secretory alveoli of the mammary gland and stimulates the smooth muscle of the uterus. Results of immunocytochemical studies have shown that vasopressin-containing neurons are most abundant in the supraoptic nucleus and oxytocin-containing neurons are most abundant in the paraventricular nucleus.

The axons of cells in the supraoptic and paraventricular nuclei constitute the **hypo-**

thalamo-hypophysial tract and terminate as expansions in contact with capillaries in the neurohypophysis (see Fig. 11-16). The secretory function of the cells is evident in the secretory granules present in the cytoplasm of the cell bodies. The granules are carried distally by axoplasmic transport, and vasopressin and oxytocin enter the blood by way of the capillary bed throughout the neurohypophysis, but principally in the infundibular process. The pituicytes change shape with the functional state of the neurohypophysis, insinuating their cytoplasmic processes between the axonal terminals and the capillaries when the rate of peptide hormone secretion is reduced.

The neurohypophysis is the only mammalian example of a **neurohemal organ**, which is a structure composed of neurosecretory axons ending on capillary blood vessels. Fishes have a histologically similar organ at the caudal end of the spinal cord. Neurohemal organs are more numerous and varied in invertebrate animals. Indeed, neurosecretory cells are phylogenetically one of the oldest neuron types.

VASOPRESSIN. The osmolarity of the blood flowing through the highly vascular supraoptic nucleus influences the activity of its neurons. A slight elevation of osmotic pressure causes these osmoreceptive cells to propagate impulses with greater frequency. The arrival of impulses at the neurohemal terminals causes the release of the antidiuretic hormone (vasopressin) into the capillary blood of the neurohypophysis. Resorption of water from the distal and collecting tubules of the kidney is then accelerated, and the osmolarity of the blood plasma returns to normal. A delicate mechanism is thereby provided to ensure homeostasis with respect to water balance. Destruction of the supraoptic nuclei, of the hypothalamo-hypophysial tract, or of the neurohypophysis results in **diabetes insipidus**, which is characterized by excretion of large quantities of dilute urine (polyuria) and excessive thirst and water intake to compensate (polydipsia). A lesion restricted to the posterior lobe of the pituitary gland is not, as a rule,

followed by diabetes insipidus because some antidiuretic hormone enters the blood from the median eminence and pituitary stalk.

OXYTOCIN. The best understood actions of oxytocin are those following reflex release of the hormone induced by a suckling infant. Contraction of the myoepithelial cells of the mammary gland causes ejection of milk into the duct system, while simultaneous contraction of the uterus contributes to the postpartum involution of this organ.

PITUITARY PORTAL SYSTEM. Secretion of hormones by the pars distalis is under the control of the hypothalamus, but by a vascular route rather than nervous connections.

The following hormones are produced in the pars distalis of the adenohypophysis:

1. Follicle-stimulating hormone (FSH), which stimulates the growth of ovarian follicles and induces their cells to secrete estradiol and other estrogens. In the male, FSH makes cells of the seminiferous tubules respond to testosterone; this effect is necessary for production of spermatozoa.
2. Luteinizing hormone (LH), which stimulates the formation of a corpus luteum in the ovary after ovulation and induces the luteal cells to secrete progesterone. FSH and LH act together to induce ovulation. LH is also known as interstitial cell-stimulating hormone in men because it induces the interstitial cells of the testis to secrete testosterone and other androgens.
3. Prolactin, which stimulates development of the mammary glands and lactation.
4. Thyrotrophic or thyroid-stimulating hormone (TSH), which stimulates the thyroid gland to synthesize and release thyroxine and triiodothyronine. The latter, which is the physiologically active thyroid hormone, also is produced from thyroxine in peripheral tissues.
5. Adrenocorticotrophic hormone (ACTH), which stimulates the cortex of the adrenal gland to produce and secrete cortisol (hydrocortisone) and other steroids that modulate carbohydrate metabolism and

protect against many effects of stress. (Secretion of aldosterone, the corticosteroid that controls sodium excretion and is necessary for life, is not under pituitary control.)

6. Growth or somatotrophic hormone (STH), which stimulates growth at the epiphyses of long bones and elsewhere.

The pituitary portal system begins with the superior hypophysial arteries, which arise from the internal carotid arteries at the base of the brain and break up into capillary tufts and loops in the median eminence (Fig. 11-17). The capillaries are drained by veins that pass along the pituitary stalk and then enter the adenohypophysis, where they empty into the large capillaries or sinusoids of the pars distalis. The preoptic area and hypothalamus contain cells that produce releasing factors and at least two release-inhibiting factors (for prolactin and STH). There is a separate releasing factor for each hormone of the pars distalis, with the exception of FSH, which is secreted in response to the same releasing factor as LH.

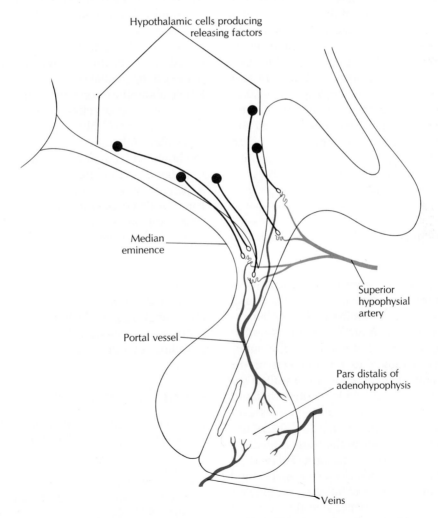

Figure 11-17. Pituitary portal system. (Arteries are red; veins are blue; neurons that secrete releasing factors are black.)

There is probably a topographical pattern of cells that produce the different factors. These factors are peptides; however, the prolactin release-inhibiting factor is dopamine, a catecholamine. The releasing factors pass distally by axoplasmic transport in the axons of the cells that produce them, and enter the capillaries of the portal system in the median eminence to reach the pars distalis. They thereby modulate the synthesis and release of the adenohypophysial hormones.

Cells that produce releasing and release-inhibiting factors are influenced by the various afferent fiber connections of the hypothalamus. Their activity is more directly regulated, however, by hormones of the target organs of pituitary hormones. For example, when the concentration of triiodothyronine in the blood is high, hypothalamic cells that produce thyrotrophin releasing hormone (TRH) are suppressed. Conversely, if the levels of thyroid hormones are low, the hypothalamic cells produce more TRH. This stimulates increased output of TSH from the adenohypophysis, and the thyroid gland, in its turn, is induced to synthesize and release more of its hormones.

Third Ventricle

The diencephalic part of the ventricular system consists of the narrow third ventricle (see Fig. 11-2). The anterior wall of this ventricle is formed by the lamina terminalis; the anterior commissure crosses the midline in the dorsal part of the lamina terminalis. The rather extensive lateral wall is marked by the hypothalamic sulcus, which runs from the interventricular foramen to the opening of the cerebral aqueduct and divides the wall of the third ventricle into thalamic and hypothalamic regions. An interthalamic adhesion (massa intermedia) bridges the ventricle in 70% of human brains. The floor of the third ventricle is indented by the optic chiasma. There is an optic recess in front of the chiasma, and behind the chiasma, the infundibular recess extends into the median eminence and the proximal part of the infundibular stem. The floor then slopes upward to the cerebral aqueduct of the midbrain, with the posterior commissure forming a slight prominence above the entrance to the aqueduct. A pineal recess extends into the stalk of the pineal gland, and the dorsal wall of the pineal stalk accommodates the small habenular commissure. Immediately ventral to the body of the fornix, the membranous roof of the third ventricle is attached along the striae medullares thalami. A small choroid plexus is suspended from the roof. The body of the fornix (see Figs. 11-11 and 11-12) is immediately above the membranous roof.

Cerebrospinal fluid enters the third ventricle from each lateral ventricle through the interventricular foramen. The foramen is bounded by the fornix and by the anterior tubercle of the thalamus and is closed posteriorly by a reflection of ependyma between the fornix and the thalamus. The **subfornical organ**, mentioned earlier in this chapter, is a small eminence on the medial side of the column of the fornix, above the interventricular foramen. It is a nucleus of nerve cells containing blood vessels that are permeable to circulating macromolecules, unlike the vessels of most parts of the brain. In laboratory animals, the nucleus responds to circulating levels of angiotensin II, a peptide whose concentration in plasma varies with circulating levels of sodium and potassium ions and with changes in blood volume. The neurons of the subfornical organ project to the zona incerta and hypothalamus, and their activity influences drinking.

Cerebrospinal fluid leaves the third ventricle by way of the cerebral aqueduct of the midbrain, through which it reaches the fourth ventricle and then the subarachnoid space surrounding the brain and spinal cord.

SUGGESTED READING

Casanova C, Nordmann JP, Molotchnikoff S: Le complexe noyau latéral postérieur-pulvinar des mammifères et la fonction visuelle. J Physiol (Paris) 85:44–57, 1991

Cassone VM: Effects of melatonin on vertebrate circadian systems. Trends Neurosci 13:457–464, 1990

Gross PM (ed): Circumventricular Organs and Body Fluids (3 vols). Boca Raton, FL, CRC Press, 1987

Hatton GI: Pituicytes, glia and control of terminal secretion. J Exp Biol 139:67–79, 1988

Hirai T, Jones EG: A new parcellation of the human thalamus on the basis of histochemical staining. Brain Res Rev 14:1–34, 1989

Hofman MA, Swaab DF: The sexually dimorphic nucleus of the preoptic area in the human brain: A comparative morphometric study. J Anat 164: 55–72, 1989

Ikeda H, Suzuki J, Sasani N, Niizuma H: The development and morphogenesis of the human pituitary gland. Anat Embryol 178:327–336, 1988

Jones EG: The Thalamus. New York, Plenum Press, 1985

Mark MH, Farmer PM: The human subfornical organ: An anatomic and ultrastructural study. Ann Clin Lab Sci 14:427–442, 1984

McEntree WJ, Mair RG: The Korsakoff syndrome: A neurochemical perspective. Trends Neurosci 13:340–344, 1990

Nieuwenhuys R, Voogd J, van Huijzen C: The Human Central Nervous System. A Synopsis and Atlas, 3rd ed. Berlin, Springer-Verlag, 1988

Parent A, Smith Y: Organization of efferent projections of the subthalamic nucleus in the squirrel monkey as revealed by retrograde labeling methods. Brain Res 436:296–310, 1987

Paxinos G (ed): The Human Nervous System. New York, Academic Press, 1990

Reiter RJ: Pineal function in the human: Implications for reproductive physiology. J Obstet Gynaecol 6 (Suppl 2):577–581, 1986

Scheithauer BW, Horvath E, Kovacs K: Ultrastructure of the neurohypophysis. Microsc Res Tech 20:177–186, 1992

Willis WD: Central neurogenic pain: Possible mechanisms. In Nashold BS, Ovelmen-Levitt J (eds): Deafferentation Pain Syndromes: Pathophysiology and Treatment, pp. 81–102. New York, Raven Press, 1991

Twelve

The Human Nervous System: An Anatomical Viewpoint, *Sixth Edition,* Murray L. Barr and John A. Kiernan. J.B. Lippincott Company, Philadelphia, © 1993.

Corpus Striatum

Important Facts

The corpus striatum is the telencephalic gray matter associated with the lateral ventricle. It comprises the striatum (caudate nucleus and putamen) and the pallidum (globus pallidus).

In clinical and physiological usage, "basal ganglia" refers collectively to the corpus striatum, subthalamic nucleus, and substantia nigra.

The striatum, subthalamic nucleus, and substantia nigra receive excitatory afferents from the cerebral cortex. Dopaminergic neurons in the substantia nigra excite some striatal neurons and inhibit others.

Major output of the striatum is to the pallidum, and it is inhibitory. Excitatory input to the pallidum comes from the subthalamic nucleus.

The major output of the pallidum, to the anterior division of the ventral lateral nucleus (VLa) of the thalamus, is inhibitory. The VLa projects to and excites the premotor and supplementary areas of the cerebral cortex.

Other pallidal efferents inhibit the subthalamic nucleus and the pedunculopontine nucleus.

At rest, the neurons in the striatum are quiescent and those in the pallidum are active, thereby inhibiting the thalamic excitation of the motor cortex. Before and during a movement, the striatum becomes active and inhibits the pallidum, thereby allowing more excitation of the VLa and cortex.

The corpus striatum may normally be the site in which instructions for parts of learned movements are remembered and from which they are transmitted to the motor cortex for assembly and eventual execution by corticospinal and reticulospinal pathways to the motor neurons.

Typical disorders of the basal ganglia (dyskinesias) include Parkinson's disease (degeneration of nigral dopaminergic neurons), Huntington's chorea (degeneration in the striatum), and ballism (damage to subthalamic nucleus).

The basal cholinergic nuclei of the forebrain are ventral to the corpus striatum, within the anterior perforated substance. Their axons are distributed to the whole cerebral cortex. These cells are among several populations of subcortical neurons that degenerate in Alzheimer's disease and some other forms of dementia.

The corpus striatum is a substantial region of gray matter near the base of each cerebral hemisphere. It consists of the **caudate nucleus** and the **lentiform nucleus**, with the latter divided into the **putamen** and the **globus pallidus**. Sometimes the corpus striatum, claustrum, and amygdaloid body are referred to by anatomists as the basal "ganglia" of the telencephalon. The **claustrum** is a thin sheet of gray matter of obscure significance situated lateral to the putamen, and the **amygdaloid body** in the temporal lobe is a component of the olfactory and limbic systems. *Clinically, the term basal ganglia is usually applied to the corpus striatum, subthalamic nucleus, and substantia nigra.* These neuronal populations are grouped under the common heading because they are interconnected to form a functional unit, and destructive lesions in any of the components result in disorders of motor control characterized by akinesia (a poverty of voluntary movement), rigidity, or dyskinesias (in which there are purposeless involuntary movements).

Phylogenetic Development

The topography of the human corpus striatum is best understood against a phylogenetic background. In amphibians, the telencephalon is formed into two tubular "hemispheres," each with a central ventricular cavity. The dorsal wall of the ventricle is the pallium, the forerunner of all the cortical structures of the mammalian cerebrum. The medial wall is the septum, which persists in mammals as the septal area, a component of the limbic system. The ventrolateral wall is the corpus striatum. In reptiles, the corpus striatum forms a thickening that bulges into the floor of the lateral ventricle. In mammals, the large corpus striatum has two distinct zones. They are the paleostriatum (homologous with the whole corpus striatum of amphibians and reptiles) and the neostriatum. The expansion of the pallium to form the extensive cerebral cortex in mammals caused the corpus striatum to be displaced from the ventrolateral wall of a tubu-

lar structure into the center of the hemisphere, where it still bulges into the floor of the lateral ventricle. In mammals, the neostriatum is much larger than the paleostriatum. The neostriatum is more often called the **striatum**, and the globus pallidus is then referred to as the **pallidum**.

In the human brain, the extensive cerebral cortex and its associated white matter are responsible for a partial separation of the striatum into two components. Fibers that connect the cortex with subcortical centers traverse the striatum and run along the medial side of the smaller pallidum (**globus pallidus**) as the internal capsule. The striatum is thereby divided into the **caudate nucleus** on the medial side of the itinerant fibers and the **putamen** lateral to the globus pallidus (Fig. 12-1). The globus pallidus and the putamen constitute the **lentiform nucleus**.

The following correlations may be helpful in understanding the terminology of the corpus striatum and "basal ganglia":

---

corpus striatum = lentiform and caudate nuclei

lentiform nucleus = putamen + globus pallidus

striatum = neostriatum = putamen + caudate nucleus

pallidum = paleostriatum = globus pallidus

basal ganglia (anatomical usage) = caudate and lentiform nuclei, amygdala and claustrum

basal ganglia (clinical usage) = corpus striatum, substantia nigra and subthalamic nucleus

---

Lentiform and Caudate Nuclei

The configuration and relations of the lentiform and caudate nuclei contribute to the topography of the lateral ventricle and the cerebral white matter, which are described in Chapter 16. This anatomy is best appreciated by dissection. For understanding the afferent and efferent connections of the corpus striatum,

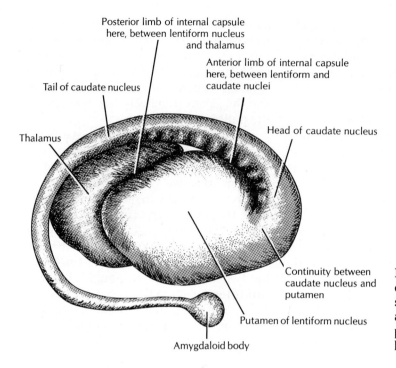

Posterior limb of internal capsule here, between lentiform nucleus and thalamus

Anterior limb of internal capsule here, between lentiform and caudate nuclei

Tail of caudate nucleus

Thalamus

Head of caudate nucleus

Continuity between caudate nucleus and putamen

Putamen of lentiform nucleus

Amygdaloid body

Figure 12-1. Lateral aspect of the right corpus striatum, showing also the thalamus and amygdala. The globus pallidus is concealed by the larger putamen.

the pallidum and striatum are the more functionally relevant divisions.

LENTIFORM NUCLEUS

The lentiform nucleus is wedge-shaped and has been described as having the approximate size and form of a Brazil nut (Figs. 12-2 and 12-3). The narrow part of the wedge facing medially, is occupied by the **globus pallidus**, which is divided into medial and lateral parts by a lamina of nerve fibers. The **putamen** forms the lateral portion of the lentiform nucleus and extends beyond the globus pallidus in all directions except at the base of the nucleus. The two components of the lentiform nucleus are separated by another lamina of nerve fibers.

The lentiform nucleus is bounded laterally by a thin layer of white matter that constitutes the **external capsule** (see Figs. 12-2 and 12-3). This is followed by the claustrum, which is a thin sheet of gray matter coextensive with the lateral surface of the putamen. Its functional significance is unknown. The best documented connections of the claustrum are

reciprocal connections with the cortices of the frontal, parietal, and temporal lobes. The **extreme capsule** separates the claustrum from the **insula** (island of Reil), an area of cortex buried in the depths of the lateral sulcus of the cerebral hemisphere. The medial surface of the lentiform nucleus lies against the internal capsule. The ventral surface is close to structures at the base of the hemisphere, such as the anterior perforated substance, optic tract, and amygdaloid body (see Fig. 12-3).

CAUDATE NUCLEUS

The caudate nucleus consists of an anterior portion or **head**, which tapers into a slender **tail** extending backward and then forward into the temporal lobe (see Fig. 12-1). The extension of the caudate nucleus into the temporal lobe, which consists only of an attenuated interrupted strand of gray matter in some human brains, terminates at the amygdaloid body, with which the caudate nucleus has no functional relation.

The head of the caudate nucleus bulges into the frontal horn of the lateral ventricle,

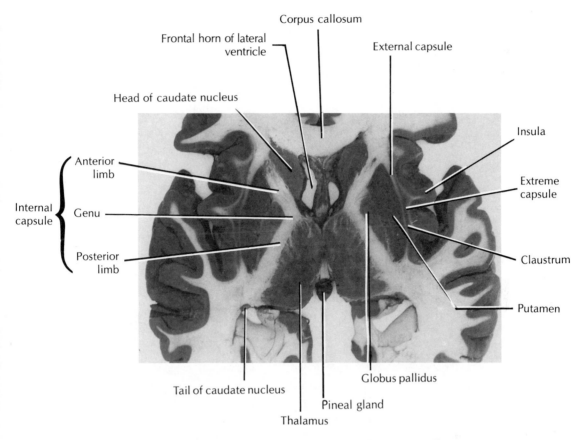

Figure 12-2. Horizontal section of the cerebrum stained to differentiate gray matter (*dark*) from white matter (*light*), showing the components and relations of the corpus striatum. ($\times$ 0.8)

and the first part of the tail lies along the lateral margin of the central part of the ventricle (see Figs. 12-2 and 12-3). The tail follows the contour of the lateral ventricle into the roof of its temporal horn. Two structures lie along the medial side of the tail of the caudate nucleus. These are the **stria terminalis**, a bundle of fibers that originates in the amygdaloid body, and the **thalamostriate vein (vena terminalis)**, which drains the caudate nucleus, thalamus, internal capsule, and nearby structures (see Fig. 11-12).

The anterior limb of the internal capsule intervenes between the head of the caudate nucleus and the lentiform nucleus. The tail of the caudate nucleus is medial to the internal capsule as the latter merges with the medul-

lary center of the hemisphere. The cortical afferent and efferent fibers that constitute the internal capsule do not completely separate the two components of the striatum. The head of the caudate nucleus and the putamen are continuous with each other through a bridge of gray matter beneath the anterior limb of the internal capsule (see Fig. 12-1). In addition, numerous strands of gray matter that join the caudate nucleus with the putamen cut across the internal capsule (see Fig. 12-3). The most ventral part of the striatum in this region is called the **nucleus accumbens**, also known as the ventral striatum. Ventral to the nucleus accumbens is the substantia innominata, which is described at the end of this chapter.

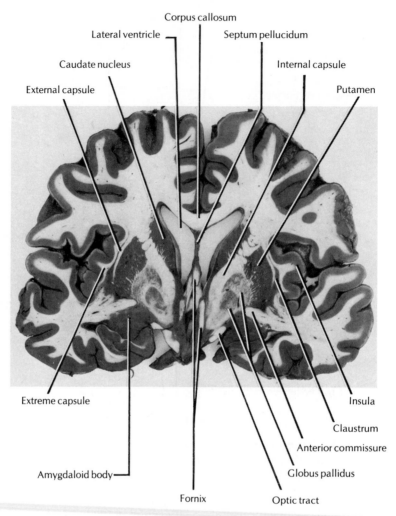

Corpus callosum

Lateral ventricle   Septum pellucidum

Caudate nucleus   Internal capsule

External capsule   Putamen

Extreme capsule   Insula

Claustrum

Anterior commissure

Amygdaloid body   Globus pallidus

Fornix   Optic tract

Figure 12-3. Coronal section of the cerebrum anterior (rostral) to the thalamus, stained to differentiate gray matter (*dark*) from white matter (*light*), showing the components and relations of the corpus striatum. (× 0.8)

Connections

The major neuronal connections of the parts of the corpus striatum are summarized in Figures 12-4 and 12-5 and explained in the following paragraphs.

STRIATUM

The striatum receives fibers from the cerebral cortex, thalamus, and substantia nigra (see Fig. 12-4). **Corticostriate** fibers originate in widespread areas of cortex, including that of all four lobes, but especially the frontal and parietal lobes. The corticostriate fibers are topographically organized, with the somatosensory and motor areas projecting to the putamen and the association cortex to the caudate nucleus. Most of these fibers enter the striatum from the internal capsule, though a substantial number enter the putamen from the external capsule. **Thalamostriate** fibers originate in the intralaminar nuclei of the thalamus, es-

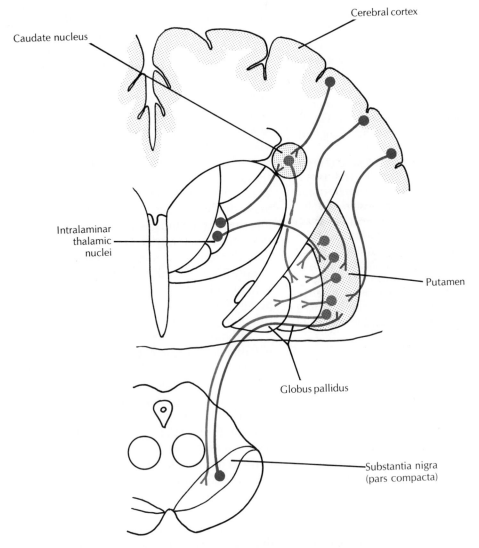

Figure 12-4. Afferent (*blue*) and efferent (*red*) connections of the striatum.

pecially the centromedian nucleus. **Nigro-striate** fibers from the pars compacta of the substantia nigra constitute a particularly important afferent connection. The nigral neurons use dopamine as a transmitter so that in Parkinson's disease, which involves degeneration of neurons in the pars compacta, the striatum is deprived of its dopaminergic input.

The fibers that leave the striatum are **striopallidal**, bringing both segments of the globus pallidus under the influence and con-

trol of the striatum, and **strionigral**, which pass through the globus pallidus before entering the midbrain and terminating in both parts of the substantia nigra.

The caudate nucleus and the putamen are similar histologically, as is to be expected. They contain great numbers of medium-size neurons with spiny dendrites that receive synaptic input from the afferent fibers and have axons that project to the globus pallidus and to the substantia nigra. Branches of these axons also form local connections in the striatum. The neurotransmitter of the medium-size spiny cells is gamma-aminobutyric acid (GABA). This inhibitory amino acid is associated with various peptides in different neurons. The striatum also contains interneurons, which use GABA, acetylcholine, and several peptides as their neurotransmitters.

Histochemical studies reveal a patchy organization of the striatal neuropil. The dopaminergic afferents from the substantia nigra end in islands of low acetylcholinesterase activity that contain clusters of neurons containing certain peptides. These areas, known as "striosomes," are surrounded by a "matrix," which stains strongly for acetylcholinesterase activity and contains a different assortment of peptides. Afferent fibers from the intralaminar thalamic nuclei end in the matrix, whereas corticostriate fibers end both in the matrix and in the striosomes.

PALLIDUM

The globus pallidus contains the myelinated axons of its own neurons together with great numbers of myelinated striopallidal and strionigral fibers. The abundance of myelin accounts for the somewhat pale appearance of the region in fresh sections and for the name "globus pallidus." Conversely, the globus pallidus is darker than the putamen and caudate nucleus in Weigert-stained sections.

The **striopallidal** fibers noted previously are the principal afferents to the globus pallidus (Fig. 12-5). They end in the external and internal segments. The pars reticulata of the substantia nigra is functionally similar to the medial segment of the pallidum and also receives afferents from the striatum.

Efferent fibers of the globus pallidus take either of two routes initially (see Fig. 12-5). Some fibers cross the internal capsule and appear as the **lenticular fasciculus** (field H_2 of Forel) in the subthalamus, dorsal to the subthalamic nucleus. Other fibers curve around the medial edge of the internal capsule, forming the **ansa lenticularis**. These fasciculi consist mainly of **pallidothalamic** fibers, which

originate in the internal segment of the globus pallidus. They enter the prerubral area of the subthalamus (field H of Forel), turn laterally into the thalamic fasciculus (field H_1 of Forel), and terminate in the anterior division of the **ventral lateral nucleus (VLa) of the thalamus**. This nucleus projects to the premotor area of cortex in the frontal lobe, including the portion of the area on the medial surface of the hemisphere that is designated the supplementary motor area (see Chs. 15 and 24). A few pallidofugal fibers accompany the main outflow to the thalamus but continue into the stria medullaris thalami and terminate in the habenular nuclei. Through this connection, the corpus striatum is potentially able to modify the descending output of the limbic system. Other pallidofugal fibers go to the superior colliculus, which is involved in the control of eye movements.

Although the efferent fasciculi of the internal (medial) segment of the globus pallidus project principally to the VLa nucleus of the thalamus, some fibers turn caudally and end in the **pedunculopontine nucleus**, which is one of the cholinergic group of reticular nuclei (see Ch. 9) in the brain stem. Fibers from the pedunculopontine nucleus proceed caudally to the central nuclei of the reticular formation and rostrally to the subthalamic nucleus and to the pallidum. The external segment of the globus pallidus has an important projection to the subthalamic nucleus; it consists of fibers that pass across the internal capsule, in the **subthalamic fasciculus** (see Fig. 12-5). This bundle also contains the axons of neurons of the subthalamic nucleus, which end in the internal segment of the globus pallidus and in the closely related pars reticulata of the substantia nigra.

Physiology and Neurochemistry of the Basal Ganglia

Knowledge of the excitatory and inhibitory synapses in the basal ganglia may explain some clinical features of disorders of the system and has provided indications for therapy

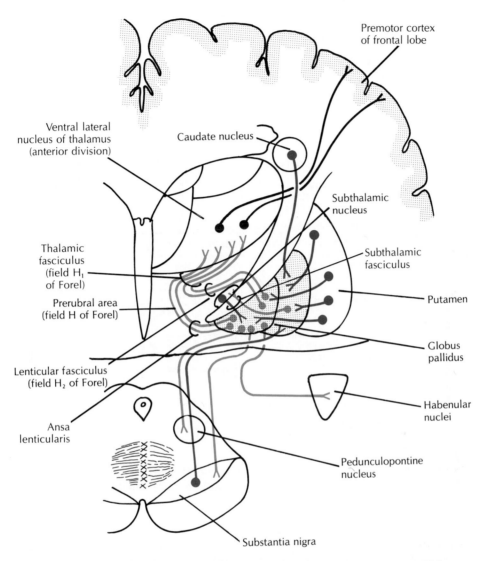

Figure 12-5. Afferent (*blue*) and efferent (*red*) connections of the pallidum. (The projection to the superior colliculus is not included in the diagram.)

with drugs that mimic or inhibit the neurotransmitters. Figure 12-6 shows some of the connections with their actions and the known or suspected transmitters.

Fibers from motor and other areas of the cerebral cortex end in the striatum (corticostriate fibers), the subthalamic nucleus (corticosubthalamic fibers), and the pars compacta of the substantia nigra (corticonigral fibers). These cortical afferents are probably all excitatory, with glutamate as the neurotransmitter.

Excitatory drive to the pallidum comes mainly from the glutamatergic neurons of the subthalamic nucleus, which stimulates the medial segment of the pallidum and substantia nigra pars reticulata, which in their turn inhibit the VLa thalamic nucleus and the superior colliculus.

The striatum inhibits the pallidum, and the pallidum inhibits the thalamocortical neurons. In both cases, the inhibitory transmitter is GABA. Electrical recordings in animals indi-

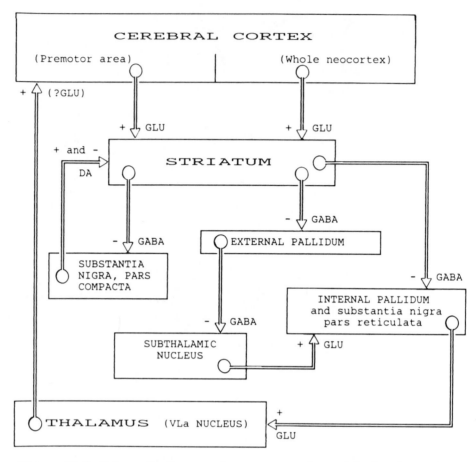

Figure 12-6. Schematic diagram of some connections of the basal ganglia, showing excitatory and inhibitory synapses and neurotransmitters.

cate that the neurons of the striatum are quiescent and those of the pallidum are active when no movements are being made. Shortly before and during a movement, the situation is reversed. Removal of pallidal inhibition allows the ventral lateral (VLa) thalamic nucleus to be stimulated by other afferent fibers, most of which come from the premotor area of the cerebral cortex. The thalamocortical neurons are excitatory to the premotor cortex. The nigrostriatal dopaminergic neurons are active all the time, though their rates of firing increase with activity of the contralateral musculature. Their transmitter stimulates some striatal neurons but inhibits others, depending on the types of dopamine receptor on their surfaces.

Clinical observations and animal experiments indicate that the corpus striatum is probably a repository of instructions for fragments of learned movements. When a movement is to be carried out, the instructions encoded by the corpus striatum are presumably transmitted from the pallidum to the thalamus (VLa) and then on to the premotor cortex. Corticospinal, corticoreticular, and reticulospinal projections would then modulate the motor neurons. The pallidal projection to the pedunculopontine nucleus provides another functional connection with the central nuclei of the reticular formation, which are the source of the reticulospinal tracts.

The great size of the human corpus striatum may indicate collaboration with the cerebral cortex in aspects of memory and thought more complex than the component parts of movements. Memory in birds, which learn most of their behavioral patterns by a process of "imprinting" soon after hatching, requires the integrity of the **hyperstriatum**, which is an avian counterpart of both the neostriatum and much of the cerebral cortex of mammals.

Dyskinesias and the Corpus Striatum

Despite the central position of the corpus striatum in the neural circuitry of motor control (see Ch. 23), lesions in the basal ganglia do not cause paralysis. They result in unwanted involuntary movements.

Types of Dyskinesia

The involuntary movements seen in the dyskinesias related to the corpus striatum take various forms. **Choreiform** movements are brisk, jerky, and purposeless, resembling fragments of voluntary movements. They are irregularly timed and often most pronounced in the distal limb musculature and the face. There may be hypotonia of the affected muscles. **Athetoid** movements are also irregular but are slow and sinuous, involving the proximal and distal musculature of the limbs. The movements blend together in a continuous mobile spasm and are usually associated with varying degrees of paresis and spasticity. The muscles of the face, neck, and tongue may be affected, with grimacing, protrusion and writhing of the tongue, and difficulty in speaking and swallowing. The term **choreoathetosis** is applied to involuntary movements with both choreiform and athetoid features. Choreoathetosis overlaps with **dystonia**, in which there are sustained involuntary muscle contractions. In **myoclonus** there are sudden, strong contractions which may be isolated, repetitive, or rhythmic. Regularly alternating movements of small amplitude constitute **tremor**. Stereotyped purposeless movements that occur at random are called **tics** or habit spasms, whereas a generalized inability to be still, with constant motion of the limbs, is sometimes called **akathisia**. The largest involuntary movements are those of **ballism**. This is an exagge-

rated form of chorea in which limbs make large, irregular flinging movements caused by contractions of muscles acting on the shoulder or hip joints.

The lesions responsible for dyskinesias are poorly understood. In chorea, there is extensive damage in the striatum. In dystonia, any of the components of the corpus striatum may be involved, but more often than not, no pathology can be identified. Ballism is usually attributed to a small destructive lesion in the contralateral subthalamic nucleus. The uncontrolled movements may be due to loss of excitatory input to the pallidum, which then fails to inhibit the anterior division of the ventral lateral thalamic nucleus. Excessive activity in the VLa stimulates the premotor area of the cerebral cortex, causing excessive movement at the proximal joints of the limbs. The most common type of ballism is **hemiballismus**, described in Chapter 11. Lesions in the pars compacta of the substantia nigra are responsible for the characteristic tremor and other features of **Parkinson's disease**, described in Chapter 7.

Diseases

There are numerous conditions in which choreiform movements are a cardinal sign. **Sydenham's chorea** (St. Vitus' dance) typically occurs in childhood after an infectious disease caused by hemolytic streptococci. Because the disease is seldom fatal, the pathology of Sydenham's chorea is poorly understood. The commonest findings are microscopic hemorrhages and emboli in the corpus striatum. **Huntington's chorea** is a dominant hereditary disorder with onset of clinical signs in middle life. Neuronal degeneration is most marked in the striatum. Concurrent loss of neurons in the cerebral cortex leads to progressive mental deterioration. Athetosis and choreoathetosis often form part of a congenital complex of neurological signs (including those of cerebral palsy) that result from metabolic disorders of the developing brain or from birth injury. Athetoid movements are most frequently associated with pathological changes in the striatum and the cerebral cortex, although lesions are sometimes also present in the globus pallidus and the thalamus.

Wilson's disease (hepatolenticular degeneration) is caused by a genetically determined error in copper metabolism. The signs of Wilson's disease usually appear between ages 10 and 25; they include muscle rigidity, dystonia, tremor, impairment of voluntary movements (including those of speech), and loss of facial expression. There may be uncontrollable laughing or crying without apparent cause, and dementia ensues if the condition is left untreated. The degenerative changes are most pronounced in the putamen and progress to cavitation of the lentiform nucleus. There may also be cellular degeneration in the cerebral cortex, thalamus, red nucleus, and cerebellum. In addition to these neurological abnormalities, the patients have cirrhosis of the liver. The neurological and hepatic changes of Wilson's disease respond to treatment with drugs that enhance the urinary excretion of copper.

Dystonia musculorum deformans (also called **generalized dystonia**) is a particularly disabling motor disturbance in which slow, writhing, involuntary movements of the axial and limb musculature are sustained, sometimes leading to permanent contractures. The symptoms first appear in older children or young adults. There may be lesions in the corpus striatum and elsewhere, but the pathology is poorly understood.

Some drugs used in psychiatry inhibit the action of dopamine in the striatum. When given for a long time, in high doses, or to unusually susceptible patients, they can cause a variety of acute parkinsonian or dystonic reactions or dyskinesias.

Substantia Innominata

The substantia innominata is the territory ventral to the internal capsule, nucleus accumbens, and anterior commissure; dorsal to the anterior perforated substance; medial to the amygdala; and lateral to the hypothalamus. The region contains the **basal forebrain nuclei**, comprising three groups of large cholinergic neurons: the **nucleus basalis of Meynert**, the **nucleus of the diagonal band**, and part of the **septal area**. These groups of cells receive afferent fibers from the cortex of the limbic system, the hypothalamus, and the central and noradrenergic nuclei of the reticular formation. The cholinergic neurons in the basal forebrain nuclei project to all areas of the cerebral cortex as well as to the hippocampus

and the amygdaloid body. They constitute the sole source of cholinergic innervation of the cortex, perhaps providing an important link between the limbic system and the neocortex.

The magnocellular basal forebrain nuclei are among several parts of the brain that have been implicated in the pathogenesis of **Alzheimer's disease**. This disorder, the first manifestation of which is the failure of memory for recent events, is a common cause of mental deterioration (dementia) in elderly people. The large cholinergic neurons at the base of the forebrain degenerate, and the cortex loses its cholinergic afferent fibers. Severe degenerative changes are also seen in the hippocampus and the locus coeruleus. In advanced Alzheimer's disease, there is also considerable neuronal loss, with shrinkage of gyri, throughout the cerebral cortex. There are fibrillary tangles in neuronal somata in all affected parts of the brain, together with large extracellular deposits of fibrillary material known as senile plaques. Similar pathological changes are found in several other diseases that cause dementia.

SUGGESTED READING

Albin RL, Young AB, Penney JB: The functional anatomy of basal ganglia disorders. Trends Neurosci 12:366–375, 1989

Butcher LL, Semba K: Reassessing the cholinergic basal forebrain. Trends Neurosci 12:483–485, 1989

Crosby EC, Schnitzlein HN (eds): Comparative Correlative Neuroanatomy of the Vertebrate Telencephalon. New York, Macmillan, 1982

Doucette R, Fisman M, Hachinski VC, Mersky H: Cell loss from the nucleus basalis of Meynert in Alzheimer's disease. Can J Neurol Sci 13:435–440, 1986

Hedreen JC, Struble RG, Whitehouse PJ, Price DL: Topography of the magnocellular basal forebrain system in the human brain. J Neuropathol Exp Neurol 43:1–21, 1984

Horn G: Neural bases of recognition memory investigated through an analysis of imprinting. Phil Trans R Soc Lond 329:133–142, 1990

Mesulam M-M, Geula C: Nucleus basalis (Ch4) and cortical cholinergic innervation in the human brain: observations based on the distribution of acetylcholinesterase and choline acetyltransferase. J Comp Neurol 275:216–240, 1988

Mesulam M-M, Mufson EJ: Neural inputs into the nucleus basalis of the substantia innominata (Ch 4) in the rhesus monkey. Brain 107:253–274, 1984

Perry RH, Candy JM, Perry EK, Thompson J, Oakley AE: The substantia innominata and adjacent regions in the human brain: Histochemical and biochemical observations. J Anat 138:713–732, 1984

Sarnat HB, Netsky MG: Evolution of the Nervous System, 2nd ed. New York, Oxford University Press, 1981

Ulfig N: Configuration of the magnocellular nuclei in the basal forebrain of the human adult. Acta Anat 134:100–105, 1989

Thirteen

The Human Nervous System: An Anatomical Viewpoint, Sixth Edition, Murray L. Barr and John A. Kiernan. J.B. Lippincott Company, Philadelphia, © 1993.

Topography of the Cerebral Hemispheres

Important Facts

The large surface area of the human cerebral cortex results in a pattern of gyri and sulci. Some of these convolutions are important anatomical landmarks or functional areas.

Five lobes (including the insula) are recognized in each cerebral hemisphere.

On the medial surface of the hemisphere, the parieto-occipital sulcus separates the parietal from the occipital lobe.

In the occipital lobe, the calcarine sulcus is the site of the primary visual cortex.

In the parietal lobe, the postcentral gyrus corresponds to the first general sensory area. The supramarginal and angular gyri are parts of the receptive language area, which extends onto the superior temporal gyrus.

The central sulcus is between the parietal and frontal lobes, separating the first somesthetic from the primary motor area.

In the frontal lobe, the precentral gyrus corresponds to the primary motor area. The olfactory bulb and tract are applied to the orbital surface of the frontal lobe.

The lateral sulcus (sylvian fissure) separates the frontal and parietal lobes from the temporal lobe.

The insular lobe (insula), in the floor of the lateral sulcus, is a landmark for part of the corpus striatum.

The superior surface of the superior temporal gyrus includes the primary auditory area.

The parahippocampal gyrus includes the uncus (a primary olfactory area) and the entorhinal area, which has olfactory and limbic functions.

The "limbic lobe" includes the parahippocampal and cingulate gyri. It is part of the limbic system, which is involved in memory.

The complicated folding of the surface of the cerebral hemispheres substantially increases the surface area and, therefore, the volume of cerebral cortex. The folds or convolutions are called **gyri**, and the intervening grooves are called **sulci**. About two-thirds of the cortex forms the walls of the sulci and is, therefore, hidden from surface view. Although some gyri are constant features of the cerebral surface, others vary from one brain to another and even between the two hemispheres of the same brain. Subtler depressions in the cerebral cortex are grooves and notches unrelated to the pattern of gyri and sulci. They are made by extracerebral structures such as the bones of the skull and the venous sinuses of the dura mater.

A sulcus is a groove on the surface of a cerebral hemisphere, whereas a **fissure** is a cleft that separates large components of the brain. Despite the different definitions of sulci and fissures, the two terms often are used interchangeably for the deepest sulci.

At an early stage in studying human neuroanatomy, the student should be able to delineate the lobes of the cerebral hemispheres and to recognize the major sulci, fissures, and gyri, which commonly are referred to as landmarks. Of the smaller sulci and gyri, some are of great functional importance, whereas others have no known significance. They are described and illustrated in the later sections of this chapter.

Major Sulci and the Fissures

The lateral and parieto-occipital sulci appear early in fetal development and are especially deep in the mature brain. These, together with the central and calcarine sulci, are the boundaries for division of the cerebral hemisphere into the frontal, parietal, temporal, and occipital lobes (Figs. 13-1 and 13-2).

The **lateral sulcus** (fissure of Sylvius or sylvian fissure) begins as a deep furrow on the inferior surface of the hemisphere. This is the **stem** of the sulcus, which extends laterally between the frontal and temporal lobes and divides into three rami on reaching the lateral surface. The **posterior ramus** is the main part of the sulcus on the lateral surface of the hemisphere, whereas the **anterior** and **ascending rami** project for only a short distance into the frontal lobe. An area of cortex called the **insular lobe** or **insula** (island of Reil) lies at the bottom of the lateral sulcus and is hidden from surface view. This cortex appears to have been bound to the underlying corpus striatum dur-

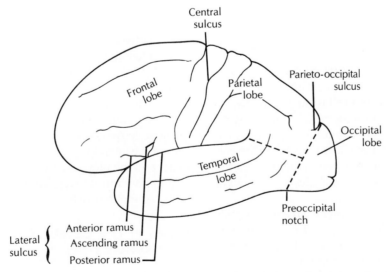

Figure 13-1. Lobes of the cerebral hemisphere (lateral surface).

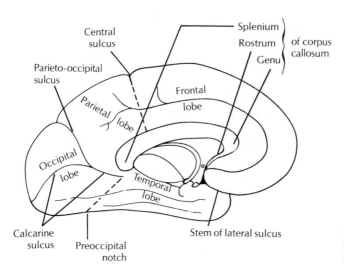

Figure 13-2. Lobes of the cerebral hemisphere (medial and inferior surfaces).

ing late embryonic and early fetal development; growth of the surrounding cortex would then produce the deep lateral sulcus.

The **central sulcus** (sulcus of Rolando; rolandic sulcus) is an important landmark for the sensorimotor cortex because the general sensory area is immediately behind the sulcus and the motor area is immediately in front of it. The central sulcus indents the superior border of the hemisphere about 1 cm behind the midpoint between the frontal and occipital poles. The sulcus slopes downward and forward at an angle of 70° to the vertical, stopping just short of the lateral sulcus, and there usually are two bends along its course. The central sulcus is about 2 cm deep, and its walls, therefore, constitute much of the sensorimotor cortex.

The **calcarine sulcus** on the medial surface of the hemisphere begins under the posterior end of the corpus callosum and follows an arched course to the occipital pole. In some brains, the sulcus continues over the pole for a short distance on the lateral surface. The calcarine sulcus is an important landmark for the visual cortex, most of which lies in the walls of the sulcus.

The **parieto-occipital sulcus** extends from the calcarine sulcus to the superior border of the hemisphere, which it intersects about 4 cm from the occipital pole.

The longitudinal and transverse cerebral fissures are external to the hemispheres and are, therefore, in a different category from the foregoing surface markings. The **longitudinal cerebral fissure** separates the hemispheres, and a dural partition called the falx cerebri extends into the fissure. The corpus callosum, which constitutes the main cerebral commissure, crosses from one hemisphere to the other at the bottom of the longitudinal fissure. The **transverse cerebral fissure** intervenes between the cerebral hemispheres above and the cerebellum, midbrain, and diencephalon below. The posterior part of this fissure is between the cerebral hemispheres and the cerebellum; it contains a dural partition known as the tentorium cerebelli. The anterior part of the transverse fissure intervenes between the corpus callosum and the diencephalon. It is triangular in outline, tapering anteriorly, and contains the tela choroidea, which consists of vascular connective tissue derived from the pia mater that covers the brain. The tela choroidea is continuous with the connective tissue core of the choroid plexuses of the lateral ventricles and the third ventricle, and the plexuses are completed by choroid epithelium derived from the ependymal lining of the ventricles.

Lobes of the Cerebral Hemispheres

Each cerebral hemisphere has lateral, medial, and inferior surfaces on which the extent of the lobes of the hemisphere are now defined (see Figs. 13-1 and 13-2).

The **frontal lobe** occupies the entire area in front of the central sulcus and above the lateral sulcus on the lateral surface. The medial surface of the frontal lobe envelops the anterior part of the corpus callosum and is bounded posteriorly by a line drawn between the central sulcus and the corpus callosum. (Such lines are drawn elsewhere; they have no functional significance and can be ignored after serving their initial purpose.) The inferior surface of the frontal lobe rests on the orbital plate of the frontal bone.

The natural boundaries of the **parietal lobe** on the lateral surface are the central and lateral sulci. The other boundaries consist of two lines; the first of these is drawn between the parieto-occipital sulcus and the preoccipital notch, and the second line runs from the middle of the one just established to the lateral sulcus. (The preoccipital notch is an inconspicuous landmark consisting of a shallow indentation of the brain formed by the petrous portion of the temporal bone.) On the medial surface, the parietal lobe is bounded by the frontal lobe, corpus callosum, calcarine sulcus, and parieto-occipital sulcus.

The **temporal lobe** is outlined on the lateral surface by the lateral sulcus and the lines previously noted. The inferior surface of the temporal lobe extends to the temporal pole from a line drawn between the anterior end of the calcarine sulcus and the preoccipital notch. Most of the **occipital lobe** appears on the medial surface of the hemisphere, where it is separated from the temporal lobe, as already described, and from the parietal lobe by the parieto-occipital sulcus. On the lateral surface, the occipital lobe consists of the small area posterior to the line that joins the parieto-occipital sulcus and preoccipital notch.

The portion of the great cerebral commissure in and near the midline is known as the **trunk of the corpus callosum**, and the fibers of the commissure that spread out within the medullary centers of the hemispheres constitute the **radiations of the corpus callosum**. Names are assigned to certain regions of the trunk of the commissure (see Fig. 13-2);

these regions are used as reference points further on. The enlarged posterior portion of the trunk is called the **splenium**. The anterior portion, or **genu**, curves ventrally and thins out to form the **rostrum**. This is continuous with the lamina terminalis, which limits the third ventricle anteriorly.

Gyri and Sulci

Some surface markings of the hemisphere are landmarks for important functional areas; the central sulcus for the sensorimotor cortex and the calcarine sulcus for the visual cortex are examples. For the most part, the sulci and gyri serve only as a rough frame of reference for cortical areas whose functions may or may not be known. The markings can be identified according to lobes for the lateral surface, but this is not practicable for the medial and inferior surfaces.

The text and illustrations that follow apply to sulci and gyri of varying functional significance. The student may need to refer to this material when studying the localization of functions in the cerebral cortex (see Ch. 15).

Lateral Surface

Frontal Lobe

The **precentral sulcus** (often broken into two or more parts) runs parallel to the central sulcus; these sulci outline the **precentral gyrus**, which is a landmark for the primary motor area of the cerebral cortex (Fig. 13-3). The remainder of the lateral surface of the frontal lobe is divided into **superior, middle**, and **inferior frontal gyri** by the **superior** and **inferior frontal sulci**. The anterior and ascending rami of the lateral sulcus divide the inferior frontal gyrus into **opercular, triangular**, and **orbital portions**. In the left hemisphere, the opercular and triangular portions consist of cortex of Broca's expressive or motor speech area. In the frontal lobe, as in the other lobes of the hemisphere, there are secondary gyri and sulci that contribute to the variable topography of different brains.

Parietal Lobe

The **postcentral sulcus** runs parallel to the central sulcus; these sulci bound the **postcentral**

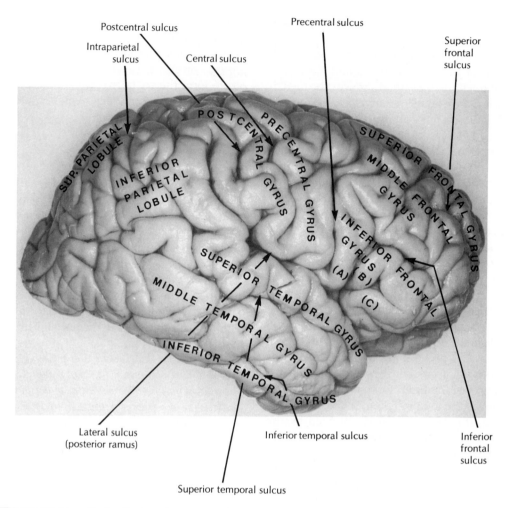

Figure 13-3. Gyri and sulci on the lateral surface of the right cerebral hemisphere. (**A**), (**B**) and (**C**) indicate the opercular, triangular, and orbital portions of the inferior frontal gyrus, respectively. (× 0.63)

gyrus, which is the landmark for the first general sensory (somesthetic) area of cortex. The **intraparietal sulcus** extends posteriorly from the postcentral sulcus and divides that part of the surface not occupied by the postcentral gyrus into **superior** and **inferior parietal lobules.** Those portions of the inferior parietal lobule that surround the upturned ends of the lateral sulcus and superior temporal sulcus are called the **supramarginal gyrus** and the **angular gyrus,** respectively. In the left hemisphere, these gyri consist of cortex included in the receptive language area, which is necessary for perception and interpretation of spoken and written language.

Temporal Lobe

Superior and **inferior temporal sulci** divide the lateral surface of the temporal lobe into **superior, middle,** and **inferior temporal gyri.** Among variations in the temporal lobe, the inferior temporal sulcus may be discontinuous, making it difficult to identify. The superior temporal gyrus has a large surface that forms the floor of the lateral sulcus. On this surface, **transverse temporal gyri** (also known as **Heschl's convolutions**) extend to the bottom of the lateral sulcus and mark the location of the auditory area of cortex. The posterior part of the left superior temporal gyrus forms part of the receptive language area, which extends onto the parietal lobe.

Occipital Lobe

In the brains of primates other than humans and in some human brains, the calcarine sulcus continues for a short distance over the occipital pole. There is then a curved **lunate sulcus** around the end of the calcarine sulcus. Except for this inconstant marking, the small area of the occipital lobe on the lateral surface has minor grooves and folds of no special significance.

Insular Lobe (Insula)

The regions that conceal the insula are known as the **frontal, parietal,** and **temporal opercula;** they must be spread apart or cut away to expose the insula (Fig. 13-4). The insula is outlined by a **circular sulcus** and is divided into two regions by a central sulcus. Several short gyri lie in front of the central sulcus, and one or two long gyri lie behind it. The inferior part of the insula in the region of the stem of the lateral sulcus is known as the **limen insulae.**

The insula is an important landmark for certain structures inside the cerebral hemisphere. The lentiform nucleus, a component of the corpus striatum, is separated from the insula by two layers of white matter (the extreme and external capsules) and an intervening layer of gray matter (the claustrum).

Medial and Inferior Surfaces

The **cingulate gyrus** begins beneath the genu of the corpus callosum and continues above the corpus callosum as far back as the splenium (Fig. 13-5). The gyrus is separated from the corpus callosum by the **sulcus of the corpus callosum** (callosal sulcus). The superior surface of the corpus callosum is covered by a very thin layer of cortical gray matter known as the **indusium griseum.** The **cingulate sulcus** intervenes between the cingulate gyrus and the **medial frontal gyrus,** which is continuous with the superior frontal gyrus on the lateral surface of the hemisphere. The cingulate sulcus gives off a **paracentral sulcus** and then divides into **marginal** and **subparietal sulci** in the parietal lobe. The region bounded by the paracentral and marginal sulci, which surrounds the indentation made by the central sulcus on the superior border, is called the **paracentral lobule.** The anterior and posterior parts of the paracentral lobule are, respectively, extensions of the precentral and postcentral gyri of the lateral surface of the hemisphere. The area above the subparietal sulcus is called the **precuneus** and is continuous with the superior parietal lobule on the lateral surface. The parieto-occipital and calcarine sulci bound the **cuneus** of the occipital lobe.

On the medial surface of the frontal lobe, underneath the rostrum of the corpus cal-

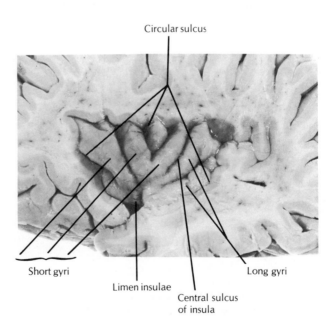

Circular sulcus

Short gyri

Limen insulae

Central sulcus of insula

Long gyri

Figure 13-4. The insula (island of Reil) of the left cerebral hemisphere, exposed by cutting away the frontal, parietal, and temporal opercula. ($\times$ 1.8)

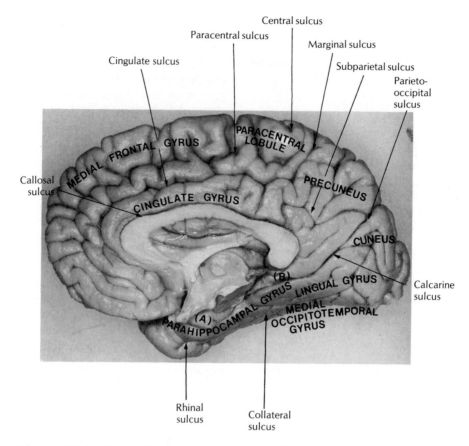

Figure 13-5. Gyri and sulci on the medial and inferior surfaces of the right cerebral hemisphere. (**A**) Uncus. (**B**) Isthmus (retrosplenial cortex) connecting the cingulate and parahippocampal gyri. (× 0.63)

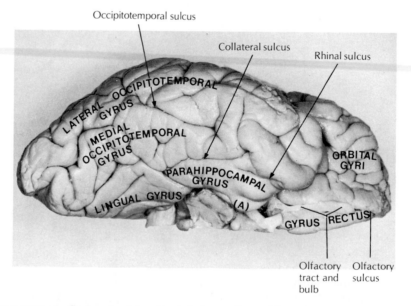

Figure 13-6. Gyri and sulci on the inferior surface of the right cerebral hemisphere. (**A**) Uncus. (× 0.63)

losum, is the **subcallosal gyrus**, also known as the parolfactory area. This is not cortex, but it is part of the **septal area**, a component of the limbic system (see Ch. 18).

On the inferior surface of the hemisphere (Figs. 13-5 and 13-6), a convolution extends from the occipital pole almost to the temporal pole. The posterior part of the convolution consists of the **lingual gyrus**. The anterior part forms the **parahippocampal gyrus**, which hooks sharply backward on its medial aspect as the **uncus**, a region in which fibers of the olfactory tract end. The **collateral sulcus** defines the lateral margin of the lingual and parahippocampal gyri. The short **rhinal sulcus**, at the lateral edge of the parahippocampal gyrus anteriorly, delimits the **entorhinal area**, which belongs to the olfactory and limbic systems. The **medial occipitotemporal gyrus**, which is inconstant in morphology and broken up by irregular sulci, lies along the lateral side of the collateral sulcus. The **occipitotemporal sulcus** intervenes between the medial occipitotemporal gyrus and the **lateral occipitotemporal gyrus**. The latter is continuous with the inferior temporal gyrus on the lateral surface of the hemisphere.

The **olfactory bulb** and **olfactory tract** on the orbital surface of the frontal lobe (see Fig. 13-6) conceal most of the **olfactory sulcus**. The **gyrus rectus** is medial to the olfactory sulcus, and the large area lateral to the olfactory sulcus consists of irregular **orbital gyri**. The cingulate and parahippocampal gyri are connected by a narrow **isthmus** (retrosplenial cortex) beneath the splenium of the corpus callosum and form the "**limbic lobe**" of the cerebral hemisphere, which also includes the hippocampus. The limbic lobe is part of the **limbic system** of the brain, which incorporates several additional structures, most prominently the dentate gyrus and amygdaloid body (both in the temporal lobe), hypothalamus (especially the mamillary bodies), septal area, and anterior and some other nuclei of the thalamus. The limbic system, which is involved in memory and certain aspects of behavior, is described in Chapter 18.

SUGGESTED READING

Bisaria KK: Grooves on the occipital lobe of Indian brains. J Anat 139:779–582, 1984

Haines DE: Neuroanatomy. An Atlas of Structures, Sections and Systems, 3rd ed. Baltimore, Urban & Schwarzenberg, 1991

Montemurro DG, Bruni JE: The Human Brain in Dissection, 2nd ed. New York, Oxford University Press, 1988

Nieuwenhuys R, Voogd J, van Huijzen C: The Human Central Nervous System. A Synopsis and Atlas, 3rd ed. Berlin, Springer-Verlag, 1988

Fourteen

The Human Nervous System: An Anatomical Viewpoint, Sixth Edition, Murray L. Barr and John A. Kiernan. J.B. Lippincott Company, Philadelphia, © 1993.

Histology of the Cerebral Cortex

Important Facts

The pallium of the telencephalon consists of the archicortex (hippocampal formation), paleocortex (olfactory and some limbic areas), and the neocortex, which has six layers and, in the human brain, contains some 10^{10} neurons.

The cortex contains principal (pyramidal) cells, which are most conspicuous on layers 3 and 5, and several types of interneuron. Brodmann's numbered areas are based on regional variations in microscopic appearance of the cortex.

The six layers are most distinct in association areas. In primary sensory areas, stellate cells are prominent in layer 4. These interneurons are rarely seen in motor areas. The primary motor area contains giant pyramidal (Betz) cells.

Afferent fibers are from other cortical areas, the thalamus, the basal forebrain cholinergic nuclei, and the noradrenergic and serotonergic neurons of the brain stem. Thalamic and cholinergic afferents excite the pyramidal cells; the aminergic fibers are inhibitory.

The cortex is a mosaic of columns of neurons, each influenced by a single thalamic neuron and responding only to a specific type of signal. Maturation of the columnar organization requires exposure to sensory experiences early in postnatal life.

The electroencephalogram is due to differences of membrane potentials between the proximal and distal ends of the apical dendrites of pyramidal cells. These potentials fluctuate as a result of changes in activity of thalamocortical and corticocortical neurons.

Each cerebral hemisphere has a mantle of gray matter, the cortex or pallium, with a characteristic structure that consists of nerve cells and nerve fibers arranged in layers. There are three types of cortex according to phylogenetic development and histological characteristics.

In amphibians, the pallium constitutes the dorsal surface of each tubular "hemisphere" of the telencephalon and does not have the layered structure of cerebral cortex. The pallium consists of two regions; the lateral one receives afferent fibers from the olfactory bulb and the medial region receives most of its afferents from the septum or medial wall of the hemisphere. Because of their phylogenetic ages, the cortices derived from the lateral and medial parts of the pallium are called the **paleocortex** and **archicortex**, respectively. Their locations in the human brain are described in subsequent chapters dealing with the olfactory and limbic systems.

In the reptilian brain, there are three cortical zones because of the first appearance of an area of **neocortex** between the paleocortex and archicortex. The amount of neocortex has increased during mammalian evolution and constitutes most of the cortex in the human brain. In addition to its important sensory and motor functions, the abundant neocortex has an important bearing on human intellectual capabilities. Sometimes paleocortex and archicortex are referred to as **allocortex**, in contrast to **isocortex**, which is a synonym for neocortex.

The number of layers evident histologically in paleocortex and archicortex varies according to region. There may be as many as five layers in paleocortex, although the more superficial ones are indistinct, and the largest number in archicortex is three. In the neocortex, which is the subject of this chapter, six layers are always recognizable at some stage in its development, but the typical six-layered structure is absent in some areas of the adult brain.

Cortical Neurons

Values obtained for the number of nerve cells in the human cerebral cortex vary widely because of the technical difficulties in their enumeration. They range from 2.6×10^9 to 1.6×10^{10}, and the number of cortical neurons is, therefore, enormous. The principal cells (neurons with long axons) are known as **pyramidal cells**. Their cell bodies range in height from 10 to 50 μm for most cells. Giant pyramidal cells, also known as **Betz cells**, have cell bodies up to 100 μm high. These are present only in the primary motor area of the frontal lobe, where they are conspicuous but not numerous. Each pyramidal cell (Fig. 14-1) has conspicuous apical and lateral dendrites, with branches that are covered with dendritic spines (see Ch. 2). The axon emerges from the base of the pyramid or from one of the larger dendrites and gives off many collateral branches before it enters the subcortical white matter. About two-thirds of cortical neurons are pyramidal cells, but the proportion is higher in motor areas of the frontal lobe and lower in the primary sensory areas. The axons of pyramidal neurons are excitatory at their synapses and are thought to use glutamate as their neurotransmitter. **Fusiform cells**, which are located in the deepest layer of the cortex, are atypical principal cells with irregularly elliptical cell bodies.

In addition to their local intracortical branches, the axons of the principal cells connect with other neurons in three ways. **Projection neurons** transmit impulses to subcortical centers, such as the corpus striatum, the brain stem, the spinal cord, or the thalamus (which receives the axons of the fusiform cells). **Association neurons** establish connections with cortical nerve cells elsewhere in the same hemisphere. Axons of **commissural neurons** proceed to the cortex of the opposite hemisphere. Most of the commissural fibers constitute the corpus callosum; smaller numbers connect cortical areas of the temporal lobes through the anterior commissure.

Several types of cortical **interneuron** are recognized on the basis of dendritic architecture. A few are shown in Figure 14-1. The **stellate cell**, which occurs only in the fourth cortical layer (see next section of this chapter), has dendritic spines and is the only type of excitatory interneuron in the cortex, with glutamate as its suspected transmitter. All the other types of interneuron are inhibitory, and probably all secrete gamma-aminobutyric acid (GABA) at their synapses. **Basket cells** have axons that branch laterally and embrace the cell bodies of pyramidal cells. The **Retzius-Cajal cells** are confined to the most superficial layer of the cortex, and the **cells of Martinotti** are more deeply placed, with axons that project toward the pial surface.

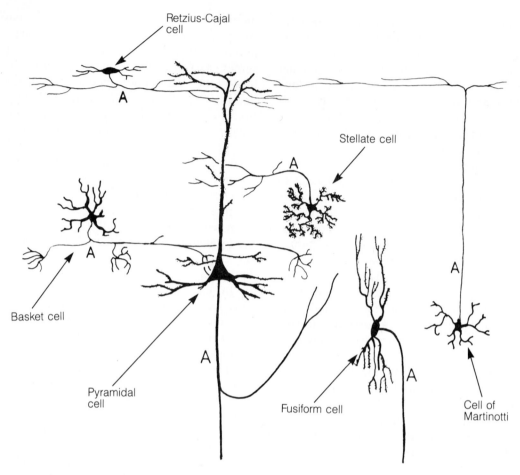

Figure 14-1. Cortical neurons. In reality, the dendrites are more numerous and more richly branched than shown in this drawing. (The letter **A** identifies the axon of each type of neuron.)

Cortical Layers

The thickness of the neocortex varies from 4.5 mm in the primary motor area of the frontal lobe to 1.5 mm in the visual area of the occipital lobe. The cortex is thicker over the crest of a gyrus than in the depths of a sulcus. The cerebral cortex has its full complement of neurons by the 18th week of intrauterine life, and six layers, which differ in the density of cell population and in the size and shape of constituent neurons, can be recognized by about the 7th month. The layers, starting at the surface and omitting regional differences for the present, are as follows (Fig. 14-2*A*):

1. **Molecular layer**. The superficial layer consists predominantly of terminal branches of dendrites and axons, which give a punctate or "molecular" appearance in sections stained for nerve fibers. Most of the dendritic branches come from pyramidal cells. The axons originate in cortex elsewhere in the same hemisphere, in that of the opposite hemisphere, and in the thalamus. Cells of Martinotti in any deeper layer also contribute axons to layer 1. The infrequent horizontal cells of Cajal intervene between some axons and dendrites. The

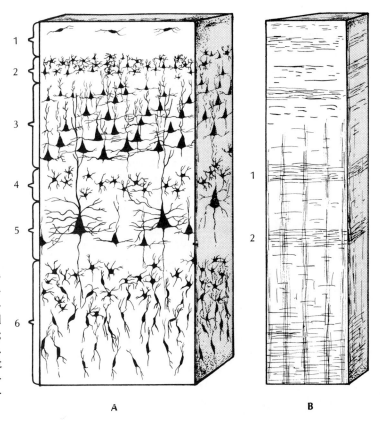

Figure 14-2. Cortical histology. (**A**) Golgi method: 1. molecular layer; 2. external granular layer; 3. external pyramidal layer; 4. internal granular layer; 5. internal pyramidal layer; 6. multiform layer. (**B**) Weigert method: 1. outer line of Baillarger; 2. inner line of Baillarger.

molecular layer is essentially a synaptic field of the cortex.

2. **External granular layer**. This layer contains many small pyramidal cells and interneurons.

3. **External pyramidal layer**. The neurons are typical pyramidal cells that increase in size from the external to the internal borders of the layer.

4. **Internal granular layer**. This layer is dominated by closely arranged stellate cells, although smaller numbers of other interneurons and pyramidal cells also are present.

5. **Internal pyramidal layer**. This layer contains pyramidal cells, which are larger than those of layer 3, intermingled with interneurons. The giant pyramidal cells (of Betz) in the primary motor area of cortex in the frontal lobe are in layer 5.

6. **Multiform layer**. Although fusiform cells are typical of this layer, there are also pyramidal cells and interneurons of various shapes.

Layers 5 and 6, which are the infragranular layers, are phylogenetically older than the more superficial layers 1 to 4 (the supragranular layers). The latter contain many small neurons that provide for complex intracortical circuitry. Layers 5 and 6 are also ontogenetically older, being derived from the first cortical neuroblasts to migrate out from the germinative epithelium of the neural tube of the telencephalon. The neuroblasts destined to form layers 2, 3, and 4 migrate through the infragranular layers to take up their more superficial positions.

The layers described are evident in sections stained by the Nissl and Golgi techniques. With silver staining methods for axons or the Weigert method for myelin sheaths, nerve fibers within the neocortex are seen to accumulate in radial bundles and in tangential bands

(Fig. 14-2*B*). The radial bundles are close together; they include axons entering and leaving the cortex. The tangential bands consist largely of collateral and terminal branches of afferent fibers. They leave the radial bundles and run parallel to the surface for some distance, branching again and making synaptic contacts with large numbers of cortical neurons. The most prominent tangential bands are the **outer** and **inner lines of Baillarger**, located in layer 4 and in the deep portion of layer 5, respectively. Fibers originating in the thalamic sensory nuclei contribute heavily to the lines of Baillarger, especially the outer one, and they are, therefore, prominent in the primary sensory areas. In the visual area in the walls of the calcarine sulcus, the outer line of Baillarger on the cut surface is thick enough to be just visible to the unaided eye. In this location, it is known as the **line of Gennari** (Fig. 14-3), having been first described by Francesco Gennari, an 18th-century Italian medical student. Because of the presence of the line of Gennari, the primary visual cortex is known alternatively as the striate area.

Variations in Cytoarchitecture

The foregoing description of cortical histology establishes the general pattern. Six layers can be identified throughout most of the neocortex, which is said to be **homotypical** cortex. In some areas, known as **heterotypical** cortex, it is not possible to identify six layers. For example, in the visual area and in parts of the auditory and general sensory areas, there are many interneurons in layer 4 and the adjoining layers, so that layers 2 to 5 merge into a single layer of small cells. This type of heterotypical cortex is called **granular cortex** or **koniocortex** (from the Greek *konis*, dust). The opposite extreme is found in the primary motor and premotor areas of the frontal lobe. Here the pyramidal cells are much more numerous than interneurons, and layers 2 to 6 appear as a single zone consisting almost entirely of pyramidal cells of different sizes, with the larger ones more deeply located. This is called **agranular cortex**.

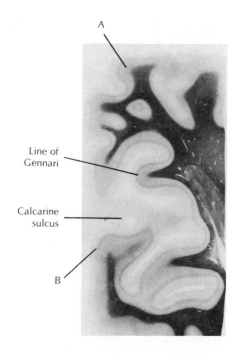

Figure 14-3. Vertical section through the medial surface of the occipital lobe at the site of the calcarine sulcus. The line of Gennari, extending from **A** to **B**, identifies the primary visual area: the striate cortex. (Weigert stain, × 2)

The cerebral cortex has been divided into cytoarchitectural areas based on differences in the thickness of individual layers, neuronal morphology in the layers, and the details of nerve fiber lamination. Such studies require great patience and attention to detail. The few investigators who have undertaken meticulous analyses of cortical cytoarchitecture hoped to establish bases for structural and functional correlations. The attempt has been only partially successful because of differing histological criteria and an incomplete understanding of the functional significance of many parts of the cerebral cortex. Different investigators have divided the cortex into 20 to 200 areas, depending on the criteria used. Brodmann's numbered map, which was published in 1909 and consists of 52 areas, provides the most widely used scheme of cortical cytoarchitectural areas.

More recent studies agree that heterotypical areas may be easily identified. For example, the anterior portion of the general sensory cortex in the postcentral gyrus is granular heterotypical cortex (area 3 of Brodmann); the visual cortex around the calcarine sulcus (area 17) and the central part of the auditory cortex in the superior temporal gyrus (area 41) also consist of granular cortex. The primary motor and premotor areas of the frontal lobe (areas 4 and 6) are agranular heterotypical cortex. Area 4 is distinguished by the presence of giant pyramidal (Betz) cells. In view of the obvious difficulties in establishing boundaries between areas with rather subtle histological differences, it is not surprising that the cytoarchitectural areas described for the large expanse of association cortex have met with some skepti-

cism. The concept has considerable appeal, however, and has resulted in the widespread use of the numbering system based on cortical histology. Some areas of Brodmann's map referred to later in the text are shown in Figures 15-1 and 15-2.

Intracortical Circuits

Investigations of cortical neurons using the Golgi technique, electron microscopy, and immunohistochemical methods, combined with electrical recording from microelectrodes placed in the cortex, have yielded much information concerning intrinsic circuits. These are summarized in simplified form in Figure 14-4.

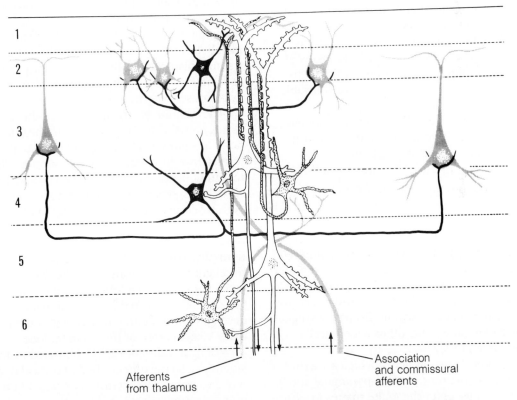

Figure 14-4. Some intracortical connections. Impulses arriving from other cortical areas directly excite the apical dendrites of pyramidal cells. Afferents from specific thalamic nuclei excite the stellate cells (stippled) in layer 4, which in turn excite pyramidal cells (white) in the same column. Also in layer 4, collateral branches of pyramidal cells excite basket cells (black), which inhibit pyramidal cells in adjacent columns (gray). (*With permission, from Martin JH: Chap. 50 in Kandel ER, Schwartz JH, Jessell TM (eds): Principles of Neural Science, 3rd ed., p. 781. New York, Elsevier, 1991*)

AFFERENT AND EFFERENT FIBERS

The major sources of afferent fibers entering the cortex are as follows:

Other cortical areas in the same and the opposite hemisphere; corticocortical fibers are the most numerous afferents. They are excitatory, being the axons of probably glutamatergic or aspartatergic cortical pyramidal cells.

The thalamus, which is the best understood source of subcortical afferents. These also are excitatory, but the transmitter has not yet been identified.

The claustrum (see Ch. 12), about which little is known.

The basal cholinergic forebrain nuclei of the substantia innominata (see Ch. 12), which send their much branched axons to all areas of the neocortex, where they have excitatory effects.

Branches of the far-reaching axons of noradrenergic neurons in the locus coeruleus (see Ch. 9), which inhibit cortical neurons.

The even more abundant serotonergic axons from the more rostral of the raphe nuclei of the brain stem (see Ch. 9), which are also inhibitory.

The axons from the ventral thalamic nuclei (VL, VP, and the geniculate bodies; see Ch. 11) are major components of motor and sensory pathways. Within the cortex, these fibers divide into branches that synapse mainly with the stellate cells (cortical excitatory interneurons) in the region of the outer line of Baillarger in layer 4. Most of the fibers from elsewhere in the thalamus, from other regions of cortex, and from other subcortical nuclei terminate in layers 1, 2, and 3.

Cortical efferent fibers, which are axons of the larger neurons, notably pyramidal and fusiform cells, enter the white matter for distribution as projection, association, or commissural fibers.

COLUMNAR ORGANIZATION

Recordings from microelectrodes inserted into the cortex have shown that it is organized functionally as minute vertical units that include nerve cells of all layers. This has been demonstrated best in sensory areas. All neurons in the unit are activated selectively by the same peripheral stimulus, whether it originates in a particular type of cutaneous receptor at a particular location or in a specific point on the retina. Each unit is 200 to 500 μm in diameter with its height the thickness of the cortex. Each column of neurons receives synaptic input from the axon of a single thalamic neuron.

Vertically organized functional units corresponding to those detected with microelectrodes can also be defined by autoradiography (see Ch. 4). To do this, a labeled amino acid is injected into the appropriate thalamic nucleus, or labeled 2-deoxyglucose is given systemically while a sensory system is receiving stimuli. Columns with increased metabolic activity can also be made visible by staining histochemically for the activity of cytochrome oxidase, the enzyme that enables cells to use oxygen.

The columnar organization of the neocortex is established in fetal life, but the synaptic connections increase in number postnatally in response to external sensory stimuli. This maturation occurs in an **early critical period**, in response to adequate sensory stimulation. If sensory stimuli are lacking in number and variety during the first year of life, the functions of the cerebral cortex fail to develop normally. For example, if refractive errors or misalignment (strabismus) of the eyes is not corrected early in childhood, visual acuity is permanently impaired because of inadequate development of neuronal circuitry in the primary visual cortex of the occipital lobe.

Visual stimuli are easily controlled in the laboratory, so the organization of cortical neurons has been most intensively studied in the primary visual cortex. There, distinct columns of cells respond to neural input associated with one or both eyes (ocular dominance columns) and to meaningful features in the observed image, such as edges, horizontal lines, and right angles. Populations of the different kinds of cell column form stripes that extend across the surface of the calcarine cortex. The Nobel Prize for Medicine and Physiology was awarded in 1981 to D. H. Hubel and T. N. Wiesel for their discovery of the distribution and development of columnar functional units in the primate visual cortex.

ELECTROENCEPHALOGRAPHY

Changes in electrical potential recorded from a point on the surface of the scalp are due to summed membrane potentials in the apical dendrites of thousands of underlying pyramidal cells. Activity in thalamic afferents to the cortex stimulates (depolarizes) the pyramidal cell dendrites in layer 4, whereas input from association and commissural fibers causes depolarization in layer 1 (see Fig. 14-4). The magnitude and direction of flow of electric current across the thickness of the cortex depend on the differences in membrane potential of the proximal and distal ends of the apical dendrites.

Electroencephalography (EEG) is informative in the clinical investigation of **epilepsy**, a group of maladies in which there are episodes of abnormal spread of neuronal excitation through the brain, typically leading to loss of consciousness and convulsions. Abnormalities in the EEG characterize the different types of epilepsy and can help to localize the epileptogenic focus in which the abnormal discharges begin. The EEG is also useful in the study of sleep (see Ch. 9).

A ''flat'' EEG 2 days or more after cardiac arrest and resuscitation is associated with halving of the cortical oxygen consumption and is an almost certain indicator of permanent loss of function of the cerebral cortex. The diagnosis of **brain death** in a comatose patient is made on the basis of absence of functions of the brain stem: failure of spontaneous respiration and absence of reflexes mediated by any of the cranial nerves. This must not be confused with **vegetative states**, in which there is no communication between the brain stem and the cerebrum, although breathing, swallowing, chewing, and cranial nerve reflexes are largely preserved. Recovery from a vegetative state of long duration can occur, but there is no reliable way to distinguish those patients who will recover from the majority in whom the condition is permanent.

SUGGESTED READING

Braak H: Architectonics of the Human Telencephalic Cortex. Berlin, Springer-Verlag, 1980

Dinopoulos A, Dori I, Parnevelas JG: Immunohistochemical localization of aspartate in corticofugal pathways. Neurosci Lett 121:25–28, 1991

Douglas RJ, Martin KAC: Neocortex. In Shepherd GM (ed): The Synaptic Organization of the Brain, 3rd ed, pp 389–438. New York, Oxford University Press, 1990

Hubel TH, Wiesel TN: Functional architecture of macaque monkey visual cortex. Proc R Soc Lond [Biol] 198:1–59, 1977

Jones EG: Neurotransmitters in the cerebral cortex. J Neurosurg 65:135–153, 1986

Jones EG, Friedman DP, Endry SHC: Thalamic basis of place- and modality-specific columns in monkey somatosensory cortex: A correlative anatomical and physiological study. J Neurophysiol 48:545–568, 1982

Ong WY, Garey LJ: Neuronal architecture of the human temporal cortex. Anat Embryol 181:351–364, 1990

Peters A, Jones EG (eds): Cerebral Cortex. Vol 1. Cellular Components. New York, Plenum Press, 1984

Young B, Blume W, Lynch A: Brain death and the persistent vegetative state: Similarities and contrasts. Can J Neurol Sci 16:388–393, 1989

Zilles K: Cortex. In Paxinos G (ed): The Human Nervous System, pp. 757–802. San Diego, Academic Press, 1990

Fifteen

The Human Nervous System: An Anatomical Viewpoint, Sixth Edition, Murray L. Barr and John A. Kiernan. J.B. Lippincott Company, Philadelphia, © 1993.

Functional Localization in the Cerebral Cortex

Important Facts

Stimulation and ablation, electrophysiological recording, and measurement of regional blood flow and associated metabolic changes have all contributed to knowledge of the localization of functions in the cerebral cortex.

Each of the main primary sensory areas (somesthetic, visual, auditory) is surrounded by a larger zone of association cortex.

The primary areas, which are topographically organized, are necessary for conscious recognition and localization of sensory stimuli.

Association cortex is necessary for the understanding of more complex features. Various types of agnosia result from damage to sensory association cortex.

There are at least three motor areas. The supplementary motor area is involved in the planning and initiation of movements. The premotor cortex controls movements at proximal joints. The primary motor area (precentral gyrus) is involved in movements of all parts of the body, with a large proportion of its extent being devoted to the hand and face.

The frontal eye field controls conjugate saccadic eye movements. The occipital eye field controls slower, involuntary movements of the eyes.

In most people, there is a motor or expressive speech area in the left frontal lobe and a large receptive or ideational language area in the left parietal and temporal lobes. Various types of aphasia result from lesions that damage the language areas.

The right cerebral cortex contains (in most people) areas necessary for appreciation of three-dimensional shapes, for awareness of the positions of parts of the body, and for musical ability.

The rostral parts of the frontal lobes are involved in some higher mental functions, including judgment, foresight, and socially proper behavior.

Development of the Concept of Cortical Localization

Results of clinicopathological studies and animal experiments conducted over more than a century have provided information concerning functional specialization in different regions of the cerebral cortex. For example, three main sensory areas have been found; they are for general sensation, vision, and hearing. Smaller areas exist for taste, smell, and vestibular sensation (awareness of position and movement of the head). There also are motor areas from which contraction of groups of skeletal muscles can be elicited by electrical stimulation. The remainder of the neocortex is usually referred to as association cortex, which may be closely related functionally to the sensory areas or to more complex levels of behavior, communication, and the intellect. The trend in mammalian evolution has been toward increasing amounts of association cortex.

The first indications of functional localization came from clinical observations. Paul Broca, in 1861, examined post mortem the brain of a patient who had suffered from a speech defect (expressive aphasia). A lesion was found in the inferior frontal gyrus, and the region is still known as Broca's motor speech area. On the basis of clinicopathological findings, Hughlings Jackson concluded in 1864 that a form of localized epilepsy, now known as jacksonian epilepsy, was caused by focal irritation of the precentral gyrus. This study drew attention to the probable existence of a somatotopically organized motor area. An area from which motor responses could be elicited on weak electrical stimulation was demonstrated by Fritsch and Hitzig (1870) in the dog and by Ferrier (1875), Horsley and Beevor (1894), and Sherrington and Grünbaum (1901) in the monkey and chimpanzee.

The identification of sensory areas has a similar history. In 1870, Gudden showed that removal of the eyes from young animals interfered with full development of the occipital lobes, and in 1873, Ferrier found that an animal's ears would rise on stimulation of a particular region of the temporal lobe. The latter region included the auditory area, and stimulation produced a movement normally made in response to a sound. Similarly, Dusser de Barenne (1916) showed that application of strychnine to a small area of the monkey's postcentral gyrus resulted in scratching of the skin in one place or another, depending on the precise point at which cortical neurons were stimulated. He was able to map the somesthetic cortex of the monkey with this technique. (Strychnine, a convulsant poison, is now known to block postsynaptic receptors that respond to glycine, an inhibitory transmitter.)

Meticulous studies were made of patients who survived penetrating bullet wounds of the brain during the Russo-Japanese War by Tatsuji Inouye, and during World War I by Henry Head, Gordon Holmes, and others. These researches aided greatly in understanding the topographical organization of the visual and other sensory areas of the human cerebral cortex.

Studies of cortical stimulation were extended from subhuman primates to the human brain by neurosurgeons, notably Harvey Cushing, Otfrid Foerster, and Wilder Penfield. In certain surgical procedures, it is essential to identify the motor area, a sensory area, or even a particular region within these areas. Identification of sensory areas requires operating on a conscious patient under local anesthesia, a procedure made possible because the brain itself is insensitive to injuries that would be painful elsewhere in the body. Electrical stimulation of the human cerebral cortex has provided information more detailed than that obtainable by observing the effects of destructive wounds.

Since 1980, the classical studies of functional localization have largely been confirmed by means of modern noninvasive techniques. Mapping of regional cerebral blood flow and of oxygen and glucose uptake (see Ch. 16) provide information about cortical activity in the normal brain and are also used to detect abnormal function. Noninvasive experimental procedures include electrical stimulation of the cortex by an externally applied magnetic field and the recording from the scalp of potentials evoked by transcutaneous stimulation of peripheral nerves.

Parietal, Occipital, and Temporal Cortex

GENERAL SENSATION

The **first somesthetic area** (general sensory area) occupies the postcentral gyrus on the lateral surface of the hemisphere and the posterior part of the paracentral lobule on the medial surface (Figs. 15-1 and 15-2). It consists of areas 3, 1, and 2 of the Brodmann cytoarchitectural map. Electrical stimulation of the general sensory area elicits modified forms of the tactile sense, such as a tingling sensation. It is possible to elicit motor responses by stimulating the first somesthetic area, as well as eliciting sensory responses from the motor area in the precentral gyrus. The functions of the two areas, therefore, overlap to some extent, and they should be considered as a **sensorimotor strip** that surrounds

the central sulcus. The postcentral gyrus and its extension in the paracentral lobule are designated as the first sensory area because they have the highest density of points that produce localized sensations on electrical stimulation.

The ventral posterior nucleus of the thalamus is the main source of afferent fibers for the first sensory area. This thalamic nucleus is the site of termination of all the fibers of the medial lemniscus and of most of the fibers of the spinothalamic and trigeminothalamic tracts. The thalamocortical fibers traverse the internal capsule and medullary center, conveying data for the various modalities of general sensation. Fibers for cutaneous sensibility end preferentially in the anterior part of the area, and those for deep sensibility, in the posterior part.

The contralateral half of the body is represented as inverted. The pharyngeal region, tongue, and jaws are represented in the most

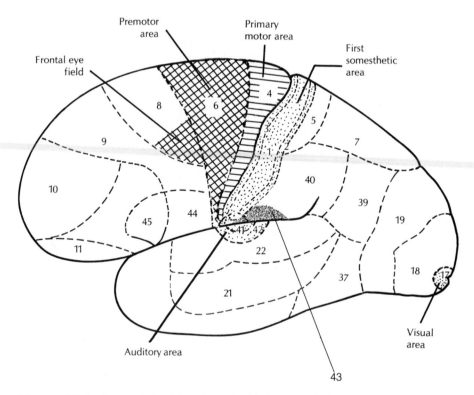

Figure 15-1. Areas of functional localization on the lateral surface of the left cerebral hemisphere. Numbers from Brodmann's cytoarchitectural map shown here and in Figure 15-2 are those mentioned in the text.

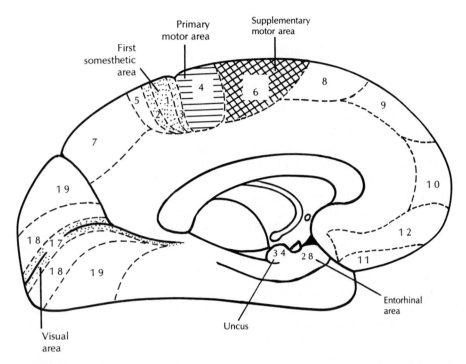

Figure 15-2. Areas of functional localization on the medial surface of the left cerebral hemisphere.

ventral part of the somesthetic area, followed by the face, hand, arm, trunk, and thigh. The area for the remainder of the leg and the perineum is in the extension of the somesthetic cortex on the medial surface of the hemisphere. The size of the cortical area for a particular part of the body is determined by the functional importance of the part and its need for sensitivity. The area for the face, especially the lips, is, therefore, disproportionately large, and a large area is assigned to the hand, particularly the thumb and index finger. A picture of the body with the proportions of its cortical map is known as a **homunculus**.

A crude form of awareness persists for pain, heat, and cold sensations on the affected opposite side of the body if this first somesthetic area has been destroyed. There is poor localization of the stimulus, for which qualitative and quantitative interpretations are diminished or absent. The somesthetic cortex must be intact for any appreciation of the more discriminative sensations of fine touch, position, and movement of the parts of the body.

An additional or **second somesthetic area** has been demonstrated in primates, including humans. This small area is in the dorsal wall of the lateral sulcus, in line with the postcentral gyrus, and may extend onto the insula. The parts of the body are represented bilaterally, although contralateral representation predominates. The second sensory area receives input from the intralaminar nuclei and from the posterior group of nuclei of the thalamus. The afferent fibers to these nuclei come, respectively, from the reticular formation and from the spinothalamic and trigeminothalamic tracts. Consequently the area is involved mainly in the less discriminative aspects of sensation. An intact second somesthetic area probably explains such residual sensibility as exists after destruction of the first sensory area. No clinical disorder has been ascribed to a lesion in the second somesthetic area.

The **somesthetic association cortex** is mainly in the superior parietal lobule on the lateral surface of the hemisphere and in the precuneus on the medial surface. Much of it coincides with Brodmann's areas 5 and 7. This association cortex receives fibers from the first somesthetic area, and its thalamic connections are with the lateral posterior nucleus and the pulvinar. Data pertaining to the general senses are integrated in this association area, permitting, for example, a comprehensive assessment of the characteristics of an object held in the hand and its identification without visual aid.

A destructive lesion in the somesthetic association cortex may leave the somesthetic area itself intact. There is then a defect in understanding the significance of sensory information, called **agnosia**. In this disorder, awareness of the general senses persists, but the significance of the information received on the basis of previous experience is elusive. There are several types of agnosia, depending on the sense that is most affected. A lesion that destroys a large portion of the somesthetic association cortex causes **tactile agnosia** and **astereognosis**, which are closely related. They combine when a person is unable to identify a common object, such as a pair of scissors, held in the hand while the eyes are closed. It is impossible to correlate the surface texture, shape, size, and weight of the object or to compare the sensations with previous experience. Astereognosis includes a loss of awareness of the spatial relations of parts of the contralateral side of the body. The most extreme form of the condition is **cortical neglect**, in which the patient ignores and even denies the existence of one side of the body and of the corresponding visual field. The condition most often is due to large lesions in the superior part of the right parietal lobe.

VISION

The **visual area** surrounds the calcarine sulcus on the medial surface of the occipital lobe, extending over the occipital pole in some brains (see Fig. 15-2). The area is more extensive than the illustration suggests because most of it is in the walls of the deep calcarine sulcus, in which there also are secondary folds. The visual cortex, which corresponds to area 17 of Brodmann's map, is called the **striate area** because it contains the line of Gennari (see Ch. 14), which is just visible to the unaided eye. The chief source of afferent fibers to area 17 is the lateral geniculate body of the thalamus, by way of the geniculocalcarine tract.

The visual cortex, through a synaptic relay in the lateral geniculate body, receives data from the lateral (temporal) half of the ipsilateral retina and the medial (nasal) half of the contralateral retina. The dividing line runs vertically through the fovea centralis at the posterior pole of the eye. The left half of the field of vision is, therefore, represented in the visual area of the right hemisphere and vice versa (see also Ch. 20). There are spatial patterns within the striate area. The lower retinal quadrants (upper field of vision) project on the lower wall of the calcarine sulcus, and the upper retinal quadrants (lower field of vision) project on the upper wall of the sulcus. Another pattern is related to central and peripheral vision. The macula lutea (which includes the fovea centralis) is represented at the occipital pole, in the posterior part of area 17; the remaining retina is represented more anteriorly. The macula is responsible for central vision of maximal discrimination. Consequently the part of area 17 that receives data for central vision accounts for a disproportionately large amount (one-third) of the visual cortex.

A destructive lesion that involves the visual cortex of a hemisphere causes an area of blindness in the opposite visual field. The size and location of the defect are determined by the extent and location of the lesion. Examination of the visual fields may show that central vision is intact after a unilateral lesion in the occipital lobe (eg, an infarction caused by a thrombus in the posterior cerebral artery). This clinical observation, known as macular sparing, cannot be explained on the basis of bilateral cortical representation of the macula. It has been suggested that anastomoses between branches of the middle and posterior cerebral arteries may partially maintain the large part of area 17 concerned with central vision after occlusion of the posterior cerebral artery. It has also been suggested that macular sparing is an artifact of testing caused by slight movements of the patient's eyes during examination of the visual fields.

The **visual association cortex** corresponds to areas 18 and 19 of Brodmann, which surround the visual area on the medial and lateral surfaces of the hemisphere (see Figs. 15-1 and 15-2). These areas receive fibers from area 17 and have reciprocal connections with other cortical areas and with the pulvinar of the thalamus. The role of this association cortex includes, among other complex aspects of vision, the relating of present to past visual experience, recognition of what is seen, and appreciation of its significance. A substantial lesion that involves areas 18 and 19, therefore, results in **visual agnosia**. Bilateral lesions that involve the superior parts of area 19 cause **visual disorientation**, loss of coordination of eye movements, and inability to carry out visually guided movements of the hands.

The inferolateral surface of the temporal lobe (inferior temporal and lateral occipitotemporal gyri) is also visual association cortex. Electrical stimulation of this region evokes vivid hallucinations of scenes from the past, indicating a role of this cortex in the storage or recall of **visual memories**. Bilateral destruction of the inferior surfaces of the occipital and temporal lobes can cause **prosopagnosia**, a rare condition in which there is impaired recognition of previously known familiar faces.

Corticotectal fibers connect the visual cortex and visual association cortex with the superior colliculus of the midbrain, which, through indirect connections, controls the oculomotor, trochlear, and abducens nuclei (see Ch. 8). This is part of a pathway for fixation of gaze and for tracking of a moving object in the field of vision. It also functions in the accommodation–convergence reaction on directing attention to a near object. These motor aspects of the occipital cortex are related to those of the frontal eye field, described later in this chapter.

HEARING

The **auditory area** (acoustic area) is concealed because it is in the ventral wall of the lateral sulcus (Fig. 15-3; see also Fig. 15-1). The surface of the superior temporal gyrus, forming the floor of the sulcus, is marked by transverse temporal gyri. The two most anterior of these, called **Heschl's convolutions**, are the classic landmarks for the auditory area, which corresponds to areas 41 and 42 of Brodmann. Recordings made from neurosurgical patients indicate that only the posteromedial part of this region is primary auditory cortex.

The medial geniculate body of the thalamus is the principal source of fibers that end in the auditory cortex, with these fibers constituting the auditory radiation in the medullary center. There is a spatial representation in the auditory area with respect to the pitch of sounds. Impulses for low frequencies impinge on the anterolateral part of the area, and impulses for high frequencies impinge on the posteromedial part. Although the medial geniculate body receives signals that originate mainly in the spiral organ (organ of Corti) of the opposite side, an additional ipsilateral pathway ensures that there also is substantial input from the ear of the same side (see Ch. 21). Sometimes a unilateral destructive lesion involving the auditory area results in difficulty with the interpretation of complex combinations of sounds, but it causes almost no impairment of hearing in the contralateral ear. Large bilateral lesions in the temporal lobes are rare, but they can cause bilateral deafness among other symptoms.

The **auditory association cortex** for more elaborate perception of acoustic information occupies the floor of the lateral sulcus behind the auditory area (the region labeled planum temporale in Fig. 15-3) and the posterior part of Brodmann's area 22 on the lateral surface of the superior temporal gyrus. The region of cortex thus defined, also known as **Wernicke's area**, is of major importance in language functions.

TASTE

The **taste area** (gustatory area) is adjacent to the general sensory area for the tongue at the inferior end of the postcentral gyrus (see Fig. 15-1) and extends onto the insula and then anteriorly to the frontal operculum. Nerve im-

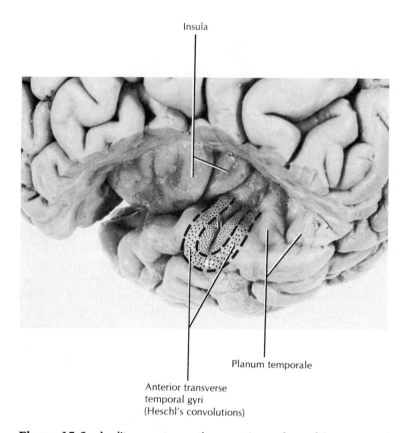

Insula

Planum temporale

Anterior transverse
temporal gyri
(Heschl's convolutions)

Figure 15-3. Auditory cortex on the superior surface of the temporal lobe, exposed by removing the frontal and parietal opercula. (× 0.8)

pulses from taste buds reach the gustatory nucleus in the brain stem (ie, the rostral part of the solitary nucleus; see Chs. 7 and 8). Fibers from the gustatory nucleus travel in the ipsilateral central tegmental tract to the most medial part of the medial division of the ventral posterior nucleus of the thalamus. The pathway is completed by thalamocortical fibers.

OLFACTION

Most of the fibers of the olfactory tract (see Ch. 17) end in the region of the limen insulae and the uncus (area 34); some end in the entorhinal cortex (area 22), which also is a major component of the limbic system (see Ch. 18). The proximity of olfactory and gustatory areas in the region of the insula suggests that this may be a site of integration of the two functionally related special senses.

VESTIBULAR REPRESENTATION

The location of a vestibular cortical area is still uncertain. In monkeys, electrical stimulation of the vestibular nerve has been shown to evoke potentials in a cortical area that corresponds to the inferior parietal lobule of the human brain. Electrical stimulation of the same region in conscious patients occasionally has produced dizziness and vertigo. Examination of regional cortical blood flow in the human brain does not support the idea of a primary vestibular area in the parietal lobe. When the kinetic labyrinth is stimulated by warm water in the external ear (see Ch. 22), increased blood flow is detected only in the superior temporal gyrus, posterior to the auditory area. Some earlier clinical observations had indicated a vestibular function for the anterior end of the superior temporal gyrus. The cortical projection from the vestibular labyrinth, wherever directed, presumably contributes information for motor regulation and awareness of spatial orientation. The ascending fibers from the vestibular nuclei are almost entirely crossed and travel near the medial lemniscus. The thalamic relay is thought to be in or near the medial division of the ventral posterior nucleus, which receives fibers for general sensation from the head.

ASSOCIATION CORTEX

Areas of association cortex adjacent to the main sensory areas and closely related functionally to them have already been described. There is additional association cortex in the parietal lobe and in the posterior part of the temporal lobe. Data reaching the sensory areas and analyzed in the adjacent association cortex are presumably correlated in this intervening region to yield a comprehensive assessment of the immediate environment. The association cortex of the three "sensory" lobes has abundant connections with cortex of the frontal lobe through fasciculi in the medullary center. Complex and flexible behavioral patterns are formulated on the basis of experience, emotional tones are added, and overt expression may follow through the motor system.

The anterior part of the temporal lobe, like the area for visual memory on its inferolateral surface, appears to have special properties related to thought and memory. Electrical stimulation of this region in the conscious subject may elicit recall of objects seen, music heard, or other experiences in the recent or distant past. A patient with a temporal lobe tumor may have auditory or visual hallucinations that reproduce earlier events.

The total expanse of association cortex in the parietal, occipital, and temporal lobes is responsible (along with association cortex in the frontal lobe) for many of the unique qualities of the human brain. Engrams, or memory traces, are laid down over the years, possibly as macromolecular changes in neurons throughout the cerebral cortex. These form the basis of learning at an intellectual level. The complex neuronal circuitry of the cortex permits the coalescence of memory traces in the form of ideas and conceptual, abstract thinking. Recently acquired information is not consolidated into long-term memory if there are bilateral lesions in the limbic system, which is necessary for short-term memory (see Ch. 18). There is probably no disease that causes loss of established memories, indicating that the engram is contained in many parts of the brain. Rare instances of permanent amnesia that follow head injury are probably due to failure of the recalling mechanisms because most amnesic patients eventually recover their memories. The eventual failure of all intellectual function in advanced cases of Alzheimer's disease and other types of dementia is attributed to the loss of enormous numbers of neurons throughout the cerebral cortex and in various subcortical nuclei.

Frontal Cortex

The neocortex of the frontal lobe has a special role in motor activities, in the attributes of judgment and foresight, and in determining mood or affect.

MOTOR AREAS

The **primary motor area** has been identified on the basis of elicitation of motor responses at a low threshold of electrical stimulation. The area is located in the precentral gyrus, including the anterior wall of the central sulcus, and in the anterior part of the paracentral lobule on the medial surface of the hemisphere (see Figs. 15-1 and 15-2). This cortex (area 4 of Brodmann) is thick agranular heterotypical cortex. Neurons other than pyramidal cells are not easily recognized, and the six layers are difficult to define, although giant pyramidal cells of Betz are present in layer 5.

The main sources of input to area 4 are the premotor cortex (area 6), somesthetic cortex, and posterior division of the ventral lateral thalamic nucleus (VLp), which in turn receives input from the cerebellum. Although area 4 contributes fibers to several motor pathways, the efferents that give it a special significance are those included in the **pyramidal system** (comprising the corticospinal and corticobulbar tracts). About 30% of these fibers arise in area 4; another 30% come from area 6. The remainder arise in the parietal lobe, with the largest proportion having their cell bodies in the first somesthetic area. These include fibers that are not motor in function, but that terminate in relay nuclei of general sensory pathways and thereby modulate transmission of sensory data to the thalamus and cortex. The motor and sensory functions of the corticospinal and corticobulbar tracts are discussed in Chapters 23 and 19, respectively.

There is agreement between the number of Betz cells in the region of area 4 that contributes fibers to the corticospinal tract and the number of large, thickly myelinated axons (about 10 μm in diameter) in the tract. The number is about 30,000, which accounts for some 3% of the fibers in the medullary pyramid. These axons of Betz cells conduct particularly rapidly and probably have some terminal branches that synapse with motor neurons.

Electrical stimulation of the primary motor area elicits contraction of muscles that are mainly on the opposite side of the body. Although cortical control of the skeletal musculature is predominantly contralateral, there is some ipsilateral control of most of the muscles of the head and of the axial muscles of the body. The body is represented in the motor area as inverted, with the pattern or homunculus being similar to that of the somesthetic cortex. The sequence from below upward is pharynx, larynx, tongue, and face; the region for muscles of the head comprises about one-third of the whole of area 4. Continuing dorsally, there is a small region for muscles of the neck, followed by a large area for muscles of the hand; this is consistent with the importance of manual dexterity in humans. Next in order are small areas for the arm, shoulder, trunk, and thigh, continuing with an area on the medial surface of the hemisphere for the remainder of the leg and the foot.

The primary motor area has a lower threshold of excitability than other areas from which contraction of skeletal muscles can be elicited by electrical stimulation. Contractions of contralateral muscles usually are elicited, as has been noted, and the muscles responding depend on the particular part of area 4 that is stimulated. The response usually involves muscles that make up a functional group, although occasionally there is contraction of a single muscle. In laboratory animals, small clusters of neurons that control individual muscles have been recognized in the primary motor cortex.

Destructive lesions of area 4 result in voluntary paresis of the affected part of the body. The muscles involved are flaccid if the damage is restricted to the precentral gyrus.[1] The much more common condition of spastic voluntary paralysis characteristically follows lesions that spread beyond area 4 or that interrupt projection fibers in the medullary center or internal capsule. There is considerable recovery with time, with the residual deficit being most evident as weakness in the distal parts of the limbs.

A **second** and a **supplementary motor area** have been identified by cortical stimulation in primates, including humans. The second motor area is ventral to the sensorimotor strip in the dorsal wall of the lateral sulcus, overlapping the second somesthetic area. The supplementary motor area is in the part of area 6 that lies on the medial surface of the hemisphere (see Fig. 15-2).

Electrical stimulation in humans indicates a somatotopic organization of the supplementary motor area, with the face represented rostrally and the lower limb in the caudal part of the region. The effects of stimulation are predominantly contralateral and are preceded by a conscious urge to make the movements.

---

[1] Destruction of part of the primary motor area without involvement of adjacent cortex or the underlying white matter seldom is encountered clinically. Deficits resulting from damage to area 4 are inferred from results of experiments on subhuman primates and from isolated instances in which a region of area 4 was removed in humans as a therapeutic procedure, as in the treatment of Jacksonian epilepsy.

Increased regional blood flow in the supplementary motor area can be demonstrated during the mental processes that precede the execution of a movement.

Results of experiments in monkeys indicate that loss of function of the supplementary motor area may cause the spasticity of muscles paralyzed as the result of an "upper motor neuron" lesion. Bilateral lesions that involve this area cause profound paralysis as well as mutism.

PREMOTOR AREA

The premotor area, which coincides with Brodmann's area 6, is anterior to the primary motor area on the lateral surface of the hemisphere (see Fig. 15-1). The cytoarchitecture of area 6 is similar to that of area 4, except that Betz cells are lacking. In addition to connections with other cortical areas, the premotor cortex receives fibers from the anterior division of the ventral lateral nucleus of the thalamus, which in turn receives input from the corpus striatum.

The premotor area contributes to motor function by its direct contribution to the pyramidal and other descending motor pathways and by its influence on the primary motor cortex. With respect to the latter, area 6 (including the supplementary motor area) elaborates programs for motor routines necessary for skilled voluntary action, both when a new program is established and when a previously learned program is altered. In general, the primary motor area is the cortex through which commands are channeled for the *execution* of movements. In contrast, the premotor and supplementary motor areas program skilled motor activity and thus *direct* the primary motor area in its execution.

The term **apraxia** refers to the result of a cerebral lesion characterized by impairment in the performance of learned movements in the absence of paralysis. One form of apraxia follows a lesion that involves the premotor area. The disability includes functional impairment of muscles that work on the proximal joints of the limbs, especially the shoulder. The ability to carry out tasks at arm's length is then severely impaired. Other forms of apraxia are caused by lesions that involve the somesthetic association cortex, proprioception being a necessary background for motor proficiency. When the disability affects writing, it is called **agraphia**.

The **frontal eye field** is in the lower part of area 8 on the lateral surface of the hemisphere. It controls voluntary conjugate movements of the eyes. Electrical stimulation of the frontal eye field causes deviation of the eyes to the opposite side. Destruction of the frontal eye field causes conjugate deviation of the eyes toward the side of the lesion. The patient cannot voluntarily move the eyes in the opposite direction, but this movement still occurs involuntarily when the eyes follow an object moving across the field of vision. Convergence of the eyes also can be accomplished without the frontal eye fields. The involuntary tracking movement and convergence are directed by the visual and visual association cortex of the occipital lobe.

PREFRONTAL CORTEX

The large expanse of cortex in the frontal lobe from which motor responses are not elicited on stimulation falls under the heading of association cortex. This region envelops the frontal pole and is called the prefrontal cortex. Corresponding to Brodmann's areas 9, 10, 11, and 12, it is well developed only in primates, especially so in humans. The prefrontal cortex has extensive connections through fasciculi in the medullary center with cortex of the parietal, temporal, and occipital lobes, thus gaining access to contemporary sensory experience and to the repository of data derived from past experience. There also are reciprocal connections with the amygdaloid body in the temporal lobe and with the mediodorsal thalamic nucleus, forming a system that determines affective reactions to present situations on the basis of past experience. The prefrontal cortices also monitor behavior and exercise control based on such higher mental faculties as judgment and foresight.

The prefrontal cortex can be damaged by appropriately placed tumors or penetrating injuries or by the operation of **prefrontal leukotomy** (or lobotomy), introduced by de Egas Moniz in 1935. This simple surgical procedure, which interrupts the connections between the thalami and the cortices of the orbital surfaces of the frontal lobes, formerly was performed as treatment for various mental disorders. A person with bilateral loss of function of the prefrontal cortex typically becomes rude, inconsiderate to others, incapable of accepting advice, and unable to anticipate the consequences of rash or reckless words or actions.[2] The patient no longer suffers from anxiety or depression, or even from severe pain, although there is no loss of awareness of pain. The awarding of a share of the Nobel prize for medicine and physiology to de Egas Moniz in 1949 recognized prefrontal leukotomy as a major advance in the relief of suffering, but perhaps without due concern for the importance of the accompanying personality changes. By the 1960s, the operation was reserved for patients with severe affective disorders that did not respond to drugs and psychotherapy, and since the 1970s, it seldom has been deemed justifiable. Stereotaxic lesions beneath the head of the caudate nucleus may relieve affective disorders with fewer adverse effects than complete prefrontal leukotomy, but the consequences of the operation are still permanent.

Bilateral damage to extensive areas of prefrontal cortex occurs in **general paralysis of the insane**, which is a manifestation of syphilis of the central nervous system, and in **Pick's disease**, the cause of which is unknown. The same areas degenerate in some cases of **Alzheimer's disease** (see also Ch. 12). These are diseases in which there is **dementia** or generalized deterioration of the memory and intellect, but the involvement of the frontal lobes causes additional behavioral abnormalities similar to those that follow leukotomy.

Language Areas

The use of language is a peculiarly human accomplishment, requiring special neural mechanisms in association areas of the cerebral cortex. Areas of cortex that have particular roles with respect to language have been identified by the study of patients in whom these areas were damaged by occlusion of blood vessels. The infarcted regions of the brain can be identified post mortem, but more accurate information is obtained by scanning the brain of the living patient to detect the distribution of an intravenously injected radioactive tracer or by computed tomography, nuclear magnetic resonance imaging, or positron emission tomography. These modern imaging techniques are reviewed in Chapters 4 and 16.

Two cortical areas have specialized language functions (Fig. 15-4). The **receptive language area** (also called the sensory or ideational language area) consists of the auditory association cortex (Wernicke's area) and adjacent parts of the parietal lobe, notably the supramarginal and angular gyri. The **expressive speech area** (Broca's area, or motor speech area) occupies the opercular and trian-

---

[2] The classic case of prefrontal lobe damage was that of Phineas Gage, an American railroad construction worker injured in 1848 by the premature explosion of a blasting charge, which drove an iron tamping rod (105 cm long and 3 cm in diameter) through his head. The missile entered through the left cheek and emerged from the right frontal bone, anterior to the coronal suture, having passed through the left orbit and the anterior parts of both frontal lobes of the brain. The motor and speech areas were spared by the injury, and the most conspicuous abnormalities were the changed personality and feckless behavior, which persisted until his death nearly 20 years later.

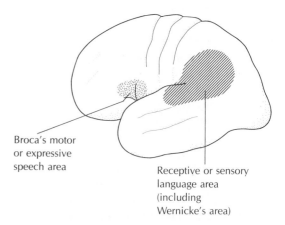

Broca's motor or expressive speech area

Receptive or sensory language area (including Wernicke's area)

Figure 15-4. The language areas.

gular portions of the inferior frontal gyrus, corresponding to areas 44 and 45 of Brodmann. The integrity of the **supplementary motor area** on the medial surface of the hemisphere is also necessary for normal speech. The language areas are situated in the left hemisphere with few exceptions, and this is, therefore, the dominant hemisphere as a rule with respect to language. The receptive and expressive language areas are in communication with each other through the **superior longitudinal (arcuate) fasciculus** in the medullary center.

Aphasia

Damage to the language areas or their connections results in aphasia; there are several types, depending on the location of the lesion. **Receptive aphasia** (Wernicke's aphasia), in which auditory and visual comprehension of language, naming of objects, and repetition of a sentence spoken by the examiner are all defective, is caused by a lesion in the receptive language area, notably in Wernicke's area. A lesion involving Wernicke's area and the superior longitudinal or arcuate fasciculus results in **jargon aphasia**, with fluent but unintelligible speech. Interruption of the arcuate fasciculus connecting Wernicke's and Broca's areas causes **conduction aphasia**, in which there is poor repetition of a sentence spoken by the examiner but relatively good comprehension and spontaneous speech. Infarcts that isolate the sensory language area from surrounding parietal and temporal cortex may cause **anomic aphasia** (isolation syndrome), characterized by fluent but circumlocutory speech caused by word-finding difficulties.

Alexia refers to loss of the ability to read and occurs with or without other aspects of aphasia. Pure alexia may result from a lesion that involves the white matter of the occipital lobe of the dominant hemisphere and the splenium of the corpus callosum. Such a lesion severs connections between both visual cortices and the unilaterally located language areas. **Dyslexia** is incomplete alexia and is characterized by an inability to read more than a few lines with understanding. **Expressive aphasia** (Broca's aphasia), caused by a lesion in Broca's area of the frontal lobe, is characterized by hesitant and distorted speech with relatively good comprehension. The term **global aphasia** refers to a virtually complete loss of the ability to communicate following destruction of the cortex on both sides of the lateral sulcus. This is one of the consequences of occlusion of the middle cerebral artery (see Ch. 25).

There usually is some recovery of function, even in severe cases of aphasia. This is attributed to assumption of linguistic functions by the intact contralateral cerebral hemisphere.

Hemispheral Dominance

Memory traces established in one hemisphere (eg, in the cortex of the left hemisphere as a result of some particular activity involving the right hand) are transferred to the cortex of the other hemisphere through the corpus callosum. There are, therefore, bilateral cortical memory patterns for previous experience.

LEFT HEMISPHERE FUNCTIONS

In right-handed people and in most who are left-handed, language is a function of the left hemisphere. The "talking" hemisphere is said to be dominant relative to the "nontalking" hemisphere. A left-sided cerebral lesion is, therefore, more serious than one in the right hemisphere because aphasia may be added to other neurological deficits. The reverse is true for those few whose right hemisphere is dominant for linguistic functions.

Although factors that determine hemispheral dominance for speech are not well known, heredity is almost certainly involved to some extent. The **planum temporale** posterior to the auditory area on the dorsal surface of the superior temporal gyrus (see Fig. 15-3) is larger in the left than in the right hemisphere in 65% of human brains and larger on the right side in only 11% of brains. This indicates that the dominance with respect to language may be reflected in structural asymmetry because the planum temporale constitutes a large part of Wernicke's area.

About 75% of the population is right-handed, preferring the right hand for skilled tasks. In these, the right hand is controlled by the left cerebral hemisphere, which also is the dominant hemisphere for language. Handedness is not always correlated with linguistic dominance because 70% of those who are left-handed have their language areas in the left hemisphere, rather than in the one that controls the left hand.

RIGHT HEMISPHERE FUNCTIONS

For some activities, the right hemisphere is the dominant one in most people. The most notable faculty residing in the right hemisphere is three-dimensional, or spatial, perception. The evidence is derived from studies of patients in whom the corpus callosum had been sectioned as a therapeutic measure in severe epilepsy. After commissurotomy, these patients were able to copy drawings and arrange blocks in a desired position more efficiently with the left hand than with the right hand. The right hemisphere is, therefore, better equipped to direct such acts.

Spatial awareness extends to the whole body and its surroundings, and this awareness is lost contralaterally in the condition of cortical neglect discussed in connection with the somesthetic association cortex. Severe cortical neglect most often follows a right-sided lesion.

Other abilities for which the right hemisphere dominates are singing and the playing of musical instruments. Musical skills commonly are lost following vascular occlusions in the right hemisphere, and it is not unusual for a patient severely aphasic from a lesion in the left hemisphere to retain the ability to sing.

SUGGESTED READING ——————

Allison T, and 5 others: Human cortical potentials evoked by stimulation of the median nerve. I and II. J Neurophysiol 62:694–722, 1989

Asanuma H: The Motor Cortex. New York, Raven Press, 1989

Damasio AR, Geschwind N: The neural basis of language. Annu Rev Neurosci 7:127–147, 1984

Damasio AR, Tranel D, Damasio H: Face agnosia and the neural substrate of memory. Annu Rev Neurosci 13:89–109, 1990

Fox PT, Burton H, Raichle ME: Mapping human somatosensory cortex with positron emission tomography. J Neurosurg 67:34–43, 1987

Friberg L, Olsen IS, Roland PE, Paulson OB, Lassen NA: Focal increase of blood flow in the cerebral cortex of man during vestibular stimulation. Brain 108:609–623, 1985

Frith CD, Friston K, Liddle PF, Frackowiak RSJ: Willed action and the prefrontal cortex in man: A study with PET. Proc R Soc Lond [Biol] 244: 241–246, 1991

Fuster J: The Prefrontal Cortex. Anatomy, Physiology, and Neuropsychology of the Frontal Lobe, 2nd ed. New York, Raven Press, 1989

Geschwind N: Specializations of the human brain. Sci Am 241:180–199, 1979

Kartsounis LD, Poynton A, Bridges PK, Bartlett JR: Neuropsychological correlates of stereotactic subcaudate tractotomy: A prospective study. Brain 114:2657–2673, 1991

Kertesz A: Aphasia and Associated Disorders. Taxonomy, Localization and Recovery. New York, Grune & Stratton, 1979

Kurata K: Somatotopy in the human supplementary motor area. Trends Neurosci 15:159–160, 1992

Lemon R: The output map of the primate motor cortex. Trends Neurosci 11:501–506, 1988

Liegeois-Chauvel C, Musolino A, Chauvel P: Localization of the primary auditory area in man. Brain 114:139–153, 1991

Narici L, and 7 others: Neuromagnetic somatosensory homunculus: A non-invasive approach in humans. Neurosci Lett 121:51–54, 1991

Penfield W, Rasmussen T: The Cerebral Cortex of Man: A Clinical Study of Localization of Function. New York, Macmillan, 1950

Springer SP, Deutsch G: Left Brain, Right Brain, rev ed. San Francisco, WH Freeman & Co, 1985

Stein JF: Representation of egocentric space in the posterior parietal cortex. Q J Exp Physiol 74: 583–606, 1989

Sixteen

The Human Nervous System: An Anatomical Viewpoint, Sixth Edition, Murray L. Barr and John A. Kiernan. J.B. Lippincott Company, Philadelphia, © 1993.

Medullary Center, Internal Capsule, and Lateral Ventricles

Important Facts

The medullary center (white matter of the cerebral hemisphere) consists of association, commissural, and projection fibers.

Most named association bundles (superior longitudinal, arcuate, inferior longitudinal, inferior occipitofrontal, uncinate, and superior occipitofrontal fasciculi) interconnect lobes.

The cingulum, fornix, longitudinal striae, and stria terminalis are association bundles of the limbic system.

The corpus callosum and anterior commissure, which interconnect symmetrical cortical regions, exchange information between the left and right sides.

After transection of the commissures, a task newly learned with one hand cannot be performed by the other. Sensory data that enter only the right hemisphere cannot be put into words because of disconnection from the language areas in the left hemisphere.

Most projection fibers pass through the internal capsule.

All parts of the internal capsule contain thalamocortical and corticothalamic fibers.

Motor fibers, including those of the pyramidal system, descend in the posterior limb of the internal capsule. A small infarct there can cause contralateral hemiplegia.

The geniculocalcarine tract is in the retrolentiform part of the internal capsule. Some of its fibers loop into the temporal lobe.

The frontal and central parts of the lateral ventricle have the corpus callosum for the roof, the thalamus and fornix as the floor, the caudate nucleus in the lateral wall, and the septum pellucidum in the medial wall.

The temporal horn is indented by the amygdala and hippocampus. The occipital horn is indented by the calcarine sulcus.

The interventricular foramen is bounded by the column of the fornix and the anterior tubercle of the thalamus.

Diagnostic images of the brain can be made with X-rays. Computed tomography has largely supplanted pneumoencephalography and ventriculography. Nuclear magnetic resonance imaging provides superior anatomical resolution. Positron emission tomography and regional cerebral blood flow studies can localize metabolically active regions of the brain.

Each cerebral hemisphere includes a large volume of white matter that constitutes the medullary center and accommodates the vast number of fibers running to and from all parts of the cortex. The medullary center is bounded by the cortex, lateral ventricle, and corpus striatum. Nerve fibers that establish connections between the cortex and subcortical gray matter continue from the medullary center into the internal capsule. The lateral ventricles, one in each hemisphere, are the largest of the four ventricles of the brain and are important in the dynamics of the cerebrospinal fluid system.

The cerebral white matter and the lateral ventricle account for much of the volume of the human brain, so this chapter is a conve-

nient place to introduce the reader to some of the methods by which pictures of the living brain can be obtained. These imaging methods are important tools of clinical neurology. Some related diagnostic techniques are reviewed in Chapters 4 and 25.

Medullary Center

The nerve fibers of the medullary center are of three types, depending on the nature of their connections (Fig. 16-1). **Association fibers** are confined to a hemisphere and connect one cortical area with another. Many of these fibers accumulate in longitudinally running bundles that can be displayed by dissection and that have been assigned names. **Com-**

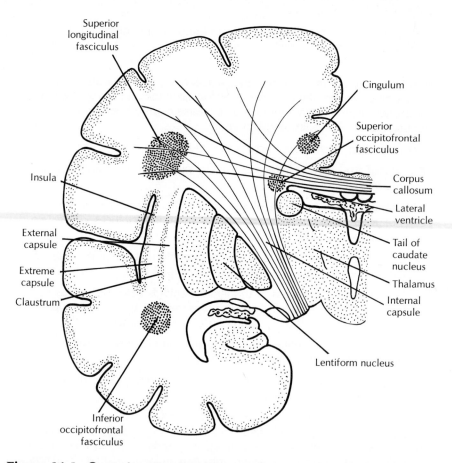

Figure 16-1. Coronal section through a cerebral hemisphere, indicating the positions of the larger bundles of association, commissural, and projection fibers.

missural fibers connect the cortices of the two hemispheres; most of the neocortical commissural fibers comprise the corpus callosum, with the remainder included in the anterior commissure. **Projection fibers** establish connections between the cortex and such subcortical structures as the corpus striatum, thalamus, nuclei of the brain stem, and spinal cord. They are afferent (corticipetal) or efferent (corticofugal) with respect to the cortex; most of the former originate in the thalamus.

Association Fasciculi

Association fibers are the most numerous of the three types of fiber noted. Operative procedures, vascular accidents, or other lesions that involve the fasciculi may lead to dysfunction by disconnecting functionally related regions of the cerebral cortex.

The **cingulum**, which is most easily displayed by dissection in the cingulate gyrus (Figs. 16-2 and 16-3), is an association fasciculus of the limbic lobe. The fibers of this longitudinal bundle run in both directions and interconnect the cingulate gyrus, parahippocampal gyrus of the temporal lobe, and septal area below the genu of the corpus callosum.

The **superior longitudinal fasciculus** (see Figs. 16-2 and 16-3), also known as the **arcuate fasciculus**, runs in an anteroposterior direction above the insula, and many of the fibers turn downward into the temporal lobe. This, like the other large association bundles, consists of fibers of various lengths that enter or leave the fasciculus at any point along its course. The superior longitudinal fasciculus provides important communications between cortices of the parietal, temporal, and occipital lobes and the cortex of the frontal lobe, including the sensory and motor language areas. An **inferior longitudinal fasciculus** has been described as running superficially beneath the lateral and ventral surfaces of the occipital and temporal lobes. This thin sheet of association fibers is difficult to demonstrate by dissection or to distinguish from other fibers at a deeper level, in particular from projection fibers of the geniculocalcarine tract.

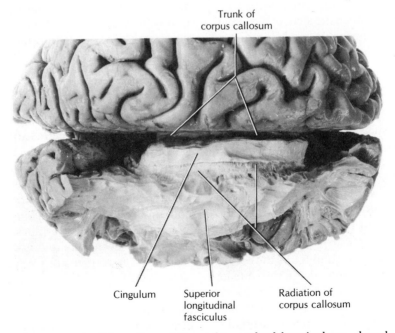

Trunk of corpus callosum

Cingulum · Superior longitudinal fasciculus · Radiation of corpus callosum

Figure 16-2. Dissection of the right cerebral hemisphere, dorsal view with frontal pole at the right. (× 0.65)

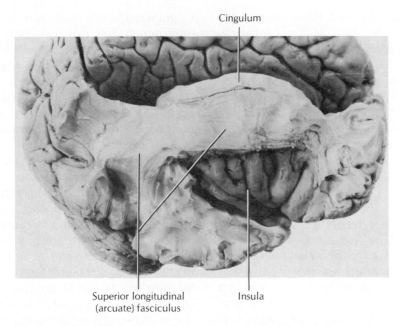

Figure 16-3. Dissection of the right cerebral hemisphere, dorsolateral view with frontal and temporal poles at the right. (× 0.65)

The **inferior occipitofrontal fasciculus** and **uncinate fasciculus** are components of a single association system (Figs. 16-4 and 16-5). The fibers are compressed into a well-defined bundle between the stem of the lateral sulcus below and the insula and lentiform nucleus above. The longer part of the fiber system, extending the length of the hemisphere, is the inferior occipitofrontal fasciculus. The uncinate fasciculus is the part that hooks around the stem of the lateral sulcus to connect the frontal lobe, especially cortex on its orbital surface, with cortex in the region of the temporal pole.

The **superior occipitofrontal fasciculus**, also called the **subcallosal bundle**, is located deep in the hemisphere and, therefore, cannot be dissected from a lateral approach. The fasciculus is compact in the middle of the hemisphere, where it is bounded by the corpus callosum, internal capsule, tail of the caudate nucleus, and lateral ventricle (see Fig. 16-1). The fibers spread out to cortex of the frontal lobe and to cortex in the posterior part of the hemisphere.

Large numbers of **arcuate fibers** connect adjacent gyri. These short subcortical association fibers are oriented at right angles to the gyri and bend sharply under the intervening sulci. Spread of activity along a gyrus or sulcus is provided by other subcortical association fibers and by axons within the cortex.

Commissures

CORPUS CALLOSUM

Most of the neocortical commissural fibers constitute the **corpus callosum**; the remainder are included in the anterior commissure, along with fibers of other than neocortical origin. There are about 300 million fibers in the corpus callosum; however, the commissure normally varies considerably in size. The posterior part of the corpus callosum (the splenium) has been reported to be larger in women than in men, but measurements of large numbers of specimens have shown that this apparent difference is not real. In laboratory animals, commissural fibers from an area of cortex in one hemisphere have been shown to terminate in the corresponding area, and in cortex closely related functionally with that

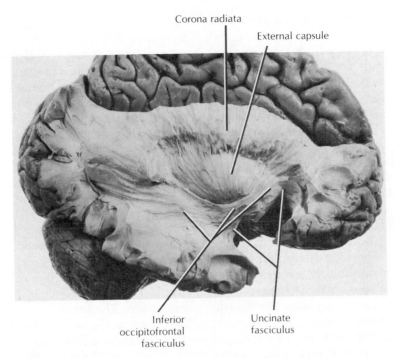

Figure 16-4. Medullary center of the right cerebral hemisphere after removal of the superior longitudinal fasciculus, insula, and underlying structures down to the external capsule. ($\times$ 0.65)

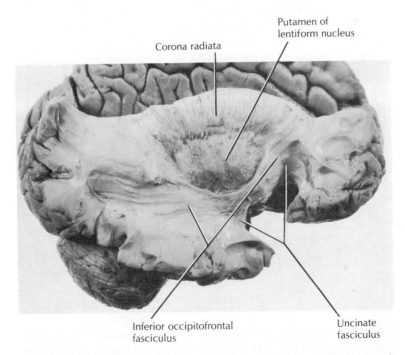

Figure 16-5. Dissection shown in Figure 16-4 continued by removal of the external capsule to expose the lentiform nucleus. ($\times$ 0.65)

area, in the other hemisphere. The hand areas of the primary somatosensory cortices and large parts of the primary visual areas are notable in that they are not directly connected by commissural fibers. They communicate functionally, however, through callosal fibers that connect the adjacent association areas. Much of the cortex of the temporal lobe makes its commissural connections by way of the anterior commissure rather than through the corpus callosum.

The **trunk** of the corpus callosum is the compact portion of the commissure in and near the midline (see Fig. 16-2). Variations in size of the trunk of the corpus callosum may be related to handedness. On entering the medullary center, the fibers constitute the **radiation** of the corpus callosum, which intersects association bundles and projection fibers. The trunk of the corpus callosum is considerably shorter than the hemispheres; this accounts for the enlargements of the ends, which are the **splenium** posteriorly and the **genu** ante-

riorly (see Fig. 13-2). The splenium and the radiations that connect the occipital lobes comprise the **forceps occipitalis** (forceps major) (Fig. 16-6), and the genu and the radiations that connect the frontal lobes form the **forceps frontalis** (forceps minor). The genu tapers into the **rostrum** of the corpus callosum, which is continuous with the lamina terminalis forming the anterior wall of the third ventricle. Some fibers of the radiation form a thin sheet, called the **tapetum**, over the temporal horn of the lateral ventricle (see Fig. 16-6). These fibers provide some of the communication between the cortices of the ventral surfaces of the temporal lobes.

Certain relations of the corpus callosum are partly the result of invasion of phylogenetically older parts of the brain by this neocortical commissure. The dorsal surface of the trunk of the corpus callosum is clothed by the **indusium griseum**, a thin layer of gray matter in which are embedded two delicate strands of fibers on each side called the **medial** and **lat-**

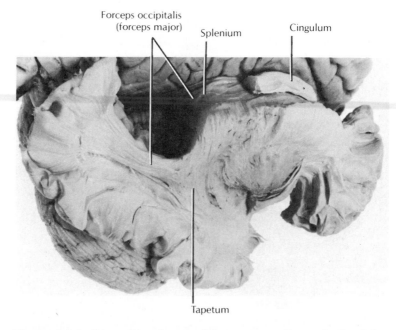

Forceps occipitalis (forceps major)   Splenium   Cingulum

Tapetum

Figure 16-6. Dissection of parts of the corpus callosum in the right hemisphere. The posterior half of the cingulum has been removed, and the longitudinal striae are visible on the upper surface of the exposed corpus callosum. (× 0.65)

eral longitudinal striae (of Lancisi). The longitudinal striae consist of fibers that proceed from the septal area on the medial surface of the frontal lobe to the hippocampus in the temporal lobe. As dorsally displaced remnants of the archicortex of the hippocampal formation and of the fornix, the indusium griseum and longitudinal striae are minor parts of the limbic system, which is discussed in Chapter 18.

The ventral surface of the corpus callosum forms the roof of the lateral ventricles and has relations with the fornix and septum pellucidum in the midline. The **fornix**, consisting of symmetrical halves, is a robust fiber system that connects the hippocampal formation of each temporal lobe with the hypothalamus (see Fig. 18-2) and the septal area of the forebrain. The crura of the fornix begin at the posterior end of each hippocampus; they curve forward and merge to form the body of the fornix, which is in contact with the undersurface of the trunk of the corpus callosum. The body of the fornix divides into two columns that turn ventrally away from the corpus callosum; they form the anterior boundaries of the interventricular foramina and continue to the hypothalamus. The resulting interval between the fornix and corpus callosum is bridged by the **septum pellucidum** (see Fig. 11-2), a thin sheet of neuroglial tissue that contains scattered groups of neurons at its anterior end and is covered on each side by ependyma. The septum pellucidum separates the frontal horns of the lateral ventricles; it is a double membrane containing a slit-like cavity, the cavum septi pellucidi, which does not communicate with the ventricular system or with the subarachnoid space.

A large hole in the septum pellucidum is often present in the brains of professional boxers. No functional disability is known to result from this perforation, but boxers commonly have numerous other small lesions that transect axons in the medullary centers of their cerebral hemispheres. The resulting generalized reduction in the number of cortical connections leads to the condition known as **chronic traumatic enceph-**

alopathy or **dementia pugilistica**, popularly called "punch-drunkenness." Deterioration of the personality, impairment of memory, and features of parkinsonism are attributable to functional disconnections in the cerebrum, whereas dysarthria and ataxia may be due to similar multiple interruptions of cerebellar connections.

ANTERIOR COMMISSURE

The **anterior commissure** is a bundle of fibers that crosses the midline in the lamina terminalis; it traverses the anterior parts of the corpora striata and provides for additional communication between the temporal lobes (Fig. 16-7). The anterior commissure includes fibers that connect the middle and inferior temporal gyri of the two sides; this is a neocortical component similar to the corpus callosum. Other fibers run between olfactory cortex of the temporal lobes (the lateral olfactory areas), for which the uncus is a landmark. There also are fibers that connect the olfactory bulbs, but these are a minor component of the human anterior commissure.

FUNCTIONS OF THE CEREBRAL COMMISSURES

The interhemispheric connections provided by the corpus callosum and anterior commissure contribute to the bilaterality of memory traces. All knowledge that arrives from the senses is collected by both cerebral hemispheres. The role of the neocortical commissures in interhemispheric transfer has been studied by assessing the effect of transection of the corpus callosum and anterior commissure in the monkey and chimpanzee (split-brain preparation). In normal, unoperated animals, a training exercise learned with one hand is performed efficiently by the other hand because of interhemispheric transfer of the neural basis of learning. In the case of the split-brain monkey or chimpanzee, a previously unfamiliar task learned by use of one hand cannot be performed by the other hand unless training in the exercise is repeated with that hand.

Similar observations, with an extension in

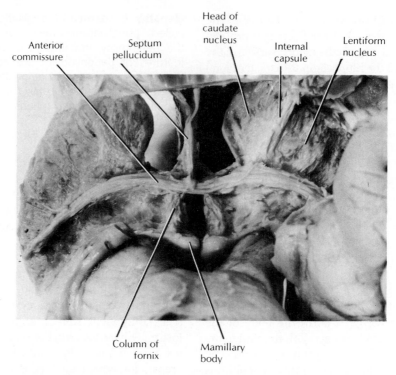

Anterior commissure • Septum pellucidum • Head of caudate nucleus • Internal capsule • Lentiform nucleus • Column of fornix • Mamillary body

Figure 16-7. Dissection exposing the anterior commissure, photographed by a camera anterior to the left frontal pole of the dissected brain. (× 1.65)

the area of language, are available for humans. In some people with severe epilepsy, the corpus callosum has been transected to confine the epileptic discharge to one hemisphere and the seizures to one side of the body. This operation leads to no significant changes in intellect, behavior, or emotional responses that can be attributed to commissurotomy. A task newly learned with one hand, however, is no longer transferable to the other hand, as is to be expected from the results of experiments on other primates.

A particularly significant result of commissurotomy in humans is related to language. Let us say that the linguistic faculties reside in the left hemisphere, as usually is the case. After recovering from the operation, the patient is unable to describe an object held in the left hand (with the eyes closed) or seen only in the left visual field, although the nature of the object is understood. There is no such diffi-

culty when the sensory data reach the left hemisphere. After commissurotomy, the right hemisphere is rendered mute and agraphic because it has no access to memory for language in the left hemisphere. However; the hemisphere that is subordinate with respect to language is superior in certain other activities. These include copying drawings that include perspective and arranging blocks in a prescribed manner. The nonlinguistic hemisphere is, therefore, the more proficient side of the brain in functions that require special competence in three-dimensional perspective. Another activity dependent on the right cerebral hemisphere is the production of music, as when singing or playing an instrument.

The Nobel prize for medicine and physiology in 1981 was shared by Hubel and Wiesel (see Ch. 15) with R. W. Sperry. The latter award was made chiefly for studies of the functions of the cerebral commissures.

Internal Capsule and Projection Fibers

The projection fibers are concentrated in the internal capsule and fan out as the **corona radiata** in the medullary center (see Fig. 16-5). The internal capsule consists of an **anterior limb**, a **genu**, a **posterior limb**, a **retrolentiform part**, and a **sublentiform part**, all of which have topographic relations with adjacent gray masses (Fig. 16-8). The anterior limb is bounded by the lentiform nucleus and by the head of the caudate nucleus. The genu is medial to the apex of the lentiform nucleus, and the posterior limb intervenes between the lentiform nucleus and the thalamus. The retrolentiform part of the internal capsule occupies the region behind the lentiform nucleus, and the sublentiform part consists of fibers that pass beneath the posterior part of the lentiform nucleus.

THALAMIC RADIATIONS

Many of the projection fibers establish reciprocal connections between the thalamus and the cerebral cortex. The **anterior thalamic radiation**, in the anterior limb of the internal capsule, consists mainly of fibers connecting the mediodorsal thalamic nucleus and prefrontal cortex. The **middle thalamic radiation** is a component of the posterior limb of the internal capsule. This radiation includes the somatosensory projection from the ventral posterior thalamic nucleus to the somesthetic area in the parietal lobe; these fibers run in the posterior part of the posterior limb, where they are partly intermingled with motor projection fibers. Other fibers of the middle thalamic radiation establish reciprocal connections between the thalamus and the association cortex of the parietal lobe. Fibers from the two divisions of the ventral lateral nucleus of the thalamus

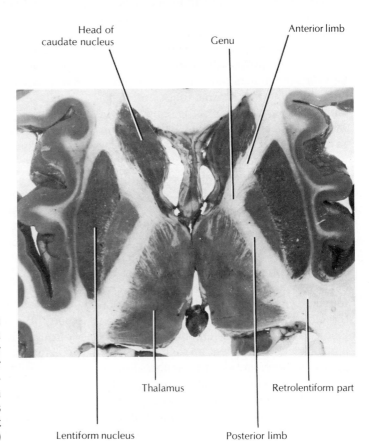

Figure 16-8. Horizontal section of the cerebrum stained by a method that differentiates gray matter (*dark*) and white matter (*light*), showing regions of the internal capsule. The sublentiform part is ventral to the plane of this section, below the posterior part of the lentiform nucleus. (× 1)

Head of caudate nucleus

Genu

Anterior limb

Thalamus

Retrolentiform part

Lentiform nucleus

Posterior limb

reach the motor and premotor areas of the frontal lobe by traversing the genu and adjacent region of the posterior limb of the internal capsule.

The **posterior thalamic radiation** establishes connections between the thalamus and cortex of the occipital lobe. The **geniculocalcarine tract** that ends in the visual cortex is a particularly important component of this radiation. Originating in the lateral geniculate body, the geniculocalcarine tract first traverses the retrolentiform and sublentiform parts of the internal capsule. The constituent fibers then spread out into a broad band bordering the lateral ventricle and turn backward into the occipital lobe. Some of the fibers, constituting **Meyer's loop**, proceed forward for a considerable distance into the temporal lobe above the temporal horn of the lateral ventricle before turning back into the occipital lobe (see Fig. 20-7). The posterior thalamic radiation also contains fibers that establish reciprocal connections between the pulvinar of the thalamus and the cortex of the occipital lobe. The **inferior thalamic radiation** consists of fibers directed horizontally in the sublentiform part of the internal capsule that connect thalamic nuclei with cortex of the temporal lobe. Most of the fibers are included in the **auditory radiation**, which originates in the medial geniculate body and terminates in the auditory area, on the superior surface of the superior temporal gyrus.

MOTOR PROJECTION FIBERS

The remaining projection fibers are corticofugal, and many of them have motor functions. The **corticobulbar (corticonuclear)** and **corticospinal tracts**, which together constitute the pyramidal motor system, originate in the motor and premotor areas in the frontal lobe and in the rostral (anterior) parts of the parietal lobe. These fibers are probably accompanied by motor corticoreticular fibers (see below). The descending axons converge as they traverse the corona radiata and enter the anterior half of the posterior limb. In their passage caudally through the internal capsule, the motor fibers are shifted into the posterior half of

the posterior limb by frontopontine fibers that have already traversed the anterior limb. Corticobulbar fibers are most anterior, followed in sequence by corticospinal fibers related to the upper limb, trunk, and lower limb. There is considerable overlap of the territories occupied by fibers for the major regions of the body, so a small destructive lesion in the internal capsule has serious effects.

Corticopontine fibers originate in widespread areas of cortex but in greatest numbers in the frontal and parietal lobes. They terminate in the nuclei pontis, in the basal portion of the pons. Fibers of the **frontopontine tract** traverse the anterior limb of the internal capsule and the anterior portion of the posterior limb. Most of the fibers of the **parietotemporopontine tract** originate in the parietal lobe and traverse the retrolentiform part of the internal capsule.

Corticostriate fibers originate in all parts of the neocortex, most profusely in the sensorimotor strip, and end in the striatum. The caudate nucleus and putamen receive these fibers from the internal capsule; the putamen receives some from the external capsule as well.

Other projection fibers pass to the red nucleus, reticular formation, and inferior olivary complex. **Corticorubral fibers** arise from the motor and premotor areas of the frontal lobe; some of them are collateral branches of corticospinal axons. The **corticoreticular fibers** begin in the motor cortex and in cortex of the parietal lobe, especially the somesthetic area. They terminate mainly in the central group of reticular nuclei. **Corticoolivary fibers**, mainly from the motor areas, terminate in the nuclei of the inferior olivary complex. These descending pathways accompany the fibers of the pyramidal system through the internal capsule and basis pedunculi into the pons and medulla. Along with the corticospinal and corticobulbar tracts, they are severed by destructive lesions in the internal capsule. Such lesions also involve the thalamocortical fibers from the ventral lateral thalamic nucleus to the motor and premotor areas of the cortex.

An infarction in the posterior part of the internal capsule results in serious neurological deficits. These include the effects of an "upper motor neuron lesion" (see Ch. 23) caused mainly by interruption of pyramidal and corticoreticular fibers. **Hemiparesis** is weakness of all the muscles of the opposite side of the body, and **hemiplegia** is complete paralysis of the affected side. A lesion in the internal capsule also may cause general sensory deficits by involvement of the thalamocortical projection to the somesthetic area and a visual field defect by interruption of geniculocalcarine fibers.

The composition of the **external capsule** is incompletely understood, but it is known that this thin layer of white matter between the putamen and claustrum consists mainly of projection fibers. These include some of the corticostriate fibers that end in the putamen and some of the corticoreticular fibers.

Lateral Ventricles

The lateral ventricles, one in each cerebral hemisphere, are roughly C-shaped cavities lined by ependyma and filled with cerebrospinal fluid. Each lateral ventricle consists of a central part in the region of the parietal lobe from which horns extend into the frontal, occipital, and temporal lobes. The principal features of the ventricular walls are shown in Figures 16-9 and 16-10. The configuration of the entire ventricular system of the brain is shown in Figure 16-11.

The **central part** of the lateral ventricle has a flat roof formed by the corpus callosum. The floor includes part of the dorsal surface of the thalamus, of which the anterior tubercle is a boundary of the interventricular foramen (of Monro) that leads to the third ventricle. The tail of the caudate nucleus forms a ridge along

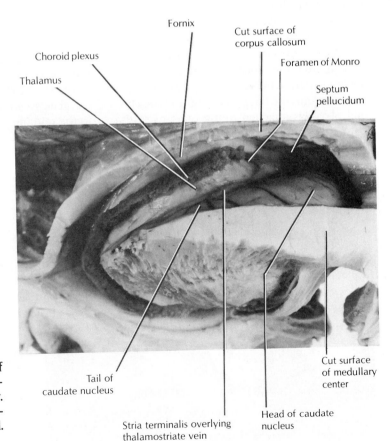

Figure 16-9. Dissection of the right cerebral hemisphere, dorsolateral view. The roof of the lateral ventricle has been removed. (× 1.25)

Fornix

Cut surface of corpus callosum

Choroid plexus

Foramen of Monro

Thalamus

Septum pellucidum

Cut surface of medullary center

Tail of caudate nucleus

Head of caudate nucleus

Stria terminalis overlying thalamostriate vein

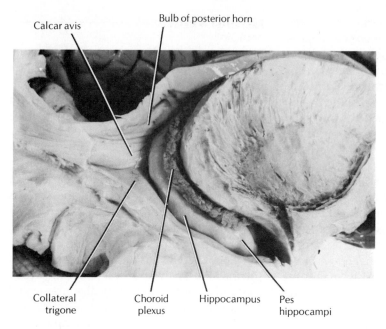

Calcar avis

Bulb of posterior horn

Collateral trigone

Choroid plexus

Hippocampus

Pes hippocampi

Figure 16-10. Dissection of the right cerebral hemisphere (lateral view), showing the occipital and temporal horns of the lateral ventricle. (× 1.25)

the lateral border of the floor. The stria terminalis, a slender bundle of fibers originating in the amygdaloid body in the temporal lobe, lies in the groove between the tail of the caudate nucleus and the thalamus, along with the thalamostriate vein (vena terminalis). The fornix completes the floor medially, and the choroid plexus is attached to the margins of the **choroid fissure**, which intervenes between the fornix and thalamus.

The **frontal horn** (formerly called the anterior horn) extends forward from the region of the interventricular foramen. The corpus callosum continues as the roof, and the genu of the corpus callosum limits the frontal horn in front. The septum pellucidum bridges the interval between the fornix and corpus callosum in the midline, separating the frontal horns of the two lateral ventricles. The **occipital horn** (posterior horn), which is of variable length, is

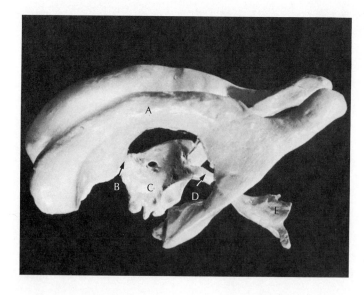

Figure 16-11. A cast of the ventricular system of the brain. (**A**) Left lateral ventricle. (**B**) Interventricular foramen. (**C**) Third ventricle. (**D**) Cerebral aqueduct. (**E**) Fourth ventricle. (*Prepared by Dr. D. G. Montemurro*)

surrounded by white matter of the medullary center. There are two elevations on the medial wall of the occipital horn. The more dorsal prominence, for which the forceps occipitalis is responsible, is called the **bulb of the occipital horn**; the lower prominence, formed by the calcarine sulcus, is called the **calcar avis**.

The slender **temporal horn** (formerly known as the inferior horn) extends to within about 3 cm of the temporal pole. There is a triangular area, called the **collateral trigone**, in the floor of the ventricle where the occipital and temporal horns diverge from the central part of the ventricle. The collateral sulcus on the external surface of the hemisphere is at the site of the trigone and may produce a **collateral eminence**. The tail of the caudate nucleus, now considerably attenuated, extends forward in the roof of the temporal horn as far as the amygdaloid body. This latter nucleus is above the anterior end of the temporal horn, which places it close to the uncus on the external surface. The stria terminalis and thalamostriate vein run along the medial side of the tail of the caudate nucleus.

The floor of the temporal horn includes an important structure, the **hippocampus** (see Fig. 16-10). The hippocampus may be visualized as an extension of the parahippocampal gyrus on the external surface that has been "rolled into" the floor of the temporal horn. The slightly enlarged anterior end of the hippocampus is known as the **pes hippocampi** because it resembles an animal's paw. Efferent fibers from the hippocampus form a ridge, the **fimbria**, along its medial border. The fimbria continues as the **crus of the fornix** after the hippocampus terminates beneath the splenium of the corpus callosum. The choroid plexus of the central part of the ventricle continues into the temporal horn, where it is attached to the margins of the choroid fissure above the fimbria of the hippocampus.

Imaging Techniques for the Brain

The brain, ventricles, and subarachnoid space are not seen in ordinary X-ray pictures but can be demonstrated by special methods, which are important diagnostic tools in clinical neurology.

RADIOGRAPHIC METHODS

In **pneumoencephalography**, some of the cerebrospinal fluid was replaced by air (Fig. 16-12). This procedure, which was painful and, in some circumstances, hazardous to the patient, has been almost completely replaced by the use of **computed tomography** (CT scan). This application of X-ray imaging is based on scanning the head with a narrow, moving beam of X-rays and measuring the attenuation of the emerging beam. The density readings from thin "sections" of the head are processed by a computer to generate an image whose brightness depends on the absorption values of the tissues (Fig. 16-13). The CT scan is so sensitive that the information obtained extends beyond that provided by air studies. The technique is valuable in clinical diagnosis because the density of many cerebral lesions is greater or less than the density of normal brain tissue. CT scanning also has largely replaced **ventriculography**, a surgical procedure in which a liquid contrast medium was introduced into the ventricular system by way of a needle passed through the cortex of the frontal or parietal lobe into a lateral ventricle.

To avoid irradiation of the eyes, the "axial" plane of the sections pictured by CT is oblique, being somewhat closer to horizontal than to coronal. Special neuroanatomical atlases are available in which CT scans are compared with photographs of slices of the brain cut in the same plane.

Other diagnostic radiographic techniques for the central nervous system include **myelography**, in which the spinal cord is outlined by contrast medium injected into the lumbar cistern, and **cerebral angiography**, which is reviewed in Chapter 25.

NUCLEAR MAGNETIC RESONANCE IMAGING

Nuclear magnetic resonance imaging (NMRI, or simply MRI) was developed from a physical method used in chemical analysis. In a strong magnetic field, the nuclei of atoms absorb radio-

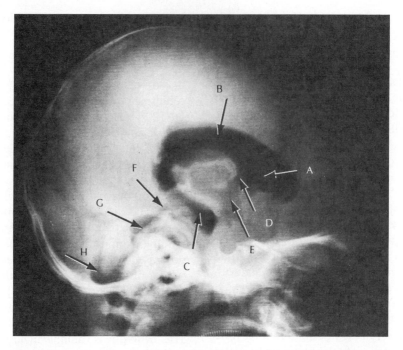

Figure 16-12. Pneumoencephalogram of a 9-month-old child (lateral view). The head was in the brow-up position, so the occipital horn contains cerebrospinal fluid. Air appears black; bone is white. (**A**) Frontal horn of lateral ventricle. (**B**) Central part of lateral ventricle. (**C**) Temporal horn of lateral ventricle. (**D**) Interventricular foramen. (**E**) Third ventricle. (**F**) Cerebral aqueduct. (**G**) Fourth ventricle. (**H**) Cisterna magna. (*Courtesy of Dr. J. M. Allcock*)

frequency energy. The absorbed frequency is characteristic of the element and of the immediate molecular environment of its atoms. In diagnostic NMRI, a frequency is chosen that is absorbed mainly by the nuclei of the hydrogen atoms of water. The patient's head is put into a magnetic field and irradiated with the radiofrequency radiation for protons. The measured energy absorptions are integrated in a computer, which generates a series of pictures of sections through the head. The sections may be reconstructed in any plane. Horizontal sections (parallel to the plane passing through the anterior and posterior commissures), as well as sagittal and coronal sections, are commonly presented. The reconstructed slices are typically 4 or 5 mm thick.

Images commonly are prepared in three ways. A **T1-weighted image** emphasizes the difference between central nervous tissue and other fluids and tissues but does not clearly distinguish gray from white matter (Figs. 16-14 and 16-15A). A **T2-weighted image** emphasizes the cerebrospinal fluid in the subarachnoid space and ventricles (Fig. 16-15B), and a **proton density image** (Fig. 16-15C) emphasizes the difference between gray and white matter.

The advantages of NMRI are that no potentially harmful radiation is used and that the anatomical resolution (Fig. 16-16) is greatly superior to that obtainable with X-rays. Bone and flowing blood are invisible in NMRI pictures. Gray and white matter and cerebrospinal fluid have different densities, and sometimes it is possible to identify regions of white matter that contain degenerating axons. A special contrast medium (a gadolinium compound) can be introduced into the circulation to reveal regions of the brain with abnormally

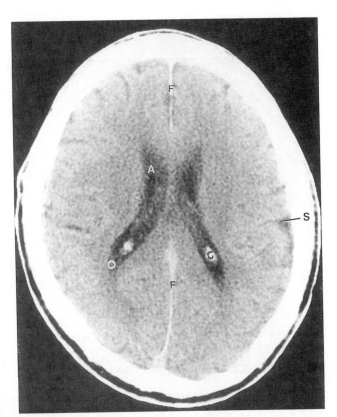

Figure 16-13. Computed tomography (CT) scan at a level showing the lateral ventricles. (**C**) Choroid plexus in the region of the collateral trigone (visible because it contains calcified deposits). (**F**) Falx cerebri. (**A**) Frontal (anterior) horn. (**O**) Occipital horn. (**S**) Subarachnoid space. The temporal horn is invisible or almost so in a normal CT scan. (*Courtesy of Dr. D. M. Pelz*)

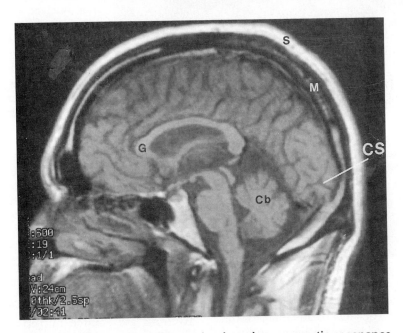

Figure 16-14. Sagittal T1-weighted nuclear magnetic resonance image of the normal brain. (**CS**) Calcarine sulcus. (**Cb**) Cerebellum. (**G**) Genu of corpus callosum. (**M**) Marrow in parietal bone. (**S**) Scalp. Note that compact bone and flowing blood are not visible. Many other neuroanatomical features can be seen, including the paracentral lobule, the fornix, a mamillary body, the cerebral aqueduct, the pons, and the medulla. Compare with Figure 1-3. (*Courtesy of Dr. D. M. Pelz*)

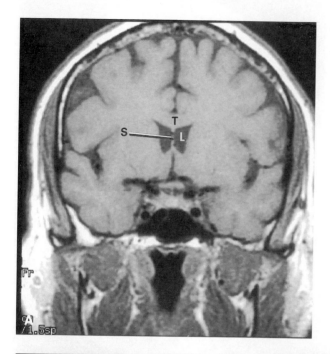

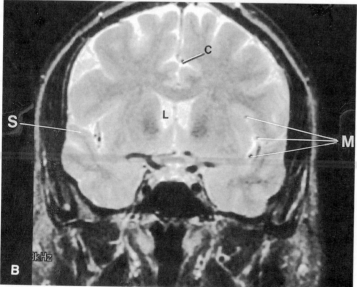

Figure 16-15. Shows coronal nuclear magnetic resonance images of a plane that contains the insula, lentiform nucleus, internal capsule, and head of caudate nucleus. (**A**) Coronal T1-weighted image. (**C**) Trunk of corpus callosum. (**L**) Lateral ventricle. (**S**) Septum pellucidum. (*Courtesy of Dr. D. M. Pelz*) (**B**) T2-weighted image. (**C**) Cingulate sulcus with callosomarginal artery. (**L**) Lateral ventricle. (**M**) Middle cerebral vessels in subarachnoid space. (**S**) Superior temporal gyrus. (*Courtesy of Dr. D. M. Pelz*)

(continued)

permeable blood vessels, which often occur at sites of disease. The chief disadvantage is that NMRI is a slow process, requiring about 1 hour to obtain information that CT can provide in a few minutes. The disadvantage of NMRI and CT in comparison to positron emission tomography, discussed in the next section, is that the two former techniques fail to distinguish living from dead tissue.

POSITRON EMISSION TOMOGRAPHY

Positrons are emitted by certain short-lived radioactive isotopes, of which ^{15}O, ^{13}N, ^{11}C, and ^{18}F are the most useful clinically. Positron emission tomography (PET) is a computerized scanning procedure for building pictures of the brain based on the detection of emitted positrons. The isotopes have half-lives of less than 2 hours, during which time they must be

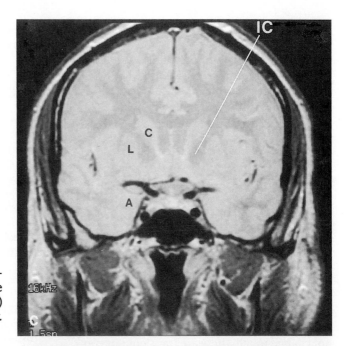

Figure 16-15 (*continued*)
(**C**) Proton density image. (**A**) Amygdaloid body. (**C**) Head of caudate nucleus. (**IC**) Internal capsule. (**L**) Lentiform nucleus. (*Courtesy of Dr. D. M. Pelz*)

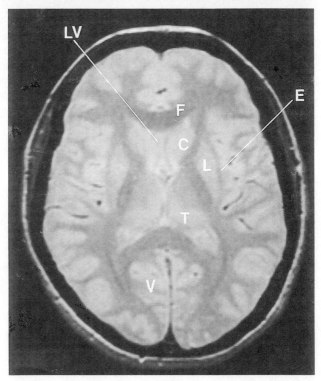

Figure 16-16. Horizontal "section" of proton density nuclear magnetic resonance image through the level of the insula. (**C**) Head of caudate nucleus. (**E**) External capsule. (**F**) Forceps frontalis. (**LV**) Lateral ventricle, (**L**) Lentiform nucleus. (**T**) Thalamus. (**V**) Visual cortex. (*Courtesy of Dr. D. M. Pelz*)

made, incorporated into suitable compounds, and administered to the patient. This technique can be used only in a hospital equipped with a cyclotron and a laboratory for radiochemical syntheses. Images produced by PET show the distribution of metabolic processes, such as the utilization of oxygen, the uptake of glucose, and the binding of drugs to receptors on the surfaces of cells. These pictures, some of which display the distributions of neurons that use or respond to particular synaptic transmitters, can be more informative to the physician than the purely anatomical images obtained with CT and NMRI. The anatomical resolution of a PET scan (5–10 mm) is inferior to that attainable with CT (2 mm) or NMRI (0.5–1.0 mm).

REGIONAL CEREBRAL BLOOD FLOW MONITORING

To monitor regional cerebral blood flow, a radioactive tracer such as ^{133}Xe that circulates in the blood is administered, and the intensities of the emitted gamma rays are measured at the surface of the patient's head. The intensity of the radiation at any point varies with the rate of vascular perfusion of the underlying tissues. The method is most valuable for examining different parts of the cerebral cortex. Although the flow of blood through the whole brain does not change much, there are transient but conspicuous local increases in flow associated with activity of the cortical neurons. Computerized synthesis of the measurements of radioactivity provides anatomical pictures of the functioning areas. Clinicians use this method to identify regions in which the circulation is inadequate. Regional cerebral blood flow can also be studied by PET, using [^{15}O]carbon dioxide as the tracer.

SUGGESTED READING

Danek A, Bauer M, Fries W: Tracing of neuronal connections in the human brain by magnetic resonance imaging in vivo. Eur J Neurosci 2: 112–115, 1990

Demeter S, Ringo JL, Doty RW: Morphometric analysis of the human corpus callosum and anterior commissure. Hum Neurobiol 6:219–226, 1988

Gazzaniga MS, Sperry RW: Language after section of the cerebral commissures. Brain 90:131–148, 1967

Kretschmann H-J: Localization of the corticospinal fibres in the internal capsule in man. J Anat 160:219–225, 1988

Montemurro DG, Bruni JE: The Human Brain in Dissection, 2nd ed. New York, Oxford University Press, 1988

Tredici G, Pizzini G, Bogliun G, Tagliabue M: The site of motor corticospinal fibres in man. A computerized tomographic study of restricted lesions. J Anat 134:199–208, 1982

Witelson SF, Goldsmith CH: The relationship of hand preference to anatomy of the corpus callosum in men. Brain Res 545:175–182, 1991

Seventeen

The Human Nervous System: An Anatomical Viewpoint, Sixth Edition, Murray L. Barr and John A. Kiernan. J.B. Lippincott Company, Philadelphia, © 1993.

Olfactory System

Important Facts

The olfactory receptor cells are unique in being neurons located in an epithelium and in being regularly replaced from a population of precursor cells.

The unmyelinated axons of the olfactory neurosensory cells constitute about 20 olfactory nerves on each side. These nerves pass through the cribriform plate of the ethmoid bone and end in the overlying olfactory bulb.

A fracture of the cribriform plate is likely to be followed by cerebrospinal fluid rhinorrhea.

The principal neurons of the olfactory bulb have axons that form the olfactory tract. This follows the ventral surface of the frontal lobe and ends in the olfactory trigone, anterior (rostral) to the anterior perforated substance.

Most of the axons of the olfactory tract follow the lateral olfactory stria and end in the lateral olfactory area, which comprises the cortex of the uncus, the limen insulae, the entorhinal area, and the corticomedial nuclei of the amygdaloid body.

Smaller numbers of olfactory tract fibers end in the anterior olfactory nucleus and in various nuclei in the region of the anterior perforated substance. Some of these cell groups give rise to fibers that pass centrifugally in the olfactory tracts and terminate in the olfactory bulbs of both sides, providing a mechanism for modulation of the input from the olfactory apparatus.

The regions in which fibers of the olfactory tract terminate are connected, directly and indirectly, with the limbic system, hypothalamus, and reticular formation of the brain stem. These connections provide for visceral and behavioral responses to different odors.

The olfactory system consists of the olfactory epithelium, olfactory nerves, olfactory bulbs, and olfactory tracts, together with functionally associated cerebral cortex and subcortical structures.

Lower vertebrates and many mammals rely heavily on the sense of smell. They are said to be macrosmatic; in the mammalian class, the dog is a familiar example. Humans are microsmatic, with smell being much less important than the other senses, especially sight and hearing. The study of comparative anatomy contributes much to an understanding of those parts of the brain involved in olfaction, which constitute the **rhinencephalon**. Thus, in macrosmatic animals, the rhinencephalic structures are large and prominent, whereas in humans, they are small by comparison with the remainder of the brain. Even in humans, however, olfaction is a significant sense that conjures up memories and arouses emotions. Smell also contributes to alimentary pleasures. Those who have lost their sense of smell complain of impairment of taste, stating that everything is bland and tastes alike, and they may be unaware of their inability to smell. Much of our enjoyment of taste is in fact an appreciation of aromas through the olfactory system. Some chemical stimuli, notably those from foods with "hot" flavors, excite general sensory fibers of the trigeminal nerve in the nose and mouth. The olfactory, gustatory, and general sensory responses to chemical stimuli in the nose may be integrated in the insula, where the primary cortical areas for the three systems are in proximity.

Olfactory Epithelium and Olfactory Nerves

The olfactory epithelium is derived from an ectodermal thickening, the **olfactory placode**, at the rostral end of the embryonic head. The cells of this placode give rise to the cells of the epithelium, the glial cells of the olfactory nerves, and probably some of the glial cells of the most superficial layer of the olfactory bulb. In the adult, the olfactory epithelium (Fig. 17-1) covers an area of 2.5 cm^2 in the roof of each nasal cavity and extends for a short distance on the lateral wall of the cavity and the nasal septum. The olfactory sensory cells are contained in a pseudostratified columnar epithelium, which is thicker than that lining the respiratory passages elsewhere. Olfactory glands (glands of Bowman) beneath the epithelium bathe the surface with a layer of

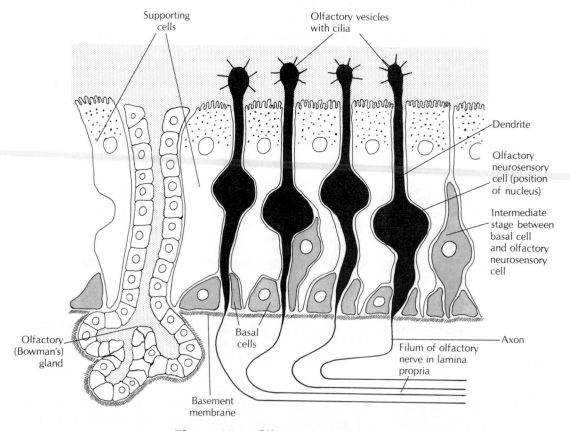

Figure 17-1. Olfactory epithelium.

mucous fluid, in which odoriferous substances are dissolved. The **olfactory neurosensory cells** (also known as primary olfactory neurons or simply as olfactory cells) are bipolar neurons that serve as sensory receptors as well as conductors of impulses. The major modification consists of specialization of the dendrite; this process extends to the surface of the epithelium, where it ends as an exposed bulbous enlargement known as an olfactory vesicle, bearing cilia that are exceptional in that they may be up to 100 μm long. A minority of human neurosensory cells have apical tufts of microvilli and resemble the sensory neurons of the vomeronasal organ, a chemical sense organ of lower mammals and submammalian vertebrates (see end of this chapter).

Unmyelinated axons of the olfactory cells are gathered into about 20 bundles on each side, which are the **olfactory nerves**. These enter the cranial cavity by passing through the foramina of the cribriform plate of the ethmoid bone and then enter the **olfactory bulb**. The axons form a superficial fibrous layer in the olfactory bulb, then continue more deeply, and terminate in specialized synaptic configurations, the **glomeruli**. The olfactory axon terminals release an excitatory neurotransmitter that has not yet been identified. (The dipeptide carnosine has been suspected.)

The few neurosensory cells shown in Figure 17-1 represent some 25 million such cells in each half of the olfactory epithelium. The olfactory cells are continuously being produced by mitosis and differentiation of some of the basal cells of the olfactory epithelium, and lost by desquamation. Observations in animals indicate that although some cells die without reaching maturity, olfactory neurons probably are lost by wear and tear rather than because of an innately short life span. In the human nose, each receptor neuron survives probably for about 2 months. Consequently there are always new axons growing along the olfactory nerves and into the olfactory bulbs.

The olfactory system is exquisitely sensitive to minute amounts of excitants in the air. Direct stimulation of the receptors, convergence of many neurosensory cells on the principal neurons of the olfactory bulb, and facilitation by neuronal circuits in the bulb are among the factors responsible for the low threshold. Smell is a chemical sense, as is taste. For a substance to be smelled, it must enter the nasal cavity as a gas or as an aerosol and then dissolve in the fluid that covers the olfactory epithelium. The secretory product of Bowman's glands contains glycoproteins that can bind odoriferous substances that are not otherwise soluble in water, for presentation to receptor molecules on the surfaces of the sensory cilia. That a large range of odors and aromas can be appreciated may be due in part to the existence of neurosensory cells with different chemical specificities.

The olfactory system adapts rather quickly to a continuous stimulus, so that the odor becomes unnoticed. A physiological mechanism that allows the receptors to recover is a cyclic alternation of mucosal blood flow in the left and right sides of the nose. At any instant, the side with the higher flow of blood presents greater resistance to the flow of air because of swelling of the mucosa. The nasal cavity with lower air flow consequently receives smaller amounts of the ambient odoriferous substances. Most older people have a reduced acuity of smell, probably caused by a progressive reduction in the population of neurosensory cells in the olfactory epithelium.

Olfactory Bulb, Tract, and Striae

The olfactory bulb is ventral to the orbital surface of the frontal lobe. It is connected by the olfactory tract to a central point of attachment in front of the anterior perforated substance (see Fig. 17-3).

The olfactory bulb has a characteristic cyto-architecture in animals that rely heavily on the sense of smell. There are five layers (Fig. 7-2):

1. Nerve fiber layer (olfactory axons) on the surface
2. Layer of glomeruli
3. External plexiform layer

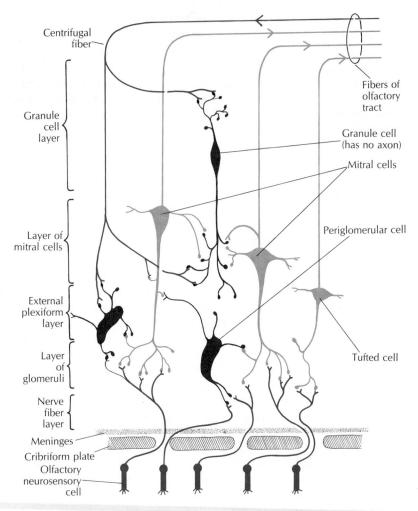

Figure 17-2. Neuronal circuitry of the olfactory bulb.

4. Layer of mitral cells
5. Granule cell layer, which in its deeper parts also contains the myelinated axons that comprise the medullary center of the olfactory bulb

The center contains nests of ependymal cells, which are vestiges of the extension of the lateral ventricle into the bulb in embryonic life. The layers are irregular and indistinct in the adult human olfactory bulb, although they are obvious in the fetal stages of development. The nerve fiber layer is of interest because it continuously admits newly growing axons from the olfactory nerves into the central nervous system. A mixture of neuroglial cells (astrocytes from the neural tube and cells of probable placodal

origin that ensheath the olfactory nerve axons) may account for this unique circumstance of axonal growth into the adult mammalian central nervous system.

The principal cells of the olfactory bulb are the **mitral cells**, whose cell bodies form a single layer. Their dendrites extend into the glomeruli, where they are contacted by axons of neurosensory cells, and into the external plexiform layer, where they receive input from centrifugal fibers of the olfactory tract. The axons of the mitral cells run in the olfactory tract and constitute the main output of the bulb. **Tufted cells** are similar to the mitral cells, but their somata lie in the external plexiform layer. Both these cell types have axonal terminals that are excitatory to the neurons with which they synapse, and the transmitter probably is glutamate.

The olfactory bulb contains interneurons of two types. **Periglomerular cells** have dendrites that receive synaptic input from olfactory neuroepithelial cells and from centrifugal fibers of the olfactory tract. There are also dendrodendritic synapses with the mitral cells. The axons of the periglomerular cells enter the external plexiform layer to contact the dendrites of mitral cells associated with other glomeruli, which they may excite or inhibit, depending on the postsynaptic receptors. Periglomerular cells secrete dopamine, γ-aminobutyric acid (GABA), and certain peptides. The most numerous interneurons are the GABAergic **granule cells**, which have no axons and are located in the deepest layer of the olfactory bulb. Their dendrites receive axodendritic contacts from mitral cells and from the centrifugal fibers. Other dendrites form dendrodendritic synapses with mitral cell dendrites. Some of these synaptic arrangements are shown in Figure 17-2. The complex circuitry of the olfactory bulb recalls that of the retina and indicates that, as is the case with visual images, sensory data are partially analyzed and edited before reaching the cerebral olfactory areas.

Three small groups of nerve cells make up the **anterior olfactory nucleus**. One is situated at the transition between the olfactory bulb and olfactory tract; the others are deep to the lateral and medial olfactory striae described in the next paragraph. Collateral branches of axons of mitral and tufted cells terminate in this nucleus. Fibers that originate in the anterior olfactory nucleus pass through the anterior commissure to the contralateral olfactory bulb. This is only one of the populations of centrifugal fibers that project to the olfactory bulb. Centrifugal fibers synapse principally with the dendrites of the interneurons.

Impulses from the olfactory bulb are conveyed to olfactory areas for subjective appreciation of odors and aromas. These areas also establish connections with other parts of the brain for emotional and visceral responses to olfactory stimuli. The olfactory tract expands into the **olfactory trigone** at the rostral margin of the anterior perforated substance. Most of the axons of the tract pass into the **lateral olfactory stria** (Fig. 17-3), which goes to the lateral olfactory area. Other axons of the olfactory tract, traditionally named the **intermediate olfactory stria**, leave the olfactory trigone to enter the anterior perforated substance, which is part of the intermediate olfactory area. The name "medial olfactory stria" is applied to a ridge that was once thought to carry olfactory fibers to the septal area. It is now known that no such connection exists.

Olfactory Areas of the Cerebral Hemisphere

RHINENCEPHALON

The "nose brain" was once thought to include a much larger proportion of the forebrain than that now known to be devoted to the sense of smell. The term is now restricted to those regions that receive afferent fibers from the olfactory bulbs. The **lateral olfactory area** receives afferents from the olfactory bulb through the lateral olfactory stria (Fig. 17-4; see also Fig. 17-3). The area consists of the paleocortex of the **uncus**, cortex of the **entorhinal area** (the anterior part of the parahippocampal gyrus) in the temporal lobe, and cortex in the region of the limen insulae (see Fig. 17-3). The uncus, entorhinal area, and limen insulae are collectively known as the **pyriform cortex** (or lobe) because the homologous area has a pear-shaped outline in macrosmatic animals. Part of the **amygdaloid body** (amygdala) also is included in the lateral olfactory area; the uncus is its landmark on the medial surface of the temporal lobe. The dorsomedial part of the amygdala consists of the **corticomedial group of nuclei**. It receives olfactory fibers, whereas the larger ventrolateral portion, a component of the limbic system, is considered in Chapter 18. The lateral olfactory area is the principal region for awareness of olfactory stimuli and is, therefore, the **primary olfactory area**.

The anterior perforated substance, situated between the olfactory trigone and the optic tract (see Fig. 17-3), derives its name from the penetration of many small blood vessels into the brain in this region. It contains several

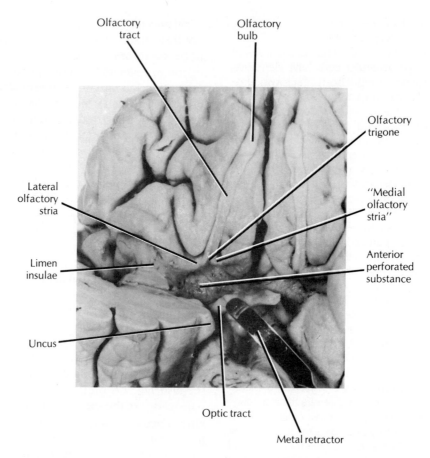

Figure 17-3. Some components of the olfactory system seen on the ventral surface of the brain. The right temporal pole has been cut away to give a clear view of the olfactory trigone, anterior perforated substance, and limen insulae. ($\times$ 1)

groups of neurons that receive fibers from the olfactory trigone and together constitute the **intermediate olfactory area**. The **diagonal band of Broca**, immediately in front of the optic tract and beneath the gray matter, connects the ventrolateral portion of the amygdala with the septal area and is, therefore, a fiber bundle of the limbic system. The adjacent **nucleus of the diagonal band**, however, is a major source of centrifugal fibers to the olfactory bulb, the other source being the contralateral anterior olfactory nucleus. The septal area, on the medial surface of the frontal lobe ventral to the rostrum of the corpus callosum, was formerly known as the "medial olfactory area", but it does not receive

any fibers of the olfactory tract. The septal area is a component of the limbic system of the brain and can no longer be assigned a role in olfaction as well.[1]

Olfactory stimuli induce visceral responses by modulating the activities of the autonomic nervous system. Examples are salivation when there are pleasing aromas from the prepara-

---

[1] The nomenclature of the olfactory areas of the human brain is decidedly unsatisfactory. Even though a "medial" olfactory area is no longer recognized in the mammalian brain, we have retained the old "intermediate olfactory area" for want of a better term. A detailed account of its components is beyond the scope of the present text.

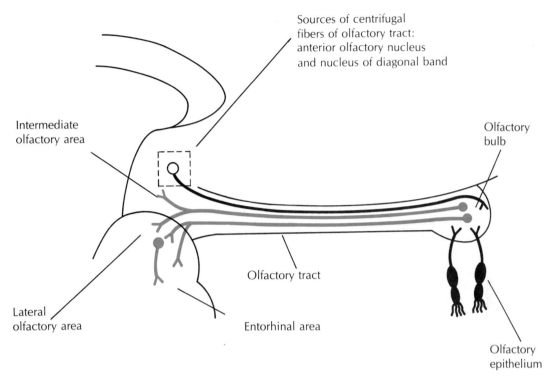

Sources of centrifugal
fibers of olfactory tract:
anterior olfactory nucleus
and nucleus of diagonal band

Intermediate
olfactory area

Olfactory
bulb

Lateral
olfactory area

Olfactory tract

Entorhinal area

Olfactory
epithelium

Figure 17-4. Components of the olfactory tract.

tion of food, and nausea or even vomiting evoked by an offensive stench. The olfactory system shares the entorhinal cortex with the limbic system, and the limbic system has extensive connections with the septal area and the hypothalamus. Most of the fibers that connect the septal area and hypothalamus with autonomic nuclei are in the **medial forebrain bundle**. This bundle, which contains fibers projecting rostrally as well as caudally, traverses the lateral part of the hypothalamus. Descending fibers from the hypothalamus proceed to autonomic nuclei in the brain stem and spinal cord. Other descending fibers of the medial forebrain bundle end in raphe reticular nuclei and in the solitary nucleus.[2]

---

[2] The autonomic nuclei are associated with cranial nerves III, VII. IX, and X (see Ch. 8) and with spinal nerves T1–L2 and S2–S4 (see Ch. 5). The organization and functions of the autonomic nervous system are discussed in Chapter 24.

Clinical Considerations

Fractures of the floor of the anterior fossa of the skull often involve the cribriform plate of the ethmoid bone, damaging the olfactory nerves and causing **anosmia**. The same injury may result in leakage of cerebrospinal fluid from the subarachnoid space into the nasal cavity, so that the fluid runs from the nose (cerebrospinal fluid rhinorrhea). This abnormal communication with the external environment is dangerous because it provides a route whereby bacteria may enter and attack the meninges and the brain.

A tumor, usually a meningioma, in the floor of the anterior cranial fossa may interfere with the sense of smell because of pressure on the olfactory bulb or olfactory tract. It is necessary to test each nostril separately because the olfactory loss is likely to be unilateral.

An irritating lesion that affects the lateral olfactory area may cause "uncinate fits," characterized by an imaginary disagreeable odor, by involuntary movements of the lips and tongue, and often by other features of disturbed function of the temporal lobe (see Ch. 18).

Terminal and Vomeronasal Nerves

Two small cranial nerves associated with the olfactory system were discovered after the 12 main cranial nerves were given their numbers. The terminal nerve (nervus terminalis) is present, although of microscopic size, in the adult human brain. Sometimes it is called cranial nerve zero because it is medial (and therefore perhaps rostral) to the olfactory nerves. The vomeronasal system appears only transiently in human embryonic development, but in most other terrestrial vertebrates, it has important functions in adult life.

Terminal Nerve

The fibers of the tiny **terminal nerve** lie along the medial side of the olfactory bulb and olfactory tract. Bipolar neuronal cell bodies are present in small ganglia along the course of the nerve. Their distal processes pass through the cribriform plate and are distributed to the nasal septum. In animals, the proximal processes have been traced experimentally to the septal and preoptic areas.

Vomeronasal System

In most mammals other than humans and in many submammalian vertebrates, there is a **vomeronasal organ**, which is a blind-ended tube lined by sensory epithelium in the ventral part of each side of the nasal septum. The receptor neurons are similar to those in the olfactory epithelium, but they have microvilli rather than cilia at their apical poles. Vascular connective tissue with sympathetic vasomotor innervation separates the vomeronasal epithelium from the rigid cartilaginous wall of the tube. The neurosensory cells of the epithelium give rise to axons that constitute the **vomeronasal nerve**. This passes through the cribriform plate alongside the olfactory nerves and ends in a part of the forebrain called the accessory olfactory bulb. In lower mammals and reptiles, the entrance to the vomeronasal organ is immediately dorsal to the nasopalatine foramen, through

which the oral and nasal cavities communicate behind the incisor teeth. Activity of the sympathetic nervous system causes constriction of the blood vessels of the vomeronasal organ, making the connective tissue layer thinner because it contains less blood. The resulting enlargement of the lumen sucks in tiny drops of liquid that have been either sniffed into the nostrils or deposited by the tongue into the nasopalatine foramen.

The vomeronasal system is for the detection of chemical messages from other members of the same species. The compounds (**pheromones**) used as sexual attractants and for marking territory may be secreted by specialized sweat or sebaceous glands, or they may be excreted in the urine. In animals with well-developed vomeronasal systems, such as snakes and rodents, transection of the vomeronasal nerves impairs reproductive behavior but does not interfere with feeding.

SUGGESTED READING

Doucette JR, Kiernan JA, Flumerfelt BA: The re-innervation of olfactory glomeruli following transection of primary olfactory axons in the central or peripheral nervous system. J Anat 137:1–19, 1983

Doucette R: PNS-CNS Transitional zone of the first cranial nerve. J Comp Neurol 312:451–466, 1991

Eccles R, Jawad MSM, Morris S: Olfactory and trigeminal thresholds and nasal resistance to airflow. Acta Otolaryngol (Stockh) 108:268–273, 1989

Graziadei PPC, Karlan MS, Monti Graziadei GA, Bernstein JJ: Neurogenesis of sensory neurons in the primate olfactory system after section of the fila olfactoria. Brain Res 186:289–300, 1980

Halpern M: The organization and function of the vomeronasal system. Annu Rev Neurosci 10: 325–362, 1987

Hinds JW, Hinds PL, McNelly NA: An autoradiographic study of the mouse olfactory epithelium: Evidence for long-lived receptors. Anat Rec 210:375–383, 1984

Mackay-Sim A, Kittel W: On the life span of olfactory receptor neurons. Eur J Neurosci 3:209–215, 1991

Morrison EE, Costanzo RM: Morphology of olfactory epithelium in humans and other vertebrates. Microsc Res and Technique 23:49–61, 1992

Scalia E, Winans SS: The differential projections of the olfactory bulb in mammals. J Comp Neurol 161:31–56, 1975

Shepherd GM, Greer CA: Olfactory bulb. In Shepherd GM (ed): The Synaptic Organization of the Brain, 3rd ed, pp 133–169. New York, Oxford University Press, 1990

Wysocki CJ, Meredith M: The vomeronasal system. In Finger TE, Silver WL (eds): Neurobiology of Taste and Smell, pp 125–150. New York, Wiley-Interscience, 1987

Eighteen

The Human Nervous System: An Anatomical Viewpoint, Sixth Edition, Murray L. Barr and John A. Kiernan. J.B. Lippincott Company, Philadelphia, © 1993.

Limbic System

Important Facts

The limbic system comprises the limbic lobe, hippocampal formation, amygdaloid body, and their connections.

Hippocampal afferents include fibers from the entorhinal area of the parahippocampal gyrus, cholinergic fibers from the septal area and substantia innominata, dopaminergic fibers from the ventral tegmental area, noradrenergic fibers from the locus coeruleus, and serotonergic fibers from the raphe nuclei.

Hippocampal efferent fibers enter the circuit of Papez, which includes the hippocampus, fornix, mamillary body, anterior thalamic nuclei, and cingulate and parahippocampal gyri. Association fibers connect the parahippocampal and cingulate gyri with extensive areas of the neocortex.

The acquisition of new memories requires the integrity of the circuit of Papez in at least one cerebral hemisphere.

The amygdala receives input from the temporal and prefrontal neocortex, and from the cholinergic and catecholaminergic nuclei that also project to the hippocampal formation.

The amygdala sends fibers to the mediodorsal thalamic nucleus and, through the stria terminalis and the diagonal band, to the hypothalamus and septal area.

The septal area projects through the stria medullaris thalami to the habenular nuclei, through the fornix to the hippocampus, and through the medial forebrain bundle to the hypothalamus.

The major descending pathways from the limbic system and hypothalamus are the mamillotegmental fasciculus, fasciculus retroflexus, medial forebrain bundle, and dorsal longitudinal fasciculus.

Stimulation of the amygdala results in fear, generalized irritability, and increased activity of the sympathetic nervous system. Destructive lesions in both temporal lobes can lead to docility, abnormal sexual behavior, and loss of short-term memory.

Anxiolytic drugs mimic the inhibitory action of γ-aminobutyric acid in the amygdala. Antidepressive drugs enhance the actions of noradrenaline and serotonin, and drugs used to treat schizophrenia antagonize the action of dopamine in the limbic system.

Certain components of the cerebral hemispheres and diencephalon are brought together under the heading of the limbic system of the brain. The notion of such a system developed from comparative neuroanatomical and neurophysiological investigations, but the terminology is rather vague and not used consistently by all authors. The **"limbic lobe"** was defined by Broca in 1878 as a ring of gray matter on the medial aspect of each hemisphere. The largest components of the lobe are the hippocampus, parahippocampal gyrus, and cingulate gyrus. The term **limbic system** is less precise. The broadest interpretation, which is probably the most useful, includes the aforementioned structures together with the dentate gyrus, amygdaloid body, septal area, hypothalamus (especially the mamillary bodies), and anterior and some other nuclei of the thalamus. Bundles of myelinated axons that interconnect these regions (fornix, mamillothalamic fasciculus, stria terminalis, and stria medullaris thalami) are also parts of the system.

The limbic system is concerned with visceral and motor responses involved in defense and reproduction and with processes involved in memory. The limbic system also has been called the **visceral brain** because of its substantial influence on visceral functions through the autonomic nervous system. Connections with the thalamus and cerebral cortex are used for the acquisition of new memories.

Hippocampal Formation

The hippocampal formation consists of the hippocampus, the dentate gyrus, and most of the parahippocampal gyrus.

INTRINSIC ORGANIZATION AND CIRCUITRY

The **hippocampus** develops in the fetal brain by a process of continuing expansion of the medial edge of the temporal lobe in such a way that the hippocampus comes to occupy the floor of the temporal horn of the lateral ventricle (Figs. 18-1 and 18-2; see also Fig. 16-10). In the mature brain, therefore, the parahippocampal gyrus on the external surface is continuous with the concealed hippocampus. The hippocampus is C-shaped in coronal section. Because its outline bears some resemblance to a ram's horn, the hippocampus is also called Ammon's horn (cornu ammonis), Ammon being the name of an Egyptian deity with a ram's head. The ventricular surface of the hippocampus is a thin layer of white matter called the **alveus**, which consists of fibers that enter and leave the hippocampal formation. These fibers form the **fimbria** of the hippocampus along its medial border and then

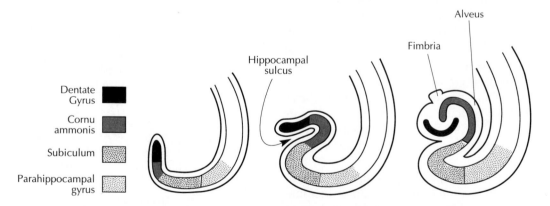

Figure 18-1. Stages in the embryonic development of the hippocampal formation at the margin of the pallium, showing how the external surfaces of the dentate gyrus and cornu ammonis become fused as a result of growth and folding.

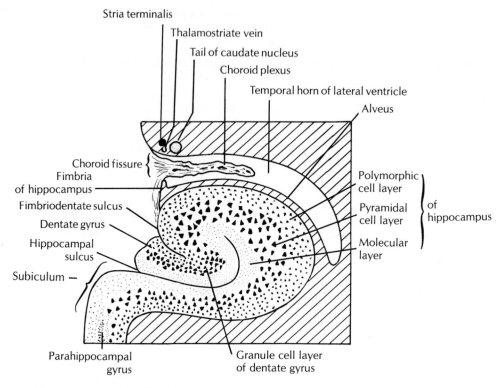

Figure 18-2. Simplified coronal section through the hippocampal formation (medial surface at the left).

continue as the crus of the fornix after the hippocampus terminates beneath the splenium of the corpus callosum (Fig. 18-3).

Continued growth of the cortical tissue composing the hippocampus is responsible for the **dentate gyrus** (see Figs. 18-1 and 18-2). This gyrus occupies the interval between the fimbria of the hippocampus and the parahippocampal gyrus; its surface is toothed or beaded, hence the name. The **hippocampal sulcus** is a groove between the parahippocampal and dentate gyri, and the **fimbriodentate sulcus** lies between the dentate gyrus and the fimbria. The **choroid fissure** in this location is dorsal to the fimbria of the hippocampus.

Although the parahippocampal gyrus is included in the limbic lobe as defined anatomically, most of its cortex is of the six-layered type or nearly so. In the region of the gyrus known as the **subiculum** (see Figs. 18-1 and

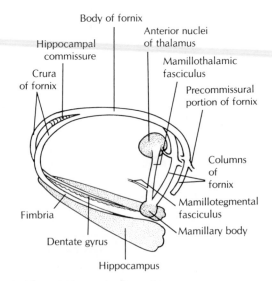

Figure 18-3. Fornix and related parts of the limbic system.

18-2), there is a transition between neocortex and the archicortex of the hippocampus.

The hippocampus, as seen in transverse (coronal) section has three areas or sectors: **CA1**, **CA2**, and **CA3**. (CA stands for cornu ammonis.) Area CA1 is adjacent to the subiculum, and CA3 is nearest to the dentate gyrus (Fig. 18-4). Three layers are recognized in the hippocampal cortex.

1. The **molecular layer** consists of interacting axons and dendrites. It is in the center of the hippocampal formation, surrounding the hippocampal sulcus. This synaptic layer is continuous with the molecular layers of the dentate gyrus and neocortex.
2. The prominent **pyramidal cell layer** (stratum pyramidale) is composed of large neurons, many of them pyramidal in shape, which are the principal cells of the hippocampus. The dendrites of these cells extend into the molecular layer, and their axons traverse the alveus and fimbria on their way to the fornix. Branches, called **Schaffer collaterals**, pass through the polymorphic and pyramidal cell layers to synapse in the molecular layer with the dendrites of other pyramidal neurons. The pyramidal cell layer is continuous with layer five (internal pyramidal) of the neocortex.

The large pyramidal cells in area CA1 are exceptionally sensitive to oxygen deprivation and die after only a few minutes without a supply of fresh arterial blood. Pathologists call area CA1 **Sommer's sector**. The hippocampal pyramidal cells are among the first to be affected in a variety of conditions that lead to loss of memory and intellectual functions, including Alzheimer's disease (see also Ch. 12).

3. The **polymorphic layer** (or stratum oriens)

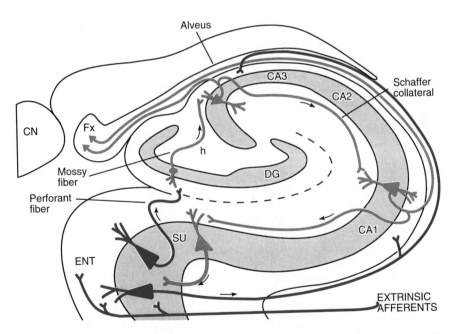

Figure 18-4. Some neuronal circuits within the hippocampal formation. The zone occupied by principal cells is shaded. Neurons of the hippocampus and dentate gyrus are *red* and afferent neurons (not all shown) are *blue*. Small black arrows indicate a loop of connections formed by mossy fibers and Schaffer collaterals. CA1, CA2, and CA3 = sectors of the hippocampus; CN = tail of caudate nucleus; DG = dentate gyrus; Ent = entorhinal cortex; Fx = fimbria; h = hilus of dentate gyrus; Su = subiculum.

is similar to the innermost layer (layer six) of the neocortex. This layer, which is beneath the alveus, contains axons, dendrites, and interneurons.

The dentate gyrus also has three layers. The cytoarchitecture differs from that of the hippocampus in that the pyramidal cell layer is replaced by a **granule cell layer** of small neurons, which are the principal cells of the region. The polymorphic layer of area CA3 of the hippocampus is continuous with the **hilus** of the dentate gyrus. The hilus contains interneurons and the axons of the granule cells. Efferent fibers from the dentate gyrus are known as **mossy fibers**. They travel in the hilus and the polymorphic layer, giving off many branches that synapse with the principal cells of areas CA3 and CA2 of the hippocampus.

The gross anatomy of the hippocampal formation varies greatly among different animals, reaching its greatest size (in absolute terms and as a proportion of the size of the cerebrum) in the human brain. The neuronal circuitry is essentially the same in all mammals, and it has been studied in great detail by neuroscientists attempting to identify cellular events involved in the rapid formation of new memories. One postulated mechanism is **long-term potentiation** (**LTP**), which is a property of certain synapses, including those of the Schaffer collaterals and the mossy fibers of the hippocampus. LTP is an increase in synaptic efficiency that follows a few seconds of high-frequency activity of a presynaptic terminal. "Increased synaptic efficiency" means a reduction in the number of afferent impulses and, therefore, of the amount of neurotransmitter needed to depolarize the postsynaptic cell. The effect, which lasts for several days, leads to increased activity of affected postsynaptic neurons. A suitable pattern of activity in axons afferent to the hippocampal formation may lead to LTP in certain connected pyramidal and granule cells. These will then continue to transmit impulses more frequently than before, even though the original external stimulus has ceased.

Knowledge of the extrinsic connections of the hippocampal formation is derived almost entirely from experimental observations on laboratory animals. The modern tracing methods based on axoplasmic transport have yielded particularly informative results. The organization of the major pathways is evidently the same in all mammalian species that have been studied, so it is reasonable to conclude that equivalent neural circuitry also exists in the human brain.

AFFERENT CONNECTIONS

The hippocampal formation has four main sources of afferent fibers: the cerebral neocortex, the septal area, the contralateral hippocampus, and various nuclei in the reticular formation of the brain stem.

The largest contingent of fibers is from the entorhinal area. There are two populations of such fibers (see Fig. 18-4). The axons of the **perforant path** from the entorhinal area pass through the subiculum and across the base of the hippocampal sulcus to end in the dentate gyrus. The **alvear path** traverses the subcortical white matter and the alveus to end in the hippocampus. Olfactory information comes from the entorhinal area, which is part of the lateral olfactory area. The entorhinal area receives association fibers from the neocortex of the temporal lobe, which in turn communicates with widespread areas of neocortex, including the sensory association areas. Through these connections, as well as through others that involve the parahippocampal cortex generally, the perforant and alvear paths keep the hippocampal formation informed of all forms of sensation and of the higher activities of the brain.

Afferent fibers for the hippocampal formation also are present in the fornix and fimbria. They come from the contralateral hippocampus and from the septal area and the closely related basal cholinergic nuclei of the substantia innominata (see Ch. 12). The commissural fibers cross the midline in the hippocampal commissure, which is described in the next section of this chapter. Some of the septal afferents travel in the longitudinal striae (of Lancisi), which are embedded in the indusium griseum, an attenuated layer of archicortex on the dorsal surface of the corpus callosum.

Other hippocampal afferent fibers in the fornix are from various thalamic nuclei (anterior group, medioventral), the posterior part of the hypothalamus, the ventral tegmental area (dopaminergic), the locus coeruleus (noradrenergic), the raphe nuclei (serotonergic), and the parabrachial nuclei.

EFFERENT CONNECTIONS

The connections through which the hippocampal formation receives information from the entorhinal area and neocortex are paralleled by connections that provide for spread of activity from the hippocampal formation to the same cortex, and there also are descending projections to the diencephalon and brain stem. The fornix contains numerous afferent fibers, as described in the previous section of this chapter, but it also is the largest efferent pathway of the hippocampal formation.

The **fornix**, which consists of more than 1 million fibers in humans, contains myelinated axons that originate in the hippocampus and in the subiculum of the parahippocampal gyrus. As described previously, the axons first traverse the alveus on the ventricular surface of the hippocampus on their way to the fimbria. The fimbria continues as the **crus** of the fornix, which begins at the posterior limit of the hippocampus beneath the splenium of the corpus callosum (see Fig. 18-3). The crus curves around the posterior end of the thalamus and joins its partner to form the **body** of the fornix. The small **hippocampal commissure** (or psalterium) at the convergence of the crura consists of decussating fibers that proceed from the hippocampus and entorhinal area of one hemisphere to the hippocampal formation of the opposite hemisphere. The body of the fornix separates into **columns**, each of which curves ventrally in front of the interventricular foramen. Here the anterior commissure lies immediately in front of the column of the fornix (see Fig. 16-7). Some fibers separate from the column just above the anterior commissure; these constitute the **precommissural** portion of the fornix and are distributed to the septal area, anterior part of the hypothalamus,

and substantia innominata. The **postcommissural** portion of the column of the fornix is much larger. It gives off some fibers that end in the lateral dorsal thalamic nucleus and then continues through the hypothalamus, where most of the fibers terminate in the mamillary body and the remainder end in the ventromedial nucleus of the hypothalamus.

The mamillary body projects to the anterior nuclei of the thalamus through the **mamillothalamic fasciculus** (bundle of Vicq d'Azyr), which is readily demonstrable by gross dissection (see Fig. 11-15). The anterior and lateral dorsal thalamic nuclei are in reciprocal communication with the cingulate gyrus through fibers that travel around the lateral side of the lateral ventricle. The cingulate gyrus also is in reciprocal communication with the parahippocampal gyrus through the cingulum, a prominent association bundle in the limbic lobe.

Amygdaloid Body (Amygdala)

The amygdaloid body consists of several groups of neurons situated between the anterior end of the temporal horn of the lateral ventricle and the ventral surface of the lentiform nucleus (Fig. 18-5). The dorsomedial portion of the amygdaloid body, known as the **corticomedial group** of nuclei, blends with the cortex of the uncus. It receives fibers from the olfactory bulb and is part of the lateral olfactory area. The larger ventrolateral portion consists of the **central** and **basolateral groups** of nuclei, which have no direct input from the olfactory bulb, although they connect with the dorsomedial portion and with the olfactory cortex of the entorhinal area. The central and basolateral groups are included in the limbic system on the basis of the results of experiments that involve stimulation and ablation in laboratory animals and clinical observations in humans. They are in communication with the septal area through the diagonal band of Broca.

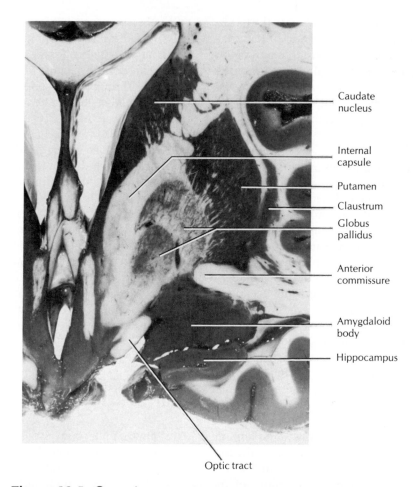

Caudate nucleus

Internal capsule

Putamen

Claustrum

Globus pallidus

Anterior commissure

Amygdaloid body

Hippocampus

Optic tract

Figure 18-5. Coronal section through the amygdaloid body and neighboring parts of the brain, stained by a method that differentiates gray matter (*dark*) and white matter (*light*). This is an enlargement of part of the section shown in Figure 12-3. (× 2)

The basolateral group has widespread connections, most of which are not in the form of well-defined fiber bundles. Using the shortest routes, there are reciprocal connections with cortex of the frontal and temporal lobes and the cingulate gyrus. Afferent fibers come from the thalamus (especially its mediodorsal nucleus), and the catecholamine nuclei and raphe nuclei of the reticular formation. Afferents also have been traced from the substantia nigra, the ventral tegmental area, and the substantia innominata. The most discrete efferent bundle of the amygdala is the **stria terminalis**. This slender fasciculus follows the curvature of the tail of the caudate nucleus, continuing along the groove between the caudate nucleus and thalamus in the floor of the central part of the lateral ventricle. Most of the constituent fibers terminate in the septal area and in the anterior part of the hypothalamus, but some enter the medial forebrain bundle and go to various parts of the brain stem, including the dorsal nucleus of the vagus nerve and the solitary nucleus.

The central nuclei of the amygdala receive afferent fibers from the corticomedial and basolateral nuclei and have projections similar to those of the basolateral group.

Circuits of the Limbic System

HIPPOCAMPAL CONNECTIONS

The largest components of the limbic system contain a ring of interconnected neurons.[1] It is named after Papez (the circuit of Papez), who postulated in 1937 that these parts of the brain

---

[1] The sequence of components of Papez' circuit is as follows: Entorhinal area of parahippocampal gyrus, *perforant and alvear paths*, hippocampus, *fimbria and fornix*, mamillary body, *mamillothalamic fasciculus*, anterior thalamic nuclei, *internal capsule*, cingulate gyrus, *cingulum*, entorhinal area. (Names of fiber tracts are italicized.)

"constitute a harmonious mechanism which may elaborate functions of central emotion, as well as participate in emotional expression." The input to the circuit of Papez (Fig. 18-6) is from the neocortex, thalamus, septal area, raphe nuclei, ventral tegmental area, and catecholamine nuclei of the reticular formation. The output is partly to the neocortex but also to regions of the reticular formation that indirectly influence the autonomic nervous system. The largest descending pathway is the **mamillotegmental fasciculus**, which consists of collateral branches of axons in the mamillothalamic fasciculus. These descending fibers terminate in the raphe nuclei of the retic-

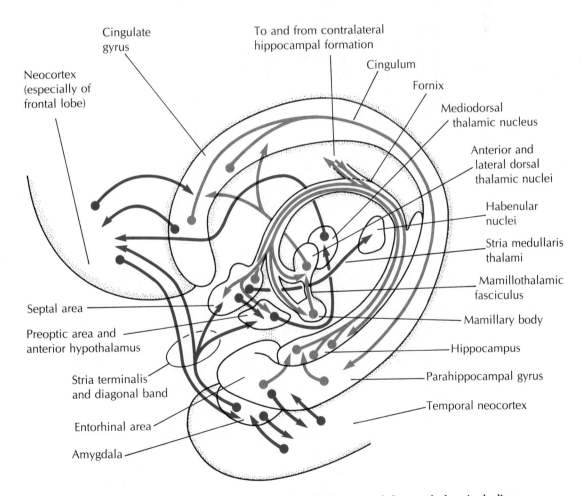

Figure 18-6. Limbic connections in the forebrain and diencephalon, including the circuit of Papez (*red*) and other connections (*blue*).

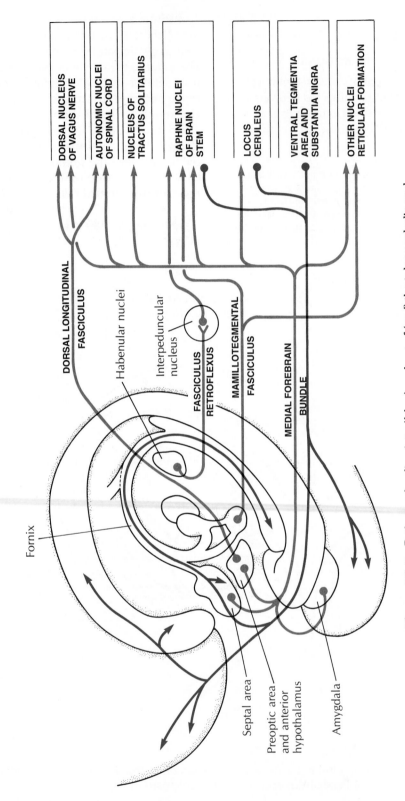

Figure 18-7. Pathways leading into (*blue*) and out of (*red*) the telencephalic and diencephalic components of the limbic system.

ular formation of the midbrain (Fig. 18-7). When thinking of the circuit of Papez, with its inputs and outputs, it is important to remember that there also are ring-like circuits of neurons within the hippocampal formation itself (see Fig. 18-4).

CONNECTIONS OF THE AMYGDALA

The principal connections of the basolateral and central groups of nuclei of the amygdala are shown in Figures 18-6 and 18-7. Here again, reciprocal connections with neocortical areas are prominent. A major descending output is through the **stria terminalis**, whose axons end in the septal area and in the anterior part of the hypothalamus. The septal area sends fibers in the stria medullaris thalami to the **habenular nuclei**. These project through the **fasciculus retroflexus** to the **interpeduncular nucleus**, and the pathway continues through the reticular formation to autonomic nuclei. The habenular nuclei also receive some afferent fibers from the globus pallidus, providing a pathway through which the neocortex and the corpus striatum can influence autonomic functions. Direct hypothalamospinal fibers in the **dorsal longitudinal fasciculus** comprise another pathway whereby the limbic system is able to influence preganglionic autonomic neurons.

The septal area and amygdala are also connected with lower levels of the neuraxis through the **medial forebrain bundle**. This bundle contains both ascending and descending fibers and interconnects the septal area, hypothalamus, and raphe nuclei of the reticular formation. Some of its fibers reach the dorsal nucleus of the vagus and the solitary nucleus.

Functional Considerations

Stimulation or ablation of parts of the limbic system in monkeys and other laboratory animals provides some indication of its function. Destructive lesions must be bilateral to affect behavior. Behavioral and emotional changes are chiefly associated with the amygdala,[2] and memory, with the hippocampal formation and the circuit of Papez.

Effects of Destructive Lesions in the Temporal Lobes

In the monkey, complete removal of both temporal lobes leads to the **Klüver-Bucy syndrome**, consisting of docility, loss of the ability to learn, excessive exploratory behavior, visual agnosia, and (in males) abnormal sexual activity. Smaller lesions have less bizarre consequences, with dysfunction attributable in part to the loss of individual parts of the limbic system.

Removal of the temporal poles, including the hippocampal formations and amygdaloid bodies, is followed by docility and lack of emotional responses such as fear or anger to situations that normally arouse those responses. Male animals exhibit increased sexual activity, and the sexual drive may be perverted, being directed toward either sex, a member of another species, or even inanimate objects. Lesions confined to the amygdaloid bodies produce similar changes in behavior, although sexual behavior is less affected. With lesions that also include the hippocampi, the animals can no longer be trained to perform tricks or carry out tasks, having evidently lost the ability to learn anything new.

When bilateral ablations extend to the posterior parts of the temporal lobes, the animal has all the abnormalities mentioned above and also is unable to recognize things that it sees. It compensates by exploring objects with its mouth. This visual agnosia, described by Klüver and Bucy in 1937 as "psychic blindness," is now attributed not to limbic dysfunction, but to loss of visual association cortex,

---

[2] In ordinary speech, the word emotion refers to subjective feelings that are difficult to define. Neuroscientists use the same word for activities of the brain evoked by incentives for survival. Emotional responses, therefore, include running away from a potential predator, drinking when thirsty, sweating when hot, and conduct in the presence of a potential mate or rival.

concerned with formed images, in the posterior part of the inferior temporal gyrus (see Chs. 16 and 20). The excessive oral exploration leads to excessive eating.

In humans, removal of both temporal lobes results in a voracious appetite, increased (sometimes perverse) sexual activity, and flattened affect. These abnormalities, together with visual agnosia, also can occur after head injury, in viral infections of the brain, and as complications of Alzheimer's disease.

Emotional Responses

Experimental and clinical studies have led to the view that the normal limbic system, especially the amygdala, is responsible for such strong affective reactions as fear and anger and the emotions associated with sexual behavior. Changes in visceral and somatic motor function accompany these emotions, and electrical stimulation of the amygdala has been shown to produce similar responses. These include increased heart rate, suppression of salivation, increased gastrointestinal movements, and pupillary dilation. Respiratory and facial movements also are changed, and there is generalized irritability, typically manifest as sudden movement (startle reaction) in response to a slight sensory stimulus. Electrical stimulation of the amygdala in humans induces feelings of fear or anger. These observations may indicate that activity in the amygdala gives rise to the autonomic and somatic accompaniments of fear and anxiety.

Anxiety States

Inappropriate activity of the amygdala may occur in abnormal mental states with excessive symptoms of anxiety. There may be severe episodes (panic attacks) of excessive activity of the sympathetic nervous system or a generalized condition dominated by subjective feelings of worry with motor manifestations such as muscle tension and jitteriness. Anxiolytic drugs (useful for the treatment of anxiety states) include the benzodiazepines, such as chlordiazepoxide, diazepam, and several others with names ending in -azepam. These drugs mimic the action of the inhibitory neurotransmitter γ-aminobutyric acid at a type of postsynaptic receptor that occurs abundantly on the surfaces of neurons in the amygdala and other parts of the limbic system.

Depression

In several psychiatric disorders, great suffering results from depression, which is an abnormal condition quite different from the sadness anyone can experience in appropriate circumstances. Drugs that relieve depression enhance the synaptic actions of noradrenaline and serotonin, either by inhibiting the enzyme monoamine oxidase (MAO inhibitors) or by blocking the reuptake of the amines into presynaptic terminals (tricyclic antidepressants such as amitriptyline and imipramine). Most of the neurons that use amines as transmitters are in the brain stem (see Ch. 9). Their greatly branched axons end in gray matter throughout the forebrain, including all parts of the limbic system.

Schizophrenia

Abnormalities of the limbic system also have been found in **schizophrenia**. In this disease, the processes of thinking are profoundly disturbed, with delusions, auditory hallucinations, inability to make associations between ideas, and reduced emotional expression. Careful anatomical measurements show that the hippocampal formation, amygdala, and parahippocampal gyrus are smaller than normal in the brains of schizophrenics, possibly as a result of abnormal growth of these parts of the brain. Drugs that alleviate the clinical features of schizophrenia antagonize the actions of dopamine, which is the principal neurotransmitter of the neurons in the ventral tegmental area that project to the limbic structures of the forebrain.

Memory

SHORT-TERM MEMORY

Impairment of memory is evident after bilateral temporal lobectomy or lesser degrees of injury that affect both hippocampal formations or their associated pathways. The hippocampal formation and its connections are necessary for the consolidation of new or short-term memories. The evidence for this function comes from many clinical observations, which generally agree with experimental results obtained in animals.

Bilateral damage to the hippocampus can occur when a head injury causes the temporal poles to strike the greater wings of the sphenoid bone, which form the anterior wall of the middle cranial fossa. Loss of hippocampal function also can occur if an arterial occlusion has caused an infarction in the hippocampal formation of one side and is followed at a later time by a similar infarction in the other hemisphere. More commonly the intact hippocampus is deprived of oxygen for only a short time, after which the patient suddenly becomes unaware of the events of the preceding few hours and is temporarily unable to form new memories. The condition is known as **transient global amnesia**. Cerebral anoxia from any cause can, as mentioned earlier, cause death of the principal neurons of Sommer's sector of the hippocampus bilaterally. Many patients resuscitated after cardiac arrest of more than a few minutes' duration are left with defective memory for this reason.

These bilateral hippocampal lesions all interrupt the major circuit of the limbic system. Interruptions of the same pathway outside the hippocampal formation, such as occurs when both mamillary bodies are involved in a lesion, also results in a memory defect. Amnesia also may follow bilateral lesions in the mediodorsal nuclei of the thalamus. The mediodorsal nuclei are connected with the prefrontal cortices, and these are involved in higher mental functions, although not specifically with memory. However, such lesions in the thalamus are likely to interrupt the mamillothalamic fibers as well. Bilateral surgical transection of the fornix, performed in attempts to limit the spread of epileptic discharges or in the course of removing tumors from the region of the third ventricle, has caused severe amnesia.

Animal experiments indicate that the cholinergic neurons of the substantia innominata in the basal forebrain also are involved in memory. The axons of these cells terminate in all parts of the cerebral cortex, including the hippocampal formation and parahippocampal gyrus. The inability to form new memories in **Alzheimer's disease** may be due in part to loss of these cholinergic projections (see Ch. 12), but degenerative changes in the entorhinal cortex and hippocampus also occur early in the course of this disorder, and in the late stages, there is extensive neocortical atrophy.

Patients with any of these lesions forget information obtained recently but retain the ability to recall old memories. When the hippocampi or the circuits of Papez are no longer functional, memories of earlier events are retained because these have already been established. There is amnesia for events that occurred more recently than the lesion because the mechanism for retention or consolidation of new or short-term memory is no longer operating. Most lesions in the diencephalon (thalamus and mamillary bodies) are due to metabolic disturbances caused by alcoholism. In the resulting syndrome (**Korsakoff's psychosis**), the patient inserts remembered events from the remote past into fluent but blatantly untrue stories, attempting to compensate for the absence of more recent memories.

LONG-TERM MEMORY

Some facts and experiences are forgotten soon (less than 1 hour) after they are learned, whereas others are incorporated into long-term memory. Localized lesions do not affect old memories, although these eventually are lost along with other mental capabilities when there is advanced dementia due to severe and widespread degeneration of the cerebral cortex. The traces representing permanent memory must be present throughout the cerebral cortex, and some investigators suspect that the corpus striatum, thalamus, and cerebellum also are involved. Synaptic long-term potentiation was mentioned earlier as a postulated mechanism for the storage of recent memories by the hippocampus. The formation of permanent memory traces may involve the synthesis of new proteins and the formation of new synapses.

The consolidation of recent memories may occur during sleep, when the serotonergic raphe neurons that project to the hippocampal formation are active. In deep sleep, when the electroencephalogram (EEG) recorded over the neocortex shows regular, synchronized rhythms, the hippocampal EEG (recorded with a needle electrode) is desynchronized. In the waking state, the neocortical record is desynchronized and the hippocampus generates a slow, regular rhythm.

SUGGESTED READING ──────────

Amaral DG, Insausti R, Cowan WM: Entorhinal cortex of the monkey: I, II and III. J Comp Neurol 264:326–408, 1987

Davis M: The role of the amygdala in fear and anxiety. Annu Rev Neurosci 15:333–375, 1992

Gaffan D, Gaffan EA: Amnesia in man following transection of the fornix: A review. Brain 114: 2611–2618, 1991

Kandel ER: Cellular mechanisms of learning and the biological basis of individuality. In Kandel ER, Schwartz JH, Jessell TM: Principles of Neural Science, 3rd ed, pp 1009–1031. New York, Elsevier, 1991

Kiernan JA: The limbic system. In Kiernan JA: Introduction to Human Neuroscience, pp 187–193. Philadelphia, JB Lippincott, 1987

Klüver H, Bucy PC: "Psychic blindness" and other symptoms following bilateral temporal lobec-tomy in rhesus monkeys. Am J Physiol 119: 352–353, 1937

Lilly R, Cummings JL, Benson F, Frankel M: The human Klüver-Bucy syndrome. Neurology 33: 1141–1145, 1983

Papez JW: A proposed mechanism for emotion. Arch Neurol Psychiatry 38:725–734, 1937

Penfield W, Milner B: Memory deficit produced by bilateral lesions in the hippocampal zone. Arch Neurol Psychiatry 79:475–497, 1958

Roberts GW: Schizophrenia: The cellular biology of a functional psychosis. Trends Neurosci 13: 207–211, 1990

Seitz R, Roland PE, Bohm C, Greitz T, Stone-Elander S: Motor learning in man: A positron emission tomographic study. NeuroReport 1:57–60, 1990

Shepherd GM: Neurobiology, 2nd ed. New York, Oxford University Press, 1988

Van Hoesen GW, Hyman BT, Damasio AR: Entorhinal cortex pathology in Alzheimer's disease. Hippocampus 1:1–8, 1991

von Cramon DY, Hebel N, Schuri U: A contribution to the anatomical basis of thalamic amnesia. Brain 108:993–1008, 1985

Review of the Major Systems

Nineteen

The Human Nervous System: An Anatomical Viewpoint, Sixth Edition, Murray L. Barr and John A. Kiernan. J.B. Lippincott Company, Philadelphia, © 1993.

General Sensory Systems

Important Facts

Neuronal signals from skin and deeper structures are segregated in the spinal cord. Transmission to the thalamus and cerebral cortex may occur through the spinothalamic tract or through the dorsal funiculi and medial lemniscus.

For pain, temperature, and the less discriminative aspects of touch, neurons in the dorsal horn have axons that cross the midline in the spinal cord and ascend as the spinothalamic tract, which is laterally situated in the spinal cord and brain stem.

For discriminative touch and conscious proprioception (except from the lower limb), the axons of primary sensory neurons ascend ipsilaterally in the dorsal funiculus and end in the gracile or cuneate nucleus. Fibers arising in these nuclei cross in the medulla and ascend in the medial lemniscus, which is near the midline in the medulla and shifts to a lateral location in the midbrain.

For conscious proprioception from the lower limb, there is a different pathway, involving the dorsal spinocerebellar tract and nucleus Z.

Both the spinothalamic tract and the medial lemniscus end in the VPl nucleus of the thalamus. This thalamic nucleus projects to the primary somesthetic cortex of the postcentral gyrus, where the contralateral half of the body is represented as an upside-down homunculus.

The somesthetic pathways for the head include the trigeminal sensory nuclei and their projections to the contralateral VPm thalamic nucleus. Primary afferent fibers for touch end in the pontine trigeminal nucleus. Pain and temperature fibers descend in the spinal trigeminal tract before ending in the caudal part of its nucleus.

Lesions in the spinal cord and brain stem can affect the somesthetic pathways separately, causing dissociated sensory loss.

The main pathways are supplemented by others, especially for pain, with relays in the reticular formation and thalamic nuclei other than the VPl or VPm.

The cerebral cortex is necessary for localizing the source of a painful stimulus and recognizing objects by touch.

Descending projections influence transmission in the ascending somatosensory pathways. These include the raphespinal tract, which inhibits the perception of stimuli that would be painful.

This chapter deals with the pathways from the general sensory receptors to the thalamus and thence to the cerebral cortex, where the sensations are appreciated subjectively. With an understanding of the anatomy of these pathways, an appraisal of sensory deficits provides information concerning the location of a lesion in the central nervous system.

Sensory fibers that enter the spinal cord in dorsal roots of spinal nerves segregate in such a way that there are two main general sensory systems. The first of these, regarded as the more primitive, includes one or more synaptic relays in the dorsal gray horn. Spinal neurons give rise to axons that cross the midline and ascend in the ventrolateral white matter to the thalamus. This is the **spinothalamic system** for pain and temperature. It also is the main pathway for the less discriminative form of touch usually referred to as light touch and probably also for some modified forms of touch, notably firm pressure.

The second system includes large numbers of primary afferent fibers that turn rostrally in the ipsilateral dorsal funiculus of the spinal cord and do not end until they reach the medulla. Smaller numbers of fibers in the dorsal funiculus, together with fibers in the dorsal part of the lateral funiculus, arise ipsilaterally from neurons in the dorsal horn. All of these fibers terminate in certain nuclei in the lower medulla, from which axons cross the midline and then ascend as the medial lemniscus to the thalamus. Hence this second pathway is called the **medial lemniscus system**. It is concerned primarily with discriminative aspects of sensation, especially the awareness of position and movement of parts of the body and the tactile recognition of shapes and textures and of changes in the positions of stimuli that move across the surface of the skin. The medial lemniscus system is often called the **posterior column system**, especially in clinical usage, because it includes the dorsal funiculi ("posterior columns") of the spinal cord.

The **spinoreticulothalamic pathway**, which includes relays in the reticular formation of the brainstem, conducts some of the ascending signals generated by cutaneous sen-

sation. It is, therefore, closely related functionally to the spinothalamic system. The association is seen especially in central conduction for pain. In fact, the spinothalamic pathway and the less direct spinoreticulothalamic pathway, with their projections to the cerebral cortex, may be combined under the term **ventrolateral (or anterolateral) system**. The comparable term **dorsomedial system** is then used for the medial lemniscus system. The various names for the pathways for general sensation are summarized in Table 19-1. Unfortunately all the terms are in fairly widespread use by anatomists, physiologists, and clinicians. The **trigeminothalamic** pathways serve the same functions as the spinothalamic and medial lemniscus systems, but for the head. They also were mentioned in Chapter 8 in connection with the central connections of the trigeminal, facial, glossopharyngeal, and vagus nerves.

The general sensory pathways are said to consist of primary, secondary, and tertiary neurons, with cell bodies in sensory ganglia, the spinal cord or brain stem, and the thalamus, respectively. The concept of a simple relay of three neurons is not accurate, however, because interneurons commonly are interposed between the major neurons of a pathway. In addition, the activity of the secondary neurons is influenced by descending fibers that originate in the cerebral cortex and the brain stem.

Spinothalamic System

The spinothalamic (or ventrolateral) system also is known as the "pathway for pain and temperature" because these modalities of sensation are transmitted to the brain in the spinothalamic tract. It also is concerned with tactile sensation, as has already been noted.

Receptors

The **receptors for pain (nociceptors)** consist of unencapsulated endings of peripheral nerve fibers; these fibers are the smaller components of group A, with thin myelin sheaths

TABLE 19-1 ▆▆▆▆▆▆▆▆▆▆▆▆▆▆▆▆
Names Used for the Somatic Sensory Pathways Concerned
with Parts of the Body Below the Head

Medial Lemniscus System	*Spinothalamic System*
Dorsomedial system	Ventrolateral system
Posterior column system	Anterolateral system
Dorsal column system	
Includes:	*Includes:*
Dorsal (posterior) funiculi	Dorsal horn of spinal gray matter
Dorsal (posterior) columns	Ventral white ''commissure'' of
Each consisting of:	cord
Gracile fasciculus	Spinothalamic tract (also spinoretic-
Cuneate fasciculus	ular tracts)
Gracile and cuneate nuclei	Spinal lemniscus (= spinothalamic
Nucleus Z	fibers in the brain stem)
Medial lemniscus	Reticulothalamic fibers
Ventral posterior nucleus of	Ventral posterior nucleus of
thalamus	thalamus (also other thalamic
Internal capsule	nuclei: intralaminar: posterior)
Primary somatosensory cortex	Internal capsule
	Primary somatosensory cortex

(group Aδ), and unmyelinated group C fibers. These simple endings are not exclusively concerned with pain, but they appear to be the only receptors that respond to painful stimuli. Pain may be felt as two waves separated by an interval of a few tenths of a second. The first wave is sharp and localized, with conduction by group A fibers. The second wave, which is rather diffuse and still more disagreeable, depends on group C fibers, with a slow conduction speed. The two waves are most easily noticed in the feet (as when treading on something sharp) because of the greater lengths of the conducting axons in the nerves of the lower limb.

The mechanism of perception of pain is inseparable from that of the initiation of **inflammation**, which is the response of living tissue to any kind of injury. Injured cells release several substances known as mediators, which act on venules and nerve endings. The venules dilate, causing redness of the affected area, and become permeable to blood plasma, which leaks out to cause swelling of the tissue. Simultaneous stimulation of the nociceptive endings results in perception of pain. Nerve impulses, however, do not pass solely to the central nervous system: they also are propagated antidromically along other peripheral branches of the afferent fiber. In the case of cutaneous group C fibers, the impulses cause a peptide neurotransmitter known as substance P to be released into the interstitial tissues of the dermis. This results in degranulation of mast cells (which thereby release more mediators), dilation of arterioles, and, sometimes, edema in the area surrounding the injury. In the skin, the total result constitutes the **triple response** (of Lewis): a red mark and a wheal, surrounded by a flare of neurogenic arteriolar vasodilation. A neurally mediated phenomenon such as this, which does not involve any synapses, is called an **axon reflex**. Other examples are known experimentally, but the axon reflex just described is the only one of clinical interest.

The question of identity of **receptors for temperature** has not yet been resolved. They are probably morphologically nondescript free nerve endings, similar to those for pain. The axons are of similar caliber to those that conduct impulses for pain. The receptors for light touch are unencapsulated nerve endings, Merkel and peritrichial endings, and Meissner's corpuscles. Ruffini endings and pacinian corpuscles respond to firm pressure on the skin, a modified form of touch. Conduction for light touch and pressure in peripheral nerves is by myelinated group A fibers of medium diameter. (Descriptions of the specialized sensory nerve endings can be read in Ch. 3.)

Ascending Central Pathway

SYNAPSES AND INTERNEURONS IN THE DORSAL HORN

Cell bodies of small and intermediate size in the dorsal root ganglia have central processes that constitute the lateral divisions of the dorsal rootlets. These fibers conduct impulses from pain and temperature receptors (Fig. 19-1). Afferents for light touch and pressure enter the dorsal gray horn through the medial division of the dorsal rootlets. The pain and temperature fibers enter the **dorsolateral tract** (of Lissauer) of the spinal cord, in which ascending and descending branches travel, in most instances, for lengths that correspond to one segment. A few of the axons travel as far as four segments rostral or caudal to their levels of entry.

The terminals and the collateral branches of the fibers in the dorsolateral tract enter the dorsal horn, where they branch profusely (see Fig. 5-6). Lamina II (the **substantia gelatinosa** of Rolando), near the tip of the dorsal horn, is an important region in which patterns of incoming sensory impulses are modified. The dendrites of the gelatinosa cells are contacted not only by primary afferent axons, but also by reticulospinal fibers, notably those derived from the raphe nuclei of the medulla. (Descending pathways that modulate transmission in the ascending sensory pathways are discussed later in this chapter.) The axons of the cells in the substantia gelatinosa ascend and descend in the dorsolateral tract and in adjacent white matter, mostly for about the

length of one segment. Throughout its length, the axon of a gelatinosa cell gives off branches that end by synapsing with the dendrites of **tract cells**, whose axons constitute the spinothalamic tract. The dendrites of these tract cells are contacted by primary afferent fibers for pain and temperature, by axons of the gelatinosa cells, and by primary afferents for light touch and pressure. These connections are shown diagrammatically in Figure 5-7.

In summary, the tract cells receive synaptic input from primary afferent fibers and from interneurons of the dorsal horn. The most prominent of the latter group of neurons are those of the substantia gelatinosa, which are, in their turn, contacted by primary afferents and descending reticulospinal fibers.

SPINOTHALAMIC TRACT

Most of the tract cells have their cell bodies in the **nucleus proprius** (laminae IV and V-VI). The large neurons at the tip of the dorsal horn (lamina I) also contribute a small proportion of the spinothalamic fibers. The axons of the tract cells cross the midline in the ventral white commissure. Continuing through the ventral horn of gray matter, the fibers ascend in the **spinothalamic tract**, situated in the ventral part of the lateral funiculus and in the adjoining region of the ventral funiculus (see Fig. 5-9). Proceeding rostrally, fibers are continually being added to the internal aspect of the tract. At upper cervical levels, therefore, fibers from sacral segments are most superficial, followed by fibers from lumbar and thoracic segments. The fibers from cervical segments are closest to the gray matter.

The ascending tracts of the spinal cord continue into the medulla without appreciable change of position initially. At the level of the inferior olivary nucleus, the spinothalamic tract traverses the lateral medullary zone (Monakow's area) between the inferior olivary nucleus and the spinal trigeminal nucleus,

Figure 19-1. Spinothalamic system for pain, temperature, light touch, and pressure. The pathway from the lower limb is shown in *red* and from the upper limb, in *blue.*

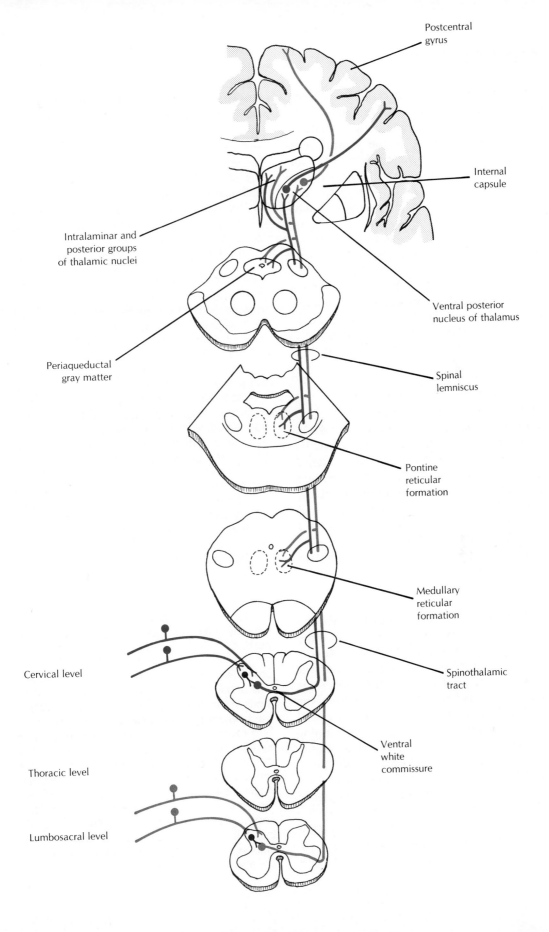

Postcentral gyrus

Internal capsule

Ventral posterior nucleus of thalamus

Intralaminar and posterior groups of thalamic nuclei

Periaqueductal gray matter

Spinal lemniscus

Pontine reticular formation

Medullary reticular formation

Cervical level

Spinothalamic tract

Ventral white commissure

Thoracic level

Lumbosacral level

where it is close to the lateral surface of the medulla. At this level and throughout the remainder of the brain stem, the spinothalamic fibers constitute most of the **spinal lemniscus**, which also includes fibers of the spinotectal (spinomesencephalic) tract destined for the superior colliculus. The spinal lemniscus continues through the ventrolateral region of the dorsal pons. In the midbrain it is close to the surface of the tegmentum, running along the lateral edge of the medial lemniscus. In their passage through the brain stem, the spinothalamic fibers give off collateral branches that terminate in the medullary and pontine reticular formation and in the periaqueductal gray matter of the midbrain. There are also spinoreticular fibers that go no further rostrally than the pons.

THALAMUS AND CEREBRAL CORTEX

Most of the spinothalamic fibers end in the **ventral posterior nucleus of the thalamus**. This nucleus consists of two parts: the ventral posterolateral division (**VPl**), in which spinothalamic fibers and the medial lemniscus terminate, and the ventral posteromedial division (**VPm**), which receives trigeminothalamic fibers. The somatotopic organization is such that the contralateral lower limb is represented dorsolaterally and the contralateral upper limb is represented ventromedially in the VPl; the opposite side of the head is represented in the VPm.

The cortical projection consists of neurons in the ventral posterior nucleus whose axons traverse the **posterior limb of the internal capsule** and corona radiata to reach the **somesthetic area** in the parietal lobe. The contralateral half of the body, exclusive of the head, is represented as inverted in the dorsal two-thirds of the somesthetic area. Beginning ventrally, the sequence is, therefore, hand, arm, trunk, and thigh, followed by representation of the remainder of the lower limb and the perineum on the medial surface of the hemisphere. The cortical area for the hand is disproportionately large, providing for maximal sensory discrimination. The somatotopic arrangement at various levels of the sensory pathways forms the basis for recognition of the site of stimulation.

Experimental tracing in monkeys reveals that the sites of origin and termination of the spinothalamic tract and the positions of the fibers in the spinal cord are more varied than the classic projections described earlier. Substantial numbers of fibers have been demonstrated in the dorsal part of the lateral funiculus, and there are some axons (mainly from regions of gray matter other than the dorsal horn) that ascend ipsilaterally. The existence of such fibers may account for the eventual recovery of sensibility to pain that follows transection of the ventrolateral pathways.

Some fibers of the spinal lemniscus end in thalamic nuclei other than the VPl, notably those of the posterior and intralaminar groups and the mediodorsal nucleus. The posterior group projects to the insula and to adjacent parietal cortex, including that of the second general sensory area, which is at the lower end of the postcentral gyrus. The intralaminar nuclei project diffusely to the frontal and parietal lobes of the cerebral cortex and to the striatum. They may be involved in the maintenance of a conscious, alert state (see Ch. 9). The mediodorsal nucleus is connected with the frontal lobes, especially their medial and orbital surfaces.

Two populations of spinothalamic fibers are recognized on the basis of experiments with various mammals and from human clinical studies. The **neospinothalamic tract**, which is prominent in primates, arises from lamina I and laminae IV-VI (nucleus proprius) in the dorsal horn. Its fibers do not have collateral branches in the reticular formation, but there are branches to the periaqueductal gray matter. The neospinothalamic fibers end in the VPl nucleus of the thalamus. The **paleospinothalamic tract**, which predominates in lower mammals, has more extensive spinal origins (including laminae VII, VIII, and X, which are not in the dorsal horn). Its axons send branches to the reticular formation and end in the intralaminar nuclei (especially the central lateral nucleus), the posterior group of nuclei, and the dorsomedial nucleus. The rather diffusely projecting paleospinothalamic tract, together with spinoreticular and reticulothalamic projections, are involved in the recognition of somatic sensory stimuli and in involuntary motor responses such as changes in facial expression. The topographically organized neospinothalamic pathway is necessary for localization of the stimuli.

Pain

Pain is a common complaint, and it is, therefore, necessary to become conversant with the anatomy, physiology, and pharmacology of this symptom. The mechanisms whereby peripheral nerve endings respond to injurious stimuli have already been reviewed. The central pathways concerned with pain are now discussed in further detail.

SPINAL MECHANISMS

Perception of pain is thought to be modified by neural mechanisms in the dorsal horn. In addition to the influence of reticulospinal and corticospinal fibers, to be discussed later, the transmission of impulses for pain to the brain is altered by dorsal root afferents for other sensory modalities. Afferent fibers of larger diameter, especially those for touch and deep pressure, have branches that synapse with the dendrites of the spinothalamic tract cells,

alongside the axons of the gelatinosa cells. Trains of impulses coming through the larger fibers are thought to cause synaptic inhibition of the tract cells concerned with nociception. This postulated mechanism, known as the **gate control theory** of pain (Fig. 19-2), enables the neurons in the spinal cord to determine, on the basis of all incoming sensory stimuli, whether a particular event should be reported to the brain as being painful. The gate mechanism probably operates when pain arising in deep structures such as muscles and joints is relieved by stimulating sensory endings in the overlying skin (for example, by rubbing or by applying warmth or a mild irritant, such as a liniment).

The simplest defensive reflex initiated by pain is the **flexor reflex**, which involves at least two synapses in the spinal cord (see Fig. 5-12) and causes withdrawal of a limb from the source of a sudden painful stimulus. In quadrupeds, there also is a **crossed extensor reflex** in which the withdrawal is assisted by extension of the contralateral limb. In normal humans, the crossed extensor reflex is largely suppressed as a result of activity in descending tracts of the spinal cord, but both it and the

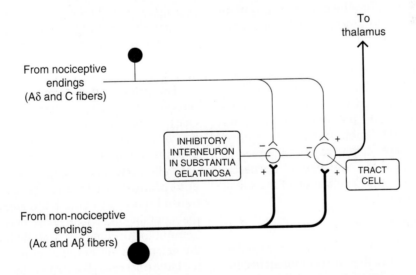

Figure 19-2. Simple illustration of the gate control theory of pain. Non-nociceptive sensory fibers stimulate the inhibitory interneurons, whereas nociceptive afferents inhibit them. An increase in non-nociceptive input will reduce the rate of firing of the spinothalamic tract neurons.

flexor reflex are conspicuous and, because of a lowered threshold, troublesome in paraplegic patients.

ASCENDING PATHWAYS

Impulses that signal pain are transmitted rostrally in the spinothalamic and spinoreticular tracts (Fig. 19-3). Additional fibers with this function appear to be present in the dorsolateral funiculus. Tractotomy or surgical transection of the ventrolateral region of the spinal cord, which contains the spinothalamic and spinoreticular tracts, results in almost complete loss of the ability to experience pain on the opposite side of the body below the level of the lesion. The sensibility usually returns gradually over several weeks. The recovery probably is a consequence of synaptic reorganization and increased usage of intact alternative pathways. A surgical cut in the midline of the spinal cord (commissural myelotomy) causes prolonged analgesia in the segments affected by the lesion.

Pain is still felt, although poorly localized, after destruction of an area of cortex that includes the primary somesthetic area. This clinical observation led to an early assumption that painful sensations reached the level of consciousness within the thalamus. It is more likely that spinothalamic and reticulothalamic afferents to the intralaminar and mediodorsal thalamic nuclei are responsible for the persistence of sensibility to pain after destruction of the primary somesthetic area. These thalamic nuclei are connected with most of the neocortex, including the prefrontal areas, and indirectly with the limbic system. The ventral posterior nucleus of the thalamus and the primary somesthetic area are undoubtedly necessary for the accurate localization of the site of the painful stimulus.

DESCENDING PATHWAYS

Descending pathways modify the activity of all ascending systems; they are prominent in controlling the conscious and reflex responses to noxious stimuli. Both the subjective awareness of pain and the occurrence of defensive reflexes may be suppressed under circumstances of intense emotional stress. This effect probably is mediated by **corticospinal fibers** that originate in the parietal lobe and terminate in the dorsal horn.

Control of a subtler kind is exerted by certain reticulospinal pathways. The best understood of these is the **raphespinal tract**, which arises from neurons in the raphe nuclei of the medullary reticular formation, mainly those of the nucleus raphes magnus. The unmyelinated axons of this tract traverse the dorsal part of the lateral funiculus of the spinal cord and are believed to use serotonin as a neurotransmitter. The highest density of serotonin-containing synaptic terminals (observable by histochemical methods) is seen in the substantia gelatinosa (lamina II). The nucleus raphes magnus is itself influenced by descending fibers from the periaqueductal gray matter of the midbrain. Electrical stimulation of the nucleus raphes magnus or the periaqueductal gray matter causes profound analgesia. This is reversed either by transection of the dorsolateral funiculus or by administration of naloxone or similar drugs that antagonize the actions of morphine and related alkaloids of opium. Furthermore, the analgesic action of opiates is suppressed by transection of the dorsolateral funiculus.

The actions of the opiates and their antagonists are attributable to selective binding molecules (**opiate receptors**) on the surfaces of neurons in several parts of the brain. The normal function of the opiate receptor is to bind naturally occurring pentapeptides, known as **enkephalins**. These serve either as neurotransmitters or as neuromodulators. Neurons that contain enkephalins have been identified immunohistochemically and include some of the gelatinosa cells of lamina II and some of the large tract cells (Waldeyer cells) of lamina I.

Figure 19-3. Ascending pathways for the appreciation of pain. The spinothalamic system is shown in *red* and the spinoreticular and reticulothalamocortical pathways are shown in *blue*.

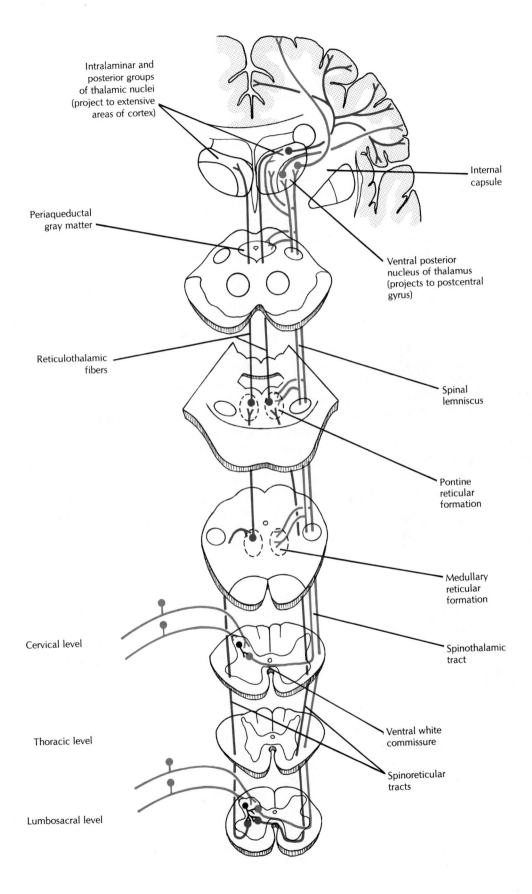

Intralaminar and posterior groups of thalamic nuclei (project to extensive areas of cortex)

Internal capsule

Periaqueductal gray matter

Ventral posterior nucleus of thalamus (projects to postcentral gyrus)

Reticulothalamic fibers

Spinal lemniscus

Pontine reticular formation

Medullary reticular formation

Cervical level

Spinothalamic tract

Thoracic level

Ventral white commissure

Spinoreticular tracts

Lumbosacral level

Enkephalins also occur in the periaqueductal gray matter and the nucleus raphes magnus. These same regions also have high concentrations of opiate receptors. The analgesic action of morphine and related opiates can be attributed to simulation of the effects of endogenously secreted enkephalins on neurons that bear opiate receptors on their surfaces. The major anatomical sites of action are evidently the periaqueductal gray matter, nucleus raphes magnus, and dorsal horn. Many other parts of the central nervous system contain enkephalins, mainly in local circuit neurons. These regions may be the sites of other pharmacological actions of the opiates, such as nausea, suppression of coughing, euphoria, and the development of addiction.

Information about the descending pathways that modulate pain has led not only to increased understanding of the sites of action of the opium alkaloids, but also to a technique for the relief of chronic pain. An electrode stereotaxically implanted into the periaqueductal gray matter enables a patient to relieve pain instantly by switching on an electrical stimulator. The analgesia often lasts for several hours after cessation of stimulation.

Medial Lemniscus System

The set of sensory pathways known as the medial lemniscus system is for proprioception, fine touch, and (although not exclusively) vibration. In contrast to the spinothalamic system, in which ascending fibers cross the midline at spinal segmental levels, the pathways that constitute the medial lemniscus system ascend ipsilaterally in the cord and cross the midline in the caudal half of the medulla.

Receptors

The medial lemniscus system is especially important in humans because of the discriminative quality of the sensations as perceived subjectively and their value in the learning process. The characteristics of fine or discriminative touch are that the subject can recognize the location of the stimulated points with precision and is aware that two points are touched simultaneously even though they are close together (two-point discrimination). These qualities accentuate recognition of textures and of moving patterns of tactile stimuli. Of the tactile receptors, Meissner's corpuscles, which have been found only in primates, have a special significance in discriminative touch. They are most abundant in the ridged, hairless skin of the palmar surface of the hands; preferential sites for Meissner's corpuscles correspond to those areas in which two-point discrimination is best developed. Several additional touch receptors, noted in connection with the spinothalamic system, also produce sensations through the medial lemniscus system. Pacinian corpuscles are the principal receptors for the sense of vibration, although this modality, once believed to be served exclusively by the dorsal funiculi, is now known to be carried also in the lateral white matter of the spinal cord.

With respect to proprioception, the dorsomedial pathway provides information concerning the precise positions of parts of the body; the shape, size, and weight of an object held in the hand; and the range and direction of movement. The proprioceptors are neuromuscular spindles, neurotendinous spindles, and endings in and near to the capsules and ligaments of joints. Conscious proprioception (kinesthesia) was once thought to depend mainly on receptors in joints, but it is now realized that the input from muscle spindles probably is of greater significance than the input from other proprioceptors.

Ascending Central Pathways

The pathways for discriminative touch and for proprioception are now known to differ with respect to conduction from the lower limbs. The pathways for the two main sensory modalities of the medial lemniscus system are, therefore, described separately.

DISCRIMINATIVE TOUCH

The primary sensory neurons for discriminative touch (and for proprioception) are the largest cells in the dorsal root ganglia; their processes are large group A fibers with thick myelin sheaths. The central processes are in the medial group of fibers of each rootlet, and they bifurcate on entering the **dorsal funiculus**. The short descending branches are described later. Most of the ascending branches proceed ipsilaterally to the medulla (Fig. 19-4). Above the midthoracic level, the dorsal funiculus consists of a medial **gracile fasciculus** and a lateral **cuneate fasciculus**. The fibers of the gracile fasciculus, which enter the spinal cord below the midthoracic level, terminate in the **gracile nucleus**; fibers of the cuneate fasciculus, coming from the upper thoracic and cervical spinal nerves, end in the **cuneate nucleus**. More precisely, there is a lamination of the dorsal funiculus according to segments. Fibers that enter the spinal cord in lower sacral segments are most medial, and fibers from successively higher segments ascend in an orderly manner along the lateral side of those already present.

Axons of neurons in the gracile and cuneate nuclei curve ventrally as **internal arcuate fibers**, cross the midline of the medulla in the decussation of the medial lemnisci, and continue to the thalamus as the **medial lemniscus**. This substantial tract is situated between the midline and the inferior olivary nucleus in the medulla, in the most ventral portion of the tegmentum of the pons, and lateral to the red nucleus in the tegmentum of the midbrain. The medial lemniscus and spinothalamic tract intermingle in the dorsal region of the subthalamus before entering the **ventral posterior nucleus of the thalamus**. The fibers of the medial lemniscus, in contrast to those of the spinothalamic tract, all terminate in the VP nucleus.

A topographic arrangement of fibers is maintained throughout the medial lemniscus. In the medulla, the larger dimension of the lemniscus is vertical as seen in cross section; fibers for the lower limb are most ventral (adjacent to the pyramid), and fibers for the upper part of the body are most dorsal. On entering the pons, the medial lemniscus "rotates" through 90 degrees; from here to the thalamus, fibers for the lower limb are in the lateral part of the lemniscus, and those for the upper part of the body are in its medial portion. This pattern conforms with the representation of the body in the ventral posterior nucleus of the thalamus (VPl). The pathway is completed by a projection from this nucleus to the **primary somesthetic cortex** of the parietal lobe.

PROPRIOCEPTION

The central pathway for conscious awareness of position and movement differs for sensory data from the lower and upper limbs (Fig. 19-5). The simpler pathway is that for the **upper limb**, which corresponds exactly with the one just described. That is, the ascending branches of primary afferent fibers terminate in the cuneate nucleus, from which the impulses are relayed through the medial lemniscus to the ventral posterior nucleus of the thalamus and thence to the first general sensory area of the cerebral cortex.

The pathway for the **lower limb** is different, being a series of four populations of neurons. The primary afferent fibers enter the cord from the lumbar and sacral dorsal roots; they bifurcate into ascending and descending branches in the dorsal funiculus, but the former only go part of the way up the spinal cord. They terminate in the **nucleus dorsalis** (nucleus thoracicus; Clarke's column), which is a column of large cells on the medial side of the dorsal horn in segments C8 through L3. The neurons in the nucleus dorsalis give rise to axons that ascend ipsilaterally as the **dorsal spinocerebellar tract** in the dorsolateral funiculus. Before entering the inferior cerebellar peduncle, some of the constituent axons give off collateral branches, which remain in the medulla. These collaterals from the dorsal spinocerebellar tract are concerned with conscious proprioception from the lower limb. They end in the **nucleus Z** of Brodal and Pompeiano. This is rostral to the nucleus gracilis, of which it may be functionally an outlying part. The cells of nucleus Z give rise to internal arcuate fibers that cross the midline and join the medial lemniscus. The remainder of the pathway is the same as for the upper limb, with a synapse in the ventral posterior thalamic nucleus (VPl) and thalamocortical fibers projecting to the leg area of the sensory cortex.

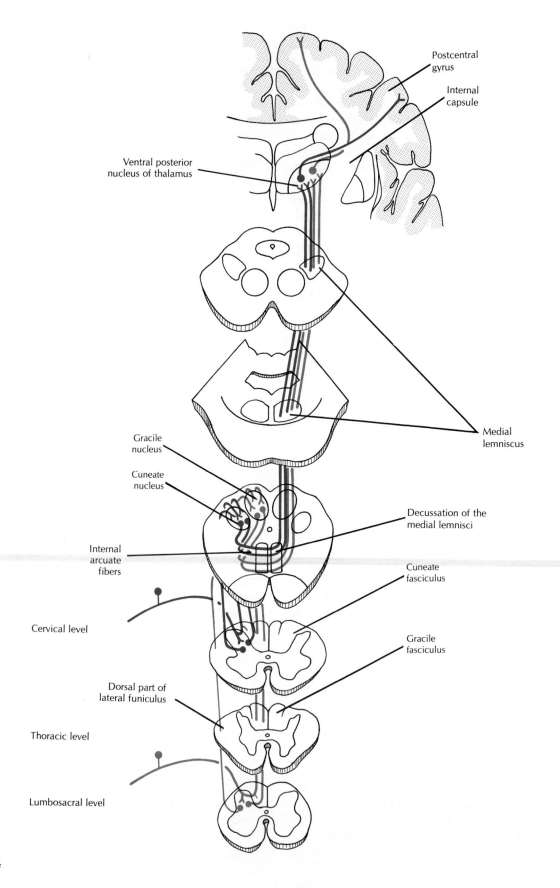

Postcentral
gyrus

Internal
capsule

Ventral posterior
nucleus of thalamus

Medial
lemniscus

Gracile
nucleus

Cuneate
nucleus

Decussation of the
medial lemnisci

Internal
arcuate
fibers

Cuneate
fasciculus

Cervical level

Gracile
fasciculus

Dorsal part of
lateral funiculus

Thoracic level

Lumbosacral level

The different neuroanatomical substrates of proprioception from the upper and lower limbs have functional consequences. Thus the dorsal funiculi do not conduct impulses concerned with proprioception in the lower limbs further rostrally than the thoracic segmental levels. The gracile nucleus, unlike the cuneate nucleus, is not concerned with proprioception. The neural pathway to the cortex for the lower limb consists of four sets of neurons, whereas that for the upper limb consists of only three. The same axons (those of the dorsal spinocerebellar tract) not only convey information that eventually reaches consciousness in the cerebral cortex, but also participate in the workings of the cerebellum (see Ch. 10), which are probably entirely unconscious.

Spinomedullary Neurons

The short descending branches of the primary neurons in the dorsal funiculus accumulate in the fasciculus septomarginalis in the lower half of the spinal cord and in the fasciculus interfascicularis in the upper half of the cord (see Fig. 5-9). They terminate in the spinal gray matter, as do some ascending branches that do not travel as far as the medulla. In addition, many of the ascending and descending branches give off collaterals to the spinal gray matter. Some of the fibers that enter the gray matter, especially those concerned with proprioception, establish connections for spinal reflexes, and the remainder terminate on tract cells. Axons of the tract cells ascend ipsilaterally, not only in the dorsal funiculus, but in the dorsolateral funiculus as well (see Fig. 19-4). All these fibers terminate in the gracile and cuneate nuclei alongside the primary ascending fibers. These spinomedullary neurons, especially those sending axons into the dorsolateral funiculus, convey some information for most modalities of cutaneous and deep sensation, including vibration and pain. This relatively small population of afferents to the gracile and cuneate nuclei broadens the role of the medial lemniscus system to some extent, beyond that of a pathway for discriminative touch and proprioception.

Spinocervicothalamic Pathway

The axons of some tract cells in the dorsal horn ascend ipsilaterally in the dorsolateral funiculus to the **lateral cervical nucleus**. This nucleus is embedded in the white matter, just lateral to the tip of the dorsal horn in spinal segments C1 and C2, and extends into the lower medulla. It projects to the contralateral thalamus by means of fibers that are included in the medial lemniscus. In some animals, this is a significant pathway for all types of cutaneous sensation. In humans, however, the lateral cervical nucleus is inconspicuous; in many instances, the nucleus cannot be identified, although it may be merged with the apex of the dorsal horn. The spinocervicothalamic pathway has to be considered as a possible supplementary pathway in humans, but its significance as a component of the medial lemniscus system has yet to be determined.

Sensory Pathways for the Head

The back of the head and much of the external ear are supplied by branches of the second and third cervical nerves, whose central connections are with the spinothalamic and medial lemniscus systems. General sensations that arise elsewhere in the head are mediated almost entirely by the trigeminal nerve. Small areas of the skin and larger areas of mucous membrane are supplied by the facial, glossopharyngeal, and vagus nerves, but the central connections of the general sensory components of these nerves are the same as for the trigeminal nerve (see Ch. 8).

Figure 19-4. Medial lemniscus system for discriminative tactile sensation. The pathway from the lower limb is shown in *red* and from the upper limb, in *blue*. (Spinomedullary fibers are shown in the dorsal and lateral funiculi. These, as opposed to the axons of primary sensory neurons, convey some information for most modalities of general sensation.)

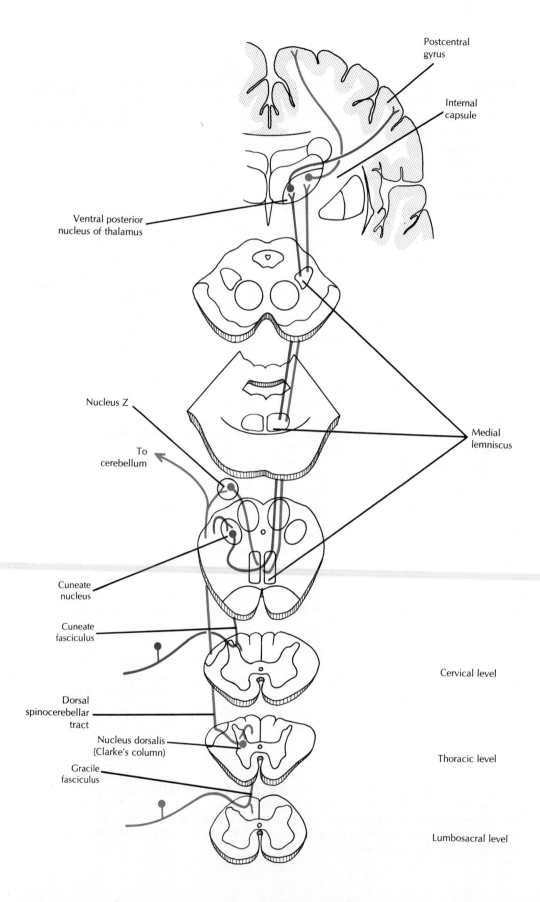

Postcentral
gyrus

Internal
capsule

Ventral posterior
nucleus of thalamus

Nucleus Z

To
cerebellum

Medial
lemniscus

Cuneate
nucleus

Cuneate
fasciculus

Cervical level

Dorsal
spinocerebellar
tract

Nucleus dorsalis
(Clarke's column)

Thoracic level

Gracile
fasciculus

Lumbosacral level

The cell bodies of primary sensory neurons of the trigeminal nerve, with the exception of those in the mesencephalic nucleus, are in the trigeminal ganglion (see Fig. 8-8). The peripheral processes have a wide distribution through the ophthalmic, maxillary, and mandibular divisions of the nerve. The central processes enter the pons in the sensory root. Some of these axons end in the pontine trigeminal nucleus, many descend in the spinal trigeminal tract and end in the associated nucleus, and still others bifurcate, with a branch ending in each nucleus.

There is a spatial arrangement of fibers in the sensory root and spinal tract that corresponds to the divisions of the trigeminal nerve. In the sensory root, ophthalmic fibers are dorsal, mandibular fibers ventral, and maxillary fibers in between. Because of a rotation of the fibers as they enter the pons, the mandibular fibers are dorsal and the ophthalmic fibers ventral in the spinal trigeminal tract. The most dorsal part of this tract includes a bundle of fibers from the facial, glossopharyngeal, and vagus nerves. The cell bodies of the primary sensory neurons are in the geniculate ganglion of the facial nerve and in the superior ganglia of the glossopharyngeal and vagus nerves. Fibers in the facial and vagus nerves supply parts of the external ear, acoustic canal, and tympanic membrane. The glossopharyngeal and vagus nerves supply the mucosa of the back of the tongue, pharynx, esophagus, larynx, auditory (eustachian) tube, and middle ear.

PAIN AND TEMPERATURE

The fibers for pain and temperature terminate in the **pars caudalis of the spinal trigeminal nucleus**; the pars caudalis is in the lower medulla and upper three cervical segments of the spinal cord. (There is some evidence that the pars interpolaris receives pain afferents from the teeth.) The portion of the pars caudalis in the cervical cord receives sensory data from areas of distribution of the trigeminal nerve and upper cervical spinal nerves. The cellular characteristics of the pars caudalis are similar to those of the tip of the dorsal gray horn of the spinal cord. The continuity of the substantia gelatinosa (lamina II) with a layer of small cells in the pars caudalis is particularly conspicuous.

Neurons in the reticular formation immediately medial to the pars caudalis of the spinal trigeminal nucleus correspond to the nucleus proprius of the spinal gray matter. The tract cells whose axons project to the thalamus are in both the spinal trigeminal nucleus and the adjacent reticular formation. The axons of these second-order neurons cross to the opposite side of the medulla and continue rostrally in the **ventral trigeminothalamic tract**. The tract terminates mainly in the **medial division of the ventral posterior nucleus of the thalamus** (**VPm**), and thalamocortical fibers complete the pathway to the ventral one-third of the **somesthetic area of cortex**. The axons of the tract cells associated with the pars caudalis, like those of the spinothalamic tract, also have branches that end in the intralaminar and posterior nuclear groups of the thalamus, thus providing for distribution of the sensory information to areas of cortex beyond the confines of the first sensory area. From the foregoing description, it is evident that the pathway for pain and temperature from the head corresponds to the spinothalamic system.

TOUCH

The central pathway for tactile sensation from the head is similar to that just described for pain and temperature, differing mainly in the sensory trigeminal nuclei involved. For light touch, the second-order neurons are in the **pars interpolaris and pars oralis** of the spinal trigeminal nucleus and in the **pontine trigeminal nucleus**. For discriminative

Figure 19-5. Pathways for conscious proprioception. The pathway from the lower limb is shown in *red* and from the upper limb, in *blue*.

touch, they are in the pontine trigeminal nucleus and the pars oralis of the nucleus of the spinal trigeminal tract. The second-order neurons project to the contralateral ventral posterior nucleus of the thalamus (VPm) through the ventral trigeminothalamic tract. In addition, smaller numbers of fibers, crossed and uncrossed, proceed from the pontine trigeminal nucleus to the VPm in the **dorsal trigeminothalamic tract**. The two sets of trigeminothalamic fibers often are named together as the **trigeminal lemniscus**.

PROPRIOCEPTION

The primary sensory neurons for proprioception in the head are unique in that most of their cell bodies are in a nucleus in the brain stem instead of in a sensory ganglion. Constituting the **mesencephalic trigeminal nucleus**, they are unipolar neurons similar to most primary sensory neurons elsewhere. The peripheral branch of the single process proceeds through the trigeminal nerve without interruption; these fibers supply proprioceptors in the trigeminal area of distribution, such as those related to the muscles of mastication. The other branch of the single process terminates in the trigeminal motor nucleus for reflex action or synapses with cells in the adjacent reticular formation, the axons of which join the **dorsal trigeminothalamic tract**. The neurons of the mesencephalic trigeminal nucleus also send peripheral branches to receptors in the sockets of the teeth. These receptors detect **pressure on the teeth**, a sense functionally related to muscle proprioception because it participates in the reflex control of the force of biting.

The only other type of sensation perceived by a tooth is **pain**, for which the sensory pathway has already been described. Pain may originate from the dentin, the pulp, or the periodontal tissues.

The innervation of proprioceptors in mus-

cles of the head that receive their motor supply from cranial nerves other than the trigeminal is discussed in Chapter 8.

Descending Pathways Involved in Sensation

The conscious perception of any sensation involves a sequence of neurons that form a pathway from the receptors to the cerebral cortex. For each of the ascending pathways described in this chapter, there are two or three levels at which synapses occur; these are sites such as the dorsal horn, gracile and cuneate nuclei, and ventral posterior nucleus of the thalamus. The synapses exist, not to delay the passage of nerve impulses, but rather to accommodate convergence in some of the pathways. They also allow the upward traffic in neurally coded information to be modified by activity in other parts of the central nervous system through descending pathways (Fig. 19-6).

The first general sensory area of the **cerebral cortex** sends fibers to all the regions in which ascending somesthetic pathways are interrupted by synapses. Thus there are projections from this part of the cortex to the ventral posterior thalamic nucleus, to the gracile and cuneate nuclei, to the sensory nuclei of the trigeminal nerve, and to the dorsal horn of the spinal cord. The corticofugal fibers destined for the medulla and spinal cord travel in the corticobulbar and corticospinal tracts (which are not entirely motor in function). Most corticospinal fibers from the first sensory area send collateral branches and cuneate to the gracile nuclei and continue to sites of termination in the dorsal horn. Fibers from the premotor and motor areas end in the ventral horn. The gracile and cuneate nuclei contribute a few descending fibers to the dorsal funiculus.

The other major source of descending fibers associated with the somesthetic pathways

Figure 19-6. Descending pathways that modulate the transmission of sensory information from the spinal cord to the cerebral cortex. (Reticulospinal and raphespinal projections are *blue*, descending fibers from the periaqueductal gray matter are *black*, other descending pathways are *red*.

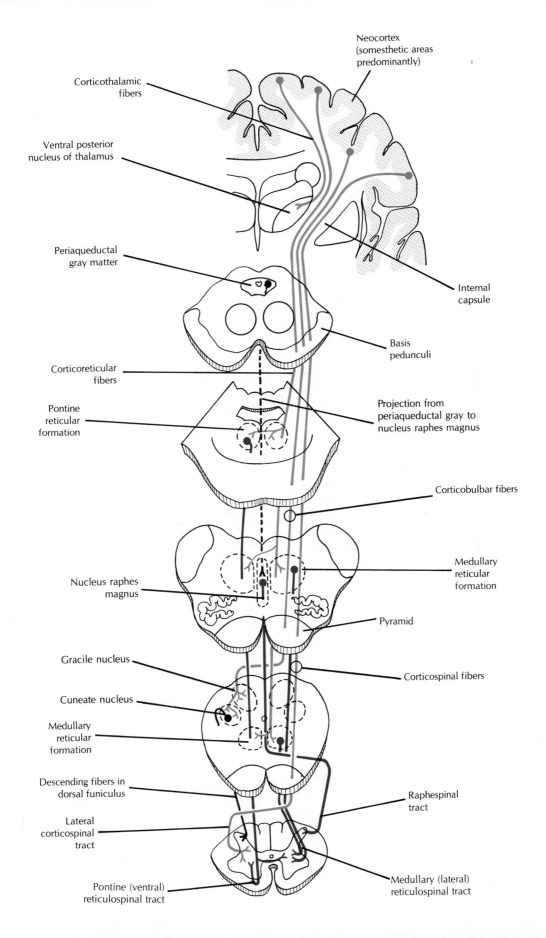

Neocortex
(somesthetic areas
predominantly)

Corticothalamic
fibers

Ventral posterior
nucleus of thalamus

Internal
capsule

Periaqueductal
gray matter

Basis
pedunculi

Corticoreticular
fibers

Projection from
periaqueductal gray to
nucleus raphes magnus

Pontine
reticular
formation

Corticobulbar fibers

Medullary
reticular
formation

Nucleus raphes
magnus

Pyramid

Gracile nucleus

Corticospinal fibers

Cuneate nucleus

Medullary
reticular
formation

Descending fibers in
dorsal funiculus

Raphespinal
tract

Lateral
corticospinal
tract

Medullary (lateral)
reticulospinal tract

Pontine (ventral)
reticulospinal tract

is the **reticular formation**. The inhibitory **raphespinal** projection to the dorsal horn from the nucleus raphes magnus of the medulla has already been discussed in connection with the neuroanatomy of pain. Other fibers comprise the **reticulospinal tracts**, which arise in the **central group of reticular nuclei** of the pons and medulla. The reticulospinal tracts terminate mostly among the interneurons in the middle regions (lamina VII) of the spinal gray matter, next to the sites of termination of corticospinal and vestibulospinal fibers, and they are concerned with the control of the motor neurons. Some reticulospinal axons, however, end in the base of the dorsal horn, and these probably synapse with dendrites of the nearby tract cells. As was seen in Chapter 9, the cells of origin of the pontine and medullary reticulospinal tracts receive synaptic input from spinoreticular fibers, from other neurons in the reticular formation, and from the cerebral cortex. The corticoreticular projection comes from many parts of the cortex but most abundantly from the motor and sensory areas of the frontal and parietal lobes.

The functions of these descending pathways are not known with certainty. It is probable that they promote attentiveness to particular stimuli. Connections are present that would enable the cerebral cortex and other parts of the brain to lower the threshold of conscious perception for a modality of sensation in any part of the body. Similarly, it would be possible to increase the thresholds for stimuli to which attention is not being paid, thereby protecting the higher levels of the ascending systems from a deluge of irrelevant information. As noted previously, corticospinal fibers are probably involved in the suppression of pain when there is intense emotional stress.

Clinical Considerations ————

Spinothalamic System

Inflammatory reactions in dorsal roots of spinal nerves or in peripheral nerves and pressure on spinal nerve roots by a **herniated intervertebral disk** stimulate pain and temperature fibers, causing painful and burning sensations in the area supplied by the affected roots or nerves. An effect opposite to that of irritation is produced by **local anesthetic** drugs. These are most effective in blocking the conduction of impulses along group C fibers, so that low doses may reduce pain perception while having little or no effect on tactile sensibility. **Ischemia** of a nerve, such as that resulting from a tight tourniquet, preferentially blocks conduction in group A fibers. Pain with a burning character is the only sensation that can be perceived before the failure of conduction in an ischemic nerve becomes complete.

Degenerative changes in the region of the central canal of the spinal cord interrupt pain and temperature fibers as they decussate in the ventral white commissure. The best example is **syringomyelia**, which is characterized by central cavitation of the spinal cord. When the disease process is most marked in the cervical enlargement, as is frequently the case, the area of anesthesia includes the hands, arms, and shoulders (yoke-like anesthesia). The typical presenting symptom is a burn that is not painful.

A lesion that includes the **ventrolateral part of the spinal cord** on one side results in loss of pain and temperature sensibility below the level of the lesion and on the opposite side of the body. If, for example, the spinothalamic and spinoreticular tracts are interrupted on the right side at the level of the first thoracic segment, the area of anesthesia includes the left leg and the left side of the trunk. Careful testing of the upper margin of sensory impairment shows that cutaneous areas supplied by the first and second thoracic nerves are spared. Some signals from these areas reach the contralateral pathways above their interruption because of the ascending branches of dorsal root fibers in the dorsolateral tract. Surgical section of the pathway for pain (tractotomy or chordotomy) may be required for **relief of intractable pain**. Tractotomy is most likely to be considered in later stages of malignant disease of a pelvic viscus; interruption of the pain pathway may be unilateral or bilateral, depending on circumstances prevailing in the particular patient. An alternative procedure is **commissural myelotomy**, in which decussating spinothalamic and spinoreticular fibers are cut by a median incision at and a few segments above the level of the source of the pain.

The spinal lemniscus may be included in an area of infarction in the brain stem. An example is provided by Wallenberg's **lateral medullary syndrome**; the area of infarction usually includes the spinal lemniscus and the spinal tract of the trigeminal nerve and its associated nucleus. The principal sensory deficit is for pain and temperature sensibility on the side of the body opposite the lesion, but on the same side for the face (see also Ch. 7).

The standard method of testing for integrity of the pain and temperature pathway is to stimulate the skin with a pin and to ask whether it feels sharp or blunt. Temperature perception usually need not be tested separately; if such testing is required, the method used is to touch the skin with test tubes containing warm or cold water. Light touch is tested with a wisp of cotton.

Medial Lemniscus System

Defective proprioception and discriminative touch result from interruption of the medial lemniscus system anywhere along its course. For example, the dorsal and dorsolateral funiculi are sites of symmetrical demyelination in **subacute combined degeneration** of the spinal cord (see Ch. 5), and conduction may be interrupted at any level by trauma, infarction, or the plaques of multiple sclerosis. The usual test for proprioception is to move the patient's finger or toe, asking him to state when the movement begins and the direction of movement. In the **Romberg test**, any abnormal unsteadiness is noted when the patient stands with the feet together and the eyes closed, thereby evaluating proprioception in the lower limbs. Another useful test is to ask the patient to identify an object held in the hand with the eyes closed. Proprioception is especially helpful in recognizing the object on the basis of shape and size (**stereognosis**) as well as weight. This is a sensitive test that the patient may perform unsuccessfully when there is a lesion in the parietal association cortex, even though the pathway to the somesthetic area is intact.

For testing of **two-point touch discrimination**, two pointed objects are applied lightly to the skin simultaneously. A suitable test object can be devised from a paper clip. Simultaneous stimuli are normally detected in a fingertip when the points are 3 to 4 mm apart, or even less. Thorough testing of two-point discrimination is a tedious procedure. A simpler test is for the examiner to ask the subject to identify simple figures "drawn" on the skin with the finger or with some other blunt object. This test relies on the ability to recognize the distance and direction of movement of the stimulus across the surface of the skin. It is highly specific for the dorsal funiculi of the spinal cord, provided there is no lesion in the cerebral cortex that is causing aphasia or agnosia.

Another sensory test is to ask the patient whether **vibration** as well as touch or pressure is felt when a tuning fork, preferably with a frequency of 128 Hz, is placed against a bony prominence such as an ankle or a knuckle. The sense of vibration often is reduced in elderly people, but even slight vibration should be felt in young people. For identifying the site of a lesion in the central nervous system, this test is less valuable than the examination of proprioception and discriminative touch. Diminished perception of vibration is often the first sign of disease affecting the largest myelinated fibers in a peripheral nerve.

Sensation from the Head

The most common sensory abnormality affecting the face and scalp is **herpes zoster**. This disease is caused by a virus (the same one that causes chicken-pox) that infects the neurons in sensory ganglia. Burning pain and itching, commonly in the field of distribution of one of the three divisions of the trigeminal nerve, is accompanied by a skin eruption. This can be a serious condition if corneal ulceration results from infection of the ganglion cells concerned with the ophthalmic division of the trigeminal nerve. The disability occasionally is prolonged, especially in elderly people, by **postherpetic neuralgia**. This may be particularly painful and recalcitrant to treatment. Relief can be obtained by applying capsaicin to the affected skin. Capsaicin first stimulates and then damages the terminal branches of nociceptive group C fibers. Herpes zoster may also affect the geniculate ganglion or the superior vagal ganglion, causing an eruption on the tympanic membrane and parts of the external auditory canal and concha of the auricle; this is classic clinical evidence for the anatomy of the dual cutaneous innervation of this region.

A less common condition that causes pain in the fields of distribution of one or more divisions of the trigeminal nerve is **trigeminal neuralgia**, described in Chapter 8.

Thalamic Lesions

Surgically or pathologically produced lesions in the ventral posterior nucleus of the thalamus cause profound loss of all sensations other than pain on the opposite side of the body. The intralaminar and posterior groups of nuclei in the thalamus are probably almost as important as the ventral posterior nucleus in the central pathway for pain.

Central neurogenic pain, which is not caused by activity in peripheral sensory fibers, can be caused by lesions that interrupt the somatosensory pathways at any level. A lesion that involves the VP nucleus of the thalamus may result in the **thalamic syndrome**, characterized by exaggerated and exceptionally disagreeable responses to cutaneous stimulation. This syndrome (see Ch. 11) may include spontaneous pain and evidence of emotional instability, such as unprovoked laughing and crying.

SUGGESTED READING

Apkarian AV, Hodge CJ: Primate spinothalamic pathways. I, II and III. J Comp Neurol 288: 447–511, 1989

Cook AW, Nathan PW, Smith MC: Sensory consequences of commissural myelotomy. A challenge to traditional anatomical concepts. Brain 107:547–568, 1984

De Broucker Th, Cesaro P, Willer JC, Le Bars D: Diffuse noxious inhibitory controls in man. Involvement of the spinoreticular tract. Brain 113:1223–1224, 1990

Hodge CJ, Apkarian AV: The spinothalamic tract. Crit Rev Neurobiol 5:363–397, 1990

McLean A: C.N.S. Neurological Examination. Toronto, Collier-Macmillan, 1980

Nieuwenhuys R, Voogd J, Van Huijzen C: The Human Central Nervous System. A Synopsis and Atlas, 3rd ed. Berlin, Springer-Verlag, 1988

Roland P: Cortical representation of pain. Trends Neurosci 15:3–5, 1992

Wall PD: The sensory and motor role of impulses travelling in the dorsal columns toward cerebral cortex. Brain 93:505–524, 1970

Wall PD, Noordenbos W: Sensory functions which remain after complete transection of dorsal columns. Brain 100:505–524, 1977

Watson CPN, Evans RJ, Watt VR: Post-herpetic neuralgia and topical capsaicin. Pain 33:333–340, 1988

Willis WD: Nociceptive pathways: Anatomy and physiology of nociceptive ascending pathways. Philos Trans R Soc Lond [Biol] 308:253–268, 1985

Willis WD, Coggeshall RE: Sensory Mechanisms of the Spinal Cord, 2nd ed. New York, Plenum Press, 1991

Twenty

The Human Nervous System: An Anatomical Viewpoint, Sixth Edition, Murray L. Barr and John A. Kiernan. J.B. Lippincott Company, Philadelphia, © 1993.

Visual System

Important Facts

In darkness, the retinal photoreceptors continuously release their excitatory synaptic transmitter substance. Absorption of light by the pigment in the rod or cone suppresses the release.

Some bipolar cells are excited; others are inhibited by illumination of the retina. Other retinal interneurons modify transmission in the two synaptic layers of the retina.

The axons of the ganglion cells of the nasal halves of the retinas cross in the optic chiasma; those from the temporal halves do not cross. Combined with the optical inversion of the retinal image, this partial decussation ensures that signals from each half of the visual field are sent to the contralateral optic tract, thalamus, and cerebral cortex.

Most fibers of the optic tract end in the lateral geniculate body, which projects to the striate area of the occipital cortex. There is topographical representation of the visual fields throughout this pathway, and destructive lesions cause visual field defects appropriate to the axonal or neuronal populations damaged.

The central parts of the retinas are represented at the occipital poles; peripheral vision is served by the more anterior parts of the primary visual cortex. The visual association cortex in the occipital and temporal lobes is necessary for recognition of colors and formed objects and for visual memory.

Some fibers of the optic tract end in the pretectal area, which forms part of the pathway for the pupillary light reflex. Others end, alongside fibers from the occipital cortex, in the superior colliculus. They are involved in the control of eye movements.

The visual pathway begins with photoreceptors in the retina from which nerve impulses reach the visual cortex in the occipital lobe through a series of neurons. There are two types of photoreceptor cell; rods have a special role in peripheral vision and vision under conditions of low illumination, whereas cones, which function in bright light, are responsible for central discriminative vision and for the detection of colors. The responses of the photoreceptors are transmitted by bipolar cells to ganglion cells within the retina, and axons of ganglion cells reach the lateral geniculate body of the thalamus through the optic nerve and optic tract. The final relay is from the lateral geniculate body to the visual cortex by way of the geniculocalcarine tract. In addition, some fibers from the retina terminate in various parts of the midbrain, in the pulvinar of the thalamus, and in the hypothalamus.

The following account of the visual system is restricted to a discussion of the neural elements and presupposes a general understanding of the structure of the eye and the optical mechanism that projects a focused, inverted image onto the retina.

Retina

Optic vesicles evaginate from the prosencephalon at an early stage of embryonic development. Each optic vesicle "caves in" to form the optic cup, which consists of two layers and is connected to the developing brain by the optic stalk. The outer layer of the optic cup becomes the pigment epithelium of the retina, and the inner layer differentiates into the complex neural layer of the retina. The optic stalk becomes the optic nerve. The cornea, lens, and other parts of the eye develop from the nearby ectoderm and mesoderm.

In addition to photoreceptors, bipolar cells, and ganglion cells, the neural layer of the retina contains association neurons and neuroglial cells. The complex neuronal pattern of the retina resembles that of the gray matter of the brain. Similarly, the optic nerve is composed of white matter and is not a peripheral nerve. The retina and the optic nerve are, therefore, outgrowths of the brain that are specialized for sensitivity to light, for encoding the sensory data, and for transmission of the resulting information to the thalamus and cerebral cortex.

Retinal Landmarks

Certain specialized regions serve as landmarks that need to be identified before the cellular components of the retina are described.

The cell layers of the retina, listed from the choroid to the vitreous body, are the pigment epithelium, rods and cones, bipolar cells, and ganglion cells (Fig. 20-1). Axons of ganglion cells run toward the posterior pole of the eye and enter the optic nerve at the **optic papilla**

or **optic disk**. The papilla is slightly medial to the posterior pole, about 1.5 mm in diameter, and pale pink. The nerve fibers are heaped up as they converge at the margin of the optic papilla and then pass through the fibrous tunic (sclera) of the eyeball into the optic nerve. The optic papilla is a blind spot because it contains only nerve fibers.

The **macula lutea**, the central area of the retina in line with the visual axis, is a specialized region about 5 mm in diameter that abuts on the lateral edge of the optic papilla. The name macula lutea (yellow spot) is derived from the presence of a diffuse yellow pigment (xanthophyll) among the neural elements in this location. The yellow color is apparent only when the retina is examined with red-free light, and the macula is, therefore, not ordinarily seen when the ocular fundus is inspected with an ophthalmoscope. The macula is specialized for acuity of vision; the probable function of the yellow pigment is to screen out some of the blue part of the visible spectrum, thereby protecting the photoreceptors from the dazzling effect of strong light.

The **fovea** (or fovea centralis) is a depression in the center of the macula; the fovea is about 1.5 mm in diameter and separated from the edge of the optic disk by a distance of about 2 mm. Visual acuity is greatest at the fovea, the center of which (the **foveola**) contains only cone receptors. The capillary network present elsewhere in the retina is absent from the center of the fovea. When the retina is viewed with an ophthalmoscope, the fovea appears darker than the reddish hue of the surrounding parts of the retina because the black melanin pigment in the choroid and the pigment epithelium is not screened by capillary blood. The visible fovea commonly is referred to as the "macula" in an ophthalmoscopic examination of the retina.

The functional retina terminates anteriorly along an irregular border, the **ora serrata**. Forward of this line, the ciliary portion of the retina consists of a double layer of columnar epithelium, with the outer layer being pigmented.

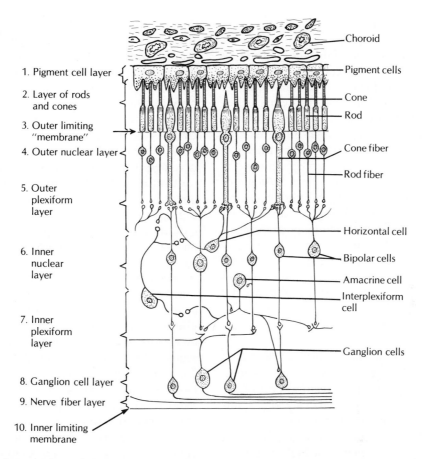

1. Pigment cell layer — Choroid
— Pigment cells
2. Layer of rods and cones — Cone
— Rod
3. Outer limiting "membrane"
4. Outer nuclear layer — Cone fiber
— Rod fiber
5. Outer plexiform layer
— Horizontal cell
6. Inner nuclear layer — Bipolar cells
— Amacrine cell
— Interplexiform cell
7. Inner plexiform layer
— Ganglion cells
8. Ganglion cell layer
9. Nerve fiber layer
10. Inner limiting membrane

Figure 20-1. Schematic representation of the neurons of the retina. The ten histological layers are identified at the left.

Pigment Epithelium

The pigment epithelium, consisting of a single layer of cells, reinforces the light-absorbing property of the choroid in reducing the scattering of light within the eye (see Fig. 20-1). Each pigment cell has a flat hexagonal base that adheres to Bruch's glassy membrane of the choroid. The basal portion of the cell contains the nucleus and a few pigment granules. Processes extending from the free surface of the cell interdigitate with the outer photosensitive regions of rods and cones. The processes, which are filled with granules of melanin pigment, isolate individual photoreceptors and enhance visual acuity. In lower verte-brates, there is a movement of pigment granules toward the tips of the processes, which also change in length and shape, in response to bright light. Such a response has not been described in mammals.

The pigment epithelium is fixed to the choroid but is not as firmly attached to the neural part of the retina. **Detachment of the retina**, which may follow a blow to the eye or occur spontaneously, consists of separation of the neural layers from the pigment epithelium. Fluid accumulates in the space thus created between the parts of the retina derived from the two layers of the optic cup. Retinal detachment can lead to blindness of the eye if untreated.

Photoreceptors

The light-sensitive part of the photoreceptor is the outer portion adjacent to the pigment epithelium. The incident light, therefore, has to pass through almost all the retina before being detected. This arrangement, known as the inverted retina, is present in all vertebrates. It does not introduce a significant barrier to light because the retina is transparent and at no point more than 0.4 mm thick. When they consist of layers of cells, the photoreceptive parts of the eyes of invertebrate animals are called retinas, but their cellular organization is always quite different from that of the vertebrate retina. The neural connections are on the opposite side to that from which the light approaches; hence, invertebrate retinas are not inverted.

RODS

The human retina contains about 130 million rods, which is 20 times the number of cones. Rods are absent from the central part of the fovea and become progressively more numerous from that point to the ora serrata. The distribution is such that rods are important for peripheral vision. There is a high density of cones along the edge of the ora serrata, possibly to provide for the recognition of objects entering the periphery of the visual field. The rods are more sensitive to dim light than the cones, and the rod-free area of the fovea is night blind. A faint point of light such as a dim star is best detected by looking slightly away from it. Each rod consists of three portions: the outer segment, inner segment, and rod fiber. The outer and inner segments are about 2 μm thick, and their combined lengths vary from 60 μm near the fovea to 40 μm at the periphery of the retina. The **rod fiber** consists of a slender filament that includes the nucleus in an expanded region and terminates as an end bulb in synaptic contact with bipolar and association neurons.

In electron micrographs, most of the light-sensitive **outer segment** is seen to be occupied by about 700 double-layered membranous disks or flattened saccules (Figs. 20-2 and 20-3). The disks contain the pigment **rhodopsin** (visual purple), which gives the retina a purplish red color when removed from the eye and viewed under dim light. Rhodopsin consists of a protein, opsin, in loose chemical combination with retinal, a derivative of vitamin A. Absorption of a quantum of light changes the configuration of a rhodopsin molecule. A subsequent series of reactions results in hyperpolarization of the surface membrane of the inner segment and rod fiber, with consequent inhibition of the release of the neurotransmitter, which is secreted continuously in darkness. It is a curious property of photoreceptors that they are inhibited by their specific stimulus.

The **inner segment** of a rod contains the organelles found in all types of cells. A region adjacent to the outer segment, known as the **ellipsoid**, contains numerous elongated mitochondria. A cilium extends into the outer segment from one of two centrioles situated at the junction of the outer and inner segments (see Fig. 20-3). The remainder of the inner segment contains neurofibrils, vesicles, and granular endoplasmic reticulum. This region is known as the **myoid** because in lower vertebrates, it contracts in response to changes in light intensity. A contractile property has not been established for the corresponding region in mammals.

CONES

The cone photoreceptors, although less numerous than the rods, are especially important because of their role in visual acuity and color vision. The cone, like the rod, consists of an outer and inner segment and a cone fiber.

The tapering **outer segment** of a cone consists principally of double-layered pigment-bearing disks, varying in number from 1000 in cones at the fovea to several hundred at the periphery of the retina (see Fig. 20-2). There are differences in detail between the disks of cones and rods, including somewhat closer stacking in cones. There are three types of cone, each containing one of three pigments that absorbs red, green, or blue light. Each cone pigment resembles rhodopsin in consist-

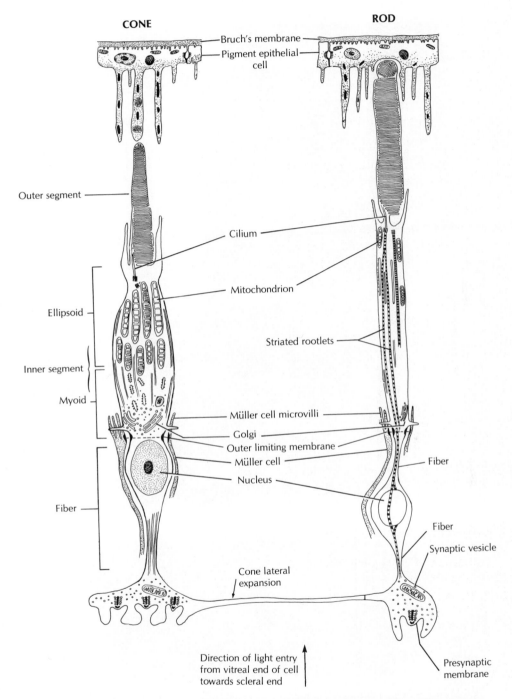

Figure 20-2. Ultrastructural components of rods and cones. The striated rootlets are prominent in the cytoplasm of rods, but their function is obscure. Other named structures are described in the text. (*Modified by permission from Enoch JM, Tobey FL [eds]: Springer Series in Optical Sciences, vol 23. Heidelberg, Springer-Verlag, 1981. Courtesy of Dr. B. Borwein*)

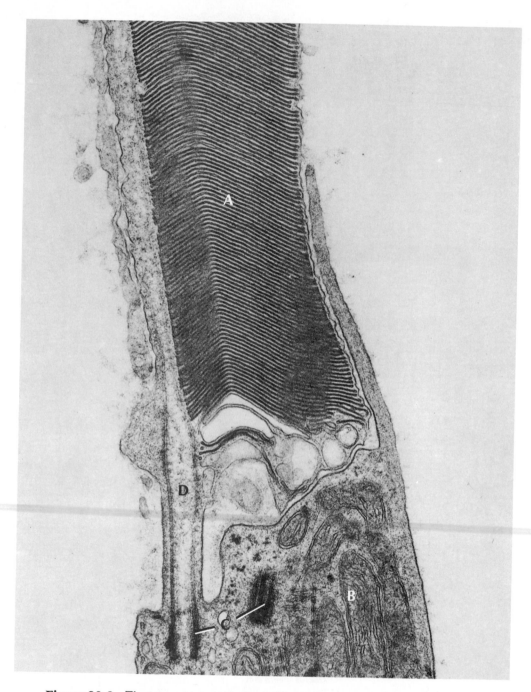

Figure 20-3. Electron micrograph of a rod from the human retina, showing part of the outer segment and the adjoining region of the inner segment. (**A**) Membranous disks in outer segment. (**B**) Mitochondria in the ellipsoid. (**C**) Centrioles. (**D**) Cilium. (× 36,000) (*Courtesy of Dr. M. Hogan*)

ing of retinal combined with a protein. Three proteins (cone opsins) are recognized, each combining with retinal in such a way as to provide maximum absorption of red, green, or blue light.

The **inner segment** of a cone is thicker than the inner segment of a rod, and it contains a larger ellipsoid and a larger amount of granular endoplasmic reticulum. The cilium of a cone is similar to that of a rod. The **cone fiber** is thicker than a rod fiber, and the nucleus is in an expansion adjacent to the inner segment. The fiber expands again terminally, establishing synaptic contact with bipolar and association neurons.

The human retina contains about 7 million cones. The central part of the fovea, the foveola, contains about 35,000 cones and no rods; there are about 100,000 cones in the whole of the fovea. The proportion of cones to rods remains high throughout the macular area for central vision, but it steadily decreases from the macula to the periphery of the retina. The cones in the fovea are longer and more slender than elsewhere (75 × 1 μm at the fovea and 40 × 6 μm at the periphery). The cone fibers and bipolar cells diverge from the center of the fovea, producing a slight concavity and reducing any slight impediment to light passing through the retina. Such scattering of light as may be caused by capillary blood flow is eliminated by the absence of a retinal capillary network at the center of the fovea. Figure 20-4 shows cone photoreceptors as they appear in a scanning electron micrograph.

Bipolar Cells

There are several types of bipolar cell according to morphological and physiological properties. These neurons are interposed between photoreceptor cells and ganglion cells (see Fig. 20-1). One bipolar cell is contacted by numerous rods (ranging from 10 near the macula to 100 at the periphery); the summation of excitation is an important factor in the sensitivity of the rod system to small amounts of light. Although there is some convergence of cones on bipolar cells in the peripheral parts of the retina, there is none at the fovea, at

which point visual acuity is greatest. There each cone fiber synapses with the dendrites of several bipolar cells. The synaptic terminals of cone fibers also have lateral expansions that contact the presynaptic parts of nearby rod fibers.

Ganglion Cells

Ganglion cells are rather large neurons with clumps of Nissl material, forming the last retinal link in the visual pathway (see Fig. 20-1). The bipolar cells contact both dendrites and somata of ganglion cells. The axons of ganglion cells form a layer of nerve fibers adjacent to the vitreous body. The fibers converge on the optic papilla from all directions, with those from the lateral part of the retina curving above or below the macula. On reaching the papilla, bundles of axons and processes of neuroglial cells pass through foramina in the sclera, which at this point is called the **lamina cribrosa**. Behind the sclera, they constitute the optic nerve. The axons acquire myelin sheaths only after traversing the sclera, although in a few people, bundles of myelinated axons are present in the retina, where they appear ophthalmoscopically as white streaks.

Excitation and inhibition of ganglion cells depend on properties of photoreceptors and bipolar cells that are atypical of most neurons elsewhere. The presynaptic part of a photoreceptor leaks its transmitter continuously in darkness. The release of transmitter is suppressed by illumination. Thus, the activity of the receptor cell is suppressed by light. This inhibition of sensory receptors by their specific stimulus, which is unique to the retina, is probably a consequence of the fact that a dark image on an illuminated background is as important biologically as an isolated source of light in an otherwise dark visual field. With respect to bipolar cells, there is no impulse conduction along these neurons. Their processes or neurites (and those of other retinal interneurons) are all called dendrites. Some bipolars respond to the transmitter from the photoreceptors with hyperpolarization of the cell membrane. Others respond to the same transmitter with partial depolarization. The

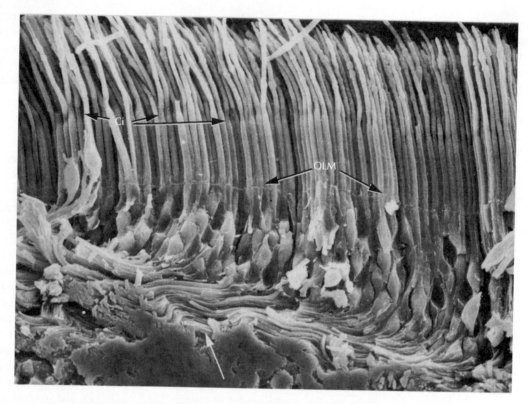

Figure 20-4. Scanning electron micrograph of foveal cones in a monkey. There is a constriction of each photoreceptor at the base of its cilium (**Ci**). The outer limiting membrane (**OLM**) appears as a thin line. The inner cone fibers (*white arrow*) turn sharply back at an angle to the photoreceptors and their nuclei. (*By permission from Enoch JM, Tobey FL [eds]: Springer Series in Optical Sciences, vol 23. Heidelberg, Springer-Verlag, 1981. Courtesy of Dr. B. Borwein*)

quantity of transmitter released by the presynaptic neurites of a bipolar neuron varies with the magnitude of the partial depolarization of the cell.

The neurotransmitters in the retina are not yet certainly identified. Several candidate substances have been detected immunohistochemically in the human retina. These include glutamate, which is present in photoreceptors, many bipolars, and ganglion cells. Glutamate is known to be the excitatory transmitter at synapses in several other parts of the central nervous system.

Association Neurons

Synaptic transmission in the retina is subject to modification by interneurons known as asso-ciation neurons (see Fig. 20-1). **Horizontal cells** are in the outer part of the zone occupied by the cell bodies of the bipolar cells. Their dendrites make contact with the synaptic terminals of the photoreceptors and with the dendrites of bipolar cells, which they inhibit. **Amacrine cells** are in the inner part of the zone occupied by the cell bodies of the bipolar cells. The dendrites of an amacrine cell all emerge from the same side of the cell to ramify and then terminate in the synaptic complexes between bipolar and ganglion cells and on cells of the type to be described next. Amacrine cells contain many putative transmitters, and there are probably inhibitory and excitatory types. The **interplexiform cells** are interspersed among the cell bodies of the bipolars. They are postsynaptic to amacrine cells and presynaptic to horizontal and bipolar cells, thus providing a feedback loop through which neural information is passed back from the inner to the outer of the two layers of retinal synapses.

Neuroglial Cells

The innermost layers of the retina contain astrocytes similar to those present in the gray matter of the brain. There also are large numbers of radial neuroglial cells, called **cells of Müller**. These extend from the interface between the nerve fiber layer of the retina and the vitreous body to the junction of the inner segments of rods and cones and the rod and cone fibers. Microvilli project from the outer end of a Müller's cell, which is connected to photoreceptor cells by zonulae adherentes. Müller's cells, therefore, extend through almost the whole thickness of the retina; lateral processes are given off that intervene between the neuronal elements of the retina and give

these neuroglial cells a supporting role, among other possible functions.

Histological Layers

In sections stained with hematoxylin and eosin (a commonly used dye combination that colors cell nuclei blue-purple and everything else pink), the retina is seen to consist of ten layers (Fig. 20-5). These can now be defined in relation to the cells that constitute the retina (see Fig. 20-1). Layer 1 is the **pigment epithelium**, and layer 2 consists of the outer and inner segments of **rods** and **cones**. Layer 3 is called the **outer limiting membrane** because it appears as a delicate line in histological sections. In fact, it is not a membrane, but rather the row of zonulae adherentes, where the outer ends of Müller's cells make contact with photoreceptor cells. Layer 4, the **outer nuclear layer**, consists of nuclei of rods and cones. Layer 5, the **outer plexiform layer**, includes principally rod and cone fibers and

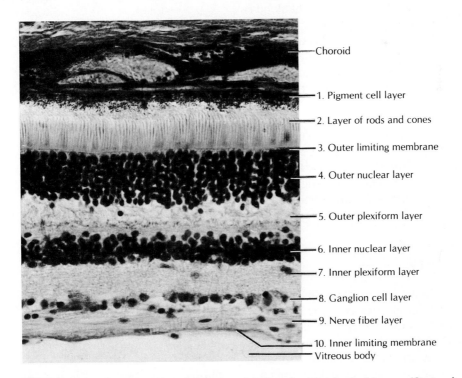

Choroid
1. Pigment cell layer
2. Layer of rods and cones
3. Outer limiting membrane
4. Outer nuclear layer
5. Outer plexiform layer
6. Inner nuclear layer
7. Inner plexiform layer
8. Ganglion cell layer
9. Nerve fiber layer
10. Inner limiting membrane
Vitreous body

Figure 20-5. Section of human retina showing the histological layers. (Stained with hematoxylin and eosin, × 350)

dendrites of bipolar cells. Layer 6 is called the **inner nuclear layer**; it contains the nuclei of bipolar cells, horizontal cells, amacrine cells, interplexiform cells, and cells of Müller. Layer 7, the **inner plexiform layer**, consists mainly of presynaptic dendrites of bipolar cells and postsynaptic dendrites of ganglion cells. The cell bodies of **ganglion cells** are in layer 8, and the axons of these cells constitute layer 9, the **nerve fiber layer**. Layer 10 is the **inner limiting membrane** formed by the expanded inner ends of Müller's cells.

Blood Supply

The retina receives nourishment from two sources. The **central artery of the retina** enters the eye through the optic disk, and its branches spread out over the inner surface of the retina. Fine branches penetrate the retina and form a capillary network that extends to the outer border of the inner nuclear layer. The capillary bed drains into retinal veins that converge on the optic papilla to form the central vein of the retina. The other source of blood is the capillary layer of the choroid, which is separated from the retina by Bruch's glassy membrane. The latter is a composite structure that consists of the basement membrane of the pigment epithelium and the innermost layer of the choroid, which is an orderly array of elastic and collagen fibrils. Soluble nutrients and metabolites of small molecular size can diffuse through Bruch's membrane, but macromolecules such as plasma proteins cannot. The outer part of the retina, extending from the pigment epithelium to the outer border of the inner nuclear layer, is devoid of capillaries.

Pathway to the Visual Cortex

There is a point-to-point projection from the retina to the dorsal nucleus of the lateral geniculate body of the thalamus, and from this nucleus to the visual cortex of the occipital lobe. There is, therefore, a spatial pattern of cortical excitation according to the retinal image of the visual field. Before discussing the components of the visual pathway, it may be useful to establish certain general rules concerning the projection from the retina to the cortex.

RETINAL PROJECTIONS

For the purpose of describing the retinal projection, each retina is divided into nasal and temporal halves by a vertical line that passes through the fovea. A horizontal line, also passing through the fovea, divides each half of the retina into upper and lower quadrants. The macular area for central vision is represented separately from the remainder of the retina. Figure 20-6 illustrates the following rules with respect to the central projection of retinal areas.

1. Fibers from the right halves of the two retinas terminate in the right lateral geniculate body, and the visual information is then relayed to the visual cortex of the right hemisphere.

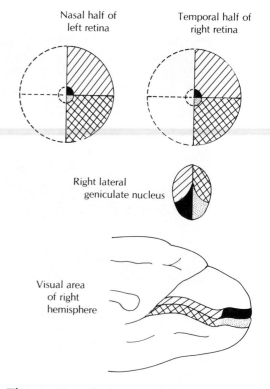

Figure 20-6. Projection of the retina on the lateral geniculate body and visual cortex.

The converse holds true, of course, for the contralateral projection.

2. Fibers from the upper quadrants peripheral to the macula end in the medial part of the lateral geniculate body, and impulses are relayed to the anterior two-thirds of the visual cortex above the calcarine sulcus.

3. Fibers from the lower quadrants peripheral to the macula end in the lateral portion of the lateral geniculate body, with a relay to the anterior two-thirds of the visual cortex below the calcarine sulcus.

4. The macula projects to a relatively large posterior region of the lateral geniculate body, which in turn sends fibers to the posterior one-third of the visual cortex in the region of the occipital pole. The macula is only 5 mm in diameter, but the proportions of the lateral geniculate body and visual cortex that receive fibers for macular vision are large because of the importance of central vision with maximal discrimination.

VISUAL FIELDS

Visual defects that result from interruption of the pathway at any point from the retina to the visual cortex are described in terms of the visual field rather than the retina. *The retinal image of an object in the visual field is inverted and reversed from right to left,* just as an image on the film in a camera is inverted and reversed. The following rules, therefore, apply to the nuclear and cortical representation of regions of the visual field.

1. The left visual field is represented in the right lateral geniculate body and in the visual cortex of the right hemisphere and vice versa.

2. The upper half of the visual field is represented in the lateral portion of the lateral geniculate body and in the visual cortex below the calcarine sulcus.

3. The lower half of the visual field is projected on the medial portion of the lateral geniculate body and on the visual cortex above the calcarine sulcus.

OPTIC NERVE, OPTIC CHIASMA, AND OPTIC TRACT

Each optic nerve contains about 1 million fibers, all myelinated; the large number of fibers is indicative of the importance of human vision. The optic nerve is surrounded by extensions of the meninges; the pia mater adheres to the nerve and is separated from the arachnoid by an extension of the subarachnoid space. The dura mater forms an outer sheath, and the meningeal extensions around the nerve fuse with the fibrous scleral coat of the eyeball. The axons are arranged in fasciculi that are separated by connective tissue septa continuous with the sheath of pia mater. Each fasciculus is further divided into small bundles by the cytoplasmic processes of fibrous astrocytes. Intimate ensheathment of the optic axons is by oligodendrocytes, whose processes penetrate between individual fibers. The myelin sheaths are formed by these oligodendrocytes.

The central artery and central vein of the retina traverse the meningeal sheaths and are included in the anterior part of the optic nerve. An increase in pressure of cerebrospinal fluid around the nerve impedes the return of venous blood. Edema or swelling of the optic disk (**papilledema**) results; this is a valuable indication of an increase in intracranial pressure. Part of the swelling is due to enlargement of the axons in the disk, attributed to partial obstruction of axonal transport within the optic nerve fibers.

The **partial crossing** of optic nerve fibers in the optic chiasma is a requirement for binocular vision. *Fibers from the nasal or medial half of each retina decussate in the chiasma and join uncrossed fibers from the temporal or lateral half of the retina to form the optic tract.* Impulses conducted to the right cerebral hemisphere by the right optic tract therefore represent the left half of the field of vision, whereas the right visual field is represented in the left hemisphere. Immediately after crossing in the chiasma, fibers from the nasal half of the retina loop forward for a short distance in the optic nerve. A lesion transecting the optic nerve close to the chiasma may, therefore, cause a temporal field defect in the opposite eye in addition to blindness in the eye whose optic nerve has been interrupted. The optic tract curves around the rostral end of the midbrain and ends in the lateral geniculate body of the thalamus.

Some of the fibers from the retina leave the optic chiasma and tract to proceed to sites other than the lateral geniculate body. These will be described after the pathway for conscious visual sensation has been discussed.

LATERAL GENICULATE BODY, GENICULOCALCARINE TRACT, AND VISUAL CORTEX

The **lateral geniculate body** is a small swelling beneath the posterior projection of the pulvinar of the thalamus. The dorsal nucleus of the lateral geniculate body, in which the great majority of the fibers of the optic tract terminate, consists of six layers of cells numbered consecutively from ventral to dorsal. Within the general pattern shown in Figure 20-6 and described previously, crossed fibers of the optic tract terminate in layers 1, 4, and 6, whereas uncrossed fibers end in layers 2, 3, and 5.

The **geniculocalcarine tract** originating in the lateral geniculate body first traverses the retrolentiform and sublentiform parts of the internal capsule. Its fibers then pass around the lateral ventricle, curving posteriorly toward their termination in the visual cortex (Fig. 20-7). Some of the geniculocalcarine fibers travel far forward over the temporal horn of the lateral ventricle. These fibers, which constitute the **temporal** or **Meyer's loop** of the geniculocalcarine tract, terminate in the visual cortex below the calcarine sulcus. It is evident from the retinal projection shown in Figure 20-6 that a temporal lobe lesion involving Meyer's loop causes a defect in the upper visual field on the side opposite the lesion. A lesion in the parietal lobe, on the other hand, may involve geniculocalcarine fibers that proceed to the visual cortex above the calcarine sulcus; the result is then a defect in the lower visual field on the side opposite the lesion.

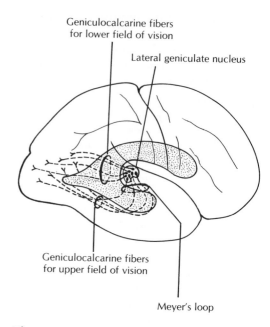

Geniculocalcarine fibers for lower field of vision

Lateral geniculate nucleus

Geniculocalcarine fibers for upper field of vision

Meyer's loop

Figure 20-7. Geniculocalcarine projection.

The **visual cortex** occupies the upper and lower lips of the calcarine sulcus on the medial surface of the cerebral hemisphere. The area is much larger than suggested by cortical maps because of the depth of the calcarine sulcus. The visual cortex is thin, heterotypical cortex of the granular type (area 17 of Brodmann); it is marked by the line of Gennari and is known alternatively as the **striate area**. There is a detailed point-to-point projection of the retina on the lateral geniculate body and on the visual cortex. The size of the retinal point is reduced to the diameter of a single cone for most acute vision in the central part of the fovea. Precise coordination of movements of the eyes ensures that the retinal patterns of excitation correspond with one another, as required for binocular vision. The **visual association cortex**, corresponding to areas 18 and 19 of Brodmann, is involved in recognition of objects, perception of color and depth, and other complex aspects of vision. Even more complex visual processing occurs in the temporal lobe, whose inferolateral surface is involved in interpreting, remembering, and recalling formed images. The organization of the visual cortex into columns of cells was reviewed in Chapter 14.

Visual Defects Caused by Interruption of the Pathway

Certain general rules governing defects in the visual field as a result of lesions in the visual pathway are indicated in Figure 20-8. The first example is an obvious one: Severe degenerative disease or injury involving an optic nerve results in blindness in the corresponding eye. Multiple sclerosis, in which central axons lose their my-

elin sheaths, can produce this effect. Example 2 refers to interruption of decussating fibers in the optic chiasma, which causes bitemporal hemianopsia if the full thickness of the chiasma is interrupted. The lesion that most commonly affects the optic chiasma is a pituitary tumor pressing on it from below. This first interrupts fibers from the inferior nasal quadrants of both retinas. The visual defect begins as a scotoma in each upper temporal quadrant of the visual field and spreads throughout the temporal fields as the chiasma is increasingly affected. Pressure on the lateral edge of the optic chiasma (example 3) happens rarely, but it may occur when there is an aneurysm of the internal carotid artery in this location. The field defect, in

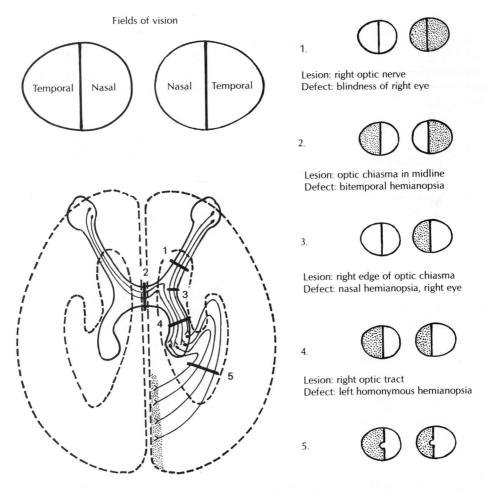

Fields of vision

1.
Lesion: right optic nerve
Defect: blindness of right eye

2.
Lesion: optic chiasma in midline
Defect: bitemporal hemianopsia

3.
Lesion: right edge of optic chiasma
Defect: nasal hemianopsia, right eye

4.
Lesion: right optic tract
Defect: left homonymous hemianopsia

5.

Figure 20-8. Visual field defects caused by lesions that affect different parts of the visual pathway.

the case of pressure on the right edge of the chiasma, is nasal hemianopsia for the right eye. Interruption of the right optic tract (example 4) causes left homonymous hemianopsia.

Example 5 refers to a lesion that involves the geniculocalcarine tract or the visual cortex. An extensive right-sided lesion results in left homonymous hemianopsia, except that central vision may remain intact (macular sparing). Decussating fibers that would provide bilateral cortical representation of the macula are lacking, and it is likely that a slight shifting of the patient's fixation or gaze during examination of the visual fields is responsible for the phenomenon known as macular sparing. Lesions that affect only a portion of the geniculocalcarine tract or the visual cortex cause field defects of lesser proportions than hemianopsia. An example is provided by the upper quadrantic defect in the opposite visual field after interruption of fibers comprising Meyer's loop in the white matter of the temporal lobe.

It is important to remember that defects in the visual field can result from lesions of the eye as well as of the central pathways or cortex. For example, chronic glaucoma and senile degeneration of the macula are common conditions that result in areas of blindness in the center of the field, often bilaterally.

Visual Reflexes

A small bundle of fibers from the optic tract bypasses the lateral geniculate body and enters the **superior brachium**. These fibers, which constitute the afferent limb of reflex arcs, terminate in the **pretectal area** and in the **superior colliculus**.

The **pupillary light reflex** is tested in the routine neurological examination; the response consists of constriction of the pupil when light, as from a pen flashlight, is directed into the eye. Impulses from the retina impinge on the pretectal area, which is immediately rostral to the superior colliculus. Impulses are relayed to the Edinger-Westphal nucleus of the oculomotor complex, then to the ciliary ganglion in the orbit, and finally to the sphincter pupillae muscle in the iris (see Fig. 8-6). Both pupils constrict in response to light entering one eye because (a) each retina sends fibers into the optic tracts of both sides and (b) the pretectal area sends some fibers across the midline in the posterior commissure to the contralateral Edinger-Westphal nucleus.

Visual signals from the retina that reach the superior colliculus collaborate with input from the occipital cortex, frontal eye field, and spinal cord, which are the sources of most of the afferent fibers to the colliculus. The layered cytoarchitecture of the superior colliculus together with its diverse sources of afferent fibers indicate that considerable integrative activity occurs in the region. Efferent fibers go to the accessory oculomotor nuclei, paramedian pontine reticular formation, and pretectal area, and a few descend to the cervical segments of the spinal cord. This last pathway is known as the tectospinal tract.

The functions of the retinal afferents of the superior colliculus cannot be easily separated from the functions of the other afferents. The efferent fibers to the accessory oculomotor nuclei and to the paramedian pontine reticular formation are part of the pathway for control of both **voluntary and involuntary movement of the eyes**, as described in Chapter 8. An indirect connection to the Edinger-Westphal nucleus by way of the pretectal area controls the contractions of the ciliary and sphincter pupillae muscles in accommodation (see below). The importance of the small tectospinal tract is not known, but this pathway is thought to influence movements of the head as required for fixation of gaze.

When attention is directed to a near object, **accommodation**, or the **accommodation-convergence reaction**, consists of three events: ocular convergence, pupillary constriction, and thickening of the lens. The reflex is tested by asking the subject to examine an object held about 30 cm in front of the eyes after looking into the distance, and noting whether or not there is pupillary constriction. When attention is directed to a near object, the medial recti muscles contract for convergence of the eyes. At the same time, contraction of the ciliary muscle allows the lens to thicken, increasing its refractive power, and pupillary constriction sharpens the image on the retina.

For accommodation to near objects, instructions from the visual association cortex reach the midbrain through fibers traversing the superior brachium and terminating in the superior colliculus. The subsequent connections to the nuclei of those cranial nerves that supply the extraocular muscles and to the Edinger-Westphal nucleus have already been described. The frontal eye field, which is necessary for voluntary conjugate movements of the eyes, is not involved in convergence. The pathways for constriction of the pupil in the light and accommodation reflexes are known to be different because they may be dissociated by disease. This occurs, for example, in central nervous system syphilis, in which there is loss of pupillary constriction in response to light but not to accommodation (the **Argyll Robertson pupil**). The lesion that causes dissociation of the responses typically is in the pretectal area, but cases have been described in which there was no abnormality in this part of the midbrain. The small size and slight irregularity of the Argyll Robertson pupil are probably caused by local disease of the iris.

There is **dilation of the pupils** in response to severe pain or strong emotional states. The pathway is presumed to begin with fibers from the amygdala, hippocampal formation, and hypothalamus, which influence the intermediolateral cell column of the spinal cord. The pathway continues to the superior cervical ganglion of the sympathetic trunk, and it is completed by postganglionic fibers in the carotid plexus to the dilator pupillae muscle in the iris (see Ch. 24). At the same time, the parasympathetic supply to the sphincter pupillae muscle is inhibited.

Other Optic Connections

Results of experimental investigations in animals have revealed that the axons of retinal ganglion cells end in several parts of the brain in addition to the lateral geniculate body, pretectal area, and superior colliculus.

The **retinohypothalamic tract** is formed by collateral branches of optic axons that leave the dorsal surface of the optic chiasma and terminate in the suprachiasmatic nucleus of the hypothalamus. The visual input synchronizes the circadian rhythm of the firing pattern of the neurons of the suprachiasmatic nucleus with the changes in ambient illumination. This is responsible for the influence of different levels of illumination on the antigonadotrophic activity of the pineal gland; in some animals, the retinohypothalamic tract regulates seasonal changes in the secretion of pituitary gonadotrophins.

The **accessory optic tract** consists of small fascicles that pass from the optic tract into the cerebral peduncle. They end in various small nuclei in the tegmentum of the midbrain. These nuclei project, both directly and through synaptic relays in the inferior olivary complex, to the flocculonodular lobe of the cerebellum. (The principal input to this part of the cerebellum is from the vestibular system.) The connections indicate that the accessory optic tract may be involved in coordination of movements of the eyes and head.

Some optic axons end in thalamic nuclei other than the lateral geniculate body. The main area of termination of such fibers is the **pulvinar**, which projects to the cortex of the occipital lobe, including the visual areas. The function of this alternative pathway from the retina to the cerebral cortex is not yet understood, but there is evidence in animals that it may permit some residue of conscious vision after destruction of the lateral geniculate body. The human condition known as **blindsight** occasionally is seen in patients with destructive lesions of the geniculostriate pathways. Despite the complete lack of conscious vision, behavioral tests can detect the perception of movements or of changes in illumination.

As is the case with other sensory systems, there are fibers that pass in directions opposite to those of the main flow of incoming visual information. Thus the primary and associational visual cortices project to the lateral geniculate body and pulvinar. There is now evidence for the existence of centrifugal fibers in the optic nerve in some mammals. They come from the pretectal area and from the ventral part of the hypothalamus. Equivalent fibers are well known in birds and fishes, in which they terminate among the amacrine cells of the retina.

SUGGESTED READING

Borwein B: The retinal receptor. A description. In Enoch JM (ed): Optics of Vertebrate Retinal Receptors, ch 2. Berlin, Springer-Verlag, 1982

Cowey A, Stoerig P: The neurobiology of blindsight. Trends Neurosci 14:140–145, 1991

Crooks J, Kolb H: Localization of GABA, glycine, glutamate and tyrosine hydroxylase in the human retina. J Comp Neurol 315:287–302, 1992

Elkington AR, Inman C, Steart PV, Weller RO: The structure of the lamina cribrosa of the human eye: An immunohistochemical and electron microscopical study. Eye 4:42–57, 1990

Haines DE: Neuroanatomy. An Atlas of Structures, Sections and Systems, 3rd ed. Baltimore, Urban & Schwarzenberg, 1991

Hubel DH, Wiesel TN: Brain mechanisms of vision. Sci Am 241:150–162, 1979

Kandel ER, Schwartz JH, Jessel TM (eds): Principles of Neural Science, 3rd ed. New York, Elsevier, 1991

Mariani AP: Biplexiform cells: Ganglion cells of the primate retina that contact photoreceptors. Science 216:1134–1136, 1982

Rodieck RW: Visual pathways. Annu Rev Neurosci 2:193–225, 1975

Van Essen DC: Visual areas of the mammalian cerebral cortex. Annu Rev Neurosci 2:227–263, 1979

Williams RW: The human retina has a cone-enriched rim. Visual Neurosci 6:403–406, 1991

Twenty-One

The Human Nervous System: An Anatomical Viewpoint, Sixth Edition, Murray L. Barr and John A. Kiernan. J.B. Lippincott Company, Philadelphia, © 1993.

Auditory System

Important Facts

The ossicles of the middle ear transfer vibrations from the air to the perilymph. Movement of the ossicles is restrained by the tensor tympani and stapedius muscles, innervated by cranial nerves V and VII, respectively.

The oscillations of the basilar membrane are detected by the inner and outer hair cells of the organ of Corti.

The outer hair cells respond with movement, which is transmitted to the tectorial membrane and thence to the inner hair cells, increasing the sensitivity of the latter to sound.

The inner hair cells respond by releasing their excitatory transmitter and stimulating the sensory terminals of the cochlear division of cranial nerve VIII.

The primary sensory neurons have their somata in the spiral ganglion of the cochlea. Their axons end in the dorsal and ventral cochlear nuclei.

Axons from the dorsal cochlear nucleus cross the midline, travel rostrally in the lateral lemniscus, and end in the inferior colliculus.

Axons from the ventral cochlear nucleus end in the superior olivary nuclei of both sides. The neurons in the superior olivary nucleus have axons that travel in the lateral lemniscus and end in the inferior colliculus.

The inferior colliculus projects (through the inferior brachium) to the medial geniculate body, which projects to the primary auditory area of the cerebral cortex.

The primary auditory cortex is on the superior surface of the temporal lobe. It is connected with auditory association cortex of the superior temporal gyrus and nearby parts of the parietal lobe.

Descending pathways modify transmission in the central auditory system. The sensitivity of the organ of Corti is actively inhibited by efferent (olivocochlear) fibers in the cochlear nerve. These inhibit both the outer hair cells and the sensory terminals.

Destructive lesions rostral to the cochlear nuclei do not cause unilateral deafness.

Hearing is second in importance among the special senses of humans, yielding first place only to sight. Their role in language accounts, to a large extent, for the reliance placed on these special senses. The auditory system consists of the external ear, middle ear, cochlea of the internal ear, cochlear nerve, and pathways in the central nervous system.

External and Middle Ear

The external ear consists of the auricle or pinna and the external acoustic meatus, with the latter being separated from the middle ear by the tympanic membrane. The function of the external ear is to collect sound waves, which cause a resonant vibration of the tympanic membrane. The vibration is transmitted across the middle ear cavity by a chain of three ossicles—the malleus, incus, and stapes. The malleus is attached to the tympanic membrane and articulates with the incus, which articulates in turn with the stirrup-shaped stapes. The foot plate of the stapes occupies the fenestra vestibuli (oval window) in the wall between the middle and internal ears; the rim of the foot plate is attached to the margin of the fenestra vestibuli by the annular ligament, composed of elastic connective tissue. The ossicles constitute a bent lever with the longer of the two arms attached to the tympanic membrane, and the area of the foot plate of the stapes is considerably less than the area of the tympanic membrane. The vibratory force of the tympanic membrane is, therefore, magnified about 15 times at the fenestra vestibuli; the substantial increase in force is important because the sound waves are transferred from air to a liquid. Protection against the effect of sudden, excessive noise is provided by reflex contraction of the tensor tympani and stapedius muscles, which are inserted on the malleus and stapes, respectively.

Inner Ear

The internal ear, which has a dual function, consists of the **membranous labyrinth** encased in the **bony labyrinth**. Certain parts of the internal ear contain sensory areas for the vestibular system, which is discussed in Chapter 22. The cochlear portion of the internal ear contains the organ of Corti (spiral organ), from which nerve impulses arise as a result of the sound waves produced in the fluid in the cochlea by vibration of the stapes. The nerve impulses are conducted to the brain stem by the cochlear division of the vestibulocochlear nerve, reaching the auditory area of the cerebral cortex through several synaptic relays, or causing reflex responses through connections in the brain stem. Although this chapter is concerned primarily with the organ of Corti and the central pathways, the main features of the bony and membranous labyrinths are reviewed as an aid in understanding how vibration of the stapes results in stimulation of sensory cells in the organ of Corti and initiation of nerve impulses traveling to the brain.

BONY AND MEMBRANOUS LABYRINTHS

The bony labyrinth (Fig. 21-1) is in the petrous portion of the temporal bone, which forms a prominent oblique ridge between the middle and posterior cranial fossae. The labyrinth is a system of tunnels within the bone. A preparation such as that represented in Figure 21-1 is made by chipping away the surrounding cancellous bone until only the walls of the tunnels (which are of compact bone) remain. The **fenestra vestibuli** (oval window), in which the foot plate of the stapes fits, is in the wall of the **vestibule**, the middle part of the bony labyrinth. The **fenestra cochleae** (round window) is below the fenestra vestibuli; it is closed by a thin membrane that makes pressure waves possible in the fluid in the internal ear. The fluid would otherwise be completely enclosed in a rigid "box," except for the source of the waves at the fenestra vestibuli. Three **semicircular canals** extend posterolaterally from the vestibule, and the **cochlea** constitutes the anteromedial portion of the bony labyrinth. The cochlea has the shape of a snail shell; its base abuts against the deep end of the internal acoustic meatus, which opens into the posterior cranial fossa.

Nerve fibers emerging from the base of the

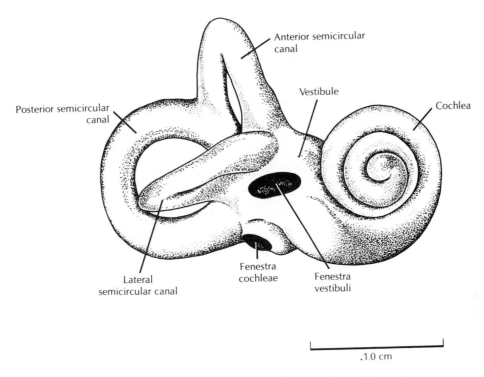

Figure 21-1. Anterolateral view of the right bony labyrinth.

cochlea constitute the cochlear nerve, whereas fibers concerned with the vestibular portion of the internal ear constitute the vestibular nerve. The two divisions of the **vestibulocochlear nerve** leave the internal acoustic meatus and are attached to the brain stem at the junction of the medulla and pons. Within the internal meatus, the vestibulocochlear nerve is accompanied by the two divisions of the facial nerve (see Ch. 8) and the **labyrinthine vessels**. The labyrinthine artery is a branch of either the anterior inferior cerebellar or the basilar artery (see Ch. 25). The labyrinthine vein accompanies the artery and drains into the superior petrosal sinus (see Ch. 26).

The delicate membranous labyrinth conforms, for the most part, to the contours of the bony labyrinth (Fig. 21-2). There are, however, two dilations, the **utricle** and the **saccule**, in the vestibule of the bony labyrinth. Three **semicircular ducts** arise from the utricle. There is a patch of sensory epithelium supplied by the vestibular nerve on the inner surface of the utricle, the saccule, and each semicircular duct. The saccule is continuous with the **cochlear duct** through a narrow channel known as the **ductus reuniens**. The cochlear duct contains a highly specialized strip of sensory epithelium along its entire length; this is the organ of Corti (spiral organ), the end organ for hearing.

The lumen of the membranous labyrinth is continuous throughout and filled with **endolymph**, whereas the interval between the membranous and bony labyrinths is filled with **perilymph**. The vestibular portion of the membranous labyrinth is suspended within the bony labyrinth by trabeculae of connective tissue. The cochlear duct is firmly attached along two sides to the wall of the cochlear canal.

COCHLEA

The **cochlear canal** makes two and one-half turns around a bony pillar or core, the **modiolus**, in which there are channels for nerve fibers and blood vessels. The cochlea is most conveniently

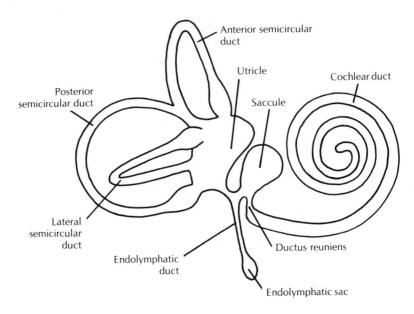

Figure 21-2. Anterolateral view of the right membranous labyrinth.

described as if it were resting on its base (Fig. 21-3), although its base in fact faces posteromedially.

The cochlear canal, the cavity of this portion of the bony labyrinth, is divided by two partitions into three spiral spaces. The middle of these is the **cochlear duct** (scala media): that is, the portion of the membranous labyrinth within the cochlea, which contains endolymph. The cochlear duct is firmly fixed to the inner and outer walls of the cochlear canal. The remaining spiral spaces are the **scala vestibuli** and the **scala tympani**, which contain perilymph. The unspecialized wall of the cochlear duct apposing the scala vestibuli is called the **vestibular** or **Reissner's membrane**, whereas the wall apposing the scala tympani constitutes the specialized **basilar membrane**, on which the organ of Corti rests.

The basilar membrane is of special importance in the physiology of hearing because it responds to vibration of the stapes in the following manner. As shown in Figure 21-4, vibration of the foot plate of the stapes produces corresponding waves in the perilymph, beginning with that of the vestibule. The vestibule opens into the scala vestibuli, which communicates with the scala tympani through a small aperture, the **helicotrema**, at the apex of the cochlea. The sound waves may be thought of as passing along the scala vestibuli and into the scala tympani through the helicotrema, causing vibration of the basilar membrane from the scala tympani. However, the helicotrema is a minute orifice, and it is more likely that the basilar membrane vibrates in response to sound waves transmitted through the endolymph in the cochlear duct from the scala vestibuli to the scala tympani. These same waves create a vibration of the membrane closing the fenestra cochleae at the base of the scala tympani; this is essential to eliminate the damping of pressure waves that would otherwise occur in bone-encased fluid.

The scala vestibuli and scala tympani are lined by a single layer of squamous cells of mesenchymal origin, with this layer resting on periosteum where the scalae are bounded by the bony labyrinth. The perilymph filling the scala vestibuli and scala tympani is a watery fluid, similar in composition to cerebrospinal fluid. In fact, there is a communication between the perilymph-filled spaces of the bony labyrinth and the subarachnoid space. It consists of a narrow channel in the petrous portion of the temporal bone, extending from the scala tympani in the basal turn of the cochlea to an extension of the subarachnoid space around cranial nerves IX, X, and XI as they traverse the jugular foramen.

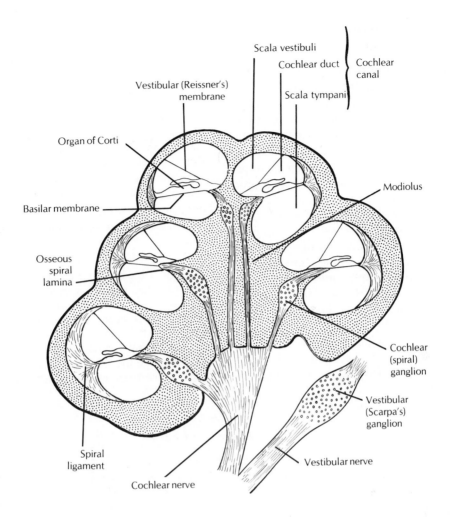

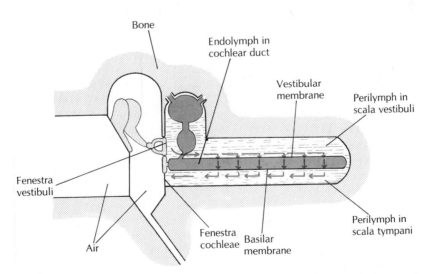

Figure 21-4. Schematic representation of the manner in which sound waves in the perilymph and endolymph cause vibration of the basilar membrane.

The **cochlear** or **spiral ganglion** consists of cells in a spiral configuration at the periphery of the modiolus (see Fig. 21-3). The primary sensory neurons of both divisions of the vestibulocochlear nerve are bipolar, rather than unipolar as in other cerebrospinal nerves, retaining this embryonic characteristic of primary sensory neurons. The peripheral processes are dendrites in the sense of conduction toward the cell bodies, but in all other characteristics, they are axons. These processes reach the organ of Corti by traversing openings in the osseous spiral lamina projecting from the modiolus, where myelin sheaths terminate. The central processes (axons) traverse channels in the modiolus, enter the internal acoustic meatus from the base of the cochlea, and continue in the cochlear division of the vestibulocochlear nerve. There is a small anastomotic connection between the vestibular and cochlear nerves within the external acoustic meatus. As will be seen, this carries efferent nerve fibers to the cochlea.

COCHLEAR DUCT

Certain specialized regions in the wall of the cochlear duct are now described (Fig. 21-5). The organ of Corti is considered separately because of its complex structure and importance as the receptor of acoustic stimuli.

Vibration of the **basilar membrane** is essential in the transduction of a mechanical stimulus (sound waves) to the electrical potential of a nerve impulse in the organ of Corti. The inner edge of the basilar membrane is attached to the **osseous spiral lamina**, which projects from the modiolus like the thread on a screw. The outer edge of the membrane is attached to the **spiral**

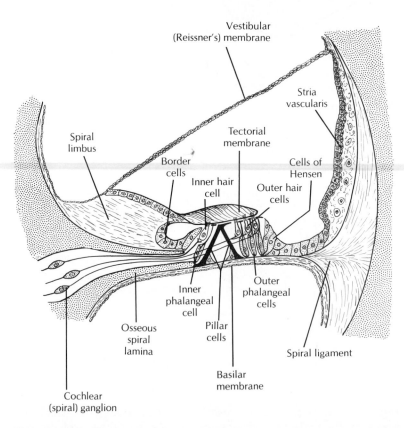

Figure 21-5. Structure of the cochlear duct and spiral organ (organ of Corti).

ligament, which is a thickening of the periosteum along the outer wall of the cochlear canal. The basilar membrane consists of collagen fibers and sparse elastic fibers embedded in a ground substance, with most of the fibers being directed across the membrane. The surface presenting to the scala tympani is covered by a thin layer of vascular connective tissue and a single layer of squamous cells. The width of the basilar membrane steadily increases from the beginning of the basal turn of the cochlea to the apex; this is made possible by a progressive narrowing of the osseous spiral lamina and spiral ligament in the same direction. The width of the membrane at any point determines the pitch of sound to which it responds maximally. *High tones, therefore, cause maximal vibration in the basal turn of the cochlea and low tones near the apex.* The range of audible frequencies in the human ear is from 20 to 20,000 Hz. The range extends over 11 octaves, of which 7 are used in musical instruments such as the piano. Ordinary conversation falls within the range of 300 to 3000 Hz. With advancing age, there is a gradual decrease in perception of high frequencies.

Persistent exposure to loud sounds causes degenerative changes in the organ of Corti at the base of the cochlea. This results in high-tone deafness, which is prone to occur in workers exposed to the sound of compression engines or jet engines and in those working for long hours on farm tractors. High-tone deafness formerly was encountered most frequently among workmen in boiler factories and is still sometimes called "boiler-makers' disease."

The **vestibular** or **Reissner's membrane** consists of two layers of simple squamous epithelium separated by a trace of connective tissue.

The outer wall of the cochlear duct is specialized as the **stria vascularis**, which consists of cuboidal epithelium overlying vascular connective tissue and produces endolymph. This is similar to intracellular fluid in respect to its high concentration of potassium ions and low concentration of sodium ions. Endolymph fills the membranous labyrinth; absorption takes place into venules surrounding the endolymphatic sac in the dura mater on the posterior surface of the petrous portion of the temporal bone. This sac is an expansion of the endolymphatic duct arising from the communication between the saccule and the utricle (see Fig. 21-2).

The epithelial lining of the membranous labyrinth, including the specialized sensory areas for the auditory and vestibular systems, is ectodermal in origin. The epithelium differentiates from the cells lining the **otic vesicle**. This is formed by an invagination of ectoderm at the level of the hindbrain of the early embryo.

ORGAN OF CORTI

The **organ of Corti** or **spiral organ** (see Fig. 21-5) consists of supporting cells and sensory cells. The latter are specialized for conversion of mechanical stimuli into the ionic and electrical events that constitute nerve impulses.

Supporting cells containing bundles of tonofibrils are of two types, pillar cells and phalangeal cells. There are two rows of **pillar cells**, inner and outer, on each side of the **tunnel of Corti**. The number in each row is of the order of 5000. Each cell consists mainly of a compact bundle of tonofibrils (the pillar), extending from the basilar membrane to the surface of the organ of Corti. The tonofibrils appear in electron micrographs as compact arrays of microtubules. The inner and outer pillars converge, and each pillar ends in a flange directed outward. The nucleus of the pillar cell is in a cytoplasmic region in the acute angle between the pillar and the basilar membrane.

The **phalangeal cells** afford intimate support for the sensory cells; they are arranged as a single row of inner phalangeal cells and three to five rows of outer phalangeal cells, with the number of rows increasing from the base to the apex of the cochlea. The base of the slender, flask-shaped phalangeal cell rests on the basilar membrane, and a bundle of tonofibrils extends the length of the cell. Some of the tonofibrils form a supporting shelf for the base of a sensory cell, and the remainder continue alongside a sensory cell. At the surface of the organ of Corti, the tonofibrils of phalangeal and pillar cells form a thin reticular plate in which holes accommodate the ends of sensory cells. The organ of Corti is completed on the inner side by **border cells** and on the outer side by **cells of Hensen**. The fluid in the tunnel of Corti and the interstitial fluid in much of the organ of Corti have a chemical composition similar to that of perilymph rather than endolymph. The high concentration of potassium ions in endolymph would prevent impulse conduction by the nerve fibers crossing the tunnel of Corti to reach the outer hair cells.

The **tectorial membrane** is a ribbon-like structure of gelatinous consistency; it is attached to the **spiral limbus**, a thickening of the periosteum on the osseous spiral lamina. The tectorial membrane extends over the organ of Corti, and the tips of the hairs of the outer hair cells are embedded in the membrane.

The sensory cells are called **hair cells** because of the hair-like projections from their free ends. There is a single row of inner hair cells, numbering about 7000; the outer hair cells, of which there are about 25,000, are arranged in three rows in the basal turn of the cochlea, increasing to five rows at the apex. The hairs project from the cell along a V- or W-shaped line, with their tips embedded in the tectorial membrane. The number of hairs per cell ranges from 50 to 150, with the largest number on hair cells at the base of the cochlea and the smallest number on cells at the apex. The hairs are microvilli of an unusual type. The **inner hair cells** are the principal sensory elements. Each one synapses with the dendrites of up to 10 rapidly conducting neurons whose myelinated axons make up at least 90% of the fibers of the cochlear nerve. No neuron is contacted by more than one inner hair cell. The **outer hair cells** synapse with branches of unmyelinated axons, which account for 5% to 10% of the fibers of the cochlear nerve. The zone of outer hair cells receives most of the efferent fibers of the cochlear nerve, which are described later. The outer hair cells are motile. Their microvilli move in response to transduced sound and produce corresponding vibrations of the tectorial membrane. This has the effect of lowering the threshold of excitation of the inner hair cells.

The cochlear nerve contains cholinergic **efferent fibers** that originate in the superior olivary nuclei in the pons. These axons terminate on the outer hair cells (where their synaptic terminals outnumber those of the afferent fibers) and on the preterminal parts of the sensory neurites that innervate the inner hair cells. The efferent axons are inhibitory to both the receptor cells and the sensory fibers. Inhibition of the outer hair cells reduces the amplitude of the vibrations of the tectorial membrane, thereby raising the threshold of excitation of the inner hair cells. Thus the efferent fibers of the cochlear nerve reduce the sensitivity of the ear.

It is basic to the physiology of the cochlea that a particular region of the basilar membrane, depending on the pitch of sound, responds by maximal vibration. Bending of the hairs reduces the membrane potential of the hair cells, causing increased release of their chemical transmitter and initiation of action potentials in the sensory nerve endings. Regardless of the pitch of sound, vibration of the basilar membrane begins at the base of the cochlea and travels along the membrane with increasing magnitude to a point determined by the pitch. At this point, the vibration suddenly dies away, and impulses reaching the brain from the place of maximal stimulation of the organ of Corti are interpreted as a particular pitch of sound. Increase in intensity of sound causes maximal vibration in a larger region of the basilar membrane, thereby activating more hair cells and neurons. Tonotopic localization is sharpened by the inhibitory effect of efferent fibers in the cochlear nerve and by feedback circuits in the central pathway to the auditory cortex.

Auditory Pathways

The **cochlear nerve** consists principally of axons or central processes of cells in the spiral ganglion, most of which are myelinated. It traverses the internal acoustic meatus in the petrous part of the temporal bone alongside the vestibular nerve. On emerging from the meatus, the cochlear nerve continues to the junction of the medulla and pons. The afferent fibers then bifurcate, one branch ending in the **dorsal cochlear nucleus** and the other branch in the **ventral cochlear nucleus** (Fig. 21-6). The cochlear nuclei are situated

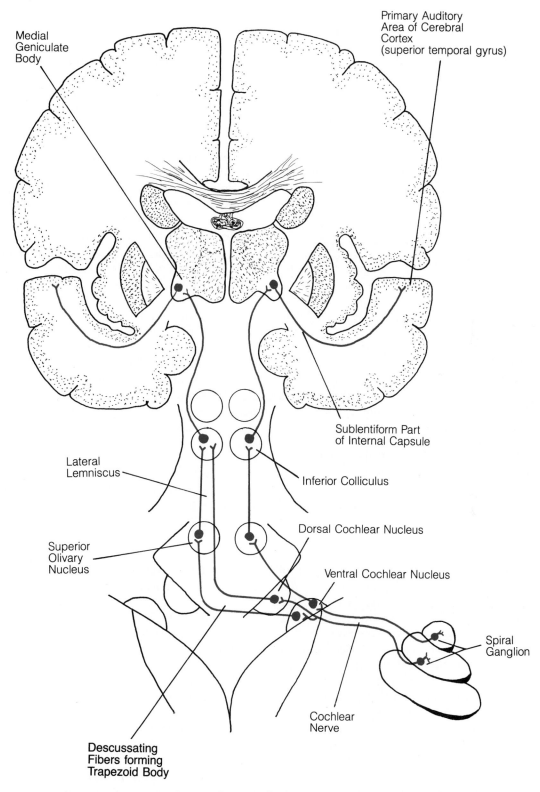

Figure 21-6. Ascending auditory pathway. (*With permission from Kiernan JA: Introduction to Human Neuroscience, p 119. Philadelphia, JB Lippincott, 1987*)

superficially in the rostral end of the medulla adjacent to the base of the inferior cerebellar peduncle (see Fig. 7-7). A tonotopic pattern of axonal endings has been demonstrated in both nuclei in laboratory animals and probably exists in humans. The dorsal and ventral cochlear nuclei differ in cellular organization, and the pattern of axonal endings in the ventral nucleus is more precise than that in the dorsal nucleus. The nuclei also differ in their contributions to the central pathways.

PATHWAY TO THE AUDITORY CORTEX

The pathway to the cerebral cortex is characterized by one or more synaptic relays between the cochlear nuclei and the specific thalamic nucleus for hearing, the medial geniculate body (see Fig. 21-6). There is a relay in the inferior colliculus, and additional synaptic interruptions may occur in the superior olivary nucleus and in the nucleus of the lateral lemniscus. The pathway also is characterized by a significant ipsilateral projection to the cortex. In view of the complicated nature of the pathway, the transmission of acoustic data to the cortex can best be described after certain components of the pathway in the brain stem have been identified.

The **superior olivary nucleus** is in the ventrolateral corner of the tegmentum of the pons at the level of the motor nucleus of the facial nerve (see Fig. 7-8). (Although considered here as a unit, the nucleus is a complex of four nuclei, whose connections differ in detail.) Auditory fibers that cross the pons in the ventral part of the tegmentum constitute the **trapezoid body**; these fibers pass ventral to the ascending fibers of the medial lemniscus or intersect them. Nerve cells situated among the transverse fibers on each side constitute the nucleus of the trapezoid body, which is the most medially situated nucleus of the superior olivary complex. (Strands of decussating auditory fibers located more dorsally in the tegmentum are named the ventral and dorsal acoustic striae, but they are not easily seen in sections of the brain stem.) The **lateral lemniscus**, the ascending auditory tract, extends from the region of the superior olivary nucleus,

through the lateral part of the pontine tegmentum, and close to the surface of the brain stem in the isthmus region between the pons and midbrain (see Fig. 7-9). The **nucleus of the lateral lemniscus** consists of cells situated among the fibers of the tract in the pons.

The projection from the cochlear nuclei to the inferior colliculus and then to the medial geniculate nucleus, through the components of the pathway just identified, is as follows (see Fig. 21-6). Fibers from the **ventral cochlear nucleus** proceed to the region of the ipsilateral superior olivary nucleus, in which some of the fibers terminate. The majority continue across the pons, with a slight forward slope; these fibers, together with others contributed by the superior olivary nucleus, constitute the trapezoid body. On reaching the region of the superior olivary nucleus on the other side of the brain stem, the fibers either continue into the lateral lemniscus or terminate in the superior olivary nucleus, from which fibers are added to the lateral lemniscus. Fibers from the **dorsal cochlear nucleus** pass over the base of the inferior cerebellar peduncle, continue obliquely to the region of the contralateral superior olivary nucleus, and then turn rostrally in the lateral lemniscus. They end in the inferior colliculus.

Impulses conveyed by the lateral lemniscus reach the **inferior colliculus** in the midbrain with or without a synaptic relay in the nucleus of the lateral lemniscus (not shown in Fig. 21-6). The complexity of neuronal organization in the inferior colliculus indicates that, far from being a simple relay station, it is capable of complex integrative activity. Fibers from the inferior colliculus traverse the inferior brachium and end in the **medial geniculate body**. The termination of axons in the ventral part of the medial geniculate nucleus of laboratory animals produces a spiral tonotopic pattern that corresponds to the spiral of the cochlea, and a similar pattern probably is present in humans.

The last link in the auditory pathway consists of the **auditory radiation** in the sublentiform part of the internal capsule, through which the medial geniculate body projects on the **auditory cortex** of the temporal lobe. This primary auditory area, corresponding to areas 41 and 42 of Brodmann, is in the floor of the lateral sulcus, extending only slightly onto the lateral surface of the hemisphere. A landmark is provided by the anterior transverse temporal gyri (Heschl's convolutions) on the dorsal surface of the superior temporal gyrus (see Fig. 15-3). The area receives afferent fibers from the tonotopically organized ventral part of the medial geniculate body. The tonotopic pattern in the auditory area is such that fibers for sounds of low frequency end in the anterolateral part of the area, whereas fibers for sounds of high frequency terminate in its posteromedial part. Analysis of acoustic stimuli at a higher neural level, notably the recognition and interpretation of sounds on the basis of past experience, occurs in the auditory association cortex of the temporal lobe (Wernicke's area). In addition to its afferents from the auditory area, the association cortex also receives projections from regions of the medial geniculate nucleus other than from its tonotopically organized ventral part. Wernicke's area, it will be recalled, makes an important contribution to sensory aspects of language in addition to being auditory association cortex.

Above the level of the cochlear nuclei, the auditory pathway is both crossed and uncrossed because significant numbers of axons ascend in the lateral lemniscus of the same side. In addition, the nuclei of the lateral lemnisci and the inferior colliculi of the two sides are connected by commissural fibers. Consequently any loss of hearing that follows a unilateral cortical lesion is so slight as to make detection difficult in audiometric testing. Most lesions in the vicinity of the auditory cortex also involve Wernicke's area and cause receptive aphasia when the dominant hemisphere for language is involved (see Ch. 15). The latter disability obscures any slight auditory deficiency.

The directions and distances of sources of sound are determined from the discrepancy in time of arrival of the stimulus in the left and right ears. Results obtained from investigations with animals indicate that the different inputs to the brain from the two cochleae are compared and analyzed in the superior olivary nuclei, although the auditory cortex is necessary if the coded information transmitted rostrally from the medulla is to have any meaning. The severest loss of ability to judge the sources of sounds is that caused by unilateral deafness resulting from disease of the ear. The condition is equivalent to the loss of binocular vision that results from blindness in one eye.

DESCENDING FIBERS IN THE AUDITORY PATHWAY

Parallel with the neurons conducting information from the organ of Corti to the auditory cortex, there are descending and efferent neurons that conduct impulses in the reverse direction. The descending connections consist of the following: corticogeniculate fibers, which originate in the auditory and adjoining cortical areas and terminate in all parts of the medial geniculate body; cortico-collicular fibers, from the same cortical areas to the inferior colliculi of both sides; colliculo-olivary fibers, from the inferior colliculus to the superior olivary nucleus; and colliculo-cochleonuclear fibers, from the inferior colliculus to the dorsal and ventral cochlear nuclei. Except for the cortico-collicular projection, which includes both crossed and uncrossed fibers, these descending pathways are ipsilateral.

As indicated earlier, control also is exerted by the central nervous system over the initiation of nerve impulses in the organ of Corti. Olivocochlear fibers, constituting the **olivocochlear bundle** (of Rasmussen), originate in the superior olivary nuclei. The axons leave the brain stem in the vestibular division of the vestibulocochlear nerve and then cross over into the cochlear division by forming an anastomotic branch, located in the internal acoustic meatus. The endings of these inhibitory fibers, which contain synaptic vesicles, are applied to the outer hair cells and to the terminal parts of the afferent neurites that supply the inner hair cells. The efferent fibers for the outer hair cells originate in both superior olivary nuclei, whereas those for neurites that supply inner hair cells come from the ipsilateral nucleus only.

The central transmission of data from the sensory hair cells is, therefore, far more than just a relay to the cortex. In the various cell stations of the pathway, there is a complex processing of acoustic data that provides for refinement of such qualities as pitch, timbre, and volume of sound perception. In particular, feedback inhibition sharpens the perception of pitch, especially through the olivocochlear bundle. This is accomplished by inhibition in the organ of Corti except for the region in which the basilar membrane is responding by maximal vibration to a particular frequency of sound waves (auditory sharpening). Central inhibition probably suppresses background noise when attention is being concentrated on a particular sound.

REFLEXES

A few acoustic fibers from the inferior colliculus pass forward to the superior colliculus, which influences motor neurons of the cervical region of the spinal cord through the tectospinal tract. The superior colliculus also influences neurons of the oculomotor, trochlear, and abducens nuclei through indirect connections in the brain stem. These pathways provide for reflex turning of the head and eyes toward the source of a sudden loud sound.

Fibers from the superior olivary nucleus, and probably from the nucleus of the lateral lemniscus, terminate in the motor nuclei of the trigeminal and facial nerves for reflex contraction of the tensor tympani and stapedius muscles, respectively. Contraction of these muscles in response to loud sounds reduces the vibration of the tympanic membrane and the stapes.

SUGGESTED READING

Altschuler RA, Bobbin RD, Clopton BM, Hoffman DW (eds): Neurobiology of Hearing: The Central Auditory System. New York, Raven Press, 1991

Celesia GG: Organization of auditory cortical areas in man. Brain 99:403–414, 1976

Clopton BM, Winfield JA, Flammino FJ: Tonotopic organization: Review and analysis. Brain Res 76:1–20, 1974

Kelly JP: Hearing. In Kandel ER, Schwartz JH, Jessell TM (eds): Principles of Neural Science, 3rd ed, pp 258–268. New York, Elsevier-North Holland, 1991

Klinke R, Galley N: Efferent innervation of vestibular and auditory pathways. Physiol Rev 54:316–357, 1974

Lim DJ: Functional structure of the organ of Corti: A review. Hearing Res 22:117–146, 1986

Masterson RB: Neural mechanisms for sound localization. Annu Rev Physiol 46:275–287, 1984

Nadol JB: Synaptic morphology of inner and outer hair cells of the human organ of Corti. J Electron Microsc Tech 15:187–196, 1990

Spoendlin H: Anatomy and physiology of cochlear innervation. Am J Otolaryngol 6:453–467, 1985

Zenner HP: Motile responses in outer hair cells. Hearing Res 22:83–90, 1986

The Human Nervous System: An Anatomical Viewpoint, Sixth Edition, Murray L. Barr and John A. Kiernan. J.B. Lippincott Company, Philadelphia, © 1993.

Twenty-Two

Vestibular System

Important Facts

The receptors in the saccule and utricle respond to the pull of gravity and to inertial movement caused by linear acceleration and deceleration.

The receptors in the ampullae of the semicircular ducts respond to rotation of the head in any plane.

The vestibular hair cells contact dendrites of neurons in the vestibular ganglion. Most of the axons of these neurons end in the vestibular nuclei, but a few go directly to the cerebellum.

Neurons in the vestibular nuclei have axons that end in the vestibulocerebellum (fastigial nucleus and flocculonodular lobe); the nuclei of cranial nerves III, IV, and VI; and the spinal cord. There also is a pathway to the thalamus and cerebral cortex.

Reflex movements of the eyes in response to stimulation of the kinetic labyrinth require the integrity of a reflex arc that includes fibers in the medial longitudinal fasciculus.

Three sources of sensory information are used by the nervous system in the maintenance of equilibrium. They are the eyes, proprioceptive endings throughout the body, and the vestibular apparatus of the internal ear. The role of the vestibular system, especially in relation to visual information, is illustrated by the person who has congenital atresia of the vestibular apparatus, usually accompanied by cochlear atresia and deaf-mutism. Such a person can orient himself satisfactorily by visual guidance but becomes disoriented in the dark or if submerged while swimming. In addition, vestibular impulses caused by motion of the head contribute to appropriate movements of the eyes to maintain fixation on an object in the visual field. These functions require the distribution of nerve impulses from the vestibular labyrinth to motor neurons through pathways in the spinal cord, brain stem, and cerebellum,

and there also is a projection to the cerebral cortex.

The static labyrinth represented by the utricle and saccule detects the position of the head with respect to gravity, whereas the kinetic labyrinth represented by the semicircular ducts detects movement of the head. Both parts of the membranous labyrinth function in the maintenance of equilibrium, and the kinetic labyrinth has a special role in coordination of eye movement with rotation of the head.

Static Labyrinth

The **utricle** and **saccule** are endolymph-containing dilations of the membranous labyrinth, enclosed by the vestibule of the bony labyrinth (see Figs. 21-1 and 21-2). Except at the maculae or specialized sensory areas, the utricle and saccule are lined by simple cuboidal epithelium derived from the otic vesicle of the embryo and supported by a thin layer of connective tissue. The utricle and saccule are suspended from the wall of the vestibule by connective tissue trabeculae, and they are surrounded by a perilymphatic space lined by a single layer of squamous cells of mesenchymal origin.

Each dilation includes a specialized area of sensory epithelium, the macula, about 2 by 3 mm in size. The **macula utriculi** is in the floor of the utricle and parallel with the base of the skull, whereas the **macula sacculi** is vertically disposed on the medial wall of the saccule. The two maculae are histologically identical (Fig. 22-1).

The columnar supporting cells of the maculae are continuous with the cuboidal epithelium that lines the utricle and saccule elsewhere. The sensory **hair cells**, of which two types have been identified in electron micrographs, are somewhat similar to hair cells in the organ of Corti (see Ch. 21). Type 1 hair cells are flask-shaped, whereas type 2 hair cells are cylindrical. From 40 to 80 hairs project from each cell, together with a long cilium (the

kinocilium) that arises from a centriole (Fig. 22-2*A*). The hairs are microvilli of an unusual type, similar to those of hair cells in the organ of Corti except for their greater length, which may be as much as 100 μm. Bundles of the hairs are the **"stereocilia"** of light microscopy. The tips of the hairs and kinocilium are embedded in the gelatinous **otolithic membrane**, in which there are irregularly shaped concretions composed of protein and calcium carbonate. These are variously known as otoliths, otoconia, statoliths, and statoconia.

Although the macula is predominantly a static organ, the higher specific gravity of the otolithic membrane with respect to the endolymph allows the macula to respond to quick, tilting movements of the head and to rapid linear acceleration and deceleration. Motion sickness is initiated by prolonged, fluctuating stimulation of the maculae. The utricle and saccule are not as efficient sensors of orientation in humans as they are in some lower animals. This is illustrated by the pilot flying a small aircraft without the aid of instruments, whose intended level flight through clouds may be altered considerably without the pilot's being aware of it.

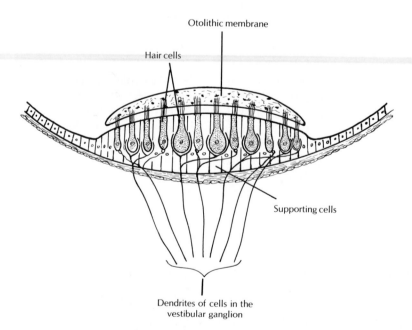

Otolithic membrane

Hair cells

Supporting cells

Dendrites of cells in the vestibular ganglion

Figure 22-1. Structure of the macula utriculi.

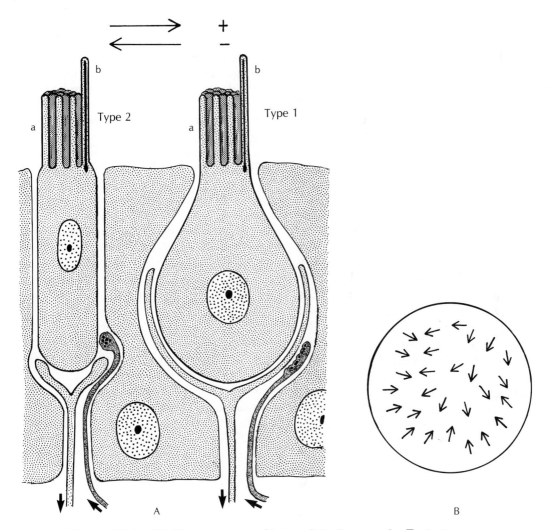

Figure 22-2. (A) The two types of hair cell in the macula. Excitation occurs when the hairs or microvilli (*a*) bend in the direction of the kinocilium (*b*), whereas inhibition of the hair cell occurs when the hairs bend in the opposite direction. (B) Surface of the macula, showing that hair cells in different regions are stimulated and different nerve fibers activated according to the direction of gravitational pull on the otolithic membrane. This pattern is caused by variations in the position of the kinocilium relative to the tuft of hairs from one region of the macula to another. Each arrow indicates the direction of gravitational pull for excitation of the hair cells in that location.

The otoliths give the otolithic membrane a higher specific gravity than the endolymph, thereby causing bending of the hairs in one direction or another except when the macula is in a strictly horizontal plane. The detailed sensory output of the macula is, however, quite complicated. In each hair cell, the kinocilium is situated at one side of the tuft of hairs, and the position of the kinocilium at the periphery of the hairs differs from one region of the macula to another. The hair cells are excited when the hairs and the kinocilium are bent in the direction of the kinocilium, and they are inhibited when the deflection is in the opposite direction (see Fig. 22-2*A*). The pattern of afferent impulses conducted by the fibers of the vestibular nerve to the vestibular nuclei and the cerebellum differs, therefore, according to the orientation of the macula to the direction of gravitational pull (see Fig. 22-2*B*). The appropriate changes in muscle tonus follow, as required to maintain equilibrium.

The cell bodies of the primary sensory neurons are in the **vestibular ganglion** (Scarpa's ganglion), situated at the bottom of the internal acoustic meatus. The peripheral processes, which are dendrites in the sense of conduction toward the cell body but are otherwise like axons, enter the maculae and end on the hair cells. The nerve terminals on type 1 hair cells take the form of chalice-like branches surrounding the cells, whereas minute terminal swellings make the synaptic contact with type 2 hair cells. In addition, efferent fibers in the vestibular nerve end as presynaptic terminals on the type 2 hair cells and on the sensory nerve endings that contact the type 1 cells. These inhibitory fibers, which are cholinergic, originate from a group of neurons in the caudal part of the pons, lateral to the abducens nucleus and medial to the superior and medial vestibular nuclei.

Kinetic Labyrinth

The three semicircular ducts are attached to the utricle and are enclosed in the semicircular canals of the bony labyrinth (see Figs. 21-1 and 21-2). The **anterior** and **posterior semicircular ducts** are in vertical planes, with the former being transverse to and the latter parallel with the long axis of the petrous portion of the temporal bone. The **lateral semicircular duct** slopes downward and backward at an angle of 30 degrees to the horizontal plane. The semicircular ducts of the two sides form spatial pairs; the lateral ducts are in the same plane, and the anterior vertical duct of one side and the posterior vertical duct of the opposite side are in the same plane. The sensory areas of the semicircular ducts respond only to move-

ment; the response is maximal when movement is in the plane of the duct.

Each semicircular duct has an expansion or **ampulla** at one end, in which the **crista ampullaris** or sensory epithelium is supported by a transverse septum of connective tissue (Fig. 22-3). Among the columnar supporting cells are the sensory **hair cells**, whose structural details and mode of innervation conform to those already described for hair cells of the static labyrinth. The hairs and kinocilium of each hair cell are embedded in gelatinous material that forms the **cupula**, in which otoliths are lacking. The cupula has the same specific gravity as the endolymph and is, therefore, not pulled on by gravity.

The cristae are sensors of rotary movement of the head, sometimes called angular movement, especially when accompanied by acceleration or deceleration. At the beginning of movement in or near the plane of a semicircular duct, the endolymph lags because of inertia, and the cupula swings like a door in a direction opposite to that of the movement of the head. The momentum of the endolymph causes the cupula to swing momentarily in the opposite direction when the movement ceases. The hairs and kinocilia of the sensory

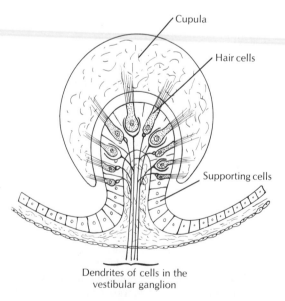

Figure 22-3. Structure of a crista ampullaris.

cells bend accordingly. Depending on the direction of movement, this may reduce the membrane potentials of the hair cells, causing release of their chemical transmitter and the initiation of action potentials in the sensory nerve endings.

The kinocilium is consistently on the side of the tuft of hairs nearest the opening of the ampulla into the utricle. The excitation of hair cells noted above occurs when the flow of endolymph is from the ampulla into the adjacent utricle, whereas there is inhibition of the hair cells when the flow is in the opposite direction. (There is a slight tonic discharge from the hair cells of both the maculae and the cristae, even in the absence of bending of the hairs.) The hair cells of the cristae, like those of the maculae, are supplied by primary sensory neurons whose bipolar cell bodies are in the vestibular ganglion. The particular fibers of the vestibular nerve that are conducting impulses to the vestibular nuclei and cerebellum at any given moment varies according to the plane in which the head is moving.

Vestibular Pathways

On entering the brain stem at the junction of the medulla and pons, most of the vestibular nerve fibers bifurcate in the usual manner of afferent fibers and end in the vestibular nuclear complex. The remaining fibers go to the cerebellum through the inferior cerebellar peduncle.

VESTIBULAR NUCLEI

The vestibular nuclei are in the rostral medulla and caudal pons, partly beneath the area vestibuli or lateral area of the floor of the fourth ventricle (Fig. 22-4). Four vestibular nuclei are recognized on the basis of cytoarchitecture and the details of afferent and efferent connections. The **lateral vestibular nucleus**, also known as **Deiters' nucleus**, consists mainly of large multipolar neurons with widely branching dendrites, long axons, and prominent Nissl bodies. The **superior, medial**, and **infe-**

rior vestibular nuclei consist of small and medium-size cells. The positions of the vestibular nuclei are described and illustrated in Chapter 7.

CONNECTIONS WITH THE CEREBELLUM

The **vestibulocerebellum**, consisting of the flocculonodular lobe, adjacent region of the inferior vermis, and fastigial nuclei, receives fibers from the superior, medial, and inferior vestibular nuclei in addition to receiving a modest number of fibers directly from the vestibular nerve. In the reverse direction, fibers from the vestibulocerebellum terminate throughout the vestibular nuclear complex (see Fig. 10-13). These afferent and efferent fibers of the vestibulocerebellum occupy the medial portion of the inferior cerebellar peduncle. The role of the cerebellum in maintaining equilibrium is exerted mainly through pathways from the vestibular nuclei to the spinal cord.

CONNECTIONS WITH THE SPINAL CORD

The connection between the vestibular nuclei and the spinal cord is through descending fibers in the vestibulospinal tract and the medial longitudinal fasciculus. (Sometimes these tracts are called the lateral and medial vestibulospinal tracts, respectively.)

The **vestibulospinal tract**, which is uncrossed, originates in the lateral vestibular or Deiters' nucleus exclusively. The fibers descend in the medulla dorsal to the inferior olivary nucleus and continue into the ventral funiculus of the spinal cord. Vestibulospinal fibers terminate for the most part in the medial part of the ventral horn (lamina VIII and parts of lamina VII) at all levels but most abundantly in the cervical and lumbosacral enlargements. A few vestibulospinal fibers synapse with motor neurons (lamina IX) that supply the axial musculature, in the medial part of the ventral horn.

The vestibulospinal tract is of prime importance in regulating the tone of muscles involved in posture, so that balance is maintained. Stimulation of the lateral vestibular nucleus causes excitation of motor neurons

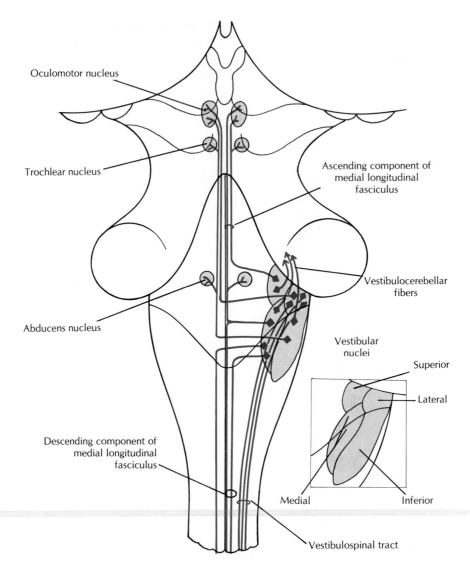

Figure 22-4. Vestibular pathways to the spinal cord and to the nuclei of the ocular motor nerves.

that supply extensor muscles of the ipsilateral lower limb. Flexors are inhibited, and the foot is pressed more firmly on the ground.

Fibers from the medial vestibular nucleus project toward the midline and turn caudally in the **medial longitudinal fasciculi** of both sides. This bundle of fibers is adjacent to the midline, close to the floor of the fourth ventricle, and ventral to the central canal of the medulla more caudally. The fibers continue into the medial part of the ventral funiculus of

the spinal cord. They influence cervical motor neurons so that the head moves in such a way as to assist in maintaining equilibrium and fixation of gaze.

CONNECTIONS WITHIN THE BRAIN STEM

The ascending portion of the **medial longitudinal fasciculus** is adjacent to the midline in the pons and midbrain, ventral to the floor of the fourth ventricle and the periaqueductal gray matter. The constituent fibers connect the vestibular nuclei with the nuclei of the abducens, trochlear, and oculomotor nerves and with the accessory oculomotor nuclei of the midbrain. Some of the ascending fibers are uncrossed; others cross the midline at the level of the vestibular nuclei. This component of the medial longitudinal fasciculus provides for conjugate movement of the eyes, coordinated with movement of the head, to maintain visual fixation. Impulses received by the vestibular nuclei from the cristae ampullares of the kinetic labyrinth are responsible for the ocular adjustments to movement of the head. A small angular rotation of the head is accompanied by movement of the eyes through the same angle but in the opposite direction: the **vestibulo-ocular reflex**.

The medial longitudinal fasciculus also contains fibers that interconnect the nuclei of the third, fourth, and sixth cranial nerves and fibers that originate in the paramedian pontine reticular formation. These connections and the effects of lesions of the medial longitudinal fasciculus are described in Chapter 8.

Excessive or prolonged stimulation of the vestibular system may cause nausea and vomiting. The connections responsible for these effects appear to be efferent fibers from vestibular nuclei, with collateral branches ending in visceral "centers" and in parasympathetic nuclei in the brain stem. Excessive input from the labyrinth to the vestibular nuclei is probably reduced to some extent by a feedback through the efferent inhibitory fibers in the vestibular nerve.

CORTICAL REPRESENTATION

Although the vestibular system functions mainly at the levels of the brain stem, cerebellum, and spinal cord, there is a significant pathway from the vestibular nuclei to the cerebral cortex. This provides for conscious awareness of position and movement of the head. The experimental and clinical evidence concerning the location of the cortical area are conflicting.

The ascending pathway from the vestibular nuclei is predominantly crossed and runs close to the medial lemniscus. The thalamic relay for the cortical projection, wherever that area may be, is thought to be in or near the medial division of the ventral posterior nucleus, which also receives somatosensory fibers for the head. The vestibular cortical field is presumed to contribute information for use in higher motor regulation and for conscious spatial orientation, but the appropriate area has not yet been identified with any certainty.

Evoked potentials have been recorded in the parietal lobe of the monkey during electrical stimulation of the vestibular nerve. The area thus identified as receiving vestibular information is adjacent to the general sensory area for the head. Sensations of turning or body displacement have been elicited in humans by stimulation of the corresponding area of cortex. It has been stated also that a vestibular area is present in the superior temporal gyrus, anterior to the auditory area. This was based on reports of vertigo or dizziness on electrical stimulation of this part of the gyrus in conscious patients and the occurrence of the same sensation in temporal lobe epilepsy. However, caloric stimulation of the kinetic labyrinth causes a regional increase in blood flow in the superior temporal gyrus posterior to the auditory area, with no such change being recorded from either of the other areas to which vestibular function has been ascribed.

Clinical Aspects of the Vestibular System

ROTATION

The vestibular projections to nuclei that supply extraocular muscles and motor neurons in the spinal cord can be demonstrated by strong stimulation of the labyrinth. This may be done by rotating a subject around a vertical axis about ten times in 20 seconds and then abruptly stopping the rotation. The responses are most pronounced if the head is bent forward 30 degrees to bring the lateral semicircular ducts in a horizontal plane. On stopping rotation, momentum acquired by the endolymph causes it to flow past (and deflect) the cupulae of the lateral semicircular ducts more suddenly and rapidly than for most movements.

The responses of the hair cells in the cristae ampullares produce the following signs immediately after rotation ceases. Impulses conveyed by the ascending fibers of the medial longitudinal fasciculus cause **nystagmus**, which is an oscillatory movement of the eyes consisting of fast and slow components. The direction of nystagmus, right or left, is designated by that of the fast component, which is opposite to the direction of rotation. The subject deviates in the direction of rotation if asked to walk in a straight line, and the finger deviates in the same direction on pointing to an object. These responses are caused by the effect of vestibulospinal projections on muscle tone. There is a subjective feeling of turning in a direction opposite to that of rotation, for which both the cortical projection and the nystagmus are, presumably, responsible. The spread of impulses to visceral centers may produce sweating and pallor, and even nausea in those who are susceptible to motion sickness.

CALORIC TESTING AND DOLL'S EYES

The caloric test is used when there is a reason to suspect a tumor of the vestibulocochlear nerve or a lesion that interrupts the vestibular pathway in the brain stem. This procedure tests the pathway from each internal ear separately. The head is positioned so that the lateral semicircular duct is in a vertical plane, and the external acoustic meatus is irrigated with warm or cold water. The ampulla of the duct is near the bone that is undergoing a change of temperature, and the endolymph "rises" or "falls," depending on whether it is warmed or cooled. In a *conscious* subject the procedure causes nystagmus if the vestibular pathway for the side tested is intact. In a *comatose* patient with intact pathways in the brain stem, caloric stimulation with warm water makes the eyes deviate to the opposite side; cold water causes a conjugate deviation toward the cooled side. The deviation is the isolated slow component of a nystagmus. The fast component, which is a voluntary compensation, is prevented by the absence of consciousness.

The **doll's eyes phenomenon**, which is a vestibulo-ocular reflex uncomplicated by voluntary eye movements, is another clinical sign useful in the diagnosis of coma. If the vestibular apparatus, nuclei, and nerve; the medial longitudinal fasciculus; and the abducens and oculomotor nuclei are all intact, movement of the head will be accompanied by conjugate movement of the eyes in the opposite direction. Loss of caloric responses and of the doll's eyes reflex are two signs that can contribute to a diagnosis of brain stem death.

LABYRINTHINE DISEASE

Labyrinthine irritation causes **vertigo**, sometimes accompanied by nausea and vomiting, pallor, a cold sweat, and nystagmus. Paroxysms of labyrinthine irritation occur in **Ménière's disease**, a condition of obscure etiology in which the endolymphatic pressure is abnormally high. There is also tinnitus (buzzing or ringing in the ears) and eventual deafness caused by degeneration of the receptor cells.

Sudden unilateral loss of vestibular function causes vertigo with considerable postural instability, and a tendency to fall toward the abnormal side. This results from undue downward pressure on one foot, perhaps due to excessive activity in the vestibulospinal tract of the normal side. The brain eventually accommodates to input from only one vestibular apparatus.

SUGGESTED READING

Carpenter MB, Chang L, Pereira AB, Hersh LB, Wu JY: Vestibular and cochlear efferent neurons in the monkey identified by immunocytochemical methods. Brain Res 408:275–280, 1987

Friberg L, Olsen IS, Roland PE, Paulson OB, Lassen NA: Focal increase of blood flow in the cerebral cortex of man during vestibular stimulation. Brain 108:609–623, 1985

Friedland RP (ed): Selected Papers of Morris B. Bender. Memorial Volume. New York, Raven Press, 1983

Highstein SM: The central nervous system efferent control of the organs of balance and equilibrium. Neurosci Res 12:13–30, 1991

Penfield W: Vestibular sensation and the cerebral cortex. Ann Otol Rhinol Laryngol 66:691–698, 1957

Twenty-Three

The Human Nervous System: An Anatomical Viewpoint, Sixth Edition, Murray L. Barr and John A. Kiernan. J.B. Lippincott Company, Philadelphia, © 1993.

Motor Systems

Important Facts

Each motor unit comprises a group of extrafusal muscle fibers and the alpha motor neuron that innervates them. Gamma motor neurons supply the intrafusal fibers of muscle spindles. The term "lower motor neuron" is applied collectively to motor neurons.

A lower motor neuron lesion (such as destruction of cell bodies or transection of axons in a ventral root or peripheral nerve) causes flaccid paralysis, loss of the stretch reflex, and considerable atrophy.

The stretch reflex is normally largely suppressed by the activity of descending pathways that end on motor neurons and nearby interneurons.

The major descending pathways are the vestibulospinal, reticulospinal, and corticospinal (pyramidal) tracts. The first of these is largely concerned with postural adjustments, and the last with voluntary movements. Most corticospinal fibers decussate at the caudal end of the medulla.

An upper motor neuron lesion (such as transection of corticospinal and corticoreticular fibers in the internal capsule) causes spastic paralysis, with exaggerated stretch reflexes and the abnormal Babinski reflex. Atrophy is not a prominent feature, except when there is prolonged disuse.

Corticobulbar and other descending fibers go to the motor nuclei of cranial nerves, in many cases bilaterally. Transection of these fibers in the internal capsule causes contralateral weakness of muscles of the lower half of the face and of the tongue, but not elsewhere in the head.

The outputs of the cerebellum and the basal ganglia are channeled through the ventral lateral nucleus of the thalamus to the motor areas of the cerebral cortex. The connections of the cerebellum are ordered such that each cerebellar hemisphere is concerned with ipsilateral muscles.

Disorders of the cerebellum cause inaccuracies in the rate, range, direction, and force of movements. Disorders of the basal ganglia cause dyskinesias or abnormalities of movement, including chorea, dystonia, hemiballismus, and parkinsonism.

Except for some visceral functions, overt expression of activity in the central nervous system depends on the somatic or skeletal musculature. The muscles are supplied by the motor neurons in the ventral horns of the spinal cord and in the motor nuclei of cranial nerves, with these neurons constituting what Sherrington termed the "final common pathway" for determining muscle action. They are collectively known as the **lower motor neu-**

ron, especially in clinical medicine. Another clinical expression is **upper motor neuron**, which embraces all the descending pathways of the brain and spinal cord involved in the volitional control of the musculature.

Components of the brain responsible for the execution of properly coordinated movements include the cerebral cortex, corpus striatum, thalamus, subthalamic nucleus, red nucleus, substantia nigra, reticular formation, vestibular nuclei, inferior olivary complex, and cerebellum. The connections of these structures have been described elsewhere in this book, but here they are reviewed with particular attention to their influence on the lower motor neuron. Although descending pathways can be traced from the motor areas of the cerebral cortex to the motor neurons, it is important to realize that the prefrontal cortex and the association areas of the parietal lobe also are importantly involved in the specification and planning stages of the formulation of motor commands by the brain.

Lower Motor Neuron and Muscles

Skeletal muscles are supplied by motor neurons of two types, named **alpha** and **gamma** after the diameters of their axons. The large alpha motor neurons innervate the extrafusal fibers that constitute the main mass of the muscle, in which the axon of each neuron branches to supply the muscle fibers. The number supplied by a single neuron varies from only a few for small muscles whose contractions are precisely controlled to several hundred for large muscles that carry out strong but crude movements. An alpha motor neuron and the muscle fibers it supplies constitute a **motor unit**.

Different types of extrafusal muscle fiber are recognized on the basis of physiological and histochemical studies. The **type I fibers** contract slowly, are resistant to fatigue, and contain little stainable myofibrillar adenosine triphosphatase (ATPase). **Type II** fibers have faster contractions, are more rapidly fatigued than those of type I, and have high concentra-

tions of ATPase in their myofibrils. Using other histochemical criteria, the type II muscle fibers are further divided into **types IIA and IIB**. All the muscle fibers in a motor unit are of the same type, and experimental evidence indicates that the type of fiber is determined by trophic influence of the innervating neuron. In addition to secreting acetylcholine to make the muscle fibers it supplies contract, a motor neuron provides trophic factors, which direct the differentiation of the muscle fibers and are necessary for their continued health. Proteins with myotrophic properties have been isolated from extracts of peripheral nerves.

The different types of muscle fiber respond differently to denervation: Type IIB fibers atrophy most rapidly, and type I fibers, most slowly.

Intrafusal muscle fibers supplied by gamma motor neurons control the length and tension of the neuromuscular spindles. The gamma motor neurons are much less numerous than the alpha motor neurons but are important because their patterns of firing determine the thresholds of the sensory nerve endings in the spindles. These endings are the receptors for the spinal stretch reflex, which is ordinarily suppressed as a result of activity in the descending tracts of the spinal cord. The muscle spindles also are receptors for the conscious awareness of position and movement.

Lower Motor Neuron Lesions

The syndrome of a lower motor neuron lesion occurs when a muscle is paralyzed or weakened as a result of disease or injury that affects the cell bodies or axons of the innervating neurons. Typical causes include **poliomyelitis**, in which a virus selectively attacks ventral horn cells or equivalent neurons in the brain stem, and **injuries** to peripheral nerves that transect some or all of the axons. The following clinical features are observed.

1. The muscle tone is reduced or absent (flaccid paresis or paralysis), owing to interruption of the efferent limb of the tonic stretch reflex.

2. The tendon-jerk reflexes are weak or absent. The cause is the same as that of the flaccidity.
3. The muscles supplied by the affected neurons atrophy progressively. The atrophy is due partly to loss of specific trophic factors normally provided by the motor nerve and partly to disuse.
4. Fibrillation potentials, caused by random contractions of isolated denervated muscle fibers, can be detected by electromyography. Fibrillation should not be confused with fasciculation, which is visible twitching that occurs at irregular intervals within a muscle. Although seen in partly denervated muscles, fasciculation is a rather unreliable diagnostic sign, being quite common in some normal muscles.
5. In a partly denervated muscle, the intact nerve fibers sprout at nodes of Ranvier and at motor end plates, with some of the new axonal branches innervating denervated muscle fibers. These changes can be seen in a suitably stained biopsy specimen, and the enlargement of the motor units can be detected by electromyography.

Signs similar to those of a lower motor neuron lesion occur in diseases of muscle in which synaptic transmission at the motor end plate is impaired (**myasthenia gravis**) or in which the contractile elements function inadequately (various forms of **dystrophy**, **myopathy**, and **myositis**). Biopsy and neurophysiological testing are used when a diagnosis cannot be made using clinical criteria.

Descending Pathways to the Spinal Cord

Motor neurons in the spinal cord are influenced by descending fibers from the cerebral cortex, central nuclei of the reticular formation, and the lateral vestibular nucleus. Large tracts of fibers from these sites descend in the lateral and ventral funiculi of the spinal cord (see Fig. 5-9). Smaller contingents of descending fibers come from certain other nuclei in the brain stem.

CORTICOSPINAL TRACTS

The corticospinal tracts (Figs. 23-1 and 23-2) consist of the axons of cells in the primary motor and premotor areas of the frontal lobe and in the parietal lobe, including the first sensory area. The corticospinal fibers pass through the medullary center, converging as they enter the posterior limb of the **internal capsule**, which is the band of white matter between the lentiform nucleus and thalamus. The internal capsule also contains fibers that descend from the cortex to the red nucleus, reticular formation, pontine nuclei, and inferior olivary complex, together with many thalamocortical, corticothalamic, and corticostriate fibers. As will be seen, all these populations of axons are involved in the control of movement.

The internal capsule continues into the **basis pedunculi** of the midbrain. At this level, some of the corticospinal axons give off branches that terminate in the red nucleus. The corticospinal fibers occupy the middle three-fifths of the basis pedunculi, flanked on each side by and partially intermingled with corticopontine fibers. On reaching the ventral (basal) portion of the **pons**, the corticospinal tract breaks up into fasciculi that pass caudally with the bundles of corticopontine fibers. At this level, some of the corticospinal fibers have collateral branches that synapse with neurons of the pontine nuclei. Such collaterals are greatly outnumbered, however, by direct corticopontine fibers. Other branches of corticospinal fibers end in the reticular formation of the pons and medulla.

At the caudal limit of the pons, the corticospinal axons reassemble to form, on the ventral surface of the medulla, the eminence known as the pyramid. The corticospinal fibers are, therefore, said to constitute the **pyramidal tract**. The term **pyramidal system** is applied to the corticospinal tracts together with the functionally equivalent **corti-**

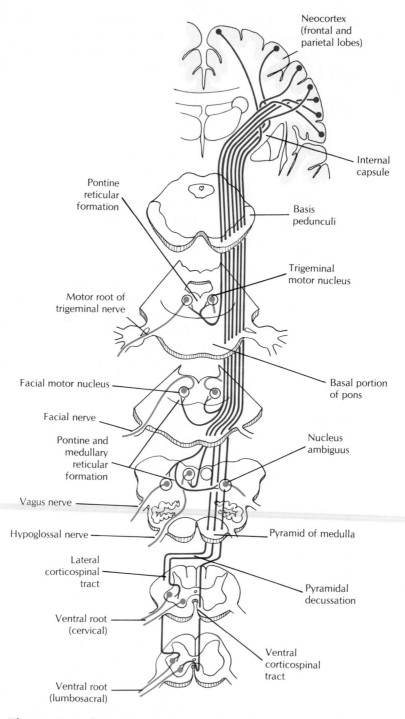

Figure 23-1. Pyramidal system. Corticobulbar and corticospinal neurons are shown in *blue*, and the motor neurons ("lower motor neuron") are shown in *red*.

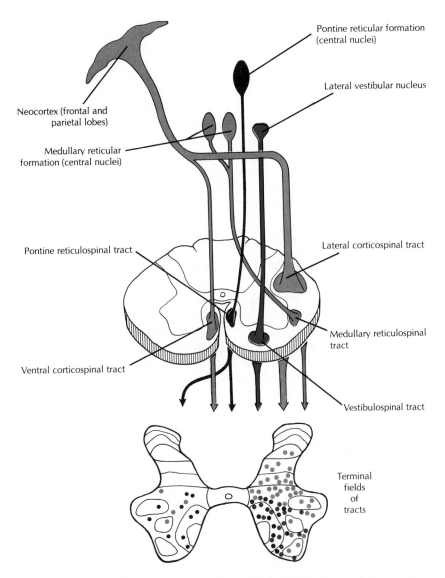

Figure 23-2. Origins, courses, and terminal distributions of the major descending pathways concerned with the control of movement.

cobulbar **(corticonuclear) fibers**, which end in and near the motor nuclei of cranial nerves. At the caudal end of the medulla in most people, about 85% of the corticospinal fibers cross the midline in the decussation of the pyramids and enter the dorsal half of the lateral funiculus of the spinal cord, where they form the **lateral corticospinal tract**. The remaining 15% of the pyramidal fibers constitute the **ventral corticospinal tract**, which descends ipsilaterally in the medial part of the ventral funiculus. The relative sizes of the two corticospinal tracts are variable. In a small percentage of the population, a much larger than usual proportion of the fibers descend ipsilaterally in the ventral tract. Most of these cross the midline at segmental levels and end in the gray matter contralateral to their hemisphere of origin.

Within the **spinal gray matter**, corticospinal axons terminate in the dorsal and ventral horns and in the intermediate gray matter. Some synapse directly with the dendrites and cell bodies of motor neurons. Most corticospinal fibers are able to influence motor neurons only through the mediation of interneurons in the spinal gray matter. Some corticospinal fibers originate in the first somesthetic area of the parietal lobe and end in the dorsal horn. These are not motor in function, but instead modulate the transmission of data through general sensory pathways (see Ch. 19).

SELECTIVE LESIONS OF THE PYRAMIDAL TRACT

Selective transection of the monkey's pyramidal tract, which can be best accomplished in the medulla, results in weakness and reduced tone in the contralateral musculature and clumsiness in actions that require discrete movements of individual fingers and toes. Recovery occurs over the course of a few months but is never complete. The hypotonia is attributed to a decreased rate of tonic discharge of gamma motor neurons, with consequent reduction of the sensory input to the cord from the muscle spindles. The stretch reflexes, however, are not abnormal. Neurosurgeons have cut through the middle part of the human basis pedunculi in attempts to relieve certain dyskinesias. The effects of this lesion are similar to those of transection of the pyramid in monkeys. These observations indicate that the most important function of the pyramidal tract is to control the precision and speed of skilled movements. The Babinski response (described later in connection with upper motor neuron lesions) probably is due to transection of corticospinal fibers, but spasticity and other "upper motor neuron" features are not so easily explained.

RETICULOSPINAL TRACTS

Each half of the spinal cord contains two reticulospinal tracts (see Fig. 23-2). Both consist of the axons of cells in the central group of nuclei of the reticular formation. The **pontine reticulospinal tract** arises ipsilaterally in the oral and caudal pontine reticular nuclei. It travels in the ventral funiculus, and its fibers terminate bilaterally, mostly in the medial part of the ventral horn (lamina VIII and adjacent part of lamina VII). The **medullary reticulospinal tract** originates in the gigantocellular reticular nuclei on both sides of the medulla. The tract descends in the ventral half of the lateral funiculus. Its fibers nearly all end bilaterally among spinal interneurons (in lamina VII); a few enter the region containing the cell bodies of motor neurons (lamina IX).

The central nuclei of the reticular formation receive afferents from all the sensory systems, from the premotor areas of the cerebral cortex, from the fastigial nucleus of the vestibulocerebellum, and from other parts of the reticular formation (see Ch. 9). The afferents from the pedunculopontine nucleus provide a descending pathway through which the corpus striatum may indirectly modulate the activities of motor neurons.

Within the brain stem, the reticulospinal axons have short branches that synapse with other neurons of the reticular formation. Longer branches ascend, often as far as the intralaminar thalamic nuclei and the cholinergic nuclei of the substantia innominata. Branching also has been demonstrated in the spinal cord, so that a single axon may have terminations in cervical, thoracic, and lumbar segments. This observation has led to the suggestion that the reticulospinal tracts control coordinated movements of muscles supplied from different segmental levels of the spinal cord, such as those of the upper and lower limbs in walking, running, and swimming. Long **propriospinal (spinospinalis)** fibers also may be important for synchronization of limb movements. Electrical stimulation of the regions that contain the cell bodies of origin of the reticulospinal tracts results in either excitation or inhibition of either alpha or gamma motor neurons, depending on the exact site of stimulation.

Information about the reticulospinal tracts is derived almost entirely from research with animals. The anatomy of the tracts is constant over a wide phylogenetic range of mammals, so it is likely to hold true also for humans. In view of what is known of other major descending pathways, it seems probable that the reticulospinal tracts mediate control over most movements that do not require dexterity or the maintenance of balance. Motor tracts from the human cerebral cortex can be studied by stimulating the motor areas electrically to evoke small movements. Normally the delay between the stimulus and the beginning of the response is short enough to be attributable to direct (monosynaptic) activation of motor neurons by the corticospinal tract. The existence of a corticoreticulospinal pathway is supported by the finding of motor responses with longer delays in patients in whom the corticospinal fibers are known to have degenerated following infarction in the internal capsule.

From the foregoing paragraphs, it can be seen that the corticospinal and cortico-reticulospinal pathways are influenced by the activities of several regions of the central nervous system that have connections with the cerebral cortex and the reticular formation. A greatly oversimplified scheme of these connections (Fig. 23-3) may help the reader to envisage the overall organization of these major parts of the motor system.

VESTIBULOSPINAL TRACT

This tract (see Fig. 23-2), which arises ipsilaterally from the large cells of the lateral

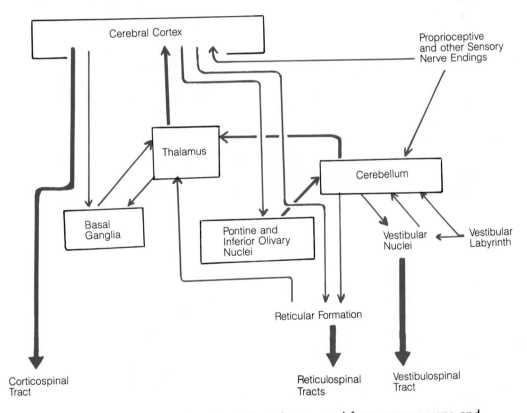

Figure 23-3. Scheme showing chains of command from sense organs and from the cerebral cortex to motor neurons, with sites at which the activities of corticospinal, reticulospinal, and vestibulospinal tracts can be modified by the basal ganglia and cerebellum. This simplified diagram omits many connections; for more details, see Figures 23-4 and 23-5. (*With permission from Kiernan JA: Introduction to Human Neuroscience. Philadelphia, JB Lippincott, 1987*)

vestibular nucleus (Deiters' nucleus), also is known as the lateral vestibulospinal tract. It is composed of myelinated axons of large caliber descending in the ventral funiculus of the spinal white matter. The fibers end in the medial part of the ventral horn (lamina VIII) of the spinal gray matter. Some vestibulospinal fibers synapse with the dendrites of both gamma and alpha motor neurons. The majority probably make contact with interneurons.

Electrical stimulation of the lateral vestibular nucleus in animals causes contraction of ipsilateral extensor muscles of the limbs and vertebral column, with relaxation of the flexors. These effects occur to a lesser extent contralaterally as well, probably because many of the neurons in lamina VIII have axons that cross the midline of the spinal cord. Transection of the brain stem above the vestibular nuclei causes a condition known as **decerebrate rigidity**, in which the extensor musculature of the whole body is in a continuous state of contraction. This condition is easily produced in laboratory animals and occasionally occurs in patients with large destructive lesions of the midbrain or upper pons. The extensor spasm is abolished by destruction of the lateral vestibular nucleus, indicating that it is caused by the unopposed excessive activity of vestibulospinal neurons. The principal sources of afferent fibers to the lateral vestibular nucleus are the vestibular nerve, fastigial nucleus of the cerebellum, and vestibulocerebellar cortex. There are no afferents from the cerebral cortex.

The physiological, pathological, and neuroanatomical data summarized above all support the view that the vestibulospinal tract is concerned with the maintenance of upright posture, which mainly results from the action of the extensor muscles in opposing gravity. Orderly functioning of the "antigravity" musculature is essential for balance, both at rest and during locomotion. Although the vestibulospinal tract does not mediate "voluntary" movements dictated by the cerebral cortex, it is essential for such highly skilled accomplishments of motor coordination as the feats of a gymnast or an acrobat. The learning of those aspects of skilled movement that in-

volve posture and balance and that are effected through the vestibulospinal tract probably occurs in neuronal circuits that include the inferior olivary complex of nuclei and the cerebellum.

OTHER DESCENDING TRACTS

The parts of the brain that connect with the cells of origin of the corticospinal, reticulospinal, and vestibulospinal tracts are summarised in Fig. 23-3. This diagram excludes some small descending tracts.

Two tracts in the medial part of the ventral funiculus terminate throughout the cervical segments of the spinal cord. These are the **tectospinal tract**, from the contralateral superior colliculus, and the descending component of the **medial longitudinal fasciculus**. The former probably is insignificantly small in humans. The latter, which also is called the medial vestibulospinal tract, arises from the medial vestibular nuclei of both sides but is mainly ipsilateral. Both tracts influence neurons that innervate the muscles of the neck, including those supplied by the accessory nerve, affecting movements of the head as required for fixation of gaze and maintaining equilibrium, respectively. The **interstitiospinal tract**, which arises from the interstitial nucleus of Cajal and the Edinger-Westphal nucleus in the midbrain, extends along the whole length of the spinal cord and probably also is involved in visuomotor coordination. It, too, is located in the medial part of the ventral funiculus. The rubrospinal tract provides a motor pathway of some importance in lower mammals. In humans, it is small, goes no further caudally than the second cervical segment, and is, therefore, of little significance.

Descending Pathways to Motor Nuclei of Cranial Nerves

Almost all the muscles supplied by the cranial nerves participate in voluntarily initiated movements, and some of them are controlled with exquisite precision.

As described in Chapter 8, the oculomotor,

trochlear, and abducens nuclei receive afferents through a complicated system of connections involving the cortex of the frontal and occipital lobes, superior colliculus, and various nuclei in the brain stem. It will be recalled that the cerebral cortex controls coordinated movements of the eyes. The frontal eye fields are necessary for changing the direction of gaze voluntarily. The occipital cortex controls involuntary conjugate movements, as when tracking a moving object, and it also is necessary for convergence of the eyes to look at a near object.

Knowledge of the afferent connections of the other motor nuclei of cranial nerves is less complete. The nuclei concerned are the trigeminal and facial motor nuclei, nucleus ambiguus, and hypoglossal nucleus. Results of studies in animals indicate that **corticobulbar (corticonuclear) fibers** from the motor areas of the cortex end mainly in the reticular formation near the motor nuclei, with a few contacting the motor neurons directly. These fibers constitute part of the pyramidal system and are equivalent to corticospinal fibers. The motor nuclei also receive afferents from the reticular formation that are equivalent to the reticulospinal tracts. Therefore, upper motor neuron paralysis or paresis, caused by a lesion in the internal capsule, for example, is due to interruption of both corticobulbar and corticoreticular fibers.

With a unilateral lesion in the motor cortex or in the posterior limb of the internal capsule, the only paralyzed muscles in the head are those of the lower half of the face (moving the lips and cheeks) and of the tongue, contralaterally. The muscles supplied by the trigeminal motor nucleus, rostral portion of the facial motor nucleus, and nucleus ambiguus are not affected on either side by a unilateral lesion in the cerebral hemisphere. It has been deduced that descending pathways are distributed bilaterally to all the motor nuclei of the brain stem except the hypoglossal nucleus and the caudal portion of the facial motor nucleus, which receive only crossed descending afferents. Partial deafferentation of the bilaterally supplied nuclei is evidently compensated for by the intact connections from the ipsilateral hemisphere. The existence of these functional connections has been confirmed by more recent studies that involve stimulation of the normal cerebral cortex.

Upper Motor Neuron Lesions

The term upper motor neuron is unsatisfactory because it refers collectively to descending pathways that make different contributions to the voluntary control of muscle action. The term is still useful in clinical medicine, however, because it often is necessary to determine whether a group of muscles is weakened or paralyzed as a result of denervation or as a consequence of some lesion in the central nervous system. An infarction in the posterior limb of the internal capsule, for example, results in the typical signs of an upper motor neuron lesion. Similar abnormalities occur below the level of a lesion that partly or completely transects the spinal cord. The clinical features of an upper motor neuron lesion are as follows.

1. Voluntary movements of the affected muscles are absent or weak.
2. Profound atrophy does not occur in the affected muscles, although there is slow wasting, and contractures may develop over several months if the condition does not improve. The muscles are not denervated,[1] so the myotrophic effect of their motor innervation is preserved. The spasticity (see below) helps to prevent atrophy caused by disuse.
3. The tone of the muscles is increased. This phenomenon, known as **spasticity**, results from the continuous operation of the stretch reflex, which normally is suppressed by the activity

---

[1] Sometimes electromyographic evidence of partial denervation is found in patients with upper motor neuron weakness caused by lesions in the cerebral hemisphere. This has not been explained, although transneuronal degeneration (see Ch. 4) is one possibility.

of the descending tracts. The tendon jerks are exaggerated. When the examining physician attempts passive extension of a flexed joint, resistance is encountered because of operation of the stretch reflex. When greater force is applied, an inhibitory reflex is initiated by the Golgi tendon organs, and the muscles relax suddenly. This phenomenon is known as "clasp knife rigidity." Alternating contractions and relaxations, known as **clonus**, also may occur when a tendon is stretched.

4. The **plantar reflex** is abnormal. There normally is plantar flexion of the big toe when the lateral margin of the sole is firmly stroked with a hard object. In the *abnormal* reflex, known as the **Babinski** sign or response, the toe is dorsiflexed. This movement typically is associated with flexion at the knee and hip joints, although similar withdrawal is seen in normal people with sensitive soles. The descending tracts involved in the normal plantar reflex probably include the pyramidal tract. An extensor plantar response is normal in children under age 1 year, and the response does not become unequivocally flexor until the 18th month. This maturation coincides with the myelination of most of the axons in the corticospinal tracts.

5. The **superficial reflexes** are suppressed or absent. These reflexes are the abdominal reflex (contraction of the anterior abdominal muscles when the overlying skin is firmly stroked) and the cremasteric reflex (withdrawal of the ipsilateral testis when the medial side of the thigh is stroked). The latter reflex usually is sluggish or absent in men but is a useful clinical test in infants. These reflexes are presumed to be mediated by long tracts to and from the cerebral cortex, but their anatomical identities are uncertain.

6. In the case of the facial muscles, only the lower half of the face is involved. For unknown reasons, muscle action expressing emotional changes usually is spared, and there often are abnormal emotional responses, such as laughter or crying on inappropriate occasions.

Systems That Control the Descending Pathways

Large numbers of pyramidal and corticoreticular fibers originate in the cortex of the frontal and parietal lobes. However, the movements elicited by electrical stimulation of the motor cortical areas (see Ch. 15) are much simpler than those that ordinarily occur either in obedience to conscious thoughts or as part of involuntary or habitual patterns of activity. The physiological output of impulses from the motor cortex must, therefore, be much more complex than its responses to simple, artificial electrical stimuli. The afferent connections of the motor areas are important with respect to their physiological complexity. The largest of these are the association and commissural fibers from other cortical areas and fibers from the thalamus, especially the two divisions of the ventral lateral nucleus. This thalamic nucleus receives projections from two other systems involved in the control of movement, the cerebellum and basal ganglia.

CEREBELLAR CIRCUITS

In connection with the motor systems, it is appropriate to review some of the afferent and efferent connections of the cerebellum (Fig. 23-4). The cortex and central nuclei of the cerebellum receive input from extensive areas of the contralateral neocortex (by way of corticopontine and pontocerebellar fibers); from ipsilateral proprioceptors in muscles, tendons, and joints (by way of the spinocerebellar tracts); and from the vestibular apparatus. The inferior olivary complex, which receives most of its afferent fibers from the neocortical motor areas, red nucleus, and spinal cord, projects to the entire cerebellar cortex. In addition to

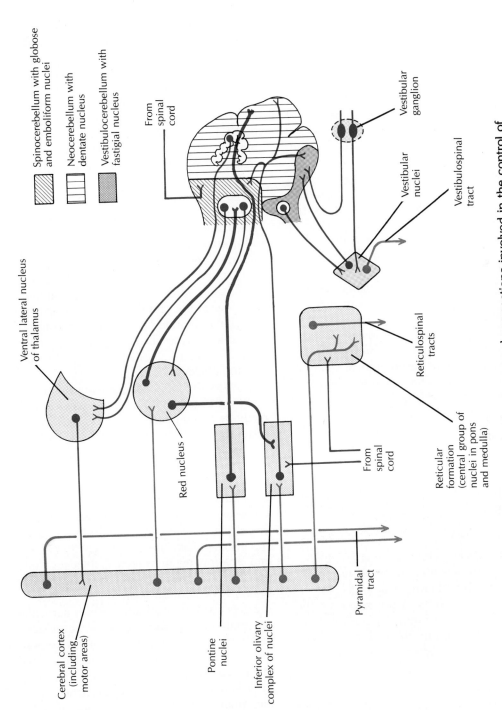

Figure 23-4. Diagram of some neural connections involved in the control of movement, with emphasis on the cerebellum (*blue* neurons) and on the major sources of descending tracts (*red* neurons). For other cerebellar connections, see Figures 10-13, 10-14, and 10-15.

Spinocerebellum with globose and emboliform nuclei

Neocerebellum with dentate nucleus

Vestibulocerebellum with fastigial nucleus

From spinal cord

Ventral lateral nucleus of thalamus

Cerebral cortex (including motor areas)

Red nucleus

Pontine nuclei

Inferior olivary complex of nuclei

Pyramidal tract

From spinal cord

Reticular formation (central group of nuclei in pons and medulla)

Reticulospinal tracts

Vestibulospinal tract

Vestibular nuclei

Vestibular ganglion

these, the precerebellar reticular nuclei relay information from the spinal cord, vestibular nuclei, and cerebral cortex. The cerebellar nuclei send their efferent fibers to the contralateral thalamus (ventral lateral nucleus) and red nucleus, as well as to the reticular formation bilaterally and the ipsilateral vestibular nuclei.

Thus the cerebellum receives information from the cerebral cortex, including motor areas, and it also is informed of changes in the lengths and tensions of muscles and of the position and angular movements of the head. These large contingents of afferent fibers are supplemented by smaller inputs that report on cutaneous, visual, and auditory sensations. The output of the cerebellar nuclei is brought to bear on the primary motor area through a relay in the posterior division of the ventral lateral thalamic nucleus (VLp). Other cerebellar efferents influence lower motor neurons through connections with reticular and vestibular nuclei.

Electrophysiological investigations indicate that the cerebellum is informed through its olivary afferents of the program of neuronal instructions for any complex movement. The pontocerebellar afferents, which are active earlier than the primary motor area, are involved in the execution of movements. The cerebellar afferents activated by proprioceptive nerve endings enable the program of instructions to be modified in the light of the changes in length and tension of muscles that are occurring.

BASAL GANGLIA

The basal ganglia, which are not ganglia but nuclei,[2] are the **corpus striatum** of the telencephalon, **subthalamic nucleus** of the diencephalon, and **substantia nigra** of the mesencephalon. The corpus striatum is functionally subdivided into the **striatum (neostriatum)** and **pallidum (paleostriatum)**.

---

[2] The unfortunate plethora of names associated with the basal ganglia and corpus striatum is explained in Chapter 12.

The largest of the nuclei that constitute the basal ganglia is the neostriatum. Its afferent fibers come from the whole neocortex, from the intralaminar thalamic nuclei, and from the substantia nigra (Fig. 23-5). The neostriatum projects to the paleostriatum, which influences the premotor and supplementary motor areas through a relay in the anterior division of the ventral lateral nucleus of the thalamus (VLa). The activity of the neostriatum is modulated by a two-way connection with the substantia nigra, and the activity of the paleostriatum is modulated by a two-way connection with the subthalamic nucleus. These connections are set out in more detail in Chapter 12.

A small contingent of pallidofugal fibers passes caudally and terminates in the **pedunculopontine nucleus** at the junction of the midbrain and pons (see Ch. 9). The pedunculopontine nucleus sends some fibers to the subthalamic nucleus, some to the pallidum, and some to the central group of nuclei of the reticular formation. A role in the timing of rhythmic activities, including locomotion and sleep, has been suggested for the pedunculopontine nucleus.

Clearly the basal ganglia comprise a large mass of gray matter influenced directly or indirectly by several parts of the central nervous system. The number and complexity of interconnections within the basal ganglia indicate that much integrative activity must be occurring. The output of the system is principally to a thalamic nucleus that projects to motor cortical areas, and electrophysiological studies indicate that in the corpus striatum, as in the cerebellar nuclei, changes in activity precede and accompany movements. It is probable, therefore, that the basal ganglia are involved in the transfer of information from the whole of the neocortex to the motor areas, in particular the premotor and supplementary motor areas, and that the corpus striatum serves as a repository of instructions for fragments of learned movements. The effects of disease also indicate a role in remembering encoded instructions for the initiation, control, and cessation of all the components of regularly made movements.

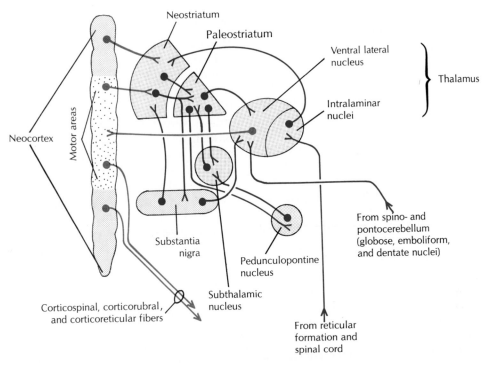

Figure 23-5. Diagram of some neural connections involved in the control of movement, with emphasis on the basal ganglia, thalamus, and motor cortex. Cortical connections are *red*; others are *blue*. For other circuitry of the basal ganglia, see Figures 12-4, 12-5, and 12-6.

It was once erroneously thought that the pyramidal system controlled all deliberate movements and that there was a parallel "extrapyramidal" system largely concerned with the habitual or automatic activities of the muscles. Unfortunately the term "extrapyramidal" has been applied not only to the reticulospinal and vestibulospinal tracts, but also to pathways that include the corpus striatum, substantia nigra, and subthalamic nucleus because some of these structures were once thought to give rise to descending fibers. From anatomical, physiologic, and clinical evidence, it is more appropriate to bracket the basal ganglia with the neocerebellum; the activity of both regions is directed through the thalamus to the motor areas of the cerebral cortex. Thus the term "extrapyramidal system" does not represent any real entity and has caused much confusion. It is mentioned here because in clinical practice, disorders in which there are abnormal spontaneous movements often still are referred to as "extrapyramidal syndromes."

Disorders of Movement

Knowledge of the neurotransmitters and their excitatory or inhibitory actions within the motor circuitry might one day make it possible to provide tidy neuroanatomical explanations for different types of disordered movement, comparable to those that account for some sensory deficits. Some progress in this direction has been made and is reviewed in Chapter 12. Some conditions with well-defined clinical features are caused by circumscribed lesions in certain regions. The most straightforward is the lower motor neuron lesion, described earlier. Some others are now reviewed. Disordered movement also is discussed in Chapters 7, 11, and 12.

UPPER MOTOR NEURON AND CORTICAL LESIONS

The clinical signs comprising the upper motor neuron lesion also were identified earlier. The syndrome occurs in its most typical form after **infarction of the posterior limb of the internal capsule**, resulting in the severance of ascending and descending tracts, including corticospinal and corticobulbar fibers, together with corticopontine, cortico-olivary, corticoreticular, corticorubral, and thalamocortical projections. **Destruction of both the primary motor and the premotor cortex**, such as often follows occlusion of the middle cerebral artery, has similar consequences.

Lesions confined to the primary motor area cause a flaccid paralysis of the part of the body appropriate to the exact position of the destroyed cortex. As with other lesions in which only small cortical areas are damaged, recovery usually occurs as the functions are taken over by adjacent areas. **Destruction of the premotor area** causes contralateral weakness of the muscles that move the shoulder and hip joints. The hand, although its own movements are unimpaired, cannot be brought into a useful position for many ordinary tasks. Locomotion also is impaired. If the **supplementary motor area** is destroyed, there is a severe contralateral motor disability in which movements cannot be initiated. Bilateral lesions cause permanent akinesia and mutism.[3] These symptoms are consonant with the normal involvement of the supplementary motor area in the initiation of movements (see Ch. 15), including those of the muscles used in speech.

---

[3] This disorder must not be confused with **akinetic mutism**, which is due to a destructive lesion in the upper pons in which the patient is apparently asleep with relaxed musculature. In response to loud sounds, the eyes open and follow moving objects, but other sensory stimuli are ineffective, and there is no other movement or speech. A related condition, seen with a midpontine lesion, is the **locked-in syndrome** in which the patient is awake but mute, with all muscles paralyzed except those that move the eyes.

DYSKINESIAS

Dyskinesias (sometimes called "extrapyramidal syndromes") are diseases in which unwanted superfluous movements occur. **Chorea**, **athetosis**, and **dystonia**, which are thought to result from lesions of the corpora striata, were discussed in Chapter 12. **Hemiballismus**, consisting of sudden flailing movements at the proximal joints of limbs, is usually due to a vascular lesion in the contralateral subthalamic nucleus (see Ch. 11). The most common dyskinesia is **Parkinson's disease**, characterized by muscular rigidity, tremor of distal muscles, and poverty of movement (bradykinesia). The primary lesion is loss of dopaminergic neurons in the pars compacta of the substantia nigra (see Ch. 7). Normally, such neurons are active at all times, irrespective of any movement being made, exerting a continuous modulating influence on the striatum and, indirectly, upon the premotor and supplementary motor areas of the neocortex. The bradykinesia of parkinsonism has been attributed to withdrawal of an excitatory action of dopamine on some striatal neurons. This releases the pallidum from inhibition by the striatum, resulting in increased pallidal inhibition of the VLa nucleus of the thalamus. This thalamic nucleus is excitatory to the premotor cortex, so in Parkinson's disease, the cortical activity is reduced. (Refer to Fig. 12-6 to follow the logic of this argument, which unfortunately does not account for the tremor and rigidity.)

Finally, **lesions of the cerebellum** lead to a variety of motor disturbances, including a specific type of ataxia, hypotonia, and a characteristic intention tremor (see Ch. 10). Cerebellar lesions may be said in general to lead to errors in the rate, range, force, and direction of willed movements. **Unilateral damage** to a cerebellar hemisphere (vascular occlusion, a tumor, or demyelination of white matter in one or more cerebellar peduncles) results in *symptoms that affect the same side of the body*. Cerebellar dysfunction, which may be bilateral, is a common feature of multiple sclerosis (MS), a disease of unknown cause in which foci of demyelination develop in white matter throughout the brain and spinal cord. Cerebellothalamic fibers commonly are affected in MS. **Lesions in the midline** of the cerebellum affect the vestibular and spinal connections, so an *ataxic gait* is the most prominent abnormality.

SUGGESTED READING

Albin RL, Young AB, Penney JB: The functional anatomy of basal ganglia disorders. Trends Neurosci 12:366–375, 1989

Brooks VB: The Neural Basis of Motor Control. New York, Oxford University Press, 1986

Brotchie P, Iansek R, Horne MK: Motor function of the monkey globus pallidus. II. Cognitive aspects of movement and phasic neuronal activity. Brain 114:1685–1702, 1991

Brouwer B, Ashby P: Corticospinal projections to upper and lower limb spinal motoneurons in man. Electroenceph Clin Neurophysiol 76:509–519, 1990

Bucy PC, Keplinger JE, Siqueira EB: Destruction of the "pyramidal tract" in man. J Neurosurg 21:385–398, 1964

Cruccu G, Berardelli A, Inghilleri M, Manfredi M: Corticobulbar projections to upper and lower facial motoneurons. A study by magnetic transcranial stimulation in man. Neurosci Lett 117:68–73, 1990

Davidoff RA: The pyramidal tract. Neurology 40:332–339, 1990

Davis HL: Trophic effects of neurogenic substances on mature skeletal muscle in vivo. In Fernandez HL, Donoso JA (eds): Nerve-Muscle Cell Trophic Communication. Boca Raton, FL, CRC Press, 1988

Freund H-J, Hummelsheim H: Lesions of premotor cortex in man. Brain 108:697–733, 1985

Fries W, Danek A, Witt TN: Motor responses after transcranial electrical stimulation of cerebral hemispheres with a degenerated pyramidal tract. Ann Neurol 29:646–650, 1991

Garcia-Rill E: The pedunculopontine nucleus. Prog Neurobiol 36:363–389, 1991

Georgopoulos AP: Higher order motor control. Annu Rev Neurosci 14:361–377, 1991

Nathan PH, Smith MC: The rubrospinal and central tegmental tracts in man. Brain 105:223–269, 1982

Nudo RJ, Masterton RB: Descending pathways to the spinal cord. II. Quantitative study of the tectospinal tract in 23 mammals. J Comp Neurol 286:96–119, 1989

Peterson BW: The reticulospinal system and its role in the control of movement. In Barnes CD (ed): Brainstem Control of Spinal Cord Function, pp 28–86. Orlando, Academic Press, 1984

Phillips CG, Porter R: Corticospinal Neurones. Their Role in Movement. Monographs of the Physiological Society, No 34. London, Academic Press, 1977

Rothwell JC: Control of Human Voluntary Movement. London, Croom Helm, 1987

Schomburg ED: Spinal sensorimotor systems and their supraspinal control. Neurosci Res 7:265–340, 1990

Seitz R, Roland PE, Bohm C, Greitz T, Stone-Elander S: Motor learning in man: A positron emission tomographic study. NeuroReport 1:57–60, 1990

Sugimoto T, Hattori T: Organization and efferent projections of nucleus tegmenti pedunculopontinus pars compactus with special reference to its cholinergic aspects. Neuroscience 11:931–946, 1984

Twenty-Four

Visceral Innervation

Important Facts

The control of smooth muscle, cardiac muscle, or secretory tissues by the central nervous system always involves a chain of at least two neurons, preganglionic and postganglionic, with the cell body of the latter being in an autonomic ganglion.

Parasympathetic ganglia are near the organs they innervate, whereas most sympathetic ganglia are paravertebral or preaortic. The enteric ganglia are in the myenteric and submucous plexuses of the alimentary canal.

Preganglionic parasympathetic neurons are present in certain nuclei of cranial nerves III, VII, IX, and X and in the intermediolateral cell columns of spinal segments S2 through S4.

Parasympathetic ganglia supply the sphincter pupillae and ciliary muscles, the lacrimal and salivary glands, thoracic and abdominal viscera (including the heart), the urinary bladder and other pelvic organs, and the erectile tissue of the genitalia.

Preganglionic sympathetic neurons are in the intermediolateral cell column of spinal segments T1 through L2. Their axons pass through the ventral roots and the white communicating rami into the sympathetic trunk. They reach paravertebral ganglia by way of the sympathetic trunk or preaortic ganglia by way of splanchnic nerves.

Gray communicating rami carry postganglionic sympathetic axons into mixed nerves to supply blood vessels, sweat glands, and piloarrector muscles. Cardiac sympathetic nerves arising in the cervical ganglia supply the heart. Mesenteric and similar nerve plexuses carry postganglionic sympathetic fibers from preaortic ganglia to abdominal organs. The adrenal medulla is a modified sympathetic ganglion, with neurons that release their transmitters directly into the blood.

The enteric nervous system can work independently, but its activities normally are modulated by preganglionic parasympathetic and postganglionic sympathetic axons. The enteric plexuses contain sensory neurons, interneurons, and cells that provide excitatory and inhibitory innervation to the gut.

Acetylcholine is the principal neurotransmitter of all preganglionic neurons and all parasympathetic postganglionic neurons. Noradrenaline is the principal transmitter of all postganglionic sympathetic neurons except those that supply sweat glands, which are cholinergic. Several peptides also occur in autonomic neurons.

The activities of the autonomic nervous system are subject to control by descending central pathways from the amygdala, septal area, hypothalamus, and reticular formation.

Fibers for visceral pain have cell bodies in dorsal root ganglia and axons that accompany the preganglionic and postganglionic sympathetic fibers. Pain often is referred to somatic structures supplied by the same spinal segments as the affected organ. The central pathway to the cerebral cortex is the spinothalamic system.

Most sensory neurons for visceral reflexes (and for conscious sensation of fullness) have cell bodies in the inferior ganglion of the vagus nerve and axons that accompany the preganglionic parasympathetic fibers. These neurons project centrally to the solitary nucleus, which is connected with the hypothalamus, various regions of the reticular formation, and preganglionic autonomic neurons.

Although viscera are the organs in the thorax and abdomen, the adjective *visceral* is applied in neurobiology to innervated smooth muscle and secretory cells in all parts of the body. The primary role of visceral innervation is to maintain optimal homeostasis in the internal environment (the *"milieu intérieur"* of Claude Bernard). This end is attained through regulation of the organs and structures concerned with digestion, circulation, respiration, excretion, reproduction, and maintenance of normal body temperature. In addition to the regulating role of visceral reflexes, the activity of smooth muscles, glandular elements, and cardiac muscle is altered by influences from the highest levels of the brain, especially in response to emotion and to the external environment.

Afferent signals of visceral origin reach the central nervous system through primary sensory neurons similar to those for general sensation. Under normal conditions, these impulses elicit reflex responses in viscera and feelings of fullness of hollow organs such as the stomach, large intestine, and urinary bladder. Visceral sensation also contributes to feelings of well-being or malaise. In the presence of abnormal function and disease, visceral afferents transmit impulses for pain. The painful sensation often is referred to a part of the body wall or a limb supplied by the same segmental nerves as the affected organ.

The motor or efferent supply of smooth muscle, cardiac muscle, and gland cells differs from that of voluntary muscles in that *the connection between the central nervous system and the viscus consists of a succession of at least two neurons* rather than a single motor neuron. The cell body of the first neuron is in the brain stem or the spinal cord; its axon terminates on a neuron in an autonomic ganglion, and the axon of the latter neuron ends either on effector cells or on a third neuron. The first and second neurons are called **preganglionic** and **postganglionic** neurons, respectively. The third neuron, when present, is part of the plexuses within the wall of the alimentary canal. Because of its involuntary nature, Langley, in 1898, assigned the term **autonomic nervous system** to the visceral efferents. He subdivided the autonomic system into the **parasympathetic**, **sympathetic**, and **enteric** nervous systems, and this classification is still in use.[1]

---

[1] The autonomic system, with its subdivisions, is exclusively efferent. Such terms as autonomic and sympathetic are frequently (though wrongly) used in a wider sense to include the functionally related afferent or sensory neurons and their axons. In the enteric nervous system, much of the neuronal circuitry is confined to the gut, and it is almost impossible to make a formal distinction between afferent and efferent neurons.

Visceral Efferent or Autonomic System

The smooth muscle and secretory cells of viscera, and also cardiac muscle, come under the dual influence of the sympathetic and parasympathetic divisions of the autonomic nervous system. In some organs, these are functionally antagonistic, and a delicate balance between the two systems maintains a more or less constant level of visceral activity. Autonomic innervation extends beyond the organs in the major body cavities to include the muscles of the iris and ciliary body in the eye, smooth muscles in the orbit, the lacrimal and salivary glands, sweat glands and arrector pili muscles of the skin, and blood vessels everywhere. In addition, the alimentary canal contains its own intrinsic nerve supply, the enteric nervous system, which is able to control at least the simpler forms of gastrointestinal motility.

AUTONOMIC GANGLIA

An autonomic ganglion receives thin, myelinated (group B) afferent fibers from the brain stem or spinal cord. Its efferent fibers, which supply visceral structures, are the axons of the principal cells of the ganglion. They are unmyelinated (group C) and more numerous than the afferent fibers. Thus the synapses in the ganglion provide for divergence in the efferent pathway, so that relatively small numbers of neurons in the central nervous system control large numbers of smooth muscle and gland cells in the periphery. The divergence is enhanced by preterminal branching of the postganglionic fibers and, in the alimentary canal, by further synapses with the neurons of the enteric nervous system.

Divergence cannot be the sole reason for the existence of autonomic ganglia; the same effect could be more simply achieved by further branching of axons. There also must be integration and comparison of the various items of information arriving in a ganglion through its preganglionic neurons. Evidence for such activity is seen in the synaptic organization of the ganglion (Fig. 24-1). Each principal cell is inhibited at the dendrodendritic synapses with nearby principal cells and from the small intrinsic neurons of the ganglion. These interneurons, whose only cytoplasmic processes are short dendrites, are excited by branches of the preganglionic axons. In at least some autonomic ganglia, sensory fibers that are passing through give off branches that synapse with the principal cells. This arrangement may provide for reflexes that do not involve the central nervous system.

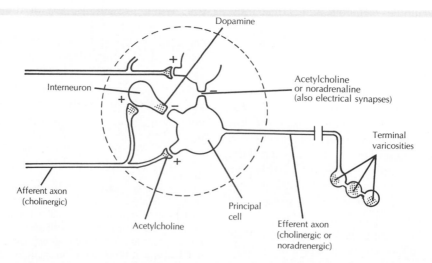

Figure 24-1. Synaptic organization of an autonomic ganglion, showing the principal transmitters and their excitatory (+) or inhibitory (−) actions.

NEUROTRANSMITTERS

The preganglionic neurons are invariably cholinergic. The principal cells are all cholinergic in parasympathetic ganglia, but only a small proportion of them are cholinergic in sympathetic ganglia. Most of the principal cells of sympathetic ganglia are noradrenergic at their peripheral synapses. The synapses between adjacent principal cells are either noradrenergic or electrical in sympathetic ganglia and either cholinergic or electrical in parasympathetic ganglia. The intrinsic neurons of the ganglia contain dopamine, which they are believed to use as a transmitter. All the neurons in autonomic ganglia also contain two or more peptides, which may serve as additional neurotransmitters or as neuromodulators. There are several clinically valuable drugs that selectively enhance or inhibit both the synthesis and the metabolism of acetylcholine, dopamine, and noradrenaline. Other drugs imitate or block the actions of these transmitters at postsynaptic sites. Information about synaptic connections in autonomic ganglia is, therefore, valuable in understanding some of the physiological effects, both therapeutic and unwanted, of these drugs.

PARASYMPATHETIC DIVISION

The actions of the parasympathetic system include a decrease in the rate and force of the heart beat, augmentation of the activity of the digestive system, emptying of the urinary bladder, and tumescence of the genital erectile tissue. As previously stated, acetylcholine is the chemical mediator at the synapses between preganglionic and postganglionic neurons and also at the contacts between postganglionic terminals and effector cells, with various peptides also being released. The parasympathetic system is, therefore, **cholinergic**. *It acts in localized and discrete regions rather than causing a mass reaction throughout the body.* The discrete nature of the response is a result of the fact that there is less divergence between preganglionic and postganglionic neurons and between the latter and effector cells than there is in the sympathetic system. Acetylcholine is rapidly inactivated by acetylcholinesterase; each

parasympathetic discharge is, consequently, of short duration.

Preganglionic parasympathetic neurons, which have long axons, are located in the brain stem and in the middle three sacral segments of the spinal cord (Fig. 24-2). The preganglionic parasympathetic nuclei and the sites of the corresponding postganglionic neurons are as follows:

1. **Edinger-Westphal nucleus** of the oculomotor complex and ciliary ganglion
2. **Superior salivatory nucleus** of the facial nerve and submandibular ganglion
3. **Lacrimal nucleus** of the facial nerve and pterygopalatine ganglion
4. **Inferior salivatory nucleus** of the glossopharyngeal nerve and otic ganglion
5. **Dorsal nucleus of the vagus nerve** and ganglia in the pulmonary plexus, cells in the myenteric and submucosal plexuses of the gastrointestinal tract (the enteric nervous system), and postganglionic neurons at other sites
6. **Nucleus ambiguus** and cardiac ganglia (see Ch. 8)
7. **Sacral parasympathetic nucleus** and postganglionic neurons in and near the pelvic viscera

SYMPATHETIC DIVISION

There are **paravertebral ganglia** associated with all the spinal nerves, although at the cervical levels, eight segments share three ganglia. The sympathetic outflow originates in the **intermediolateral cell column** (lateral horn) of all thoracic spinal segments and the upper two or three lumbar segments (Figs. 24-3 and 24-4). The axons of preganglionic neurons reach the **sympathetic trunk** by way of the corresponding ventral roots and **white communicating rami** (see Fig. 24-3). With respect to the sympathetic supply of structures in the head and thorax, the preganglionic fibers terminate in ganglia of the sympathetic trunk. For smooth muscles and glands in the head,

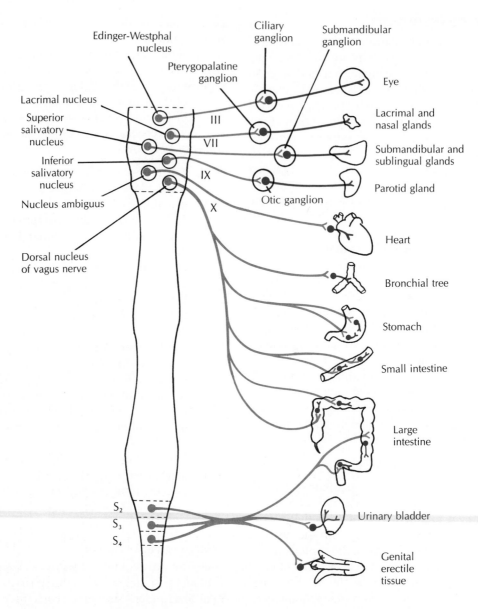

Figure 24-2. Plan of the parasympathetic nervous system. Preganglionic neurons are *red*; postganglionic neurons are *blue*.

the synapses between preganglionic and postganglionic neurons are mainly in the superior cervical ganglion of the sympathetic trunk. In the case of thoracic viscera, the synapses are in the three cervical sympathetic ganglia (superior, middle, and inferior) and the upper five ganglia of the thoracic portion of the sympathetic trunk.

Preganglionic fibers for abdominal and pelvic viscera proceed without interruption through the sympathetic trunk and into the **splanchnic nerves**. The fibers terminate on postganglionic neurons located in **preaortic ganglia**, which are in the plexuses that surround the main branches of the abdominal aorta. The largest are the **celiac plexus** and the superior and inferior **mesenteric plexuses**. The sympathetic supply to the **adrenal**

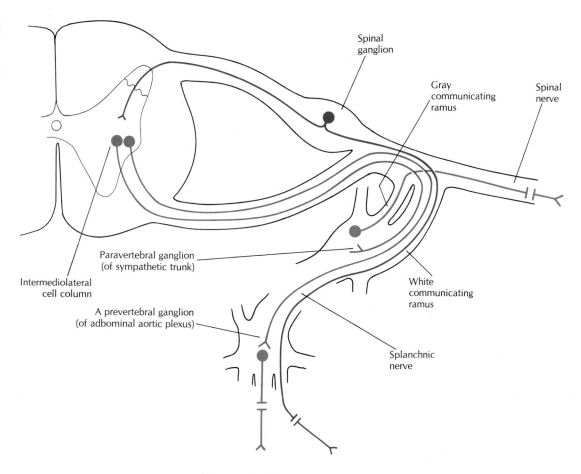

Figure 24-3. Visceral efferent and afferent neurons associated with a thoracic segment of the spinal cord. Preganglionic sympathetic neurons are *red*, and postganglionic sympathetic neurons are *green*. A sensory (pain) neuron supplying an internal organ of the abdomen is shown in *blue*. Visceral sensory fibers pass through autonomic ganglia, but their cell bodies are in dorsal root ganglia.

Labels in figure: Spinal ganglion; Gray communicating ramus; Spinal nerve; Paravertebral ganglion (of sympathetic trunk); Intermediolateral cell column; A prevertebral ganglion (of adbominal aortic plexus); White communicating ramus; Splanchnic nerve

medulla is exceptional. The secretory cells of the medulla, which are derived from the neural crest, are postganglionic sympathetic neurons that lack axons or dendrites. The adrenal medulla is, consequently, supplied directly by preganglionic sympathetic neurons. The glomus cells of the **carotid and aortic bodies** also receive preganglionic sympathetic innervation, which may control the sensitivity of these chemosensory organs. The alimentary canal is chiefly supplied by the ganglia in the celiac and mesenteric plexuses; the postganglionic fibers do not terminate directly on smooth muscle and gland cells, but the enteric upon neurons of nervous system.

For the body wall and the limbs, preganglionic fibers terminate in all ganglia of the sympathetic trunk, from which postganglionic fibers are distributed by way of **gray communicating rami**[2] and spinal nerves to blood vessels, arrector pili muscles, and sweat glands.

The sympathetic system stimulates activities that are accompanied by an expenditure of energy. These include acceleration of the heart and increase in force of the heart beat,

---

[2] White communicating rami are white because the preganglionic axons are myelinated (group B). Gray rami are gray because the postganglionic axons are unmyelinated (group C fibers).

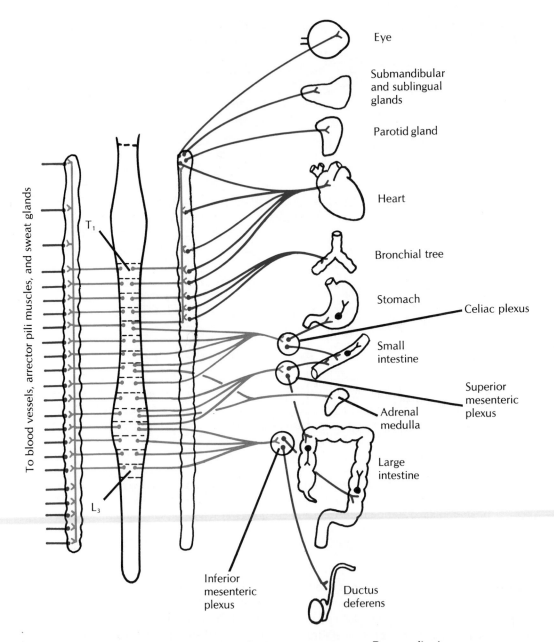

Figure 24-4. Plan of the sympathetic nervous system. Preganglionic neurons are *red*; postganglionic neurons are *blue*; enteric neurons are *black*.

rise of arterial pressure, elevation of the blood sugar level, and direction of blood flow to skeletal muscles at the expense of visceral and cutaneous circulation. Sympathetic responses are most dramatically expressed during stress and emergency situations (the fight-or-flight reaction). The neurotransmitter substance between preganglionic and postganglionic neurons is acetylcholine, as in the parasympathetic system. In the case of the sympathetic system, **noradrenaline** (also known as **norepinephrine**) is the transmitter substance between most postganglionic terminals and effector cells and between postganglionic neurons and neurons of the enteric plexuses. The sympathetic system is, therefore, said to be **noradrenergic**. The sympathetic supply to sweat glands is cholinergic, constituting an exception to the general rule. Cutaneous areas lack parasympathetic fibers; the sudomotor neurons are anatomically sympathetic but functionally similar to those of parasympathetic ganglia.

Noradrenaline has different actions in different tissues, according to the type of receptor molecule on the responding cells. **Alpha receptors** occur on the surfaces of smooth muscle cells in the dilator pupillae muscle and in the blood vessels of the skin and internal organs. These cells contract when noradrenaline is bound by their alpha receptors, with consequent pupillary dilation and cutaneous and visceral vasoconstriction. Those enteric neurons that cause closure of sphincters also bear alpha receptors. The **beta receptors** occur on cardiac muscle cells in the atrial pacemaker tissue and in the ventricles, on smooth muscle in the bronchioles, in blood vessels of skeletal muscle, and on enteric neurons that inhibit propulsive movements of the alimentary tract. Smooth-muscle cells with beta receptors relax in response to noradrenaline, so that there is dilation of the bronchioles and vasodilation in skeletal muscles. The rate and force of contraction of the heart are increased, and propulsion along the gut is inhibited. Several clinically important drugs act by stimulating or blocking the alpha or beta receptors.

Strong sympathetic stimulation produces diffuse effects because of the following factors, which are the converse of those present in the parasympathetic system. Each sympathetic preganglionic neuron synapses with many postganglionic neurons, and each of the latter supplies numerous effector cells or enteric neurons. Hence there is much divergence. Noradrenaline liberated at postganglionic terminals is deactivated by being taken up into the axonal terminals from which it was released, and this is a slower process than the enzyme-catalyzed hydrolysis of acetylcholine. As expressed by Cannon, "the sympathetics are like the loud and soft pedals, modulating all the tones together, while the parasympathetics are like the separate keys."

ENTERIC NERVOUS SYSTEM

From the esophagus to the rectum, the walls of the human alimentary canal contain some 10^8 neurons, a population comparable to the number of neurons in the spinal cord. The cell bodies occur in two zones. The **myenteric plexus** (of Auerbach) lies between the longitudinal and circular muscle layers, and the **submucous plexus** (of Meissner) lies in the connective tissue between the circular muscle layer and the muscularis mucosae. Each plexus consists of small enteric ganglia, joined to one another by thin nerves in which all the axons are unmyelinated. Similar nerves connect the two plexuses across the circular muscle layer and carry branches from the plexuses into the smooth muscle and into the lamina propria of the mucosa. Most of the neurons are multipolar, but there also are many bipolar and unipolar ones, especially in the submucous plexus. In addition to neurons, the enteric nervous system contains neuroglial cells, which ensheath the neurons and their processes. The nervous tissue is avascular and receives its nutrients by diffusion from capillary vessels outside the glial sheath.

The synaptic organization of the enteric nervous system (Fig. 24-5) is not simple. Several types of neuron are found in the plexuses. The bipolar and unipolar cells are presumed to have sensory functions, especially in initiating the peristaltic reflex. Neurons of two types have axons that end on smooth muscle and gland cells; the excitatory neurons are cholinergic. The nonadrenergic, noncholinergic inhibitory neurons may use a peptide or a nucleotide or nitric oxide; the identity of this transmitter has not yet been settled. There also are interneurons that use γ-aminobutyric acid and have inhibitory axoaxonic synapses with cholinergic neurons. Some enteric neurons send axons centripetally, in the nerves that accompany the mesenteric and other abdominal arteries, to the celiac and mesenteric sympathetic ganglia. Enteric neurons have been shown to contain many different peptides with

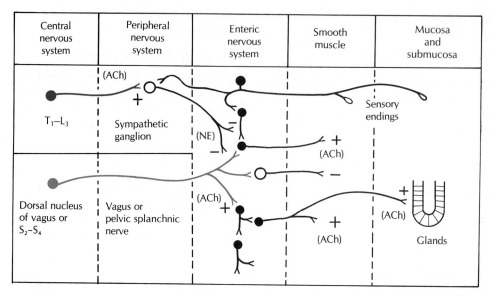

Figure 24-5. Organization of the enteric nervous system. For simplification, the myenteric and submucous plexuses have been combined. The sites of some known transmitters are shown, as are sites of synaptic excitation (+) and inhibition (−). NE = noradrenaline (norepinephrine); ACh = acetylcholine.

pharmacologically demonstrable actions on the gut, and it is considered probable that at least some of these substances serve as neurotransmitters.

The fibers afferent to the enteric nervous system are of two types. Cholinergic axons of preganglionic parasympathetic neurons terminate on the dendrites and cell bodies both of interneurons and of neurons that supply smooth muscle and glands. The noradrenergic axons of sympathetic neurons terminate in axoaxonal synapses on both parasympathetic and intrinsic fibers. They are believed to mediate presynaptic inhibition of the cholinergic neurons that stimulate contraction of the musculature and glandular secretion.

CENTRAL CONTROL OF THE AUTONOMIC NERVOUS SYSTEM

The hypothalamus has a diverse afferent input, and its efferent connections include projections to neurons that constitute the autonomic outflow. It is, therefore, an important controlling and integrating center for the autonomic system.

Through afferent connections described in earlier chapters, the hypothalamus is influenced by the neocortex, hippocampal formation, amygdala and septal area, and olfactory areas. Ascending pathways from the spinal cord and brain stem convey information of visceral and gustatory origin. There also are hypothalamic neurons that are directly sensitive to changes in the temperature, osmolarity, and levels of various substances (including hormones) in the circulating blood. Depending on specific sensitivities, these neurons are related either to the autonomic system or to the pituitary gland.

Signals that originate in the hypothalamus reach autonomic nuclei in the brain stem and spinal cord directly and through relays in the reticular formation. There also are direct projections from the amygdala and septal area to preganglionic autonomic neurons. The autonomic neurons are influenced as well by visceral "centers" and by visceral afferent nuclei, notably the solitary nucleus, in the medulla. The autonomic outflow, therefore, comes under a wide range of influences: visceral (including taste and smell), emotional (both basic drives and moods), and even mental processes at the neocortical level.

Central pathways that control the **sympathetic innervation of the head** can be interrupted by lesions in the brain stem. Horner's syndrome (see Ch. 7) and loss of thermoregulatory sweating of facial skin can follow lesions in the medulla, dorsal to the inferior olivary nucleus. The sympathetic dysfunction is part of Wallenberg's syndrome, and the position of the lesion (see Fig. 7-17) indicates that descending fibers essential for pupillary dilation and facial vasomotor control descend through the lateral part of the medullary reticular formation.

Visceral Afferents

Olfactory neurosensory cells and gustatory neurons are classified as **special visceral afferents** because these are senses especially concerned with feeding and with eliciting visceral responses. The neurons that convey sensation from the thoracic and abdominal organs and from receptors involved in cardiovascular and respiratory regulation are the **general visceral afferents**, the main features of which are now discussed.

The cell bodies of general visceral afferent neurons are situated in the inferior ganglia of the glossopharyngeal and vagus nerves and in the ganglia of spinal nerves. The peripheral processes of visceral afferent neurons traverse autonomic ganglia and plexuses without interruption to reach the organs they supply. These neurons are functionally of two kinds: physiological afferents and afferents for pain. Most physiological afferents accompany fibers of the parasympathetic (or craniosacral) division of the autonomic nervous system. The afferents for pain all accompany the fibers of the sympathetic division.

Physiological Afferents

Visceral afferents of special physiological importance are associated with the parasympathetic division of the autonomic system. The

following examples illustrate the reflex arcs of which they form the afferent limbs.

CARDIOVASCULAR SYSTEM

Terminals of sensory fibers in the aortic arch and carotid sinus (at the bifurcation of the common carotid artery) serve as **baroreceptors**, signaling changes in arterial blood pressure. The cell bodies of neurons supplying the aortic arch are in the inferior (nodose) ganglion of the vagus nerve, whereas those for the carotid sinus are in the inferior ganglion of the glossopharyngeal nerve. The central processes terminate in the solitary nucleus in the medulla, from which fibers pass to regions of the reticular formation referred to as **cardiovascular "centers."** These in turn project to the nucleus ambiguus and intermediolateral cell column of the spinal cord. Through the reflex pathways thereby established, a rapid increase in arterial pressure causes a decrease in heart rate (vagus nerve) and vasodilation through inhibition of the vasoconstrictor action of the sympathetic outflow. A fall in arterial pressure, such as occurs after hemorrhage, initiates reflex responses that are the reverse of those caused by a rise in arterial pressure. Visceral afferents in the glossopharyngeal and vagus nerves, therefore, participate in the maintenance of normal arterial blood pressure.

The cardiac output also is regulated by the **Bainbridge reflex**, which is triggered by vagally innervated receptors in the right atrium; these monitor the central venous pressure. The central connections involved are unknown, but efferent limbs of the reflex include provisions for stimulation of the sympathetic nervous system and inhibition of the vagal slowing of the heart. Thus the cardiac output is increased as the volume of the venous return rises.

RESPIRATORY SYSTEM

There are **respiratory "centers"** in the brain stem for automatic control of respiratory movements. Two such regions are situated in the reticular formation of the medulla, an inspiratory center medially and an expiratory center laterally. In addition, a pneumotaxic center at the level of the pontomedullary junction regulates the rhythmicity of inspiration and expiration.[3] Inspiration is initiated by stimulation of neurons in the inspiratory center by **carbon dioxide** of the circulating blood.[4] The chemosensory neurons, by means of reticulospinal connections, stimulate the motor neurons that supply the diaphragm and intercostal muscles.

Respiratory movements also are influenced by nerve impulses conducted centrally from the carotid bodies situated near the bifurcation of the common carotid arteries and from small aortic bodies adjacent to the aortic arch. The glomus cells of these bodies serve as **chemoreceptors** that respond to decreased **oxygen** concentration in the blood. The resulting impulses reach the solitary nucleus through neurons with cell bodies in the inferior ganglia of the glossopharyngeal and vagus nerves. Further connections with respiratory centers in the brain stem bring about an increase in the rate and depth of respiratory movements. This reflex operates in vigorous exercise, when a person is exposed to a lowered oxygen tension such as at high altitudes, or in any circumstances that produce asphyxia.

Sensory neurons in the vagus nerve constitute the afferent limb of the **Hering-Breuer reflex**, through which expiration is initiated. Nerve terminals in the bronchial tree, especially the smaller branches, discharge at an increasing rate as the lungs are inflated. These signals reach the expiratory center through a relay in the solitary nucleus. Neurons in the expiratory center then inhibit those of the inspiratory center. Expiration ensues as a passive (elastic) process when the inspiratory muscles relax.

OTHER SYSTEMS

Sensory fibers in the vagus nerve are distributed to the gastrointestinal tract at least as far as the splenic flexure at the junction of the transverse colon and descending colon. The nerve terminals are stimulated by distention of the stomach and intestine, contraction of the smooth musculature, and irritation of the mucosa. Although motility and secretion are not dependent on the extrinsic nerves, they are modified by reflex action involving vagal afferent and efferent neurons. The distal colon, rectum, and urinary bladder are supplied by splanchnic branches of the second, third, and fourth sacral nerves. Reflexes in these segments of the spinal cord and the sacral portion of the parasympathetic system stimulate emptying of the large bowel and urinary bladder, subject to voluntary control.

FULLNESS ASCENDING PATHWAYS

There are ascending visceral pathways distinct from those for pain (described in the next section). One such pathway originates in the solitary nucleus in the medulla, which receives general visceral afferents from the vagus nerve predominantly. A second pathway originates in segments T1 through L2 of the spinal cord, probably in the intermediomedial cell column of lamina VII, and in segments S2 through S4. These ascending fibers are included in the spinoreticular and spinothalamic tracts. Through the pathways from the medulla and spinal cord, impulses of visceral origin reach the reticular formation of the brain stem, hypothalamus, and ventral posterior nucleus of the thalamus. A thalamocortical projection provides for a feeling of fullness when the stomach is distended and a feeling of hunger when the stomach is empty. Feelings of fullness in the distal colon and urinary bladder are

---

[3] These "centers" as well as those for the cardiovascular system probably are fields within the network of long dendrites in the reticular formation, rather than compact collections of cell bodies. The pneumotaxic center is coextensive with the Kolliker-Fuse nucleus of the parabrachial area (see Ch. 9).

[4] Experiments in animals indicate that neurons sensitive to increased CO_2 concentration (or the associated fall in pH of extracellular fluid) are near the ventrolateral surface of the medulla. This region (see also Ch. 9) also receives afferent fibers that respond to input from the carotid and aortic baroreceptors and chemoreceptors and contains neurons that project to the hypothalamus and to respiratory motor neurons in the spinal cord.

also mediated by these spinoreticular and spinothalamic connections.

Pain Afferents

The sensory endings for pain arising in internal organs are stimulated in various ways in the presence of abnormal function or disease. The pain is most commonly caused by distention of a hollow viscus such as the intestine. This may occur proximal to localized and forcible contraction of the smooth muscle. Similarly, distention of a bile duct or a ureter occurs when the lumen is obstructed by a stone. Visceral pain also results from rapid stretching of the capsule of a solid organ, such as the liver or spleen. Peritoneal irritation contributes to the pain of inflammatory disease. In the case of angina and the pain of myocardial infarction, the effective stimulus is anoxia of cardiac muscle.

The sensory neurons for pain of visceral origin are associated only with the sympathetic nervous system. The cell bodies of the primary sensory neurons are in the dorsal root ganglia of the thoracic and upper lumbar nerves (see Fig. 24-4). The peripheral processes of these neurons reach the sympathetic trunk by way of white communicating rami (see Fig. 24-3); they run in the sympathetic trunk for variable distances and then continue to the viscera by way of the cardiac, pulmonary, and splanchnic nerves. The termination of the corresponding dorsal root fibers in the spinal gray matter is not known precisely; however, the majority probably enter the dorsolateral tract of Lissauer along with somatic pain fibers and end similarly in the dorsal horn. The ascending pathway for visceral pains in part, with the pathway for somatic pain, through crossed fibers in the spinothalamic tract. There are also bilateral spinoreticular fibers and relays in the reticular formation, as in the pathway for pain from somatic structures.

REFERRED PAIN

Visceral pain has characteristics that distinguish it from pain arising in somatic structures, notably diffuse localization and radiation to somatic areas (referred pain). The zone of reference of the pain from an internal organ coincides with the part of the body served by somatic sensory neurons associated with the same segments of the spinal cord. The principle of referred pain is illustrated by the following examples. The reader should compare the areas of reference with the distribution of segmental innervation of the skin (see Fig. 5-13).

The **heart** is supplied with pain fibers by the middle and inferior cervical cardiac nerves and by the thoracic cardiac branches of the left sympathetic trunk. Central processes of the primary sensory neurons enter segments T1 through T5. Pain of cardiac origin is, therefore, referred to the left side of the chest and the inner aspect of the left arm. Deviations from this zone of reference are common and are probably due to variations in the laterality and segmental levels of the cardiac innervation.

Pain from the **gallbladder** or **bile ducts** passes centrally in the right greater splanchnic nerve, entering the spinal cord through the seventh and eighth thoracic dorsal roots. The pain is referred to the upper quadrant of the abdomen and the infrascapular region on the right side. Disease of the liver or gallbladder may irritate the peritoneum covering the **diaphragm**. The resulting pain is referred to the shoulder because the diaphragm is supplied with sensory fibers (as well as motor fibers) by the phrenic nerve, which originates from segments C3 through C5.

Pain of gastric origin is felt in the epigastrium because the **stomach** is supplied with pain afferents that reach segments T7 and T8 by way of the left and right greater splanchnic nerves. Pain from the **duodenum**, as in duodenal ulcer, is referred to the anterior abdominal wall just above the umbilicus, with both this area and the duodenum being supplied by the ninth and tenth thoracic nerves. Afferent fibers from the **appendix** are included in the lesser splanchnic nerve, which contains axons from the T10 dorsal root ganglion. The pain of appendicitis is referred initially to the region of the umbilicus, which lies in the tenth thoracic dermatome. The pain shifts to the lower right quadrant of the abdomen when the parietal peritoneum becomes involved in the inflammatory process. (The parietal peritoneum and pleura are supplied by segmental somatic nerves.) Pain fibers from the **renal pelvis** and **ureter** are included in the least splanchnic nerve; they enter the first two lumbar segments of the spinal cord, and the pain is referred to the loin and the groin.

There is no entirely satisfactory explanation for the referral of pain. An early proposal was that afferent fibers for visceral and somatic pain synapse with the same tract cells in the spinal cord, with these cells being excited by subliminal somatic stimuli when receiving impulses of visceral origin. A more recent hypothesis is that both visceral and somatic pain from regions served by a specific segment of the spinal cord are relayed to the same group of cells in the ventral posterior nucleus of the thalamus. The topographic representation of the body in the thalamus and cerebral cortex allows recognition of the sources of ordinary somatic sensations. Localization may be in error when pain originates internally, perhaps because pain of somatic origin is a common experience compared with pain caused by visceral malfunction or disease. It is of interest that 230 years ago, John Hunter called referred pain a "delusion of the mind."

SUGGESTED READING

Brooks CMcC, Koizumi K, Sato AY (eds): Integrative Functions of the Autonomic Nervous System. Amsterdam, Elsevier, 1979

Bruce EN, Cherniak NS: Central chemoreceptors. J Appl Physiol 62:389–402, 1987

Gershon MD: The enteric nervous system. Annu Rev Neurosci 4:227–272, 1981

Grundy D: Gastrointestinal Motility. Lancaster & Boston, MTP Press, 1985

Hainsworth R: Reflexes from the heart. Physiol Rev 71:617–658, 1991

Jessen KR, Mirsky R, Hills JM: GABA as an autonomic neurotransmitter: Studies on intrinsic GABA-ergic neurons in the myenteric plexus of the gut. Trends Neurosci 10:255–262, 1987

Karczmar AG, Koketsu K, Nishi S (eds): Autonomic and Enteric Ganglia. New York, Plenum Press, 1986

Nathan PW, Smith MC: The location of descending fibres to sympathetic neurons supplying the eye and sudomotor neurons supplying the head and neck. J Neurol Neurosurg Psychiatry 49:187–194, 1986

Sanders KM, Ward SM: Nitric oxide as a mediator of nonadrenergic noncholinergic neurotransmission. Am J Physiol 262:G379–G392, 1992

Smith OA, DeVito JL: Central neural integration for the control of autonomic responses associated with emotion. Annu Rev Neurosci 7:43–65, 1984

Swanson LW, Mogenson GJ: Neural mechanisms for the functional coupling of autonomic, endocrine and somatomotor responses in adaptive behavior. Brain Res Rev 3:1–34, 1981

Blood Supply and the Meninges

The Human Nervous System: An Anatomical Viewpoint, Sixth Edition, Murray L. Barr and John A. Kiernan. J.B. Lippincott Company, Philadelphia, © 1993.

Blood Supply of the Central Nervous System

Important Facts

Blood flow through arteries in the central nervous system is kept constant by a process known as autoregulation.

Exchange through the capillaries of the central nervous system is regulated by endothelial transport mechanisms. These vessels are impermeable to large molecules, except in a few small regions that have no blood–brain barrier.

The anterior choroidal artery supplies the optic tract and parts of the internal capsule.

The anterior cerebral artery gives rise to the recurrent artery of Heubner, which supplies the corpus striatum and internal capsule, and the anterior communicating artery. It then continues, to supply the medial and superior surfaces of the frontal and parietal lobes.

The middle cerebral artery supplies the lateral surface of the frontal, parietal, and temporal lobes, including the motor and somesthetic areas for the body above the knee and (on the left) the language areas. The geniculocalcarine tract is also supplied by this vessel.

The spinal cord is supplied by branches of the vertebral and radicular arteries.

The largest branch of the vertebral artery is the posterior inferior cerebellar artery, which supplies the lateral part of the medulla and much of the cerebellum.

The anterior inferior and the superior cerebellar arteries are branches of the basilar artery. Smaller branches supply the pons and the labyrinth of the inner ear.

The posterior cerebral artery gives rise to the posterior choroidal artery, connects with the posterior communicating artery, and then supplies the occipital lobe, the inferior surface of the temporal lobe, and parts of the hippocampal formation.

Aneurysms at sites of arterial bifurcation in and near the circle of Willis are a common source of subarachnoid hemorrhage.

Superior cerebral veins drain into the superior sagittal sinus. Blood from the inferior surfaces of the cortex and from the interior of the brain eventually is collected by the great cerebral vein, which empties into the straight sinus.

The blood supply of the central nervous system is of special interest because of the metabolic demands of nervous tissue. The brain depends on aerobic metabolism of glucose and is one of the most metabolically active organs of the body. Although composing only 2% of body weight, the brain receives about 17% of the cardiac output and consumes about 20% of the oxygen used by the entire body. Unconsciousness follows cessation of cerebral circulation in about 10 seconds. Lesions of vascular origin are responsible for more neurological disorders than any other category of disease process.

Cerebrovascular Disease

Arterial occlusion by an embolus or a thrombus usually is followed by infarction of a portion of the region supplied. There are anastomotic channels between branches of the major arteries on the surface of the brain. There also are communications at the arteriolar level, and the capillary bed is continuous throughout the brain. These anastomoses, however, usually are inadequate to sustain the circulation in the region normally supplied by a major artery. The size of an infarction depends on the caliber of the occluded artery, existing anastomoses, and the time elapsing before complete obstruction. In addition to intracranial occlusions, impairment of the cerebral circulation often is the result of stenosis of a carotid or vertebral artery in the neck.

The slender, thin-walled arteries that penetrate the ventral surface of the brain to supply the internal capsule and adjacent gray masses are especially prone to rupture. Hypertension and degenerative changes in these arteries are major factors that lead to **cerebral hemorrhage**. An **aneurysm** usually occurs at the site of branching of one of the larger arteries at the base of the brain. An aneurysm may leak or rupture, in which case the bleeding typically is into the subarachnoid space; however, adhesion of the aneurysmal sac to adjacent structures can give rise to hemorrhage that is intracerebral or into a cranial nerve.

Arterial Supply of the Brain

Because of the practical importance of cerebrovascular disease and because the neurological signs depend on the site of the lesion, an understanding of the distribution of the arteries is essential. The brain is supplied by the paired internal carotid and vertebral arteries through an extensive system of branches. Descriptions of the arteries follow, with some notes on their clinical significance. Later in this chapter, there are summaries of cortical areas and deeper parts of the brain, indicating the arteries by which they are supplied.

Internal Carotid System

The **internal carotid artery**, a terminal branch of the common carotid artery, traverses the carotid canal in the base of the skull and enters the middle cranial fossa beside the dorsum sellae of the sphenoid bone. Beyond this point, the artery undergoes the following sequence of bends that constitute the "carotid siphon" in a cerebral angiogram (see Fig. 25-5). The internal carotid artery first runs forward in the cavernous venous sinus and then turns upward on the medial side of the anterior clinoid process. At this point, the artery enters the subarachnoid space by piercing the dura mater and arachnoid, courses backward below the optic nerve, and finally turns upward immediately lateral to the optic chiasma. This brings the artery under the anterior perforated substance, where it divides into the middle and anterior cerebral arteries (Fig. 25-1).

COLLATERAL BRANCHES

The following branches arise from the internal carotid artery before its terminal bifurcation.

HYPOPHYSIAL ARTERIES. These arteries originate from the cavernous and postclinoid portions of the internal carotid artery. The posterior hypophysial arteries supply the neural lobe of the pituitary gland, and the anterior

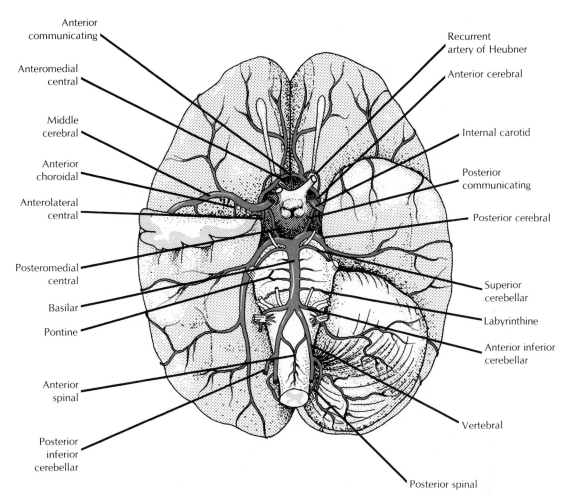

Figure 25-1. Arteries that supply the brain, as seen from the ventral surface. The right cerebral hemisphere and the tip of the right temporal lobe have been removed.

hypophysial arteries enter the median eminence of the hypothalamus. The latter blood vessels break up into capillary loops, into which hypothalamic releasing factors gain access, and the capillary loops drain through small veins into the sinusoids of the anterior lobe. This constitutes the hypophysial portal system through which the hypothalamus influences the output of pituitary hormones (see also Ch. 11).

OPHTHALMIC ARTERY. This branch comes off immediately after the internal carotid artery

enters the subarachnoid space. The ophthalmic artery passes through the optic foramen into the orbit, supplying the eye and other orbital contents, frontal area of the scalp, frontal and ethmoid paranasal sinuses, and parts of the nose.

POSTERIOR COMMUNICATING ARTERY. This slender artery arises from the internal carotid artery close to its terminal bifurcation. The posterior communicating artery runs backward to join the proximal part of the posterior cerebral artery, thereby forming part of the arterial circle (circle of Willis). Some of the postero-medial central arteries, described later, are branches of the posterior communicating artery.

ANTERIOR CHOROIDAL ARTERY. This branch comes off the distal part of the internal carotid artery or the beginning of the middle cerebral artery and has a wider distribution than its name suggests. The artery passes back along the optic tract and the choroid fissure at the medial edge of the temporal lobe. In addition to supplying the choroid plexus in the temporal horn of the lateral ventricle, the anterior choroidal artery gives off branches to the optic tract, uncus, amygdala, hippocampus, globus pallidus, lateral geniculate nucleus, and ventral part of the internal capsule. The branching is variable, and the territory supplied by this artery sometimes includes the subthalamus, ventral parts of the thalamus, and the rostral part of the midbrain (including the red nucleus). The terminal branches of the anterior choroidal artery supply the choroid plexus in the temporal horn of the lateral ventricle and anastomose there with branches of the posterior choroidal artery.

Internal Carotid Occlusion

Occlusion of the internal carotid artery has serious consequences. Blindness of the ipsilateral eye (supplied by the ophthalmic artery) and the contralateral half of the visual field of the other eye (from infarction of the optic tract and lateral geniculate body, supplied by the anterior choroidal artery) are added to the effects of occlusion of the middle and anterior cerebral arteries (principally a contralateral hemiplegia and hemianopsia, with global aphasia if the affected hemisphere is the dominant one for language).

Occlusion of the **anterior choroidal artery** alone can be asymptomatic, or it may have a variety of effects, depending on the site of the obstruction and the efficiency of the anastomoses with the posterior choroidal artery. Symptoms can include contralateral hemiplegia and sensory abnormalities (internal capsule) and contralateral homonymous hemi-

anopsia (optic tract and lateral geniculate body).

MIDDLE CEREBRAL ARTERY

Of the terminal branches of the internal carotid artery, the middle cerebral artery is the larger and more direct continuation of the parent vessel (see Fig. 25-1). This artery runs deep in the lateral sulcus between the frontal and temporal lobes. Central arteries (the anteromedial group, described later) arise from the proximal part of the middle cerebral artery, lateral to the optic chiasma. They enter the base of the hemisphere and supply internal structures, including the internal capsule. **Frontal, parietal**, and **temporal branches** emerge from the lateral sulcus of the cerebral hemisphere (Fig. 25-2) to supply a large area of cortex and subcortical white matter in the three corresponding lobes of the cerebrum.

The territory of distribution of the middle cerebral artery includes most of the primary motor and premotor cortex, the frontal eye field, and the primary somatosensory area. The motor and sensory cortex for the lower limb and the perineum are excluded. The left middle cerebral artery (in most people) supplies all the cortical areas concerned with language. These are the receptive or ideational language area in the temporal and parietal lobes and Broca's expressive speech area in the inferior frontal gyrus (see Fig. 25-2 and Ch. 15). The white matter underlying the parietal cortex contains the fibers of the geniculocalcarine tract.

Middle Cerebral Artery Occlusion

Loss of function of the cortical areas supplied by the middle cerebral artery results in contralateral paralysis most noticeable in the lower part of the face and in the arm, together with general sensory deficits of the cortical type. Involvement of the geniculocalcarine tract results in hemianopsia of the contralateral visual fields of both eyes (see Ch. 20). The auditory cortex is included in the area of distribution; however, a unilateral lesion causes no demonstrable im-

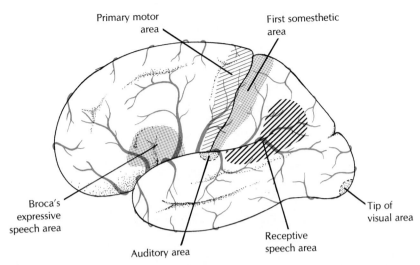

Figure 25-2. Distribution of the middle cerebral artery on the lateral surface of the cerebral hemisphere. Terminal branches of the anterior and posterior cerebral arteries are also visible (compare Fig. 25-3).

pairment of hearing because of the bilateral cortical projection from the organ of Corti. Occlusion of the middle cerebral artery of the hemisphere dominant for language causes global aphasia (see Ch. 15).

Fragments of the complete syndrome, such as monoplegia or receptive aphasia, are seen when individual cortical branches of the artery are blocked. Obstruction of the central branches can cause hemiplegia due to infarction of motor fibers in the internal capsule. A lesion in the internal capsule does not cause aphasia because the connections of the language areas with the contralateral hemisphere are intact.

ANTERIOR CEREBRAL ARTERY

The smaller terminal branch of the internal carotid artery is the anterior cerebral artery, which is first directed medially above the optic nerve (see Fig. 25-1). The two anterior cerebral arteries almost meet at the midline where they are joined together by the **anterior communicating artery**. A special branch of the anterior cerebral artery is given off just proximal to the anterior communicating artery. This is the **recurrent artery of Heubner**, which penetrates the anterior perforated substance to

supply the ventral part of the head of the caudate nucleus, adjacent portion of the putamen, and anterior limb and genu of the internal capsule. The recurrent artery of Heubner also is called the **medial striate artery** because of its contribution to the blood supply of the corpus striatum.

The anterior cerebral artery ascends in the longitudinal fissure and bends backward around the genu of the corpus callosum (Fig. 25-3). Branches given off just distal to the anterior communicating artery supply the medial portion of the orbital surface of the frontal lobe, including the olfactory bulb and olfactory tract. The artery continues along the upper surface of the corpus callosum as the **pericallosal artery**, and a large branch, the **callosomarginal artery**, follows the cingulate sulcus. The anterior cerebral artery supplies the medial portions of the frontal and parietal lobes and the corpus callosum. In addition, branches extend over the dorsomedial border of the hemisphere and supply a strip on the lateral surface (see Fig. 25-2). The supplementary motor area and the dorsal parts of the primary motor and somatosensory areas are included in its territory.

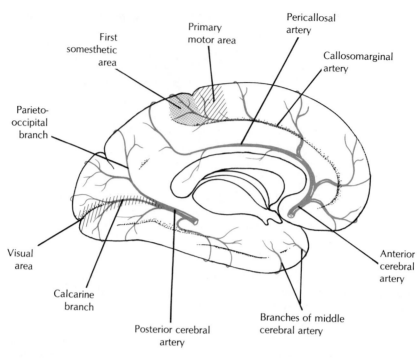

Figure 25-3. Distribution of the anterior and posterior cerebral arteries on the medial surface of the cerebral hemisphere.

Anterior Cerebral Artery Occlusion

Occlusion of the anterior cerebral artery causes paralysis and sensory deficits in the contralateral leg and perineum. There commonly is urinary incontinence due to inadequate perineal sensation and defective cortical control of the pelvic floor musculature. If the obstruction is in the proximal part of the vessel, blocking the recurrent artery of Heubner, there is contralateral upper motor neuron weakness of the face, tongue, and upper limb because of corticofugal motor fibers that are in or near the genu of the internal capsule before they pass into its posterior limb (see Ch. 16). A proximal occlusion may also cause ipsilateral anosmia due to infarction of the olfactory bulb and tract.

Anterior cerebral artery syndromes often are associated with mental confusion and dysphasia, perhaps attributable to loss of functions of the prefrontal cortex, the cingulate gyrus, and the supplementary motor area.

Vertebrobasilar System

The **vertebral artery**, a branch of the subclavian artery, ascends in the foramina of the transverse processes of the upper six cervical vertebrae. On reaching the base of the skull, the artery winds around the lateral mass of the atlas, pierces the posterior atlanto-occipital membrane, and enters the subarachnoid space at the level of the foramen magnum by piercing the dura mater and arachnoid. The vertebral artery runs forward with a medial inclination beneath the medulla, joining its fellow of the opposite side at the caudal border of the pons to form the **basilar artery**. The latter artery runs rostrally in the midline of the pons and divides into the **posterior cerebral arteries** (see Fig. 25-1).

BRANCHES OF THE VERTEBRAL ARTERY

SPINAL ARTERIES. The upper portion of the cervical cord receives blood through spinal branches of the vertebral arteries. A single **anterior spinal artery** is formed by a contribution from each vertebral artery. A **posterior spinal artery** arises on each side as a branch of either the vertebral or the posterior inferior cerebellar artery (see Fig. 25-1). The anterior and posterior spinal arteries continue throughout the length of the spinal cord. However, except for their proximal portions, the blood comes from reinforcements by the anterior and posterior radicular arteries (described below).

POSTERIOR INFERIOR CEREBELLAR ARTERY. This artery, often called "PICA," is the largest branch of the vertebral artery. It pursues an irregular course between the medulla and cerebellum. Branches are distributed to the posterior part of the cerebellar hemisphere, inferior vermis, central nuclei of the cerebellum, and choroid plexus of the fourth ventricle. There also are important **medullary branches** to the dorsolateral region of the medulla. In addition to branches from the posterior inferior cerebellar artery, fine branches arising directly from the vertebral artery supply the medulla.

BRANCHES OF THE BASILAR ARTERY

The basilar artery gives off the following branches before dividing into the posterior cerebral arteries at the rostral border of the pons.

ANTERIOR INFERIOR CEREBELLAR ARTERY. Arising from the caudal end of the basilar artery, the anterior inferior cerebellar artery (or "AICA") supplies the cortex of the inferior surface of the cerebellum anteriorly and the underlying white matter; it assists in the supply of the central cerebellar nuclei. In addition, slender twigs from the artery penetrate the upper medulla and lower pons.

LABYRINTHINE ARTERY. This artery, a branch of either the basilar artery or the anterior inferior cerebellar artery, traverses the internal acoustic meatus and ramifies throughout the membranous labyrinth of the internal ear.

PONTINE ARTERIES. These are slender branches that arise from the basilar artery along its length. They penetrate the pons and ramify in both the ventral portion of the pons and the pontine tegmentum.

SUPERIOR CEREBELLAR ARTERY. This branch arises close to the terminal bifurcation of the basilar artery, ramifies over the dorsal surface of the cerebellum, and supplies the cortex, medullary center, and central nuclei. Branches from the proximal part of the superior cerebellar artery are distributed to the pons, superior cerebellar peduncle, and inferior colliculus of the midbrain.

Vascular Lesions That Affect the Brain Stem
A substantial hemorrhage within the pons is instantly fatal. Thrombosis of the whole **basilar artery** causes coma and decerebrate rigidity (see Ch. 23), soon followed by death due to failure of the central control of respiration. An embolus that passes through a vertebral artery typically lodges at the bifurcation of the basilar artery. Infarction in the reticular formation of the midbrain causes coma, and the associated destruction of the fibers of both oculomotor nerves results in bilateral divergence of the eyes with fixed, dilated pupils. This syndrome can resemble the end stage of compression of the oculomotor nerves and midbrain due to herniation through the tentorial incisura (see Ch. 26), but the effects of an embolus are sudden, not gradual. A small embolus that lodges in one of the posteromedial central arteries can cause a small infarct in the midbrain, such as the lesion responsible for Weber's syndrome (see Ch. 7).

Some 30 syndromes (most with eponyms) have been described as resulting from occlusion of individual branches of the vertebral and basilar arteries. The positions of the lesions usually can be defined from the tracts and cranial nerve nuclei or fibers that are destroyed. A few examples are explained in Chapter 7. Of these, the most common is the **lateral medullary (Wallenberg's) syndrome**, which typically is due to obstruction of the posterior inferior cerebellar artery but is more often due to a thrombus in the vertebral artery.

Although of rare occurrence, occlusion of the **labyrinthine artery** (or of its parent vessel, the anterior inferior cerebellar artery) results in the expected deafness in the corresponding ear and vestibular dysfunction (vertigo, with a tendency to fall toward the side of the lesion).

Infarction of the ventral part of the **pons** causes paralysis of all voluntary movement, except of the eyes. The general and special sensory pathways are spared, and the patient is conscious but can communicate only by means of eye movements. This condition is called the **"locked-in" syndrome.** More dorsally located lesions in the rostral pons or caudal midbrain cause akinetic mutism (see Ch. 23), in which consciousness is severely impaired.

POSTERIOR CEREBRAL ARTERY

Central arteries (the posteromedial group) arise at and near the bifurcation of the basilar artery into the two posterior cerebral arteries. Each posterior cerebral artery then curves around the midbrain and reaches the medial surface of the cerebral hemisphere beneath the splenium of the corpus callosum (see Fig. 25-3). The artery gives off **temporal branches**, which ramify over the inferior surface of the temporal lobe, and **calcarine** and **parieto-occipital branches**, which run along the corresponding sulci. All these arteries send branches around the border of the cerebral hemisphere to supply a peripheral strip on the lateral surface (see Fig. 25-2). The calcarine branch is of special significance because it supplies the primary and association cortex for vision. Much of the parahippocampal gyrus together with parts of the hippocampus are supplied by the temporal branches.

The **posterior choroidal artery** (not seen in Fig. 25-3) comes off the posterior cerebral artery in the region of the splenium and runs forward in the transverse fissure beneath the corpus callosum. The posterior choroidal artery supplies the choroid plexus of the central part of the lateral ventricle, choroid plexus of the third ventricle, posterior part of the thalamus, fornix, and tectum of the midbrain. Its terminal branches anastomose with those of the anterior choroidal artery, within the choroid plexus of the lateral ventricle.

Posterior Cerebral Artery Occlusion

Infarction of the cortical areas supplied by the posterior cerebral artery causes blindness in the contralateral field of vision. Ischemia of the hippocampal formation can result in a disturbance of memory after the arterial occlusion, but this recovers because lesions in the limbic system must be bilateral to cause lasting disability.

If the infarct is in the hemisphere dominant for language (usually the left) and extends into the splenium of the corpus callosum, the contralateral (intact) visual cortex is disconnected from the language areas of the dominant hemisphere. This causes alexia (see Ch. 15) in addition to the homonymous hemianopsia.

Herniation of the uncus through the tentorial incisura, due to an expanding space-occupying lesion in the supratentorial compartment of the cranial cavity, can stretch and compress one or both posterior cerebral arteries over the rigid anterior edge of the tentorium (see Ch. 26). Even if the cause is treated surgically, there may be necrosis of the areas supplied by the compressed arteries. Cortical blindness results, and there also may be permanent impairment of the ability to form new memories (see Ch. 18) due to bilateral hippocampal involvement.

Cortical Branches of the Cerebral Arteries

Anastomoses between branches of the anterior, middle, and posterior cerebral arteries are concealed in the sulci. The caliber of an anastomotic vessel may be sufficient to sustain a portion of the territory of another artery if the latter is occluded. The cerebral arteries are also interconnected through an arteriolar network in the pia mater. Short cortical branches from the pial plexus supply the rich capillary network of the cortex, whereas longer branches of arteries in the subarachnoid space penetrate into the white matter and form a less profuse capillary network.

Arterial Circle (Circle of Willis)

The major arteries that supply the cerebrum are joined to one another at the base of the brain in the form of an arterial circle, or the circle of Willis (see Fig. 25-1). Starting from the midline in front, the circle consists of the anterior communicating, anterior cerebral, internal carotid (a short segment), posterior communicating, and posterior cerebral arteries; then it continues to the starting point in reverse order. There normally is little exchange of blood between the main arteries through the slender communicating vessels. The arterial circle provides alternative routes, however, when one of the major arteries leading into it is occluded. These anastomoses frequently are inadequate, especially in elderly people, in whom the communicating arteries may be narrowed because of vascular disease.

There are frequent variants of the conventional configuration of the arterial circle. The posterior cerebral artery is a branch of the internal carotid artery in the embryo. In the course of development, the posterior cerebral artery becomes a terminal branch of the basilar artery, leaving the posterior communicating artery as the vestige of the embryonic condition. About one person in three has one posterior cerebral artery as a major branch of the internal carotid artery. This type of connection of the posterior cerebral artery seldom occurs bilaterally. Often one of the anterior cerebral arteries is unusually small in the first part of its course, in which case the anterior communicating artery has a larger than usual caliber.

Aneurysms often develop at sites of branching of arteries in and near the arterial circle, and they can rupture or leak, causing **subarachnoid hemorrhage**. The commonest sites for such aneurysms are the terminal part of the internal carotid artery, the anterior communicating artery, and the proximal part of the middle cerebral artery. A subarachnoid hemorrhage causes a severe headache of sudden onset, with a stiff neck and other signs of meningeal irritation.

Central Arteries

Numerous central arteries arise from the region of the arterial circle as four groups (see Fig. 25-1). These slender, thin-walled blood vessels, also variously known as ganglionic, nuclear, striate, or thalamic perforating arteries, supply portions of the corpus striatum, internal capsule, diencephalon, and midbrain. The recurrent artery of Heubner is similar to the central arteries with respect to its distribution, as are the anterior and posterior choroidal arteries with respect to parts of their distributions.

ANTEROMEDIAL GROUP. These central arteries arise from the anterior cerebral arteries and from the anterior communicating artery. They penetrate the medial part of the anterior perforated substance and are distributed mainly to the preoptic and suprachiasmatic regions of the hypothalamus.

ANTEROLATERAL GROUP. This group of central arteries consists mainly of branches of the middle cerebral artery that enter the anterior perforated substance. They also are called **striate arteries** (or lateral striate arteries) because they supply a major portion of the corpus striatum. The region of distribution of the anterolateral central arteries includes the head of the caudate nucleus, putamen, lateral part of the globus pallidus, much of the internal capsule (anterior limb, genu, and dorsal portion of the posterior limb), external capsule, and claustrum. Several of these arteries also send twigs into the lateral area of the hypothalamus.

POSTEROMEDIAL GROUP. The posteromedial central arteries are branches of the posterior cerebral and posterior communicating arteries. After penetrating the posterior perforated substance between the cerebral peduncles, they are distributed to the anterior and medial portions of the thalamus, subthalamus, middle and posterior regions of the hypothalamus, and medial parts of the cerebral peduncles of the midbrain.

POSTEROLATERAL GROUP. These central arteries come off the posterior cerebral artery as it curves around the midbrain. They are distributed to the posterior portion of the thalamus (including the medial and lateral geniculate bodies), tectum of the midbrain, and lateral part of the cerebral peduncle.

DISTRIBUTION OF CENTRAL ARTERIES

The following summary identifies the blood supply of structures situated within the region of the brain that is nourished by the central arteries.

Head of caudate nucleus and putamen (striatum): anterolateral central arteries; recurrent artery of Heubner

Globus pallidus (pallidum): anterolateral central arteries; anterior choroidal artery

Thalamus: posteromedial and posterolateral central arteries; anterior and posterior choroidal arteries

Subthalamus: posteromedial central arteries; anterior choroidal artery

Hypothalamus: anteromedial, posteromedial, and anterolateral central arteries

Pineal gland: posterolateral central arteries

Internal capsule: anterolateral and posterolateral central arteries; anterior choroidal artery; recurrent artery of Heubner

Amygdala, uncus, and hippocampal formation: anterior choroidal artery; temporal branches of posterior cerebral artery

External capsule and claustrum: anterolateral central arteries

Tectum of midbrain: posterolateral central arteries; posterior choroidal artery; superior cerebellar artery

Cerebral peduncle: posteromedial and posterolateral central arteries; anterior choroidal artery

Vasomotor Control

The calibers of small arteries in the brain are controlled by **autoregulation**, which means that their muscular walls contract if the pressure inside rises and relax if the pressure falls, so that a constant rate of flow tends to be maintained. The increased blood flow in active areas of gray matter probably is due to vasodilator metabolites, notably carbon dioxide. Noradrenergic axons (from the sympathetic system and from the locus coeruleus) are present in the walls of many cerebral blood vessels, but their functional importance has not yet been ascertained.

Venous Drainage of the Brain

The capillary bed of the brain stem and the cerebellum is drained by unnamed veins that empty into the dural venous sinuses adjacent to the posterior cranial fossa. The cerebrum has an external and an internal venous system. The external cerebral veins lie in the subarachnoid space on all surfaces of the hemispheres, whereas the central core of the cerebrum is drained by internal cerebral veins situated beneath the corpus callosum in the transverse fissure. Both sets of cerebral veins empty into dural venous sinuses, which are described in Chapter 26.

EXTERNAL CEREBRAL VEINS

The **superior cerebral veins**, 8 to 12 in number, course upward over the lateral surface of the hemisphere. On nearing the midline, they pierce the arachnoid, run between the arachnoid and the dura mater for 1 to 2 cm, and empty into the superior sagittal sinus or into venous lacunae adjacent to the sinus. Trauma to the head may tear a superior cerebral vein as it lies between the arachnoid and dura mater, resulting in a **subdural hemorrhage**. Owing to the low venous pressure, the blood typically escapes slowly, clotting as it accumulates in the subdural space and gradually pushing the cerebrum downward.

The **superficial middle cerebral vein**

runs downward and forward along the lateral sulcus and empties into the cavernous sinus. Anastomotic channels allow for drainage in other directions. These are the superior anastomotic vein (of Trolard), which opens into the superior sagittal sinus, and the inferior anastomotic vein (of Labbé), which opens into the transverse sinus.

The **deep middle cerebral vein** runs downward and forward in the depths of the lateral sulcus to the ventral surface of the brain; the **anterior cerebral vein** accompanies the anterior cerebral artery. These veins unite in the region of the anterior perforated substance to form the **basal vein** (of Rosenthal), which runs backward at the base of the brain, curves around the midbrain, and empties into the great cerebral vein (see Internal Cerebral Veins). The basal vein receives tributaries from the optic tract, hypothalamus, temporal lobe, and midbrain.

In addition to the named veins just noted, there are numerous small vessels that drain limited areas. These have no consistent pattern and empty into adjacent dural sinuses.

INTERNAL CEREBRAL VEINS

The internal venous system forms adjacent to each lateral ventricle and continues through the transverse cerebral fissure beneath the corpus callosum (Fig. 25-4). The **thalamostriate vein (vena terminalis)** begins in the region of the amygdaloid body in the temporal lobe and follows the curve of the tail of the caudate nucleus on its medial side. The thalamostriate vein receives tributaries from the corpus striatum, internal capsule, thalamus, fornix, and septum pellucidum. The **choroidal vein**, which is rather tortuous, runs along the choroid plexus of the lateral ventricle. In addition to draining the plexus, the choroidal vein receives tributaries from the hippocampus, fornix, and corpus callosum. The thalamostriate vein and choroidal vein unite immediately behind the interventricular foramen to form the **internal cerebral vein**. The paired internal cerebral veins run posteriorly in the transverse fissure, uniting beneath the splenium of the corpus callosum to form

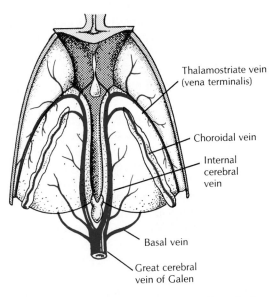

Figure 25-4. Internal cerebral system of veins, as seen from above after removal of the corpus callosum and fornix.

the **great cerebral vein** (of Galen). The latter vein, which is no more than 2 cm in length, receives the basal veins and tributaries from the cerebellum. The great cerebral vein empties into the straight sinus, which is in the midline of the tentorium cerebelli.

Blood Supply of the Spinal Cord

SPINAL ARTERIES

Three arterial channels, the **anterior spinal artery** and paired **posterior spinal arteries**, run longitudinally throughout the length of the spinal cord. The anterior spinal artery originates in a Y-shaped configuration from the vertebral arteries, as already described, and runs caudally along the ventral median fissure. Each posterior spinal artery is a branch of either the vertebral artery or the posterior inferior cerebellar artery and consists of multiple anastomosing channels along the line of attachment of the dorsal roots of the spinal nerves.

The blood received by the spinal arteries

from the vertebral arteries is sufficient for only the upper cervical segments of the spinal cord. The arteries are, therefore, reinforced at intervals in the following manner. The vertebral artery in the cervical region, the posterior intercostal branches of the thoracic aorta, and the lumbar branches of the abdominal aorta give off segmental **spinal arteries**, which enter the vertebral canal through the intervertebral foramina. In addition to supplying the vertebrae, these segmental spinal arteries give rise to **anterior** and **posterior radicular arteries**, which run along the ventral and dorsal roots of the spinal nerves. Most of the radicular arteries are of small caliber, sufficient only to supply the nerve roots and contribute to a vascular plexus in the pia mater covering the spinal cord. A variable number of anterior radicular arteries of substantial size, about 12 including both sides, join the anterior spinal artery. Similarly, a variable number of posterior radicular arteries, about 14 including both sides, join the posterior spinal arteries. These larger radicular arteries are in the lower cervical, lower thoracic, and upper lumbar regions; the largest, an anterior radicular artery known as the **spinal artery of Adamkiewicz**, usually is in the upper lumbar region. The spinal cord is vulnerable to circulatory impairment if the important contribution by a major radicular artery is compromised by injury or by the placing of a surgical ligature.

Sulcal branches arise in succession from the anterior spinal artery and enter the right and left sides of the spinal cord alternately from the ventral median fissure. The sulcal arteries are least frequent in the thoracic part of the spinal cord. The anterior spinal artery supplies the ventral gray horns, part of the dorsal gray horns, and the ventral and lateral white funiculi. Penetrating branches from the posterior spinal arteries supply the remainder of the dorsal gray horns and the dorsal funiculi of white matter. A fine plexus (the vasocorona) derived from the spinal arteries is present in the pia mater on the lateral and ventral surfaces of the cord. Penetrating branches from the vasocorona supply a narrow zone of white matter beneath the pia mater.

SPINAL VEINS

Although the pattern of spinal veins is irregular, there are essentially six of them. **Anterior spinal veins** run along the midline and along the line of ventral rootlets. **Posterior spinal veins** are situated in the midline and along the line of dorsal rootlets. The spinal veins are drained at intervals by up to 12 **anterior radicular veins** and by a similar number of **posterior radicular veins**. The radicular veins empty into an epidural venous plexus, which in turn drains into an external vertebral plexus through channels in the intervertebral foramina. Blood from the external vertebral plexus empties into the vertebral, intercostal, and lumbar veins.

Cerebral Angiography

In 1927, de Egas Moniz introduced the technique of cerebral angiography, which developed into a valuable diagnostic aid in the hands of neuroradiologists. The method consists of injecting a radiopaque solution into the artery, followed by serial x-ray photography at about 1-second intervals. The radiographs show the contrast medium in progressive stages of its passage through the arterial tree and the venous return. Injection into the common carotid artery or the internal carotid artery shows the distribution of the middle and anterior cerebral arteries (Figs. 25-5 and 25-6). Similarly, injection of the vertebral artery, which is approached with a long catheter passed through the femoral artery and aorta, permits visualization of the vertebral, basilar, and posterior cerebral arteries together with their branches (Fig. 25-7). The cerebral veins are seen in later pictures of a series.

The technique of cerebral angiography is especially useful in identifying vascular malformations and aneurysms. The method often provides valuable information concerning occlusive vascular disease and space-occupying lesions that displace blood vessels. The larger cerebral vessels also can be demonstrated by computed tomography after intravenous injection of a contrast medium and by nuclear magnetic resonance imaging.

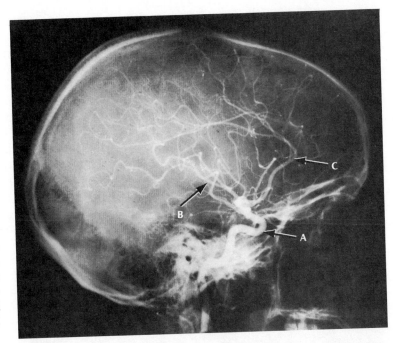

Figure 25-5. Carotid angiogram (*lateral view*). (**A**) Carotid siphon. (**B**) Branches of the middle cerebral artery. (**C**) Anterior cerebral artery. (*Courtesy of Dr. J. M. Allcock*)

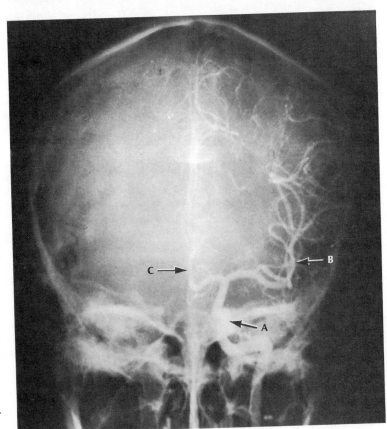

Figure 25-6. Carotid angiogram (*anteroposterior view*). (**A**) Carotid siphon. (**B**) Branches of the middle cerebral artery. (**C**) Anterior cerebral artery. (*Courtesy of Dr. J. M. Allcock*)

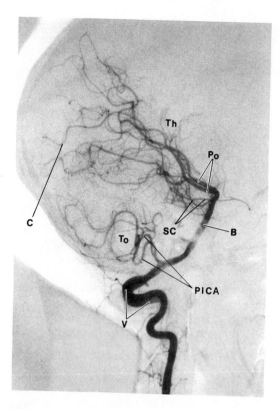

Figure 25-7. Vertebral angiogram, lateral view. This is a subtraction image made by superimposing a positive plain radiograph of the patient's skull (ie, with dark bones) on the angiogram and then photographing through the two films, so that the contrast medium now appears dark and the naturally radiopaque structures are largely eliminated. The contrast medium has flowed into the basilar artery and the contralateral vertebral artery, so the vertebrobasilar circulation is filled bilaterally. (**B**) Basilar artery. (**C**) Calcarine branch of a posterior cerebral artery. (**PICA**) Posterior inferior cerebellar arteries of both sides. (**Po**) Posterior cerebral arteries. (**SC**) Superior cerebellar arteries. (**Th**) Position of thalamus. (**To**) Position of cerebellar tonsil. (**V**) Vertebral arteries (*superimposed*). (*Courtesy of Dr. D. M. Pelz*)

Blood–Brain Barrier

Certain substances fail to pass from capillary blood into the central nervous system, although the same substances gain access to non–nervous tissues. They include dyes used in animal experimentation and some agents that would otherwise be of therapeutic value. In the blood, these substances are bound to plasma protein molecules, which are unable to leave normal cerebral blood vessels. The lumen of a capillary and the parenchyma of the brain and spinal cord are separated by endothelium, a basal lamina, and perivascular end feet of astrocytic processes. In mammals, the blood–brain barrier to proteins is formed by the internal plasma membranes of the endothelial cells and the tight junctions between them. In a few small regions (for example, the area postrema in the medulla, the subfornical organ, and the neurohypophysis), the classic blood–brain barrier is lacking.

The entry of small molecules into the brain is restricted by carrier mechanisms within the endothelial cells of the cerebral blood vessels. These regulate the transport of glucose, amino acids, and other substances from the blood to the neurons and neuroglia.

The blood–brain barrier is defective for 2 to 3 weeks after injury, and it also fails in various pathological states, such as inflammatory and neoplastic diseases. It is possible to make images of sites of abnormal vascular permeability by administering an appropriate radioactive tracer and scanning the head for the emitted radiation. Other tracers (gadolinium compounds) make permeable regions visible in images produced by nuclear magnetic resonance imaging.

SUGGESTED READING

Caronna JJ: Cerebrovascular diseases. In Kelley WN (ed): Textbook of Internal Medicine, 2nd ed, pp 2161–2168. Philadelphia, JB Lippincott, 1991

Davson H: History of the blood-brain barrier concept. In Neuwelt EA (ed): Implications of the Blood-Brain Barrier and Its Manipulation, vol 1, pp 27–52. New York, Plenum Press, 1989

Gillilan LA: The blood supply of the human spinal cord. J Comp Neurol 110:75–103, 1958

Gross PM: Morphology and physiology of capillary systems in subregions of the subfornical organ and area postrema. Can J Physiol Pharmacol 69:1010–1025, 1991

Montemurro DG, Bruni JE: The Human Brain in Dissection, 2nd ed. Philadelphia, WB Saunders, 1988

Netter FH: The Ciba Collection of Medical Illustra-tions. Vol I. The Nervous System. Pt I. Anatomy and Physiology. West Caldwell, NJ, Ciba-Geigy, 1983

Salamon G: Atlas de la Vascularization Artérielle du Cerveau chez l'Homme, 2nd ed. Paris, Sandoz Editions, 1973

Twenty-Six

The Human Nervous System: An Anatomical Viewpoint, Sixth Edition, Murray L. Barr and John A. Kiernan. J.B. Lippincott Company, Philadelphia. © 1993.

Meninges and Cerebrospinal Fluid

Important Facts

The cranial dura mater adheres to the skull, but extradural hemorrhage from the middle meningeal artery can compress the brain. The spinal epidural space contains fat, nerve roots, and veins.

Most of the cranial dura is supplied by the trigeminal nerve.

The largest dural reflections are the falx cerebri and the tentorium cerebelli.

Pressure on a cerebral hemisphere can lead to transtentorial herniation. This causes compression of the ipsilateral oculomotor nerve and uncus, either cerebral peduncle, and sometimes the posterior cerebral arteries.

Veins leaving the cerebral cortex traverse the subarachnoid and subdural spaces before entering the superior sagittal sinus. A head injury can tear these veins, which then bleed into the subdural space.

Most other cerebral veins empty into the straight sinus. All the venous blood from the brain eventually passes through the sigmoid sinuses into the internal jugular veins.

The epithelium of the arachnoid has occluding tight junctions that form a barrier between the cerebrospinal fluid and the dura. There is free exchange across the pia mater, between the cerebrospinal fluid and the extracellular spaces of the central nervous system.

The width of the subarachnoid space varies because the arachnoid adheres to the dura and the pia to the external glial limiting membrane. The widest spaces are the subarachnoid cisterns, of which the lumbar and cerebellomedullary are the largest.

The subarachnoid space accompanies the optic nerve as far as the optic disk. Raised intracranial pressure causes swelling of the disk (papilledema).

Cerebrospinal fluid is secreted by the choroid plexuses; circulates through the ventricles, the apertures of the fourth ventricle, and the subarachnoid space; and is absorbed into the dural sinuses by way of the arachnoid villi.

Hydrocephalus can be due to obstruction of the flow of cerebrospinal fluid through the ventricular system or subarachnoid space or to obstruction of the arachnoid villi. The sites of accumulation of fluid are appropriate to the position of the blockage.

The consistency of the brain is soft and gelatinous, although the spinal cord is slightly firmer. The meninges provide protection for the central nervous system in addition to the protection provided by the skull and the vertebral column and its ligaments. They consist of the thick **dura mater** externally, the delicate **arachnoid** lining the dura, and the thin **pia mater** adhering to the brain and spinal cord. The latter two layers, constituting the pia-arachnoid, bound the subarachnoid space filled with cerebrospinal fluid. The main support and protection provided by the meninges come from the dura mater and the cushion of cerebrospinal fluid in the subarachnoid space.

Dura Mater and Associated Structures

The internal surfaces of the bones enclosing the cranial cavity are clothed by periosteum, such as covers bones elsewhere. This periosteum is continuous with the periosteum on the external surface of the cranium at the margins of the foramen magnum and smaller foramina for nerves and blood vessels. The cranial dura mater is attached intimately to the periosteum, which sometimes is called incorrectly the "external layer" of the dura mater.

Periosteum and Meningeal Blood Vessels

The periosteum consists of collagenous connective tissue and contains arteries, somewhat inappropriately called meningeal arteries, which mainly supply the adjoining bone. Of these, the largest is the **middle meningeal artery**, a branch of the maxillary artery that enters the cranial cavity through the foramen spinosum in the floor of the middle cranial fossa. The artery divides into anterior and posterior branches soon after entering the middle cranial fossa; these branches ramify over the lateral surface of the cranium, producing grooves on the bones. Less extensive areas of the cranium and dura are supplied by several small arteries. These include meningeal branches of the ophthalmic artery,

branches of the occipital artery traversing the jugular foramen and hypoglossal canal, and small twigs arising from the vertebral artery at the foramen magnum.

Extradural Hemorrhage

A fracture in the temporal region of the skull may tear a branch of the middle meningeal artery. The extravasated blood accumulates between the bone and the periosteum. As in the case of any space-occupying lesion in the nonexpansile cranial cavity, intracranial pressure rises and prompt surgical intervention usually is necessary. The effects of the expanding lesion are similar to those of a subdural hemorrhage (see Ch. 25) and are discussed in this chapter under the heading "Transtentorial and Other Herniations." The deterioration is typically faster with arterial blood escaping at high pressure than with venous bleeding into the subdural space.

The meningeal arteries are accompanied by **meningeal veins**, which also are subject to tearing in fractures of the skull. The largest meningeal veins accompany the middle meningeal artery, leave the cranial cavity through the foramen spinosum or the foramen ovale, and drain into the pterygoid venous plexus. **Diploic veins**, within the cancellous bone of the vault of the skull, drain into the veins of the scalp and into the dural venous sinuses described below.

Dura Mater

The dura mater, or pachymeninx (thick membrane), is a dense, firm layer of collagenous connective tissue. The **spinal dura mater** takes the form of a tube, pierced by the roots of spinal nerves, that extends from the foramen magnum to the second segment of the sacrum. The spinal dura mater is separated from the wall of the spinal canal by an **extradural (epidural) space** that contains adipose tissue and a venous plexus. The **cranial dura mater** is firmly attached to the periosteum, as previously described, from which it receives small blood vessels. The smooth inner surface of the dura mater consists of simple squamous epithelium, and a film of fluid occupies the **subdural space** between the dura and arachnoid. The cranial dura mater has several features of importance, notably the dural reflections and dural venous sinuses.

DURAL REFLECTIONS

The dura mater is reflected along certain lines to form the dural reflections or dural septa. The intervals between the periosteum and dura along the lines of attachment of the septa accommodate dural venous sinuses (Fig. 26-1). The largest septa, the falx cerebri and the tentorium cerebelli, form incomplete partitions that divide the cranial cavity into three compartments (Fig. 26-2).

The **falx cerebri**, named from its having the shape of a sickle, is a vertical partition in the longitudinal fissure between the cerebral hemispheres. This dural reflection is attached to the crista galli of the ethmoid bone in front, to the midline of the vault as far back as the internal occipital protuberance, and to the tentorium cerebelli. The free edge is close to the splenium of the corpus callosum, but some distance from the corpus callosum further forward. The anterior portion of the falx cerebri often is fenestrated.

The **tentorium cerebelli** intervenes between the occipital lobes of the cerebral hemispheres and the cerebellum. The attachment of the falx cerebri along the midline draws the tentorium upward, giving it a shallow, tent-like configuration. The peripheral border of the tentorium is attached to the upper edges of the petrous parts of both temporal bones and to the margins of the sulci on the occipital bone for the transverse sinuses. The free border bounds the **incisura of the tentorium** (tentorial notch); the incisura is completed by the sphenoid bone, and it accommodates the midbrain.

The **falx cerebelli** is a small dural fold in the posterior cranial fossa, extending vertically for a short distance between the cerebellar hemispheres. The **diaphragma sellae** roofs over the pituitary fossa or sella turcica of the sphenoid bone and has a hole in its middle for passage of the pituitary stalk.

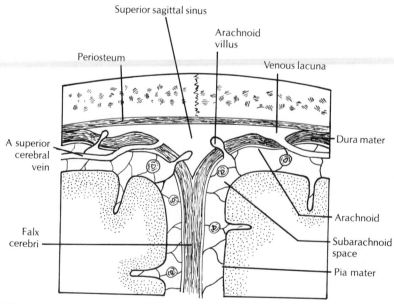

Figure 26-1. Coronal section at the vertex of the skull, including the superior sagittal sinus and the attachment of the falx cerebri.

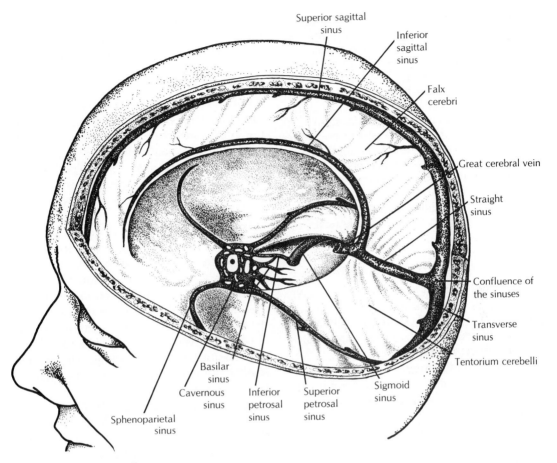

Superior sagittal
sinus

Inferior
sagittal
sinus

Falx
cerebri

Great cerebral vein

Straight
sinus

Confluence of
the sinuses

Transverse
sinus

Tentorium cerebelli

Sigmoid
sinus

Superior
petrosal
sinus

Inferior
petrosal
sinus

Cavernous
sinus

Basilar
sinus

Sphenoparietal
sinus

Figure 26-2. Dural reflections and dural venous sinuses.

Transentorial and Other Herniations

The narrow interval between the midbrain and the boundary of the tentorial incisura is the only communication between the subtentorial and supratentorial compartments of the cranial cavity. An expanding lesion in the supratentorial compartment, such as a subdural hematoma or a tumor in a cerebral hemisphere, may push the medial part of the temporal lobe (the uncus) down into the incisura of the tentorium. An uncal herniation presses on the ipsilateral oculomotor nerve. The first clinical sign of this event is impairment of the pupillary light reflex (see Ch. 8) because the preganglionic parasympathetic fibers for constriction of the pupil are superficially located in the nerve.

Further herniation can damage descending motor fibers in one or both cerebral peduncles,

causing weakness, spasticity, and exaggerated tendon reflexes on either side or bilaterally. When the midbrain is displaced toward the opposite side, the pressure of the rigid edge of the tentorium on the basis pedunculi may result in the unusual finding of upper motor neuron paresis on the same side of the body as the cerebral lesion. Sometimes the downward displacement of the brain occludes one or both posterior cerebral arteries by stretching these vessels over the free edge of the tentorium, with consequences that are explained in Chapter 25. In the later stages of transtentorial herniation, the contralateral oculomotor nerve may be affected. The pupil that dilates first is the most reliable lateralizing sign for the causative lesion.

There are other abnormal movements of parts of the brain from one dural compartment to another. A **subfalcial herniation** occurs when a space-occupying lesion pushes the cingulate gyrus of one hemisphere across the midline beneath the free edge of the falx cerebri. In an **upward transtentorial herniation**, the brain stem and cerebellum are displaced into the supratentorial compartment by a mass in the posterior fossa. Such a mass also may cause **medullary coning**, when the brain stem and part of the cerebellum descend through the foramen magnum into the spinal canal. Medullary coning can follow withdrawal of cerebrospinal fluid from the lumbar subarachnoid space in a patient with raised intracranial pressure. The tonsils of the cerebellum compress the medulla, and the condition can be quickly fatal.

NERVE SUPPLY OF THE DURA MATER

The cranial dura mater has a plentiful supply of sensory nerve fibers, mainly from the trigeminal nerve. Most of the fibers terminate as unencapsulated endings, and they are of significance in certain types of headache.

The dura lining the anterior cranial fossa is supplied by ethmoid branches of the ophthalmic nerve. The mandibular nerve supplies a large area through the nervus spinosum, which enters the middle cranial fossa with the middle meningeal artery and ramifies with the arterial branches. A meningeal branch comes off the maxillary nerve while it is still in the cranial cavity and joins the fibers of the nervus spinosum that accompany the anterior branch of the middle meningeal artery. The tentorium cerebelli and the dura mater lining the vault above it are supplied by several large branches coming off the first part of the ophthalmic nerve. These nerves run backward in the tentorium, spreading out over the vault and in the falx cerebri. The dura lining the floor of the posterior cranial fossa is supplied by the vagus nerve and upper cervical nerves. The meningeal branch of the vagus nerve arises from the superior ganglion at the level of the jugular foramen, through which it enters the posterior fossa. Sensory twigs from the first three cervical spinal nerves enter the posterior fossa through the hypoglossal canal. (The first cervical nerve lacks a sensory component in about half of individuals.) Recurrent branches of all spinal nerves enter the vertebral canal through the intervertebral foramina and give off meningeal branches to the spinal dura mater.

DURAL VENOUS SINUSES

As described in Chapter 25, the veins draining the brain empty into the venous sinuses of the dura mater, from which blood flows into the internal jugular veins. The walls of the sinuses consist of dura mater (and periosteum) lined by endothelium. The locations of most of the dural venous sinuses are shown in Figure 26-2.

The **superior sagittal sinus** lies along the attached border of the falx cerebri. It begins in front of the crista galli of the ethmoid bone, where there may be a narrow communication with nasal veins. **Venous lacunae**, which are shallow, blood-filled spaces within the dura, lie alongside the superior sagittal sinus and open into it. The superior cerebral veins drain into the sinus or into the lacunae. The superior sagittal sinus usually is continuous with the right transverse sinus.

The **inferior sagittal sinus** is smaller than the one just described; it runs along the free border of the falx cerebri and receives veins from the medial aspects of the cerebral hemispheres. The inferior sagittal sinus opens into the **straight sinus**, which lies in the attachment of the falx cerebri to the tentorium cerebelli. The straight sinus also receives the great cerebral vein; it therefore drains the system of internal cerebral veins and the territories of the cerebral hemispheres drained by the basal vein, formed by the union of the deep middle cerebral and anterior cerebral veins. The straight sinus usually is continuous with the left transverse sinus. Venous channels connect the transverse sinuses at the internal occipital protuberance; the configuration of sinuses in this location is called the **confluence of the sinuses** (torcular Herophili).

Each **transverse sinus** lies in a groove on the occipital bone along the attached margin of the tentorium cerebelli. On reaching the petrous part of the temporal bone, the transverse sinus continues as the **sigmoid sinus**; the latter follows a curved course in the posterior fossa on the mastoid portion of the petrous bone and becomes continuous with the internal jugular vein at the jugular foramen.

The **cavernous sinuses** are situated one on each side of the body of the sphenoid bone; each sinus receives the ophthalmic vein and the superficial middle cerebral vein. Venous channels in the anterior and posterior margins of the diaphragma sellae connect the cavernous sinuses; these channels and the cavernous sinuses constitute the **circular sinus**. The cavernous sinus drains into the transverse sinus through the **superior petrosal sinus**, running along the attachment of the tentorium cerebelli to the petrous part of the temporal bone. The **inferior petrosal sinus** lies in the groove between the petrous part of the temporal bone and the basilar portion of the occipital bone, providing a communication between the cavernous sinus and the internal jugular vein. Small venous channels posterior to the circular sinus constitute the **basilar sinus**, which is connected with the cavernous and inferior petrosal sinuses. Finally, the **spheno-parietal sinus** is a small venous channel under the lesser wing of the sphenoid bone, draining into the cavernous sinus, and the small **occipital sinus** in the falx cerebelli drains into the confluence of the sinuses. The sinuses at the base of the cranium receive veins from adjacent parts of the brain.

Within the orbit, the ophthalmic vein has anastomotic communications with the superficial veins of the middle part of the face. Some blood from the facial skin can, therefore, enter the cavernous sinus and pass into the internal jugular vein.

Emissary veins connect dural venous sinuses with veins outside the cranial cavity. Blood may flow in either direction, depending on venous pressures. The parietal and mastoid emissary veins are the largest of these connecting channels. The parietal emissary vein traverses the parietal foramen, joining the superior sagittal sinus with tributaries of the occipital veins. The mastoid emissary vein traverses the mastoid foramen and joins the sigmoid sinus with the occipital and posterior auricular veins.

Thrombosis in Venous Sinuses

Thrombosis in the **superior sagittal sinus** can follow a fracture that damages the dura. If the posterior part of the sinus is obstructed, blood cannot escape from much of the cerebral cortex, and areas of infarction form in the frontal and parietal lobes.

Sometimes infective particles can become dislodged from a facial lesion (such as a carbuncle of the upper lip) and pass through the veins of the orbit and the ophthalmic vein into the **cavernous sinus**. The effects of septic thrombosis of the cavernous sinus include compression of the oculomotor, trochlear, abducens, and maxillary nerves, which are in the walls of the sinus (see Ch. 8), together with swelling and protrusion of the conjunctiva and systemic signs of a serious infection. A congenital weakness in the wall of the internal carotid artery may cause a split that leaks into the cavernous sinus. Like a septic thrombosis, this **arteriovenous fistula** compresses the nerves that pass through the sinus and causes considerable venous congestion of the eye. The eyeball protrudes and pulsates, and a loud pulsating sound is heard by the patient and by anyone applying a stethoscope to the head.

Pia-Arachnoid

The **pia mater** and the **arachnoid** together constitute the **leptomeninges** (slender membranes). They develop initially as a single layer from the mesoderm surrounding the embryonic brain and spinal cord. Fluid-filled spaces form within the layer and coalesce to become the subarachnoid space. The origin of the membranes from a single membrane is reflected in the numerous trabeculae passing between them (see Fig. 26-3). The arachnoid is closely applied to the inside of the dura mater, so the **subdural space** normally contains only a film of extracellular fluid. The pia mater adheres to the external glial limiting membrane of the central nervous system (see Ch. 2).

The arachnoid contains fibroblasts, collagen fibers, and some elastic fibers. It is thick enough to be manipulated with fingers or forceps. In contrast, the pia mater is barely visible to the unaided eye, although it imparts a shiny appearance to the surface of the brain. Both surfaces of the arachnoid and the external surface of the pia are covered by simple squamous epithelium. The trabeculae crossing the subarachnoid space are delicate strands of connective tissue with squamous epithelial cells on their surfaces. Tight junctions connect adjacent arachnoid epithelial cells, preventing exchange of large molecules between the blood in the dural vasculature and the cerebrospinal fluid. There are no tight junctions between the pial cells, so there can be free exchange of macromolecules between the cerebrospinal fluid and the central nervous tissue.

The avascular arachnoid is separated from the dura mater by a film of fluid in the subdural space. The pia mater, which contains a network of fine blood vessels, adheres to the surface of the brain and spinal cord, following all their contours. The collagen fibers in the spinal pia-arachnoid run mostly in a longitudinal direction. This is accentuated along the ventromedian line of the spinal cord, where a thickened strand of fibers superficial to the anterior spinal artery is known as the **linea splendens**. The **denticulate ligament**, described in Chapter 5, also is derived from the pia-arachnoid.

PERIVASCULAR SPACES

It was formerly thought that the subarachnoid space continued around arteries and veins entering and leaving the central nervous tissue. However, electron microscopy of surgically removed human cerebral cortex reveals that where an artery enters the substance of the brain, the pia mater splits, and one leaflet forms a cellular sheath that constitutes the adventitia of the vessel. A **periarterial subpial space** separates the pia-adventitia from the external glial limiting membrane of the brain. There also is an **intrapial periarterial space** between the smooth muscle of the artery and the pia. The latter space is a continuation of the space that separates an artery from its leptomeningeal covering as it crosses the subarachnoid space (Fig. 26-3). Veins do not have pial extensions, so the **perivenular spaces**

within the brain are equivalent to the intrapial periarterial spaces. The subarachnoid space is continuous, through fenestrations in the pia, with all three types of perivascular space.

The old term **Virchow-Robin spaces** applies to all perivascular spaces seen in sections prepared for light microscopy. Capillary blood vessels in the central nervous system are surrounded by single basal laminae, against which abut the foot processes of astrocytes (see Ch. 2). Spaces are often seen around capillaries in material conventionally prepared for light microscopy, but these are artifacts caused by differential shrinkage, as are the spaces commonly seen around the cell bodies of neurons.

Subarachnoid Cisterns

The width of the subarachnoid space varies because the arachnoid rests on the dura mater, whereas the pia mater adheres to the irregular contours of the brain. The space is narrow over the summits of gyri, wider in the regions of major sulci, and wider yet at the base of the brain and in the lumbosacral region of the spinal canal. Regions of the subarachnoid space that contain more substantial amounts of cerebrospinal fluid are called **subarachnoid cisterns** (Fig. 26-4).

The **cerebellomedullary cistern (cisterna magna)** occupies the interval between the cerebellum and medulla and receives cerebrospinal fluid through the median aperture of the fourth ventricle. The basal cisterns beneath the brain stem and diencephalon include the **pontine** and **interpeduncular cisterns** and the **cistern of the optic chiasma**. The last-named cistern is continuous with the **cistern of the lamina terminalis**, which in turn continues into the **cistern of the corpus callosum** above this commissure. The subarachnoid space dorsal to the midbrain is called the **superior cistern** or, alternatively, the **cistern of the great cerebral vein**. This cistern and subarachnoid space on the sides of the midbrain constitute the **cisterna ambiens** or perimesencephalic cistern (not seen in Fig. 22-4). The **cistern of the lateral sulcus** corresponds with that sulcus. The

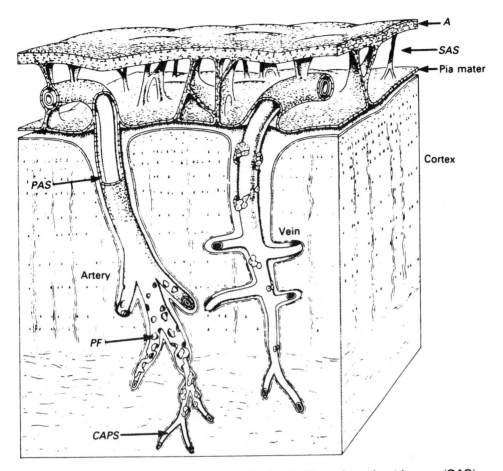

Figure 26-3. Perivascular spaces in the brain. The subarachnoid space (**SAS**) separates the arachnoid (**A**) from the pia mater. The pia splits to ensheath the artery, but not the vein. The periarterial space (**PAS**) has subpial and intrapial components, which become continuous as the pial periarterial sheath becomes perforated (**PF**). Capillaries (**CAPS**) have no pial ensheathment. (*With permission from Zhang ET, Inman CBE, Weller RO: J Anat 170:111–123, 1990*)

lumbar cistern of the spinal subarachnoid space is especially large, extending from the second lumbar vertebra to the second segment of the sacrum. It contains the cauda equina, formed by lumbosacral spinal nerve roots.

The meningeal layers and subarachnoid space extend around cranial nerves and spinal nerve roots for a distance approximately to the level of sensory ganglia when these are present. For example, an extension of the subarachnoid space, enclosed by dura mater, around the proximal part of the trigeminal ganglion in the middle cranial fossa at the tip of

the petrous portion of the temporal bone constitutes the trigeminal cave (Meckel's cave). The meningeal extension of greatest clinical importance surrounds the optic nerve to its attachment to the eyeball. The central artery and central vein of the retina run within the anterior part of the optic nerve and cross the extension of the subarachnoid space to join the ophthalmic artery and ophthalmic vein. An increase of cerebrospinal fluid pressure slows the return of venous blood, causing edema of the retina. This is most apparent on ophthalmoscopic examination as swelling of

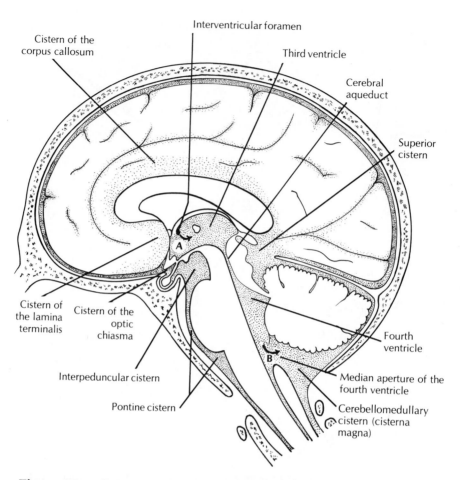

Figure 26-4. Subarachnoid cisterns. **(A)** Arrow showing flow of cerebrospinal fluid from lateral to third ventricle through the right interventricular foramen. **(B)** Arrow showing flow of fluid from the fourth ventricle, through the median aperture, into the cerebellomedullary cistern.

the optic papilla or disk **(papilledema)**. Dilation of the axons of the optic nerve, caused by impairment of the slow component of anterograde axoplasmic transport, contributes to the swelling. Inspection of the ocular fundi is an important part of every physical examination of a patient.

Cerebrospinal Fluid

PRODUCTION

The cerebrospinal fluid is produced mainly by the choroid plexuses of the lateral, third, and fourth ventricles, with those in the lateral ventricles being the largest and most important.

The **choroid plexus** of each lateral ventricle is formed by an invagination of vascular pia mater (the **tela choroidea**) on the medial surface of the cerebral hemisphere. The vascular connective tissue picks up a covering layer of epithelium from the ependymal lining of the ventricle. The choroid plexuses of the third and fourth ventricles are similarly formed by invaginations of the tela choroidea attached to the roofs of these ventricles. Each choroid plexus, which has a minutely folded surface, consists of a core of connective tissue containing many wide capillaries and a surface layer of cuboidal or low columnar epithelium (the choroid epithelium; Fig. 26-5). The surface

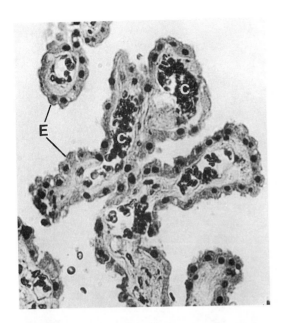

Figure 26-5. Fragment of choroid plexus, showing large capillaries (**C**) and the choroid epithelium (**E**). (Stained with alum-hematoxylin and eosin, × 400)

area of the choroid plexuses of the two lateral ventricles combined is about 40 cm².

Several features of the choroid epithelium as seen in electron micrographs are of functional interest (Fig. 26-6). The large spherical nucleus, abundant cytoplasm, and numerous mitochondria indicate that the production of cerebrospinal fluid is at least partly an active process that requires expenditure of energy on the part of these cells. The plasma membrane at the free surface is greatly increased in area by irregular microvilli. The membranes of adjoining cells are thrown into complicated folds at the base of the cells. The choroid epithelial cells bear motile cilia in the embryo, and patches of ciliated epithelium persist for varying periods postnatally. A basement membrane separates the epithelium from the subjacent stroma with its rich vascular network. The capillaries are unlike those supplying nervous tissue generally in that the endothelial cells have fenestrations or pores closed by thin diaphragms and are permeable to large molecules. The blood–cerebrospinal fluid barrier to

macromolecules is formed by the cells of the choroid epithelium and the tight junctions (zonulae occludentes) between adjacent cells.

Production of cerebrospinal fluid is a complex process. Some components of the blood plasma enter the cerebrospinal fluid readily by diffusion. Others reach the fluid with the assistance of metabolic activity on the part of the choroid epithelial cells. An important factor is active transport of certain ions (notably sodium ions) through the epithelial cells, followed by passive movement of water to maintain the osmotic equilibrium between cerebrospinal fluid and blood plasma.

CIRCULATION

The flow of cerebrospinal fluid is from the lateral ventricles into the third ventricle through the interventricular foramina and then into the fourth ventricle by way of the cerebral aqueduct. Cerebrospinal fluid leaves the ventricular system through the median and lateral apertures of the fourth ventricle, with the former opening into the cerebellomedullary cistern and the latter into the pontine cistern. From these sites, there is a sluggish movement of fluid through the spinal subarachnoid space, determined in part by movements of the vertebral column. More importantly, the cerebrospinal fluid flows slowly forward through the basal cisterns and then upward over the medial and lateral surfaces of the cerebral hemispheres. Movement of cerebrospinal fluid is assisted by the pulsation of arteries in the subarachnoid space, especially in the subarachnoid space around the spinal cord.

ABSORPTION

The main site of absorption of the cerebrospinal fluid into venous blood is through the **arachnoid villi** projecting into dural venous sinuses, especially the superior sagittal sinus and adjacent venous lacunae (see Fig. 26-1). Each arachnoid villus consists of a thin cellular layer, derived from the epithelium of the arachnoid and the endothelium of the sinus, which encloses an extension of the subarachnoid space containing trabeculae. The

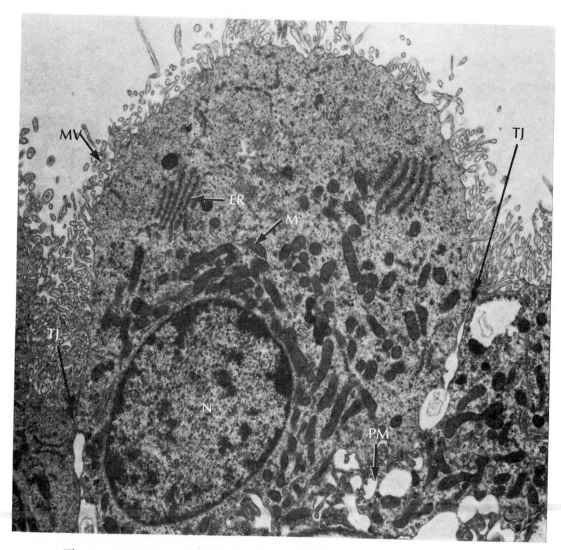

Figure 26-6. Electron micrograph of a choroid epithelial cell. (**ER**) Endoplasmic reticulum. (**M**) Mitochondria. (**MV**) Microvilli. (**N**) Nucleus. (**PM**) Folds of plasma membrane. (**TJ**) Tight junction (zonula occludens). (× 800; *courtesy of Dr. D. H. Dickson*)

absorptive mechanism depends on the hydrostatic pressure of the cerebrospinal fluid being higher than that of the venous blood in the dural sinuses, and transport through cells forming the walls of the arachnoid villi. The arachnoid cells of the villus are joined by tight junctions, and the movement of fluid occurs in large vesicles that are transported through the cytoplasm. The arachnoid villi become hypertrophied with age, when they are called **arachnoid granulations** or **pacchionian bodies**; these may be sufficiently large to produce erosion or pitting of the cranial bones.

Although the choroid plexuses are the main source of cerebrospinal fluid and the arachnoid villi of its absorption, there are exchanges between blood plasma and cerebrospinal fluid elsewhere. Results of studies using radioactive isotopes in laboratory animals show that the chemical composition of cerebrospinal fluid is determined in part by passive two-way transfer of water and solutes across the ependymal lining of the ventricles and the walls of small blood vessels in the pia mater. Some cerebrospinal fluid is absorbed into arachnoid villi that protrude into veins that pass alongside the spinal nerve roots before emptying into the epidural venous plexus. A small proportion of the fluid enters lymphatic vessels adjacent to the extensions of the subarachnoid space around the olfactory nerves, other cranial nerves, and spinal nerve roots.

PRESSURE AND PROPERTIES

The volume of the cerebrospinal fluid varies from 80 to 150 ml; these figures include the fluid in both the ventricles and the subarachnoid space. The ventricular system alone contains from 15 to 40 ml of fluid. The rate of production is sufficient to effect a total replacement several times daily. The pressure of cerebrospinal fluid is from 80 to 180 cm H_2O when a subject is recumbent; the pressure in the lumbar cistern is about twice these values when measured in a sitting position. Venous congestion in the closed space of the cranial cavity and the spinal canal, as produced by straining or coughing, is reflected in a prompt rise of cerebrospinal fluid pressure.

Cerebrospinal fluid is clear and colorless, with a density of 1.003 to 1.008 g/cm^3. The few cells present are mainly lymphocytes. These vary in number from one to eight in each cubic millimeter; a count of more than ten cells is indicative of disease. The glucose level is about one-half that of blood, and the protein content is very low (15 to 45 mg/dl).

Hydrocephalus

When there is an excess of cerebrospinal fluid, the condition is known as hydrocephalus, of which there are several types. External hydrocephalus, in which the excess fluid is mainly in the subarachnoid space, is found in senile atro-

phy of the brain. Internal hydrocephalus refers to dilation of the ventricles. All the ventricles are enlarged if the apertures of the fourth ventricle are occluded; the third and lateral ventricles, if the obstruction is in the cerebral aqueduct; and one lateral ventricle only, in the rare occurrence of occlusion of an interventricular foramen.

The term communicating hydrocephalus refers to a combination of internal and external hydrocephalus. The commonest cause is obstruction of the arachnoid villi by blood after a subarachnoid hemorrhage. If the flow of cerebrospinal fluid through the incisura of the tentorium around the midbrain is obstructed, the excess fluid accumulates in the ventricles and in the part of the subarachnoid space below the tentorium.

SUGGESTED READING ——————

Baumbach GL, Cancilla PA, Hayreh MS, Hayreh SS: Experimental injury of the optic nerve with optic disc swelling. Lab Invest 39:50–60, 1978

Dandy WE: Experimental hydrocephalus. Trans Am Surg Assoc 37:397–428, 1919

Davson H: Formation and drainage of the cerebrospinal fluid. In Shapiro K, Marmarou A, Portnoy H (eds): Hydrocephalus, pp 3–40. New York, Raven Press, 1984

Davson H: History of the blood-brain barrier concept. In Neuwelt EA (ed): Implications of the Blood-Brain Barrier and Its Manipulation. Vol 1. Basic Science Aspects, pp 27–52. New York, Plenum Press, 1989

Parkinson D: Human spinal arachnoid septa, trabeculae, and rogue strands. Am J Anat 192: 498–509, 1991

Suckling AJ, Rumsby MG, Bradbury MWB (eds): The Blood-Brain Barrier in Health and Disease. Chichester, Ellis Horwood, 1986

Yamada S, DePasquale M, Patlak CS, Cserr HF: Albumin outflow into deep cervical lymph from different regions of the rabbit brain. Am J Physiol 261:H1197–H1204, 1991

Zhang ET, Inman CBE, Weller RO: Interrelationships of the pia mater and the perivascular (Virchow-Robin) spaces of the human cerebrum. J Anat 170:111–123, 1990

Appendices

The Human Nervous System: An Anatomical Viewpoint, Sixth Edition, Murray L. Barr and John A. Kiernan. J.B. Lippincott Company, Philadelphia, © 1993.

Glossary of Neuroanatomical Terms

In this text, the standard Latin forms of anatomical names are anglicized wherever this is possible without loss of euphony. Most anatomical terms have Latin origins, and most names related to diseases are derived from Greek words.

Abbreviations

Eng. *English*; Fr. *French*; Ger. *German*; Gr. *Greek*; L. *Latin*

Abducens. L. *ab*, from + *ducens*, leading. Abducens (or abducent) nerve supplies the muscle that moves the direction of gaze away from the midline.

Adiadochokinesia. *a*, neg. + Gr. *diadochos*, succeeding + *kinēsis*, movement. Inability to perform rapidly alternating movements. Also called dysdiadochokinesia.

Agnosia. *a*, neg. + Gr. *gnōsis*, knowledge. Lack of ability to recognize the significance of sensory stimuli (auditory, visual, tactile, etc. agnosia).

Agraphia. *a*, neg. + Gr. *graphō*, to write. Inability to express thoughts in writing owing to a central lesion.

Akinesia. *a*, neg. + Gr. *kinēsis*, movement. Lack of spontaneous movement, as seen in Parkinson's disease.

Ala cinerea. L. wing + *cinereus*, ashen-hued. Vagal triangle in floor of fourth ventricle.

Alexia. *a*, neg. + Gr. *lexis*, word. Loss of the power to grasp the meaning of written or printed words and sentences.

Allocortex. Gr. *allos*, other + L. *cortex*, bark. Phylogenetically older cerebral cortex, usually consisting of three layers. Includes paleocortex and archicortex.

Alveus. L. trough. Thin layer of white matter covering the ventricular surface of the hippocampus. The name seems quite inappropriate but has become an accepted part of anatomical terminology.

Amacrine. *a*, neg. + Gr. *makros*, long + *inos*, fiber. Amacrine nerve cell of the retina.

Ambiguus. L. changeable or doubtful. Nucleus ambiguus (Chs. 7 and 8) occupies an atypically ventral position for a cranial nerve nucleus, and its limits are somewhat indistinct.

Ammon's horn. Hippocampus, which has an outline in cross section suggestive of a ram's horn. Also known as the cornu Ammonis. Ammon was an Egyptian deity with a ram's head.

Amygdala. L. *amygdalum*, from Gr. *amygdalē*, almond. Amygdala or amygdaloid body in the temporal lobe of the cerebral hemisphere.

Anopsia. *an*, neg. + Gr. *opsis*, vision. Defect of vision.

Ansa hypoglossi. L. *ansa*, handle + Gr. *hypo*, under + Gr. *glōssa*, tongue. Loop of nerves containing axons of the first three cervical roots that encircles the common carotid artery and internal jugular vein in the neck. The fibers from C1 pass within the trunk of the hypoglossal nerve before joining the ansa. Also called the **ansa cervicalis**.

Antidromic. Gr. *anti*, against + *dromos*, a running. Relating to the propagation of an impulse along an axon in a direction that is the reverse of the normal or usual direction.

Aphasia. *a*, neg. + Gr. *phasis*, speech. Defect of the power of expression by speech or of comprehending spoken or written language.

Apraxia. *a*, neg. + Gr. *prattō*, to do. Inability to carry out purposeful movements in the absence of paralysis.

Arachnoid. Gr. *arachnē*, spider's web + *eidos*, resemblance. Meningeal layer that forms the outer boundary of the subarachnoid space.

Archicerebellum. Gr. *archē*, beginning + diminutive of cerebrum. Phylogenetically old part of the cerebellum, functioning in the maintenance of equilibrium. Also spelled archeocerebellum.

Archicortex. Gr. *archē*, beginning + L. *cortex*, bark. Three-layered cortex included in the limbic system; located mainly in the hippocampus and dentate gyrus of the temporal lobe. Also spelled archeocortex.

Area postrema. Area in the caudal part of the floor of the fourth ventricle.

Astereognosis. *a*, neg. + *stereos*, solid + *gnōsis*, knowledge. Loss of ability to recognize objects or to appreciate their form by touching or feeling them.

Astrocyte. Gr. *astron*, star + *kytos*, hollow (cell). Type of neuroglial cell.

Asynergy. *a*, neg. + Gr. *syn*, with + *ergon*, work. Disturbance of the proper association in the contraction of muscles that ensures that the different components of an act follow in proper sequence, at the proper moment, and of the proper degree, so that the act is executed accurately.

Ataxia. *a*, neg. + Gr. *taxis*, order. Loss of power of muscle coordination, with irregularity of muscle action.

Atheroma. Gr. *athērē*, porridge. Thickening of the lining of an artery caused by deposition of lipid material.

Athetosis. Gr. *athetos*, without position or place. Affliction of the nervous system caused by degenerative changes in the corpus striatum and cerebral cortex and characterized by bizarre, writhing movements of the fingers and toes, especially.

Atresia. *a*, neg. + Gr. *trēsis*, perforation. Absence of a passage caused by an error in development.

Autonomic. Gr. *autos*, self + *nomos*, law. Autonomic system; the efferent or motor innervation of viscera.

Autoradiography. Gr. *autos*, self + L. *radius*, ray + Gr. *graphō*, to write. Technique that uses a photographic emulsion to detect the location of radioactive isotopes in tissue sections. Also called radioautography.

Axolemma. Gr. *axōn*, axis + *lemma*, husk. Plasma membrane of an axon.

Axon. Gr. *axōn*, axis. Efferent process of a neuron that conducts impulses to other neurons or to muscle fibers (striated and smooth) and gland cells.

Axon hillock. Region of the nerve cell body from which the axon arises; it contains no Nissl material.

Axon reaction. Changes in the cell body of a neuron after damage to its axon.

Axoplasm. Gr. *axōn*, axis + *plasm*, anything formed or molded. Cytoplasm of the axon.

Ballism. See **hemiballismus.**

Baroreceptor. Gr. *baros*, weight + *receptor*, receiver. Sensory nerve terminal that is stimulated by changes in pressure, as in the carotid sinus and aortic arch.

Basis pedunculi. Ventral part of the cerebral peduncle of the midbrain on each side, separated from the dorsal part by the substantia nigra. Also called the crus cerebri.

Brachium. L. from Gr. *brachiōn*, arm. As used in the central nervous system, denotes a large bundle of fibers that connects one part with another (eg, brachia associated with the colliculi of the midbrain).

Bradykinesia. Gr. *brady*, slow + *kinēsis*, movement. Abnormal slowness of movements.

Brain stem. In the mature human brain, denotes the medulla, pons, and midbrain. In descriptions of the embryonic brain, the diencephalon is included as well.

Bulb. Referred at one time to the medulla oblongata, but in the context of "corticobulbar tract," refers to the brain stem, in which motor nuclei of cranial nerves are located.

Bulbospongiosus muscle. L. *bulbus*, bulb or onion + *spongia*, sponge. Muscle surrounding the corpus spongiosus, the body of erectile tissue surrounding the urethra at the base of the penis.

Calamus scriptorius. L. *calamus*, a reed, therefore a reed pen. Refers to an area in the caudal part of the floor of the fourth ventricle that is shaped somewhat like a penpoint.

Calcar. L. spur, used to denote any spur-shaped structure. Calcar avis, an elevation on the medial aspects of the lateral ventricles at the junction of occipital and temporal horns. Also calcarine sulcus of occipital lobe, which is responsible for the calcar avis.

Cauda equina. L. horse's tail. Lumbar and sacral spinal nerve roots in the lower part of the spinal canal.

Caudate nucleus. Part of the corpus striatum, so

named because it has a long extension or tail.

Cerebellum. L. diminutive of *cerebrum*, brain. Large part of the brain with motor functions situated in the posterior cranial fossa.

Cerebrum. L. brain. Principal portion of the brain, including the diencephalon and cerebral hemispheres, but not the brain stem and cerebellum.

Chordotomy. Gr. *chordē*, cord + *tomē*, a cutting. Division of the spinothalamic and spinoreticular tracts for intractable pain (tractotomy). Also spelled cordotomy.

Chorea. L. from Gr. *choros*, a dance. Disorder characterized by irregular, spasmodic, involuntary movements of the limbs or facial muscles. Attributed to degenerative changes in the neostriatum.

Choroid. Gr. *chorion*, a delicate membrane + *eidos*, form. Choroid or vascular coat of the eye; choroid plexuses in the ventricles of the brain. Also spelled chorioid.

Chromatolysis. Gr. *chrōma*, color + *lysis*, dissolution. Dispersal of the Nissl material of neurons after axon section or in viral infections of the nervous system.

Cinereum. L. *cinereum*, ashen-hued, from *cinis*, ash. Refers to gray matter, but limited in usage. Tuber cinereum (ventral portion of the hypothalamus, from which the neurohypophysis arises); tuberculum cinereum (slight elevation on medulla formed by spinal tract and nucleus of trigeminal nerve); ala cinerea (vagal triangle in floor of fourth ventricle).

Cingulum. L. girdle. Bundle of association fibers in the white matter of the cingulate gyrus on the medial surface of the cerebral hemisphere.

Claustrum. L. a barrier. Thin sheet of gray matter of unknown function situated between the lentiform nucleus and the insula.

Colliculus. L. Small elevation or mound. Superior and inferior colliculi composing the tectum of the midbrain; facial colliculus in the floor of the fourth ventricle.

Commissure. L. a joining together. Bundle of nerve fibers that passes from one side to the other in the brain or spinal cord. Strictly, this term should be applied to tracts that connect symmetrical structures (cf. **decussation**).

Contracture. Persistent shortening, as in a muscle paralyzed for a long time.

Contralateral. L. *contra*, opposite + *lateris* of a side. Of the other (left or right) side of the body. Opposite of "ipsilateral."

Cornu. L. horn. See **Ammon's horn**. Horns of the lateral ventricle and of the spinal gray matter also are formally named as cornua.

Corona. L. from Gr. *korōnē*, a crown. Corona radiata (fibers radiating from the internal capsule to various parts of the cerebral cortex).

Corpus callosum. L. body + *callosus*, hard. Main neocortical commissure of the cerebral hemispheres.

Corpus luteum. L. body + *luteum*, yellow. Progesterone-secreting endocrine tissue that forms in the ovary after ovulation.

Corpus striatum. L. body + *striatus*, furrowed or striped. Mass of gray matter with motor functions at the base of each cerebral hemisphere.

Cortex. L. bark. Outer layer of gray matter of the cerebral hemispheres and cerebellum.

Crus. L. leg. Crus cerebri is the ventral part of the cerebral peduncle of the midbrain on each side, separated from the dorsal part by the substantia nigra. Also called the basis pedunculi. Crus of the fornix.

Cuneus. L. wedge. Gyrus on the medial surface of the cerebral hemisphere. Fasciculus cuneatus in the spinal cord and medulla; nucleus cuneatus in the medulla.

Cytosol. Gr. *kytos*, a hollow vessel + solution. Soluble portion of the cytoplasm, excluding all membranous and particulate components.

Decussation. L. *decussatio*, from *decussis*, the numeral X. Point of crossing of paired tracts. Decussations of the pyramids, medial lemnisci, and superior cerebellar peduncles are examples. A decussation connects asymmetrical parts of the nervous system.

Dendrite. Gr. *dendritēs*, related to a tree. Process of a nerve cell on which axons of other neurons terminate. Sometimes also used for the peripheral process of a primary sensory neuron, although this has the histological and physiological properties of an axon.

Dentate. L. *dentatus*, toothed. Dentate nucleus of the cerebellum; dentate gyrus in the temporal lobe.

Diabetes. Gr. *dia*, through + *dynein*, to go, hence *diabētēs*, a syphon. Disease with excessive production of urine. In **diabetes mellitus** (L. *mellitus*, sweet), the urine contains sugar, whereas in **diabetes insipidus** (L. *in*, not + *sapor*, flavor), the urine is watery and quite tasteless.

Diencephalon. Gr. *dia*, through + *enkephalos*, brain. Part of the cerebrum, consisting of the thalamus, epithalamus, subthalamus, and hypothalamus. The posterior of the two brain vesicles formed from the prosencephalon of the developing embryo.

Diplopia. Gr. *diploos*, double + *ōps*, eye. Double vision.

Dura. L. *dura*, hard. Dura mater (the thick external layer of the meninges).

Dyskinesia. Gr. *dys*, difficult or disordered + *kinēsis*, movement. Abnormality of motor function characterized by involuntary, purposeless movements.

Dysmetria. Gr. *dys*, difficult or disordered + *metron*, measure. Disturbance of the power to control the range of movement in muscle action.

Ectoderm. Gr. *ektos*, outside + *derma*, skin. Most dorsal layer of cells of the early embryo, which gives rise to the epidermis, neural tube, neural crest, etc.

Edema (oedema). Gr. *oidēma*, swelling. Abnormal accumulation of fluid in a tissue.

Emboliform. Gr. *embolos*, plug + L. *forma*, form. Emboliform nucleus of the cerebellum.

Embolus. Gr. *embolos*, plug. Fragment of a thrombus that breaks loose and eventually obstructs an artery.

Endoneurium. Gr. *endon*, within + *neuron*, nerve. Delicate connective tissue sheath surrounding an individual nerve fiber of a peripheral nerve. Also called the sheath of Henle.

Engram. Gr. *en*, in + *gramma*, mark. Used in psychology to mean the lasting trace left in the brain by previous experience; a latent memory picture.

Entorhinal. Gr. *entos*, within + *rhis* (*rhin-*), nose. Entorhinal area is the anterior part of the parahippocampal gyrus of the temporal lobe adjacent to the uncus. It is included in the lateral olfactory area.

Ependyma. Gr. *ependyma*, an upper garment. Lining epithelium of the ventricles of the brain and central canal of the spinal cord.

Epineurium. Gr. *epi*, upon + *neuron*, nerve. Connective tissue sheath surrounding a peripheral nerve.

Epithalamus. Gr. *epi*, upon + *thalamos*, inner chamber. Region of the diencephalon above the thalamus; includes the pineal gland.

Estrogen (oestrogen). L. *oestrus*, gadfly or frenzy + *generator*, producer. Steroid hormones (estradiol, estrone, estriol) secreted by the ovary that stimulate the secondary sex organs, especially before ovulation.

Euphony. Gr. *eu*, well + *phōnē*, sound. Agreeable sound or easy pronunciation.

Exteroceptor. L. *exterus*, external + *receptor*, receiver. Sensory receptor that serves to acquaint the individual with his or her environment (exteroception).

Extrapyramidal system. Vague and confusing term applied to motor parts of the central nervous system other than the pyramidal motor system.

Falx. L. sickle. Two of the dural partitions in the cranial cavity are the falx cerebri and the small falx cerebelli.

Fasciculus. L. diminutive of *fascis*, bundle. Bundle of nerve fibers.

Fastigial. L. *fastigium*, the top of a gabled roof. Fastigial nucleus of the cerebellum.

Fenestra. L. window. A hole. Fenestra rotunda (round) and fenestra ovale (oval) are between the middle and inner ear. Capillary blood vessels are fenestrated when their endothelial cells have pores, each closed by a diaphragm that does not prevent the egress of large molecules.

Fimbria. L. *fimbriae*, fringe. Band of nerve fibers along the medial edge of the hippocampus, continuing as the fornix.

Fistula. L. pipe. Abnormal communication between two cavities or between a cavity and the surface of the body. In an arteriovenous fistula, blood is shunted directly from an artery into a vein or venous sinus.

Forceps. L. a pair of tongs. Used for the U-shaped configuration of fibers that constitute the anterior and posterior portions of the corpus callosum (forceps frontalis and forceps occipitalis).

Fornix. L. arch. Efferent tract of the hippocampal formation, arching over the thalamus and terminating mainly in the mamillary body of the hypothalamus.

Fovea. L. a pit or depression. Fovea centralis (depression in the center of the macula lutea of the retina).

Fundus. L. bottom. Rounded interior of a hollow

organ. The ocular fundus is lined by the retina, with its blood vessels, the optic disk, and other landmarks visible through an ophthalmoscope.

Funiculus. L. diminutive of *funis*, cord. Area of white matter that may consist of several functionally different fasciculi, as in the lateral funiculus of white matter of the spinal cord.

Fusiform. L. *fusus*, spindle + *forma*, shape. Widest in the middle and tapering at both ends

Ganglion. Gr. knot or subcutaneous tumor. Swelling composed of nerve cells, as in cerebrospinal and sympathetic ganglia. Also used inappropriately for certain regions of gray matter in the brain (eg, basal ganglia of the cerebral hemisphere).

Gemmule. L. *gemmula*, diminutive of *gemma*, bud. Minute projections on dendrites of certain neurons, especially pyramidal cells and Purkinje cells, for synaptic contact with other neurons.

Genu. L. *genu*, knee. Anterior end of corpus callosum; genu of facial nerve. Also geniculate ganglion of facial nerve and geniculate bodies of thalamus.

Glia. Gr. glue. Neuroglia, the interstitial or accessory cells of the central nervous system.

Glioblast. Gr. *glia*, glue + *blastos*, germ. Embryonic neuroglial cell.

Gliosome. Gr. *glia*, glue + *soma*, body. Granules in neuroglial cells, in particular astrocytes.

Globus pallidus. L. a ball + pale. Medial part of lentiform nucleus of corpus striatum. Also globose nuclei of cerebellum.

Glomerulus. Diminutive of L. *glomus*, ball of yarn. Synaptic glomeruli of the olfactory bulb and cerebellum.

Glomus. L. ball of yarn. Applied to various small organs, including the carotid and aortic bodies, and to one of their characteristic cell types.

Glycocalyx. Gr. *glycyx*, sweet + *kalyx*, cup. Outer coating of carbohydrate molecules on the surface of cells.

Gracilis. L. slender. Fasciculus gracilis of the spinal cord and medulla; nucleus gracilis and gracile tubercle of the medulla.

Granule. L. *granulum*, diminutive of *granum*, grain. Used to denote small neurons, such as granule cells of cerebellar cortex and stellate cells of cerebral cortex. Hence granular cell layers of both cortices.

Habenula. L. diminutive of *habena*, strap or rein. Small swelling in the epithalamus adjacent to the posterior end of the roof of the third ventricle.

Haarscheibe. Ger. *haar*, hair + *scheibe*, disk. Small elevated area of skin that develops in association with specialized hair follicles and serves as a receptor for tactile stimuli.

Hemiballismus. Gr. *hēmi*, half + *ballismos*, jumping. Violent form of motor restlessness that involves one side of the body, caused by a destructive lesion involving the subthalamic nucleus.

Hemiplegia. Gr. *hēmi*, half + *plēgē*, a blow or stroke. Paralysis of one side of the body.

Hippocampus. Gr. *hippos*, horse + *kampos*, sea monster; also the zoological name for a genus of small fishes known as sea-horses. Rather inappropriate name given to a gyrus that constitutes an important part of the limbic system; produces an elevation on the floor of the temporal horn of the lateral ventricle.

Homeostasis. Gr. *homois*, like + *stasis*, standing. Tendency toward stability in the internal environment of the organism.

Hydrocephalus. Gr. *hydrōr*, water + *kephalē*, head. Excessive accumulation of cerebrospinal fluid.

Hyperacusis. Gr. *akousis*, a hearing. Abnormal loudness of perceived sounds.

Hypothalamus. Gr. *hypo*, under + *thalamos*, inner chanber. Region of the diencephalon that serves as the main controlling center of the autonomic nervous system.

Induction. L. *inducere*, to bring in. In embryology, action of one population of cells on the development of another population nearby.

Indusium. L. a garment, from *induo*, to put on. Indusium griseum, thin layer of gray matter on the dorsal surface of the corpus callosum (gray tunic).

Infarction. L. *infarcire*, to stuff or fill in. Regional death of tissue caused by loss of blood supply.

Infundibulum. L. funnel. Infundibular stem of the neurohypophysis.

Insula. L. island. Cerebral cortex concealed from surface view and lying at the bottom of the lateral sulcus. Also called the island of Reil.

Interoceptor. L. *inter*, between + *receptor*, receiver. One of the sensory end organs within viscera.

Interstitial. L. *inter*, between + *statum*, placed. Within spaces. Interstitial cells of the testis are in the spaces between the seminiferous tubules.

Ipsilateral. L. *ipse*, itself + *lateris* of a side. Of the same side (left or right) of the body. Opposite of "contralateral."

Ischemia. Gr. *ischein*, to check + *haimos*, blood. Condition of tissue that is not adequately perfused with oxygenated blood.

Ischiocavernosus muscle. Gr. *ischion*, hip joint + L. *caverna*, cave or hollow. Paired muscle associated with the bodies of erectile tissue on either side of the base of the penis.

Isocortex. Gr. *isos*, equal + L. *cortex*, bark. Cerebral cortex having six layers (neocortex).

Kinesthesia. Gr. *kinēsis*, movement + *aisthēsis*, sensation. Sense of perception of movement.

Koniocortex. Gr. *konis*, dust + L. *cortex*, bark. Areas of cerebral cortex that contain large numbers of small neurons; typical of sensory areas.

Lemniscus. Gr. *lēmniskos*, fillet (a ribbon or band). Used to designate a bundle of nerve fibers in the central nervous system (eg, medial lemniscus and lateral lemniscus).

Lentiform. L. *lens* (*lent-*), a lentil (lens) + *forma*, shape. Lens-shaped. Lentiform nucleus, a component of the corpus striatum. Also called lenticular nucleus.

Leptomeninges. Gr. *leptos*, slender + *mēninx*, membrane. Arachnoid and pia mater.

Lesion. L. *laesum*, hurt or wounded. Applied to any abnormality. In the nervous system, a lesion may be destructive (such as an infarct, injury, hemorrhage, or tumor), or it may stimulate neurons (as in epilepsy).

Limbus. L. a hem or border. Limbic lobe: C-shaped configuration of cortex on the medial surface of the cerebral hemisphere that consists of the septal area and the cingulate and parahippocampal gyri. Limbic system: limbic lobe, hippocampal formation, and portions of the diencephalon, especially the mamillary body and anterior thalamic nuclei.

Limen. L. threshold. Limen insulae: ventral part of the insula (island of Reil); included in the lateral olfactory area.

Locus coeruleus. L. place + *caeruleus*, dark blue. Small dark spot on each side of the floor of the fourth ventricle; marks the position of a group of nerve cells that contain melanin pigment.

Macroglia. Gr. *makros*, large + *glia*, glue. Larger types of neuroglial cells: astrocytes, oligodendrocytes, and ependymal cells.

Macrosmatic. Gr. *makros*, large + *osmē*, smell. Having the sense of smell strongly or acutely developed.

Macula. L. a spot. Macula lutea: spot at the posterior pole of the eye that has a yellow color when viewed with red-free light. Maculae sacculi and utriculi: sensory areas in the vestibular portion of the membranous labyrinth.

Mamillary. L. *mammilla*, diminutive of *mamma*, breast (shaped like a nipple). Mamillary bodies: swellings on the ventral surface of the hypothalamus. Also spelled mammillary.

Massa intermedia. Bridge of gray matter that connects the thalami of the two sides across the third ventricle; present in 70% of human brains. Also called the interthalamic adhesion.

Medulla. L. marrow, from *medius*, middle. Medulla spinalis: spinal cord. Medulla oblongata: caudal portion of the brain stem. In current usage, "medulla" means the medulla oblongata.

Medulloblastoma. Malignant tumor of young children, usually in the midline of the cerebellum, enlarging into the fourth ventricle and spreading by way of the subarachnoid space to other parts of the central nervous system.

Mesencephalon. Gr. *mesos*, middle + *enkephalos*, brain. Midbrain; second of the three primary brain vesicles.

Mesoderm. Gr. *mesos*, middle + *derma*, skin. Middle layer of cells of the early embryo, which gives rise to connective tissues, muscle, etc.

Metathalamus. Gr. *meta*, after + *thalamos*, inner chamber. Medial and lateral geniculate bodies (nuclei).

Metencephalon. Gr. *meta*, after + *enkephalos*, brain. Pons and cerebellum; anterior of the two divisions of the rhombencephalon or posterior primary brain vesicle.

Microglia. Gr. *mikros*, small + *glia*, glue. Type of neuroglial cell.

Microsmatic. Gr. *mikros*, small + *osmē*, smell. Having a sense of smell, but of relatively poor development.

Mimetic. Gr. *mimētikos*, imitative. Muscles of expression supplied by the facial nerve; sometimes referred to as mimetic muscles.

Mitral. L. *mitra*, a turban; later the tall, cleft hat (miter) of a bishop. Mitral cells of the olfactory bulb.

Mnemonic. Gr. *mnēmē*, memory. Pertaining to memory.

Molecular. L. *molecula*, diminutive of *moles*, mass. Used in neurohistology to denote tissue that contains large numbers of fine nerve fibers and that, therefore, has a punctate appearance in silver-stained sections. Molecular layers of cerebral and cerebellar cortices.

Mutism. L. *mutus*, silent or dumb. Inability to speak.

Myasthenia gravis. Gr. *myos*, muscle + *a*, without + *sthenos*, strength + L. *gravis*, heavy (severe). Disease in which there is failure of neuromuscular transmission (see Ch. 3).

Myelencephalon. Gr. *myelos*, marrow + *enkephalos*, brain. Medulla oblongata; posterior of the two divisions of the rhombencephalon or posterior primary brain vesicle.

Myelin. Gr. *myelos*, marrow. Layers of lipid and protein substances that form a sheath around axons.

Myotrophic. Gr. *mys*, muscle + *trephein*, to nourish. Responsible for maintaining the structural and functional integrity of muscle. (Principally by chemical agents from motor neurons, hence the earlier but ambiguous term "neurotrophic.")

Neocerebellum. Gr. *neos*, new + diminutive of cerebrum. Phylogenetically newest part of the cerebellum present in mammals and especially well developed in humans. Ensures smooth muscle action in the finer voluntary movements.

Neocortex. Gr. *neos*, new + L. *cortex*, bark. Six-layered cortex, characteristic of mammals and constituting most of the cerebral cortex in humans.

Neostriatum. Gr. *neos*, new + L. *striatus*, striped or grooved. Phylogenetically newer part of the corpus striatum that consists of the caudate nucleus and putamen; the striatum.

Neurite. Gr. *neurites*, of a nerve. Cytoplasmic processes of neurons. The term embraces both axons and dendrites.

Neurobiotaxis. Gr. *neuron*, nerve + *bios*, life + *taxis*, arrangement. Tendency of nerve cells to move during embryological development toward the area from which they receive the most stimuli.

Neuroblast. Gr. *neuron*, a nerve + *blastos*, germ. Embryonic nerve cell.

Neurofibril. Gr. *neuron*, nerve + L. *fibrilla*, diminutive of *fibra*, fiber. Filaments in the cytoplasm of neurons (see Ch. 2).

Neuroglia. Gr. *neuron*, nerve + *glia*, glue. Accessory or interstitial cells of the nervous system; includes astrocytes, oligodendrocytes, microglial cells, ependymal cells, satellite cells, and Schwann cells.

Neurokeratin. Gr. *neuron*, nerve + *keras* (*kerat-*), horn. Fibrillar material consisting of proteins that remains after lipids have been dissolved from myelin sheaths.

Neurolemma. Gr. *neuron*, nerve + *lemma*, husk. Delicate sheath surrounding a peripheral nerve fiber consisting of a series of neurolemma cells or Schwann cells. Also spelled neurilemma.

Neuron. Gr. a nerve. Morphological unit of the nervous system consisting of the nerve cell body and its processes (dendrites and axon).

Neuropil. Gr. *neuron*, nerve + *pilos*, felt. Complex net of nerve cell processes that occupies the intervals between cell bodies in gray matter.

Nociceptive. L. *noceo*, I injure + *capio*, I take. Responsive to injurious stimuli.

Nucleus. L. nut, kernel. (1) Body in a cell that contains, in the DNA of its chromosomes, the genetic information that encodes the amino acid sequences of proteins. (2) Collection of neuronal cell bodies, which may be large (like the caudate nucleus) or microscopic (like many nuclei in the brain stem).

Nystagmus. Gr. *nystagmos*, a nodding, from *nystazō*, to be sleepy. Involuntary oscillation of the eyes.

Obex. L. barrier. Small transverse fold overhanging the opening of the fourth ventricle into the central canal of the closed portion of the medulla.

Oligodendrocyte. Gr. *oligos*, few + *dendron*, tree + *kytos*, hollow (cell). Type of neuroglial cell. Forms the myelin sheath in the central nervous system in the same manner as the Schwann cell in peripheral nerves.

Olive. L. *oliva*. Oval bulging of the lateral area of the medulla. Inferior, accessory, and superior olivary nuclei.

Ontogeny. Gr. *ontos*, being + *genesis*, generation. Development of an individual. The adjective **ontogenetic**, which means much the same as "embryological" or "developmental," is used in contrast to "phylogenetic" (which see).

Operculum. L. a cover or lid, from L. *opertum*, covered. Frontal, parietal, and temporal opercula bound the lateral sulcus of the cerebral hemisphere and conceal the insula.

Oxytocin. Gr. *oxys*, sharp + *tokos*, birth. Hormone that stimulates uterine contraction and milk ejection.

Pachymeninx. Gr. *pachys*, thick + *mēninx*, membrane. Dura mater.

Paleocerebellum. Gr. *palaios*, old + diminutive of cerebrum. Phylogenetically old part of the cerebellum that functions in postural changes and locomotion.

Paleocortex. Gr. *palaios*, old + L. *cortex*, bark. Olfactory cortex consisting of three to five layers.

Paleostriatum. Gr. *palaios*, old + L. *striatum*, striped or grooved. Phylogenetically older and efferent part of the corpus striatum; the globus pallidus or pallidum.

Pallidum. L. *pallidus*, (*-um*), pale. Globus pallidus of the corpus striatum; medial portion of the lentiform nucleus comprising the paleostriatum.

Pallium. L. cloak. Cerebral cortex with subjacent white matter, but usually used synonymously with cortex.

Paralysis. Gr. *paralysis*, secret undoing; from *para*, beside + *lyein*, to loosen. Loss of the power of motion.

Paraplegia. Gr. *para*, beside or beyond + *plēgē*, a stroke or blow. Paralysis of both legs and lower part of trunk.

Parenchyma. Gr. *parenchein*, to pour in beside. Essential and distinctive tissue of an organ. (The name is from an early notion that internal organs contained material poured in by their blood vessels.)

Paresis. Gr. *parienai*, to relax. Partial paralysis.

Pathway. Eng. Route within the central nervous system consisting of interconnected populations of neurons that serve a common function. A pathway often contains one or more tracts.

Perikaryon. Gr. *peri*, around + *karyon*, nut, kernel. Cytoplasm surrounding the nucleus. Sometimes refers to the cell body of a neuron.

Perineurium. Gr. *peri*, around + *neuron*, nerve. Cellular and connective tissue sheath surrounding a bundle of nerve fibers in a peripheral nerve.

Pernicious anemia. L. *per*, through + *necis*, of murder + Gr. *an*, negative + *haimos*, blood. Disease caused by failure to absorb vitamin B_{12} (cyanocobalamin). The vitamin deficiency results in defective production of red blood cells and degeneration in the central nervous system, including subacute combined degeneration in the spinal cord (see Ch. 5).

Pes. L. foot. Pes hippocampi: anterior thickened end of the hippocampus that slightly resembles a cat's paw.

Phylogeny. Gr. *phy'lon*, race + *genesis*, origin. Evolutionary history, typically as deduced from comparative anatomy.

Pia mater. L. tender mother. Thin innermost layer of the meninges attached to the surface of the brain and spinal cord; forms the inner boundary of the subarachnoid space.

Pineal. L. *pineus*, relating to the pine. Shaped like a pine cone (pertaining to the pineal gland).

Plexus. L. plaited, interwoven. Arrangement of interwoven and intercommunicating nerve trunks or fibers or of blood vessels.

Pneumoencephalography. Gr. *pneuma*, air + *enkephalos*, brain + *graphē*, a writing. Replacement of cerebrospinal fluid by air followed by x-ray examination (pneumoencephalogram); permits visualization of the ventricles and subarachnoid space. This technique has been replaced by computed tomography (CT scan).

Pons. L. bridge. Part of the brain stem that lies between the medulla and the midbrain; appears to constitute a bridge between the right and left halves of the cerebellum.

Positron. (From *positive electron*.) Subatomic particle with the same mass as an electron and equal but opposite charge. Positrons emitted by radioactive elements combine with electrons, with elimination of matter and emission of x-rays. Detection of the latter forms the basis of positron emission tomography (PET).

Progesterone. Steroid hormone secreted by the corpus luteum and the placenta.

Projection. L. *proiectus*, thrown forwards. Applied to the axons of a population of neurons and their sites of termination. Often used when the axons do not constitute a circumscribed tract.

Proprioceptor. L. *proprius*, one's own + *receptor*, receiver. One of the sensory endings in muscles, tendons, and joints; provides information concerning movement and position of parts of the body (proprioception).

Prosencephalon. Gr. *pros*, before + *enkephalos*, brain. Forebrain, consisting of the telencephalon (cerebral hemispheres) and diencephalon; anterior primary brain vesicle.

Prosopagnosia. Gr. *prosōpon*, person or face + agnosia (*q.v.*). Inability to recognize previously familiar faces.

Ptosis. Gr. *ptōsis*, a falling. Drooping of the upper eyelid.

Pulvinar. L. a cushioned seat. Posterior projection of the thalamus above the medial and lateral geniculate bodies.

Putamen. L. shell. Larger and lateral part of the lentiform nucleus of the corpus striatum.

Pyramidal system. Corticospinal and corticobulbar tracts. So-called because the corticospinal tracts occupy the fancifully pyramid-shaped area on the ventral surface of the medulla. The term pyramidal tract refers specifically to the corticospinal tract.

Pyriform. L. *pyrum*, pear + *forma*, form. Pyriform area is a region of olfactory cortex consisting of the uncus, limen insulae, and entorhinal area; has a pear-shaped outline in animals with a well-developed olfactory system.

Quadriplegia. L. *quadri*, four + Gr. *plēgē*, stroke. Paralysis that affects the four limbs. Also called tetraplegia.

Raphe. Gr. seam. Anatomical structure in the midline. In the brain, several raphe nuclei are in the midline of the medulla, pons, and midbrain. Their names are partly latinized, as in nucleus raphes magnus (great nucleus of the raphe), etc.

Receptor. L. *receptus*, received. Word used in two ways in neurobiology: (a) Structure of any size or complexity that collects and usually also edits information about conditions inside or outside the body. Examples are the eye, the muscle spindle, and the free ending of the peripheral neurite of a sensory neuron. (b) Protein molecule embedded in the surface of a cell (or sometimes inside the cell) that specifically binds the molecules of hormones, neurotransmitters, drugs, or other substances that can change the activity of the cell.

Reticular. L. *reticularis*, pertaining to or resembling a net. Reticular formation of the brain stem.

Rhinal. Gr. *rhis*, nose, therefore related to the nose. Rhinal sulcus in the temporal lobe indicates the margin of the lateral olfactory area.

Rhinencephalon. Gr. *rhis* (rhin-), nose + *enkephalos*, brain. Obsolete term that referred to components of the olfactory system. In comparative neurology, structures incorporated in the limbic system (especially the hippocampus and dentate gyrus) were included.

Rhombencephalon. Gr. *rhombos*, a lozenge-shaped figure + *enkephalos*, brain. Pons and cerebellum (metencephalon) and medulla (myelencephalon); posterior primary brain vesicle.

Roentgenogram. After Wilhelm Konrad Roentgen (1845-1923), who discovered x-rays, + Gr. *gramma*, a letter or record. Picture made with x-rays; more often called an x-ray or a radiograph.

Rostrum. L. beak. Recurved portion of the corpus callosum, passing backward from the genu to the lamina terminalis.

Rubro-. L. *ruber*, red. Pertaining to the red nucleus (nucleus ruber), as in rubrospinal and corticorubral.

Saccadic. Fr. *saccader*, to jerk. Saccadic or quick movements of the eyes in altering direction of gaze.

Satellite. L. *satteles*, attendant. Satellite cells: flattened cells of ectodermal origin that encapsulate nerve cell bodies in ganglia. Also satellite oligodendrocytes adjacent to nerve cell bodies in the central nervous system.

Septal area. Area ventral to the genu and rostrum of the corpus callosum on the medial aspect of the frontal lobe that is the site of the septal nuclei.

Septum pellucidum. L. partition + transparent. Triangular double membrane between the frontal horns of the lateral ventricles; it fills in the interval between the corpus callosum and the fornix.

Somatic. Gr. *somatikos*, bodily. Denoting the body, exclusive of the viscera (as in somatic efferent neurons that supply the skeletal musculature).

Somatotopic. Gr. *sōma*, body + *topos*, place. Representation of parts of the body in corresponding parts of the brain.

Somesthetic. Gr. *soma*, body + *aisthēsis*, perception. Consciousness of having a body. Somesthetic senses are those of pain, temperature, touch, pressure, position, movement, and vibration. Also spelled somaesthetic.

Splenium. Gr. *splēnion*, bandage. Thickened posterior extremity of the corpus callosum.

Squint. From Middle English *asquint*, with the eyes askew. See also **strabismus**.

Stellate. L. *stella*, star. Stellate neuron has many short dendrites that radiate in all directions.

Stenosis. Gr. *stenos*, narrow. Abnormal narrowing of a tube or passage.

Strabismus. Gr. *strabismos*, a squinting. Constant lack of parallelism of the visual axes of the eyes. Also known as a **squint**. (This is the only correct usage of the word squint.)

Stria terminalis. L. a furrow, groove + boundary, limit. Slender strand of fibers running along the medial side of the tail of the caudate nucleus. Originating in the amygdaloid body, most of the fibers end in the septal area and hypothalamus.

Striatum. L. *striatus*, furrowed. Phylogenetically more recent part of the corpus striatum (neostriatum) consisting of the caudate nucleus and the putamen or lateral portion of the lentiform nucleus. In comparative anatomy, striatum refers to a region of the brain in fishes, amphibians, and reptiles that is comparable to the corpus striatum of mammals.

Subiculum. L. diminutive of *subex* (*subic-*), a layer. Transitional cortex between that of the parahippocampal gyrus and the hippocampus.

Substantia gelatinosa. Column of small neurons at the apex of the dorsal gray horn throughout the spinal cord.

Substantia nigra. L. black substance. Large nucleus with motor functions in the midbrain; many of the constituent cells contain melanin.

Subthalamus. L. under + Gr. *thalamos*, inner chamber. Region of the diencephalon beneath the thalamus, containing fiber tracts and the subthalamic nucleus.

Sudomotor. L. *sudor*, sweat + *motor*, mover. Applies to sympathetic neurons that stimulate secretion from sweat glands.

Synapse. Gr. *synaptō*, to join. Word introduced by Sherrington in 1897 for the site at which one neuron is excited or inhibited by another neuron.

Syndrome. Gr. *syndrome*, the act of running together or combining. Collection of concurring clinical symptoms and signs. A syndrome usually is due to a single cause. The word is often used incorrectly as a synonym for "disease."

Syringomyelia. Gr. *syrinx*, pipe, tube + *myelos*, marrow. Condition characterized by central cavitation of the spinal cord and gliosis around the cavity.

Tangential. L. *tangens*, touching. In the direction of a line or plane that touches a curved surface. Used in anatomy for a plane of section approximately parallel to the surface of an organ.

Tanycyte. Gr. *tanyō*, to stretch + *kytos*, hollow (cell). Specialized type of ependymal cell present in the floor of the third ventricle.

Tapetum. L. *tapete*, a carpet. Fibers of the corpus callosum sweeping over the lateral ventricle and forming the lateral wall of its temporal horn.

Tectum. L. roof. Roof of the midbrain consisting of the paired superior and inferior colliculi.

Tegmentum. L. cover, from *tego*, to cover. Dorsal portion of the pons; also the major portion of the cerebral peduncle of the midbrain, lying between the substantia nigra and the tectum.

Tela choroidea. L. a web + Gr. *chorioeidēs*, like a membrane. Vascular connective tissue continuous with that of the pia mater that continues into the core of the choroid plexuses.

Telencephalon. Gr. *telos*, end + *enkephalos*, brain. Cerebral hemispheres; anterior of the two divisions of the prosencephalon or anterior primary brain vesicle.

Telodendria. Gr. *telos*, end + *dendrion*, tree. Terminal branches of axons.

Tentorium. L. tent. Tentorium cerebelli is a dural partition between the occipital lobes of the cerebral hemispheres and the cerebellum.

Tetraplegia. Gr. *tetra-*, four + *plēgē*, a blow or stroke. Paralysis that affects the four limbs. Also called quadriplegia.

Thalamus. Gr. *thalamos*, an inner chamber; also meant a bridal couch, so that the pulvinar *(q.v.)* was its cushion or pillow. Galen made up the word thalamus, and Willis was probably the first to use the word in its modern sense.

Thrombus. Gr. *thrombos*, clot. Clotted blood in a living blood vessel. Thrombosis occurs at sites of irregularity, typically due to atheroma in arteries.

Tomography. G. *tomos*, cutting + *graphō*, to write. Production of images of sections through a part of the body. Computed tomography with x-rays and nuclear magnetic resonance imaging are valuable diagnostic techniques.

Tone, tonus. Eng. from Gr. *tonos*, pitch, tension. Normal firmness and elasticity of muscles caused by partial contraction of some of their fibers.

Torcular. L. wine press, from *torquere*, to twist. Confluence of the dural venous sinuses at the internal occipital protuberance was formerly known as the torcular Herophili.

Tract. L. *tractus*, a region or district. Region of the central nervous system largely occupied by a population of axons that all have the same origin and destination (which often form the name, as in "spinothalamic tract").

Transducer. L. *transducere*, to lead across. Structure or mechanism for converting one form of energy into another; applied to sensory receptors.

Trapezoid body. Transverse fibers of the auditory pathway situated at the junction of the dorsal and ventral portions of the pons.

Trigeminal. L. born three at a time. Trigeminal nerve has three large branches or divisions.

Trochlear. L. *trochlea*, a pulley. Trochlear nerve supplies the superior oblique muscle, whose tendon passes through a fibrous ring, the trochlea. This ring changes the direction in which the muscle pulls.

Uncinate. L. hook-shaped. Uncinate fasciculus: association fibers connecting cortex of the ventral surface of the frontal lobe with that of the temporal pole. Also a bundle of fastigiobulbar fibers (uncinate fasciculus of Russell) that curves over the superior cerebellar peduncle in its passage to the inferior cerebellar peduncle.

Uncus. L. a hook. Hooked-back portion of the rostral end of the parahippocampal gyrus of the temporal lobe, constituting a landmark for the lateral olfactory area.

Uvula. L. little grape. A part of the inferior vermis of the cerebellum.

Vagus. L. wandering. Tenth cranial nerve is so named on account of the wide distribution of its branches in the thorax and abdomen.

Vallecula. L. diminutive of *vallis*, valley. Midline depression on the inferior aspect of the cerebellum.

Velate. L. *velum*, sail, curtain, veil. Velate or protoplasmic astrocytes have flattened processes.

Velum. L. sail, curtain, veil. Membranous structure. Superior and inferior medullary vela forming the roof of the fourth ventricle.

Ventricle. L. *ventriculus*, diminutive of *venter*, belly. Lateral, third, and fourth ventricles of the brain.

Vermis. L. worm. Midline portion of the cerebellum. Its ventral surface looks a little like a folded earthworm.

Zona incerta. Gray matter in the subthalamus representing a rostral extension of the reticular formation of the brain stem.

Zonula occludens. L. diminutive of *zona*, belt + occluding. Also known as a tight junction. Form of continuous close apposition of the membranes of neighboring cells, impermeable to macromolecules.

Appendices

The Human Nervous System: An Anatomical Viewpoint, Sixth Edition, Murray L. Barr and John A. Kiernan. J.B. Lippincott Company, Philadelphia, © 1993.

Investigators Mentioned in the Text

Adamkiewicz, Albert (1850–1921) Polish pathologist who described the blood supply of the human spinal cord (an anterior radicular artery supplying the lumbar region of the spinal cord known as the artery of Adamkiewicz).

Adie, William John (1886–1935) English clinical neurologist. The Holmes-Adie pupil is large and reacts slowly to light.

Alzheimer, Alois (1884–1915) German neuropsychiatrist who also made important contributions to neuropathology. Studied presenile and senile dementia, describing in 1907 the condition now known as Alzheimer's disease.

Argyll Robertson, Douglas Moray Cooper Lamb (1837–1909) Scottish ophthalmologist. The Argyll Robertson pupil includes, among other signs, pupillary constriction in accommodation, but not in response to light.

Auerbach, Leopold (1828–1897) German anatomist. Auerbach's plexus (myenteric plexus) in the gastrointestinal tract; end bulbs of Held-Auerbach (synaptic terminals or boutons terminaux).

Babinski, Joseph François Félix (1857–1932) French clinical neurologist of Polish origin. The Babinski sign, which consists of upturning of the great toe and spreading of the toes on stroking the sole, is characteristic of an upper motor neuron lesion.

Baillarger, Jules Gabriel François (1806–1891) French psychiatrist. The lines of Bail-larger consist of two transverse strata of nerve fibers in the cerebral cortex.

Bainbridge, Francis Arthur (1874–1921) British physiologist who found that an increase of pressure on the venous side of the heart accelerates the heart rate.

Beevor, Charles Edward (1854–1908) English clinical neurologist who contributed to our knowledge of neurology, especially with respect to localization of function in the cerebral cortex.

Bell, Sir Charles (1774–1842) Scottish anatomist, clinical neurologist, and surgeon. Bell's palsy is a form of facial paralysis caused by interruption of conduction by the facial nerve. The Bell-Magendie law states that dorsal spinal roots are sensory, whereas ventral roots are motor.

Bernard, Claude (1813–1878) French physiologist and one of the great investigators of the 19th century. Established experimental physiology as an exact science. One of his contributions was the demonstration of vasomotor mechanisms.

Betz, Vladimir A. (1834–1894) Russian anatomist. Betz discovered and described the giant pyramidal cells (Betz cells) in the motor area of the cerebral cortex.

Bielschowsky, Max (1969–1940) German neuropathologist and clinical neurologist who developed Bielschowsky's silver staining method for nerve cells and fibers.

Bodian, David (b. 1910) American anatomist who developed a stain for nerve cells and fibers, using the organic silver compound protargol.

Bowman, Sir William (1816–1892) English anatomist and ophthalmologist. His name is associated with glands in the olfactory mucosa, the capsule of the renal glomerulus, and a layer in the cornea.

Breuer, Josef (1842–1925) Austrian physician and psychologist who contributed to our knowledge of reflexes controlling respiratory movements.

Broca, Pierre Paul (1824–1880) French pathologist and anthropologist. Broca localized the cortical motor speech area in the inferior frontal gyrus; also described a band of nerve fibers (the diagonal band of Broca) in the anterior perforated substance on the ventral surface of the cerebral hemisphere.

Brodal, Alf (1910–1988) Norwegian neuroanatomist who made numerous contributions to knowledge of the reticular formation, cranial nerves, cerebellum, and other aspects of neuroanatomy, including the nucleus Z of Brodal and Pompeiano (in the medulla). One of his most famous papers was, "Self-observations and neuro-anatomical considerations after a stroke," (*Brain* 96:675–694, 1973).

Brodmann, Korbinian (1868–1918) German neuropsychiatrist. Brodmann's cytoarchitectural map of the cerebral cortex is used frequently when referring to specific regions of the cortex.

Brown-Séquard, Charles Edouard (1817–1894) Physiologist and clinical neurologist. Born in the Crown Colony of Mauritius of American and French parents, he retained British citizenship even though his professional life was spent in several countries. The Brown-Séquard syndrome consists of the sensory and motor abnormalities that follow hemisection of the spinal cord.

Bruch, Karl Wilhelm Ludwig (1819–1884) German anatomist. Bruch's membrane is the innermost layer of the choroid of the eye, separating the capillary layer of the choroid from the retina.

Bucy, Paul C. (b. 1904) American neurosurgeon. The Klüver-Bucy syndrome is caused by extensive bilateral lesions of the temporal lobes. He also found that selective corticospinal tract lesions did not cause hemiplegia.

Büngner, Otto von (1858–1905) German clinical neurologist who described the endoneurial tubes containing modified Schwann cells in the distal portion of a sectioned peripheral nerve (bands of von Büngner).

Cajal See Ramón y Cajal.

Cannon, Walter Bradford (1871–1945) American physiologist who contributed much to our understanding of autonomic regulation of visceral functions. Among other contributions he demonstrated the "fight or flight" reaction to stress.

Chiari, Hans (1851–1916) Czech physician, after whom the Chiari malformation (medulla and cerebellar tonsils in the upper cervical spinal canal) is named.

Clark, Sir Wilfrid Edward Le Gros (1895–1971) English anatomist who made important contributions to comparative neuroanatomy, especially of sensory systems, and to primate paleontology.

Clarke, Jacob Augustus Lockhard (1817–1880) English anatomist and clinical neurologist. Among numerous contributions, Clarke described the nucleus dorsalis (thoracicus) of the spinal cord, known as Clarke's column.

Corti, Marchese Alfonso (1822–1888) Italian histologist who described the sensory epithelium of the cochlea (organ of Corti).

Cushing, Harvey (1869–1939) Pioneer American neurosurgeon. Cushing contributed to many basic aspects of neurology, including the function of the pituitary gland, pituitary tumors, tumors of the eighth cranial nerve, and classification of brain tumors.

Darkschewitsch, Liverij Osipovich (1858–1925) Russian clinical neurologist who discovered the nucleus of Darkschewitsch, one of the accessory oculomotor nuclei in the midbrain.

de Egas Moniz, António Caetano de Abreau Friere (1874–1955) Portuguese physician who was awarded the Nobel Prize for Medicine and Physiology in 1949 for demonstration of the therapeutic value of prefrontal leukotomy. He introduced the technique of cerebral angiography in 1927.

Deiters, Otto Friedrich Karl (1834–1863) German anatomist. The lateral vestibular nucleus, which is the origin of the vestibulospinal tract, is known as Deiters' nucleus.

Dusser de Barenne, Johannes Gregorius (1885–1940) Dutch neurophysiologist who studied cortical function and introduced the technique of physiological neuronography.

Edinger, Ludwig (1855–1918) German neuroanatomist and clinical neurologist. An outstanding teacher of functional neuroanatomy and a pioneer in comparative neuroanatomy. The Edinger-Westphal nucleus is the parasympathetic component of the oculomotor nucleus.

Eustachio, Bartolemeo (1524–1574) Italian physician, surgeon, and anatomist. The auditory tube bears his name.

Ferrier, Sir David (1843–1928) Scottish neuropathologist, neurophysiologist, and clinical neurologist, best known for his studies of the motor and sensory areas of the cerebral cortex.

Foerster, Otfrid (1873–1941) German clinical neurologist and neurosurgeon. Otfrid made important contributions to the study of epilepsy, pain, the dermatomes, brain tumors, and the cytoarchitecture and functional localization of the cerebral cortex; he also introduced the chordotomy (tractotomy) operation for intractable pain.

Forel, Auguste Henri (1848–1931) Swiss neuropsychiatrist who described certain fiber bundles in the subthalamus, which are known as the fields of Forel. The ventral tegmental decussation of Forel in the midbrain consists of crossing rubrospinal fibers. Forel proposed the Neuron Theory on the basis of the response of nerve cells to injury.

Fritsch, Gustav Theodor (1838–1927) German anthropologist and anatomist. With Hitzig, he studied localization of motor function in the dog's cerebral cortex by electrical stimulation.

Frölich, Alfred (1871–1953) Austrian pharmacologist and clinical neurologist who described the adiposogenital syndrome, which is caused by a lesion involving the hypothalamus.

Galen, Claudius (130–200) Hellenistic physician, who practiced mainly in Rome and Pergamon. Galen was the leading medical authority of the Christian world for 1400 years. His name is attached to the great cerebral vein.

Gasser, Johann Laurentius Austrian anatomist of the 18th century. The sensory ganglion of the trigeminal nerve was named for him by one of his students, A.B.R. Hirsch, in 1765.

Gennari, Francesco (1750–1796?) Italian physician who described the white line in the visual cortex, now known as the line of Gennari, while he was a medical student in Parma, Italy.

Golgi, Camillo (1843–1926) Italian histologist who introduced a silver staining method that provided the basis of numerous advances in neurohistology. Described type I and type II neurons and the tendon spindles, and the organelle now called the Golgi apparatus. Awarded the Nobel Prize for Medicine and Physiology in 1906 (with Ramón y Cajal).

Gray, Edward George (b. 1924) English biologist who has made numerous contributions to an appreciation of the ultrastructure of the nervous system. Gray's type I and type II synapses are named for him.

Grünbaum, Albert S.F. (later Leyton, A.S.F.) (1869–1921) British bacteriologist and physiologist who worked with Sir Charles Sherrington on functional localization of the cerebral cortex.

Gudden, Bernhard Aloys von (1824–1886) German neuropsychiatrist who described the partial crossing of nerve fibers in the optic chiasma together with certain small commissural bundles adjacent to the chiasma. He studied connections in the brain by observing changes subsequent to lesions made in the brains of young rabbits (the Gudden method). His pupils included Forel, Meynert, Monakow and Nissl. Gudden provided medical evidence that removed the mad king Ludwig II from the throne of Bavaria. He was allegedly murdered by his royal patient, who then committed suicide.

Hamburger, Viktor (b. 1900) American (originally German) experimental embryologist, famous for his studies on neuronal death in the developing nervous system.

Head, Sir Henry (1861–1940) English clinical neurologist. Studied the dermatomes (Head's areas), cutaneous sensory physiology, and particularly the sensory disturbances and aphasia following cerebral lesions.

Held, Hans (1866–1942) German anatomist who made extensive studies of interneuronal relationships (axonal synaptic terminals or end bulbs of Held-Auerbach).

Henle, Friedrich Gustav Jacob (1809–1885) German anatomist and pioneer in histology. The endoneurial sheath surrounding individual fibers of a peripheral nerve is known as either the sheath of Henle or sheath of Retzius.

Hensen, Victor (1835–1924) German embryologist and physiologist who studied the anatomy and physiology of the sense organs (cells of Hensen in the organ of Corti).

Hering, Heinrich Ewald (1866–1948) German physiologist, best known for his study of the reflex that initiates expiration.

Herophilus (ca. 300–250 BC) Greek physician in Alexandria. Herophilus made early observations on the anatomy of the brain and other organs. The confluence of the dural venous sinuses at the internal occipital protuberance is known as the torcular Herophili.

Herrick, Charles Judson (1868–1960) American neuroanatomist who made many contributions to the embryology and comparative anatomy of the nervous system. Herrick was editor for 54 years of the Journal of Comparative Neurology, which was founded by his brother Clarence.

Heschl, Richard (1824–1881) Austrian anatomist and pathologist who described the anterior transverse temporal gyri (Heschl's convolutions), which serve as a landmark for the auditory area of the cerebral cortex.

Heubner, Johann Otto Leonhard (1843–1926) German pediatrician who described the recurrent branch of the anterior cerebral artery.

Hilton, John (1804–1878) English surgeon. Hilton's law states that the nerve supplying a joint also supplies the muscles that move the joint and the skin covering the articular insertions of those muscles.

His, Wilhelm (1831–1904) Swiss anatomist and a founder of human embryology. Proposed the Neuron Theory on the basis of his embryological studies of the development of nerve cells.

Hitzig, Eduard (1838–1907) German physiologist and clinical neurologist. Hitzig studied localization of motor function in the cerebral cortex of dogs and monkeys by electrical stimulation.

Holmes, Gordon Morgan (1876–1965) English clinical neurologist. His contributions include mapping of the visual cortex from clinical studies of patients with gunshot wounds of the brain during the First World War. The Holmes-Adie pupil, caused by death of neurons in the ciliary ganglion, is enlarged and reacts slowly to light.

Holmes, William British zoologist. Developed the Holmes silver staining method for axons. He has also contributed to knowledge of axonal regeneration and comparative histology of the peripheral nervous system.

Horner, Johann Friedrich (1831–1886) Swiss ophthalmologist who described Horner's syndrome, caused by interruption of the sympathetic innervation of the eye, which includes pupillary constriction and ptosis of the upper eyelid.

Horsley, Sir Victor Alexander Haden (1857–1916) A founder of neurosurgery in England. Horsley studied the motor cortex and other parts of the brain by electrical stimulation and introduced the Horsley-Clarke stereotaxic apparatus.

Hubel, David Hunter (b. 1926) American neurophysiologist (born and educated in Canada), who with T.N. Wiesel mapped the columnar organization of the monkey's visual cortex. Hubel shared the Nobel Prize for Medicine and Physiology with Sperry and Wiesel in 1981.

Hunter, John (1728–1793) British anatomist and pioneer surgeon of the 18th century. His collection of anatomical and pathological specimens formed the basis of the Hunterian Museum of the Royal College of Surgeons.

Huntington, George Sumner (1850–1916) American general medical practitioner. Huntington described a hereditary form of chorea resulting from neuronal degeneration in the corpus striatum and the cerebral cortex.

Inouye, Tatsuji (1881–1976) Japanese ophthalmologist who mapped the human visual cortex by plotting the visual fields of soldiers with gunshot wounds of the brain incurred in 1905 during the Russo-Japanese war.

Jackson, John Hughlings (1835–1911) English clinical neurologist and pioneer of modern neurology. Jackson gave a thorough description of focal epilepsy (jacksonian seizures), resulting from local irritation of the motor cortex.

Kappers, C.U. Ariens (1878–1946) Dutch neuroanatomist and Director of the Central Brain Institute in Amsterdam. His many contributions include the theory of neurobiotaxis, anthropological studies of the brain, and cytoarchitectonics of the cerebral cortex.

Key, Ernst Axel Henrik (1832–1901) Swedish histologist. The lateral apertures of the fourth ventricle are sometimes called foramina of Key and Retzius.

Klüver, Heinrich (1897–1979) American psychologist. The Klüver-Bucy syndrome is caused by bilateral lesions of the temporal lobes.

Kölliker, Rudolf Albert von (1817–1905) German physiologist and comparative anatomist. Initially an opponent and later a supporter of the neuron doctrine. The Kölliker-Fuse nucleus is in the medial group of parabrachial nuclei.

Korsakoff, Sergei Sergeievich (1854–1900) Russian psychiatrist. Korsakoff's psychosis or syndrome, which is usually a sequel of chronic alcoholism, includes a memory defect, fabrication of ideas, and polyneuritis.

Krause, Wilhelm Johann Friedrich (1833–1910) German anatomist who described sensory endings in the skin, including the end bulbs of Krause.

Labbé, Léon (1832–1916) French surgeon. Studied the veins of the brain (lesser anastomotic veins of Labbé).

Lancisi, Giovanni Maria (1654–1720) An Italian physician whose patients included three successive popes. The longitudinal striae in the indusium griseum are known as the striae of Lancisi.

Langley, John Newport (1852–1925) English physiologist best known for his studies of the autonomic nervous system, a term that he introduced in 1898.

Lanterman, A. J. American anatomist of the 19th century who described the incisures of Schmidt-Lanterman in myelin sheaths of peripheral nerve fibers.

Lewis, Sir Thomas (1881–1945) British physician noted for studies of human physiology, especially as related to the heart and blood vessels, and of referred pain.

Lissauer, Heinrich (1861–1891) German clinical neurologist who described the dorsolateral fasciculus of the spinal cord (Lissauer's tract or zone).

Luschka, Hubert von (1820–1875) German anatomist. Among other contributions to anatomy, Luschka described the lateral apertures of the fourth ventricle (foramina of Luschka; also called the foramina of Key and Retzius).

Luys, Jules Bernard (1828–1895) French clinical neurologist who described the subthalamic nucleus (nucleus of Luys), whose degeneration causes hemiballismus.

Magendie, François (1783–1855) French physiologist and pioneer of experimental physiology. The sensory function of dorsal spinal nerve roots and motor function of ventral roots constitute the Bell-Magendie law. Magendie also described the median aperture of the fourth ventricle (foramen of Magendie).

Marchi, Vittorio (1851–1908) Italian physician and histologist who developed the Marchi staining method for tracing the course of degenerating myelinated fibers.

Martinotti, Giovanni (1857–1928) Italian physician and student of Golgi who described a type of neuron known as the cell of Martinotti in the cerebral cortex.

Mazzoni, Vittorio Italian physician of the 19th century. The Golgi-Mazzoni ending is a type of sensory receptor.

Meckel, Johann Friedrich (1714–1774) German anatomist especially known for his careful description of the trigeminal nerve. The trigeminal ganglion is situated in an extension of the meninges called Meckel's cave.

Meissner, Georg (1829–1905) German anatomist and physiologist. His name is associated with touch corpuscles in the dermis and the submucous nerve plexus of the gastrointestinal tract.

Ménière, Prosper (1801–1862) French otologist who described the syndrome characterized by episodes of vertigo, nausea, and vomiting occurring in some diseases of the internal ear.

Merkel, Friedrich Siegmund (1845–1919) German anatomist who described tactile endings in the epidermis, known as Merkel's disks.

Meyer, Adolph (1866–1950) American psychiatrist. The fibers of the geniculocalcarine tract that loop forward in the temporal lobe constitute Meyer's loop.

Meynert, Theodor Hermann (1833–1892) Austrian neuropsychiatrist. The habenulointerpeduncular fasciculus is also called the fasciculus retroflexus of Meynert. The dorsal tegmental decussation of Meynert in the midbrain consists of crossing tectospinal fibers. The nucleus basalis of Meynert is in the substantia innominata of the forebrain.

Monakow, Constatin von (1853–1930) Neurologist of Russian birth who lived in Switzerland. Monakow made fundamental contributions to the knowledge of the thalamus and brain stem. The dorsolateral region of the medulla is known as Monakow's area.

Moniz See de Egas Moniz.

Monro, Alexander (1733–1817) Scottish anatomist, also known as Alexander Monro (Secundus). Including tenure by his father (Primus) and son (Tertius), the Chair of Anatomy in the University of Edinburgh was occupied by Alexander Monros for over a century. The interventricular foramen between the lateral and third ventricles is known as the foramen of Monro.

Müller, Heinrich (1820–1864) German anatomist. Müller's orbital muscle and cells of Müller are in the retina.

Nissl, Franz (1860–1919) German neuropsychiatrist who made important contributions to neurohistology and neuropathology. Nissl introduced a method of staining gray matter with cationic dyes to show the basophil material (Nissl bodies) of nerve cells.

Pacchioni, Antonio (1665–1726) Italian anatomist. The arachnoid villi become hypertrophied with age and are then known as arachnoid granulations or pacchionian bodies.

Pacini, Filippo (1812–1883) Italian anatomist and histologist. Described the sensory endings known as the corpuscles of Vater-Pacini.

Papez, John Wenceslas (1883–1958) American anatomist who made important contributions to comparative neuroanatomy and in 1937 postulated the involvement of the circuitry of the limbic system in emotional feeling and expression.

Parkinson, James (1775–1824) English physician, surgeon, and paleontologist. Parkinson described "shaking palsy" or paralysis agitans, which is more frequently called Parkinson's disease.

Penfield, Wilder Graves (1891–1976) Canadian neurosurgeon who made fundamental contributions to neurocytology and neurophysiology, including functions of the cerebral cortex, speech mechanisms, and pathological changes underlying epilepsy.

Perroncito, Aldo (1882–1929) Italian histologist who described whorls of regenerating axons (spirals of Perroncito) in the central stump of a sectioned peripheral nerve.

Pompeiano, Ottavio (b. 1927) Italian physiologist who has contributed to knowledge of the physiology of the cerebellum and vestibular nuclei. Nucleus Z was first described in the cat's medulla (by Brodal and Pompeiano) and later recognized in the human brain.

Purkinje, Johannes (Jan) Evangelista (1787–1869) Bohemian physiologist, pioneer in histological techniques, and an accomplished histologist. He described the Purkinje cells of the cerebellar cortex and Purkinje fibers in the heart, among others.

Ramón y Cajal, Santiago Felipe (1852–1934) Spanish histologist, who is foremost among neurohistologists. He was awarded the Nobel Prize for Medicine and Physiology (with Camillo Golgi) in 1906. Among innumerable contributions, Cajal vigorously championed the Neuron Doctrine on the basis of his observations with silver staining methods.

Ranvier, Louis-Antoine (1835–1922) French histologist and a founder of experimental histology. Ranvier described the nodes of Ranvier in the myelin sheaths of nerve fibers.

Rasmussen, Grant Litster (b. 1904) American neuroanatomist. His numerous contributions to neuroanatomy include description of the olivocochlear bundle (of Rasmussen).

Rathke, Martin Heinrich (1793–1860) German physiologist, pathologist, zoologist and anatomist. Rathke's pouch is the outgrowth of the embryonic pharynx that becomes the adenohypophysis.

Reil, Johann Christian (1759–1813) German physician. The insula, lying in the depths of the lateral sulcus of the cerebral hemisphere, is known as the island of Reil.

Reissner, Ernst (1824–1878) German anatomist. The vestibular membrane of the cochlea is known as Reissner's membrane.

Remak, Robert (1815–1867) German physician who described "gray nerve fibers" in peripheral nerves. A Remak fiber is a Schwann cell with included unmyelinated axons.

Renshaw, Birdsey (1911–1948) American neurophysiologist. Certain interneurons in the ventral gray horn of the spinal cord are called Renshaw cells.

Retzius, Magnus Gustaf (1842–1919) Swedish histologist. The lateral apertures of the fourth ventricle are sometimes called foramina of Key and Retzius. In peripheral nerves the sheath of Retzius (also called sheath of Henle or sheath of Key & Retzius) is the endoneurial connective tissue that invests each nerve fiber.

Rexed, Bror (b. 1914) Swedish neuroanatomist who divided the gray matter of the spinal cord into regions (laminae of Rexed) on the basis of differences in cytoarchitecture.

Rio Hortega, Pio del (1882–1945) Spanish histologist who worked in his later years in England and Argentina. He is best known for his studies of neuroglial cells, especially the microglia.

Robin, Charles Philippe (1821–1885) French anatomist. The perivascular spaces of the brain are known as Virchow-Robin spaces.

Rolando, Luigi (1773–1831) Italian anatomist. Among various contributions to neurology, Rolando described the central sulcus of the cerebral hemisphere and the substantia gelatinosa of the spinal cord.

Roller, Christian Friedrich Wilhelm (1802–1878) German psychiatrist. One of the perihypoglossal nuclei is known as the nucleus of Roller.

Romberg, Moritz Heinrich (1795–1873) German clinical neurologist. Romberg's sign of impaired proprioceptive conduction in the spinal cord consists of abnormal unsteadiness when standing with the feet together and the eyes closed.

Rosenthal, Friedrich Christian (1779–1829) German anatomist who studied the veins of the brain (basal vein of Rosenthal).

Ruffini, Angelo (1864–1929) Italian anatomist who described sensory endings, especially those known as the end bulbs of Ruffini.

Russell, James Samuel Risien (1863–1939) British physician and clinical neurologist. Russell published on diseases of the nervous system and described the uncinate fasciculus of efferent cerebellar fibers.

Scarpa, Antonio (1747–1832) Italian anatomist and surgeon who made numerous contributions to anatomy, including a description of the vestibular ganglion.

Schmidt, Henry D. (1823–1888) American anatomist and pathologist. Schmidt described the incisures of Schmidt-Lanterman in myelin sheaths of peripheral nerve fibers.

Schütz, H. German anatomist of the 19th century who described the dorsal longitudinal fasciculus of the brain stem in 1891.

Schwann, Theodor (1810–1882) German anatomist who formulated the Cell Theory (with M. J. Schleiden) and described the neurolemmal cells (Schwann cells) of peripheral nerve fibers.

Sherrington, Sir Charles Scott (1856–1952) English neurophysiologist and a major contributor to basic knowledge of the function of the nervous system. His researches included studies of reflexes, decerebrate rigidity, reciprocal innervation, the synapse, and the concept of the integrative action of the nervous system.

Sömmering, Samuel Thomas von (1755–1830) German anatomist and surgeon who recognized the difference between gray matter and white matter and gave the cranial nerves the numbers that are still used.

Sperry, Roger Wolcott (b. 1913) American neurobiologist. Sperry made major contributions to the knowledge of development of specific connections in the brains of fishes and amphibians, and of the functions of the human corpus callosum. He received the Nobel Prize for Medicine and Physiology, 1981, which he shared with Hubel and Wiesel.

Sydenham, Thomas (1624–1689) English physician, known as the English Hippocrates. Described the form of chorea to which his name is attached.

Sylvius, Francis De La Boe (1614–1672) French anatomist who gave the first description of the lateral sulcus of the cerebral hemisphere.

Sylvius, Jacobus (also known as Jacques Dubois) (1478–1555) French anatomist who described the cerebral aqueduct of the midbrain (aqueduct of Sylvius).

Tinel, Jules (1879–1952) French clinical neurologist. Tinel's sign, elicited by percussion in the region of a regenerating nerve, consists of a tingling sensation in the field of sensory distribution.

Trolard, Paulin (1842–1910) French anatomist who described the venous drainage of the brain (greater anastomotic vein of Trolard).

Vater, Abraham (1684–1751) German anatomist. Among other contributions, Vater described the sensory endings known as the corpuscles of Vater-Pacini.

Vicq D'Azyr, Felix (1748–1794) French anatomist and a leading comparative anatomist. The mamillothalamic fasciculus bears his name.

Virchow, Rudolph Ludwig Karl (1821–1902) German pathologist and founder of modern (or cellular) pathology. The perivascular spaces of the brain are known as Virchow-Robin spaces.

Waldeyer, Heinrich Wilhelm Gottfried (1836–1921) German anatomist who popularized the Neuron Doctrine on the basis of studies by Cajal, Forel, His, and others. Waldeyer cells in the dorsal horn of the spinal cord are named for him.

Walker, A. Earl (b. 1907) American neurosurgeon (born and educated in Canada) who made contributions to cerebellar and cerebral cortical physiology, anatomy and physiology of the thalamus, and various clinical topics.

Wallenberg, Adolf (1862–1949) German physician who described the lateral medullary syndrome.

Waller, Augustus Volney (1816–1870) English physician and physiologist who described the degenerative changes in the distal portion of a sectioned peripheral nerve, known as wallerian degeneration.

Warwick, Roger (1912–1991) British anatomist. Among other contributions, Warwick described the organization of the oculomotor nucleus with respect to the ocular muscles that it supplies.

Weber, Sir Hermann David (1823–1918) English physician who described the midbrain lesion causing hemiparesis and ocular paralysis.

Weigert, Karl (1843–1905) German pathologist who introduced several staining methods, including a stain for myelin in sections of nervous tissue.

Wiesel, Torsten Nils (b. 1924) Swedish neurobiologist who, with Hubel, discovered the columnar organization of the visual cortex of the monkey. He shared the Nobel Prize for Medicine and Physiology with Hubel and Sperry in 1981.

Wernicke, Carl (1848–1905) German neuropsychiatrist who made a special study of disorders in the use of language. Wernicke's sensory language area and Wernicke's aphasia are named for him.

Westphal, Karl Friedrich Otto (1833–1890) German clinical neurologist. Among other contributions to neurology, Westphal described the Edinger-Westphal nucleus in the oculomotor complex.

Willis, Thomas (1621–1675) English physician who was one of the dominant figures in medicine of the 17th century and a founder of the Royal Society. Among numerous contributions to the anatomy of the brain, he described the arterial circle that bears his name. Willis also named the thalamus as the destination of the optic tract, though his intention may have been to apply the name to the lateral ventricle rather than to a solid structure.

Wilson, Samuel Alexander Kinnier (1878–1937) British clinical neurologist who described hepatolenticular degeneration, known as Wilson's disease.

Wrisberg, Heinrich August (1739–1808) German anatomist. Among other contributions to anatomy, Wrisberg described the sensory root of the facial nerve (nervus intermedius of Wrisberg).

Index